Would You Like to Know

the latest scientific facts on:

- PREGNANCY
- NATURAL CHILDBIRTH
- INFANT NUTRITION
- CHILDHOOD DISEASES
- NATURAL BIRTH CONTROL
- MENSTRUAL PROBLEMS
- BREAST CANCER

- DEPRESSION
- VARICOSE VEINS
- OVERWEIGHT PROBLEMS
- MENOPAUSAL DISTRESS
- BEAUTY SECRETS
- DIETS AND SUPPLEMENTS
- ... AND MUCH MORE!

These are just a few of the subjects covered in this monumental, fully-documented reference manual on every aspect of physical, mental, and spiritual wellbeing, written by the world's leading authority on Holistic Medicine and the most reputable and knowledgeable nutritionist of our time — Dr. Paavo Airola.

Here's what distinguished medical experts say about this book:

"Never have I read such a fascinating, exciting, and complete health manual. A truly wonderful book — the most needed book of the century." **Mary Ann Kibler, M.D.**

"A massive accomplishment... It distinguishes Dr. Airola as a giant in the field. His book deserves to be immediately read and then used as a reference by families throughout our country." **Robert S. Mendelsohn, M.D.**

"Truly a treasure chest! Each chapter is a jewel and an obvious product of thorough research." **Virginia Flanagan, M.D.**

"A masterpiece! Must be read by every woman — preferably together with her husband." **Abram Ber, M.D.**

"A great new contribution in the field of alternative medicine! I certainly will use it and recommend it to all my female patients." **Willem H. Khoe, M.D.**

*"If **Everywoman's Book** was used as a major text in the curriculum of our medical schools, we would have a healthier and stronger America."* **J. P. Hutchins, M.D.**

THIS BOOK IS A **MUST** FOR EVERY WOMAN — YOUNG AND OLD — CONCERNED WITH HER AND HER FAMILY'S HEALTH!

Other Books by Dr. Paavo Airola

HOW TO GET WELL
ARE YOU CONFUSED?
HYPOGLYCEMIA: A BETTER APPROACH
HOW TO KEEP SLIM, HEALTHY, AND YOUNG
  WITH JUICE FASTING
WORLDWIDE SECRETS FOR STAYING YOUNG
CANCER: CAUSES, PREVENTION, AND
  TREATMENT: THE TOTAL APPROACH
SWEDISH BEAUTY SECRETS
STOP HAIR LOSS
THE MIRACLE OF GARLIC
THERE *IS* A CURE FOR ARTHRITIS
SEX AND NUTRITION
HEALTH SECRETS FROM EUROPE

Dr. Airola's Practical Guide to Holistic Health

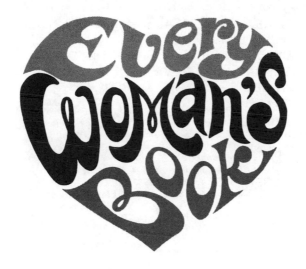

by PAAVO AIROLA, Ph.D., N.D.

Foreword by **MARY ANN KIBLER, M.D.**
Introduction by **ROBERT S. MENDELSOHN, M.D.**

HEALTH PLUS PUBLISHERS, Phoenix, Arizona

EVERYWOMAN'S BOOK
Copyright © 1979 by
Paavo Airola, Ph.D., N.D.

First Printing, April, 1979 Hard Cover Edition
Second Printing, Aug., 1979 Hard Cover Edition
Third Printing, Nov., 1979 Hard Cover Edition
Fourth Printing, April, 1980 Hard Cover Edition
Fifth Printing, Jan., 1982 Soft Cover Edition
Sixth Printing, June, 1983 Hard Cover Edition
Seventh Printing, July, 1983 Soft Cover Edition
Eighth Printing, Sept., 1988 Soft Cover Edition
Ninth Printing, Jan., 1990 Soft Cover Edition

ISBN 0-932090-10-9

Drawings by the Author

Published by
HEALTH PLUS, Publishers

Printed in the United States of America

MEDICAL EDITORS

ACKNOWLEDGEMENTS

I wish to express my heartful thanks and everlasting indebtedness to many dedicated individuals for their unselfish and invaluable contributions without which **Everywoman's Book** would never have materialized.

My grateful acknowledgement goes to all the medical editors who, although extremely busy with their own practices, gave so much of their time, assisting me with expert advice and recommendations on the multiplicity of medical and health issues dealt with in this book. Their authoritative contributions were generous, magnanimous, and of inestimable value to me.

I wish to express my deepest gratitude to members of my family: Anni, Evi, Karen, Paula, Becky, and Paul, whose love, co-operation, and encouragement helped immensely in the preparation of this book.

My warm appreciation goes to some very special friends who, in one way or another, contributed with their inspiration and assistance to the birth and completion of this work: Ilse Washington, Mary Myers, Mark Selby, and Scott Smith.

I also wish to thank Karen Jensen for her invaluable secretarial and editorial assistance in the preparation of the manuscript.

Last, but not least, I wish to acknowledge my eternal indebtedness to the Divine Source of All Wisdom for the inspiration, enlightenment, guidance, courage, and strength which enabled me to conceive and execute this book for the benefit of all those who seek knowledge, help, and direction.

Dedication

I dedicate this book to

Every Woman

who has the foresight and the wisdom to accept with joy and honor her glorious, divinely-designed role of womanhood, and, realizing that the future of mankind and the fate of civilization rests in her hands, exemplifies womanhood, with all its richness, in every facet of her life—as a wife, mother, student, or in whatever her chosen profession or field of endeavor may be.

It is my sincerest hope and prayer that the information in this book will contribute to the enhancement of the physical, emotional, and spiritual well-being of today's women and their families—and, thereby, to a healthier human race and a better quality of life.

TABLE OF CONTENTS

PART THREE: SPECIFIC FEMALE HEALTH PROBLEMS

IMPORTANT NOTE

The information in the sections of this book which deal with female, infant, and childhood health problems, is intended for use by nutritionally and biologically oriented physicians, naturopaths, and the members of the other healing professions, as well as for researchers and students engaged in scientific work in the field of nutrition and biological medicine.

In recommending certain diets, food supplements, herbs, and vitamins in large doses, we do not diagnose or prescribe, but offer this information purely for educational and experimental purposes. A patient who suffers from serious illness should use the information in this publication in cooperation with his doctor (preferably a nutritionally oriented one), and abide by his decision regarding the advisability of using the suggested therapies for a specific condition. In the event the reader of this volume uses the information without the approval of his doctor, he is prescribing for himself (which is his constitutional right to do) and he assumes the responsibility for it. The author and the publisher, however, assume no responsibility in regard to the effectiveness of, or possible harm incurred from, correct or incorrect application of therapeutic approaches described herein.

FOREWORD

by Mary Ann Kibler, M.D.

Perhaps the most remarkable feature of *Every-woman's Book* is the fact that it was so long in coming; such information has been so desperately needed. Had it been written fifty years ago, it would have eased the upbringing of generations of children and spared much suffering for millions of women.

Dr. Paavo Airola is looked upon as the foremost nutritionist in America, as well as world-renowned authority on biological medicine. One of the cornerstones of physical and mental well-being is optimal nutrition, as he demonstrates so expertly in this book. In my own practice as a physician and nutritionist, I rely heavily on the information and proven practices advocated by the author.

After reading this self-help book, the woman who is interested in health can be her own family doctor ninety-five percent of the time. She can use the programs suggested in the book without fear of adverse side effects or reactions to drugs. This book is filled with practical advice on how a woman can maintain a high level of well-being for herself and her family—in spite of the stresses, strains, and tensions of this complex world in which we live.

Dr. Airola says that women occupy a supremely important position in life. They hold the key to the future of mankind, and, therefore, must rise to their responsibilities —whether they have chosen the role of wife and mother, or a career outside the home, or a combination of both. In any case, the individual woman's lifestyle is structured upon her chosen vocation and the optimum health that it demands. In the pages of this book are the answers that women have been seeking since becoming aware of the increasing threat to their health from our denatured and polluted environment.

At the time the author asked me to write the Foreword for *Everywoman's Book*, I had already admired his expertise and had derived much benefit from his knowledge. However, with this giant undertaking, which resulted in a painstakingly researched compendium of a complete way of life, Dr. Airola has emerged not only as the nation's foremost exponent of holistic medicine, but as the greatest authority of the century on health and healing.

As an additional attraction, the author has the rare ability to write in a readable style, and presents highly technical material in a manner which both laymen and professionals can appreciate.

Never have I read such a fascinating, exciting, and complete health manual! It covers virtually all the health-related problems that women and children may encounter from infancy to maturity.

A truly wonderful, much needed book!

Mary Ann Kibler, M.D.

INTRODUCTION

by Robert S. Mendelsohn, M.D.

Paavo Airola's new book represents an authoritative and encyclopedic blend of modern science and traditional folk medicine. Covering the entire human life span, integrating nutrition and medicine in healthy states and disease, this remarkable work is a massive accomplishment by a single author. Comprehensively documented, yet not pedantic, easily understood, yet not simplistic, were this book merely a compilation of scientific and anecdotal evidence, it would still fill a void in today's health literature.

However, it is the additional, invaluable qualities of judgement, assessment, evaluation, and selectivity that dramatically silhouette Airola's book against the horizon. Thus, the collection of methods, facts, techniques, and remedies are filtered through the analytic deliberation, ethical standards, and mature wisdom that distinguishes Dr. Airola as a giant in the field.

If American medical schools ever decide to produce physicians instead of technicians, this book will occupy a position of highest priority in the curriculum. However, the people cannot afford to wait for that jubilee year; and, therefore, this book deserves to be immediately read and then used as a reference by families throughout our country, particularly those whose knowledge of historically validated truths has been obscured by the glare of contemporary medicine. The language is clear, often poetic, the directions explicit, while touches of good humor and sharp critique make for exciting reading. Furthermore, and most refreshing, this is not the kind of book that, at the end of each chapter, advises you to "see your doctor."

We will recognize true progress in creating a healthy American population when Benjamin Spock's influence of decades ago is replaced by Paavo Airola and his new book.

Robert S. Mendelsohn, M.D.

COMMENTS BY THE OTHER MEDICAL EDITORS OF
EVERYWOMAN'S BOOK

I have enjoyed each one of Dr. Airola's books, and learned a great deal from them, but this new one, *Everywoman's Book*, is truly a treasure chest. For new and experienced mothers both, I am sure, the chapters on childbirth, infant feeding, allergies, colic, and vaccination will be especially helpful. I found them most informative myself! And for young and old, men and women, the whole book is sure to be interesting. Each chapter is a jewel and an obvious product of thorough research.

Virginia Flanagan, M.D.

Everywoman's Book is the best to-date by a Holistic author placing an emphasis on the integration of the Body, Mind, and Spirit.

James H. Coyle, M.D., D. Psych.

Congratulations on a truly excellent and much-needed book! It is a superb and thorough document. I, literally, could not put the book down. The material is comprehensive, well-organized, and presented with clarity. The subject matter has not been given proper attention since Adelle Davis wrote her books in the Forties, when many mothers enthusiastically declared that their children were "raised by Adelle Davis." Now, the new-coming generations of fortunate children will be "raised by Airola."

Congratulations also on taking a stand on many controversial issues, such as circumcision and vaccination, for example. It's about time!

Michael E. Rosenbaum, M.D.

Everywoman's Book is a great new contribution in the field of alternative medicine. I am well acquainted with Dr. Airola's other excellent books and feel that this new book will be extremely helpful not only to all women, but also to doctors. I certainly will use it and recommend it to all my female patients.

Willem H. Khoe, M.D.

A masterpiece! The best thing you have ever written. It must be read by every woman—perferably together with her husband!

Abram Ber, M.D.

Everywoman's Book is magnificent! It is one of your most important works. I am continually amazed at how similarly we think on all the issues dealt with in this book, especially on topics like immunization, circumcision, treatment modalities, morality, etc. Your conclusions are well-documented by massive scientific references—this is crucial to wider acceptance in the professional health community. I commend you for it.

Michael L. Gerber, M.D.

I have read and benefited from all books written by Dr. Paavo Airola. His book, *How To Get Well*, is the "Bible of Natural Healing" in my medical practice.

Dr. Airola's new work, *Everywoman's Book*, will, without a doubt, have the greatest impact on the betterment of health on this planet. It is the result of incredible and painstaking research into the science of health and healing. It is a monument to Dr. Airola's profound knowledge, not only of nutrition and medicine, but also of the human spirit. More importantly, the book is a venerable homage and complimentary tribute to womanhood. Dr. Airola's keen understanding of and admiration for women motivated him to write a book that will be of inestimable value to them. The book is packed with practical and useful information on virtually every aspect of women's and children's health—it is an assuring beacon which illuminates the path to optimum physical, emotional, and spiritual well-being.

Finally, it is my conviction that if *How To Get Well* and *Everywoman's Book*, two of Dr. Airola's masterworks on Holistic Medicine, were used as major texts in curriculums of every medical school in this country, we would have a healthier and stronger America, and be able to halt the epidemic of degenerative diseases that is now plaguing this nation.

J.P. Hutchins, M.D.

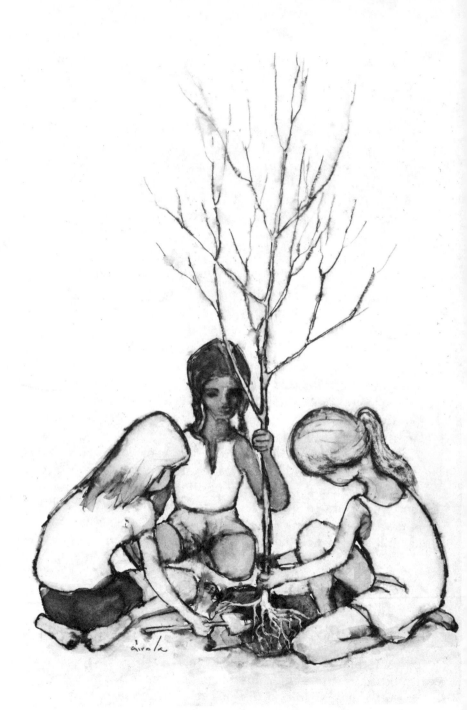

Why I Wrote This Book

For many years now, I have been writing question and answer columns on natural health and holistic healing for several magazines. I am always flooded with readers' questions on every imaginable aspect of health and disease. Naturally, only a fraction of the questions I receive can be answered in the limited space of the columns. Sometimes readers' questions stimulate me to write an article; occasionally, questions inspire me to write a book. For example, one of my most recent books, *Hypoglycemia: A Better Approach*, was written as a direct response to hundreds of questions from my readers who were dissatisfied with, and had so many negative experiences and side-effects from, the conventional high-protein diet for low blood sugar.

It would not be an overestimation to say that more than half of all the comments and questions I receive concern health problems related to *women*—specific questions dealing with various health-related issues in a woman's life. They could deal with anything from sore nipples to the pros and cons of rocking a baby, or from breast cancer to the "sudden" lack of sexual desire in an 87-year-old woman. Questions on teen-age acne, vaginal infections, natural and safe forms of birth control, estrogen-replacement therapy, pre-adolescent promiscuity, menstrual disorders, proper doses of vitamins for children and women of different ages, obesity ("tried everything and failed"), sexually transmitted diseases, menopausal distress—the list is endless!

One specific area which seems to be of much concern to many younger women is infant and child feeding. The confusion is apparently widespread as there are so many books by "experts" and so much unreliable, biased information, especially when it is coming from commercial food processing and baby food manufacturing sources.

Finally, one particular letter—one of thousands of similar letters with a desperate cry for knowledge— triggered my decision to write this book. It was from a young woman who wants to become a mother, but, wanting to insure the birth of a healthy baby by giving her "child-to-be a good start in life," feels a great sense of responsibility and has many concerns about the correct ways of going about it.

Here is her letter:

"Dear Dr. Airola,

I've just finished reading all of your books and am so thrilled that, at last, the path to glorious health is made clear! Everything you write makes so much sense to me and your books have "de-confused" me on so many questions about my health and nutrition that I have had for years.

I want to have a child, but I want to have a very healthy body before becoming pregnant. I have hypoglycemia and also kidney complications due to the extremely high-protein diet that was prescribed by my doctor to treat my hypoglycemia; so it will be a while yet before I will feel healthy enough to give my child-to-be a good start in life.

I plan to follow the basic Optimum Diet as recommended in your book, *How To Get Well*. But, I have *so many* questions, and I am sure there are many other mothers-to-be who have similar questions. Would you, *please*, someday write a book on pregnancy, natural birth, and the feeding of little children, which would be so helpful to us all?

For example:

- What special nutritional needs are there during pregnancy and how can they best be met?
- What about exercises during pregnancy?
- Are there natural means to handle complications if they arise?
- Do you know of any natural pain relievers for use during childbirth if they are needed?
- How long should I feed my baby exclusively on breast milk?
- What should I feed my baby if there is no, or not enough, milk in the breasts?
- When should I start and what solid foods should I feed my baby, and how should I prepare them?
- At what age can the child go on your Optimum Diet totally?
- When should I begin giving vitamins and supplements and in what dosages?
- What should be given in place of bone meal and fish oils if the parents are strict vegetarians?

All these and more are questions that I, and, I am sure, many other mothers and prospective mothers have. I think a book by you would be very helpful to all of us. It would mean a new generation of healthy, radiant, happy children and

eventually better health in the nation and the whole world.
May God bless you in your work!

Mrs. P.W.P., Colorado Springs, Co."

In this denatured and synthetic world, it is becoming
more and more difficult to maintain good health. In their
heroic efforts to "improve" nature, our chemically-oriented
scientists and medical inventors tell women that it is better
that the mother and child are both sedated with toxic
drugs during delivery; that it is better that the baby is
wrapped in synthetic, fire-retardant clothing and sleeps
alone, away from his mother, in a plastic crib with plastic
toys; that chemicalized bottle formula and denatured baby
food from a jar is better for the baby than mother's milk;
that baby's tonsils should be removed at the first sign of
infection; etc., etc.

The woman of today has an enormous responsibility
as a wife and mother. She is a dietician, doctor, nurse, and
teacher all combined in one. She gambles with the health
and the life of her family when she fills up her cart at the
supermarket. She can unknowingly kill her husband or
cripple her child for life by what she prepares in the
kitchen. Her understanding of proper nutrition determines
to a great degree if and when her husband suffers a heart
attack, if she will save her own breasts from mastectomy,
or if her children will develop sufficient intelligence to
succeed in school. Just as simple an issue as what kind of
water she drinks before and during pregnancy, or gives to
her young children, can mean the difference between a
mongoloid child and a healthy one. And, how many
women know what kind of water is coming from the tap?

The more letters from confused, bewildered, and
desperate women I read, the more I realized the necessity—
a crying need!—for a book that can help to give a new
orientation.

There has been during the past couple of decades a
growing dissatisfaction among women with the orthodox
synthetic version of motherhood and child-rearing, as well
as with the conventional medical approach to dealing with
female health and sex problems with the use of pills,
powerful drugs, and carcinogenic chemical hormone sub-

stitutes. There is a massive world-wide movement towards living a more natural life. People are becoming more and more aware of the grave threat to their health from increasingly chemicalized and poisoned foods, air, water, and environment.

The purpose of this book is to offer practical advice and natural non-toxic alternatives for dealing with the health problems women face throughout their lives—from before conception to menopause and old age. I will show how to complete a pregnancy without endangering the health of the mother or of the future child; how to deliver naturally—without drugs—and with a minimum of stress; how a woman can feed herself, her infant, children, and husband to achieve optimum health, long life, and absence of disease. I will offer natural, biological, herbal, and holistic alternatives for treating various diseases of childhood, as well as specific female health problems such as breast cancer, varicose veins, vaginitis, sexually transmitted diseases, depression, anemia, etc.

After having written a dozen books, some of which are used as textbooks in universities and medical schools, I feel an increasing sense of humility and responsibility with each new book project. This book, I feel, is the most important I have written. It has also been a labor of love on a subject which is very close to my heart. I am keenly aware that since it deals with child-rearing, motherhood, and womanhood, it may influence and affect the health and well-being of generations of human beings. This is why, sensing the immense responsibility towards humanity, I have solicited and enlisted the help and advice not only of the comprehensive board of medical experts, but also of my Creator—my ultimate Source of knowledge, courage, strength, and wisdom. I hope and pray that this book will fulfill my aspirations to be of help and benefit to all those who are confused and troubled and earnestly seeking help, comfort, and knowledge.

May your inherent, intuitive wisdom and the Divine Creative Power light your path and be your guide as you go through the pages of this book.

Part One
Mothering

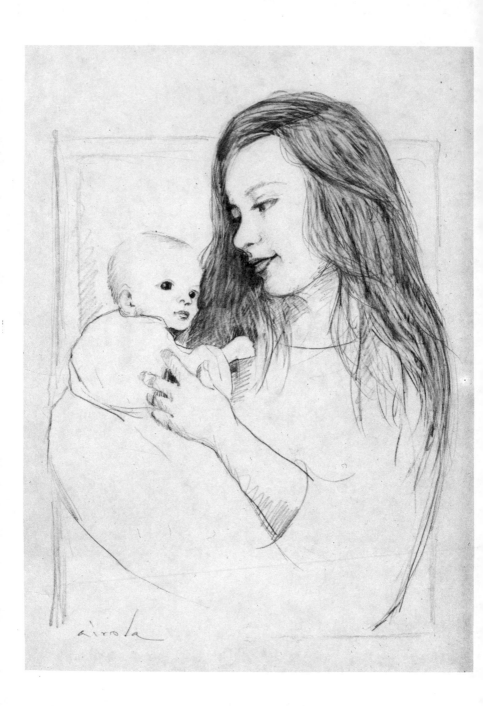

I

The Fulfilling Role of Motherhood

Currently, there is a trend toward unisex. Some misguided individuals who have lost sight of the natural order would like to erase the differences between the sexes. Masquerading as advocates of equal rights, they deliberately confuse the equality of male and female human rights with the equality of roles. Unquestionably, men and women should have the same rights and privileges as well as responsibilities under the law and in regard to education, employment, equal pay, etc. But, although men and women are entitled to equal human *rights,* their *roles* in life were not meant to be identical. Men and women were created equal in terms of human and spiritual worth in the sight of God, but different in terms of the roles they should play in the drama of life. The differences between the two sexes are essential. Biologically, physically and emotionally man was not made to function in the same manner as woman, nor vice-versa. If the Creator had meant man and woman to perform the same functions in life, why make two different models for the same job? When men and women lose the understanding of their essential differences, we find chaos, confusion and reversal of human progress. Although the so-called liberation movement dialogue has brought some women a greater understanding and appreciation of their worth as human beings, the implication that equality with men can be achieved through imitation can only bring unhappiness, despair, and disastrous confusion to women, as well as a sense of abandonment, loss of identity and rejection among children.

Divine plan

I believe that our life on this planet is not an accidental bio-cosmo-geo-chemo-physical occurrence, but is a part of a carefully designed Divine plan of eternal progression. As immortal spiritual beings, we are placed on this planet in mortal physical form to fulfill the purpose of this plan, the essence of which is perfection and refinement of our divine spirits. Our task is to develop and improve our human and divine characteristics by learning to love one another, by being more caring and compassionate in our relationships with our "neighbors" as well as with all living creatures, by being more forgiving, by renouncing and rejecting selfishness, greed, and injustice—thus preparing the way for our continued growth and perfection throughout immortality.

All human beings are created with an equal opportunity to fulfill this plan in an individual and personal way. Each of us is born with particular qualities, talents, and mental, emotional, intellectual, and physical faculties which are perfectly suited for fulfillment of the plan for our progression.

When we understand the essence and the purpose of this Divine plan, and devote ourselves to our personal responsibility within it, we find harmony, fulfillment, peace, and supreme happiness!

Motherhood: the ultimate self-realization

Woman has been given a very special position in this grand plan. She is a partner and co-creator with God in bringing life into the world. She shares this lifework with man. Man and woman must be **One** in making the Divine plan possible by bringing spirits into the world and giving them physical bodies. The family unit is the cornerstone of purposeful human existence on this earth. The progress of all humanity is dependent on the solidarity of the family. It is through the family, which was instituted by God, that the order and harmony of the universal laws are translated to the earthly experience.

I shall illustrate the essence and equality of the union between a man and a woman by the following mathematical formula which makes it visually comprehensible: $1 + 1 = 1$. The perfect union of two equal human beings, man and woman, creates **one** new separate entity—family. From this original unit, all creation is brought into being: families form communities; communities make up nations; nations fashion the world. The current attempts to eradicate the differences between the sexes are not only destroying the family—the basic unit of society—which can lead to the end of all humanity, but are belittling and disparaging the superior and glorious role of motherhood. They also destroy the opportunity for and deprive woman of her inherent right to experience the supreme joy and fulfillment which comes with motherhood.

Great responsibility

A mother has the great responsibility of determining and influencing the direction her children will take in their lives. That influence continues throughout infancy and childhood, but begins even before birth. The thoughts, the desires, and the wishes of the mother have the power to impress her forming child with the personality characteristics it will have as it grows up—this is the essence of Stirpiculture, the science of prenatal care.[1] Truly, "the hand that rocks the cradle rules the world"! Under what conditions a child is conceived and nurtured in the womb, and how he is influenced by his parent's feelings, thoughts, and actions before and after birth, predetermines to a vast degree his moral fiber, talents, mental capacity, abilities, state of health, and even longevity.[2]

Heredity modified

We have been told by cell-probing scientists that the physical and mental attributes and capabilities of a child are predetermined by the heredity-carrying genes in male spermatozoa and female ovum. These scientists, who usually comprehend only what they see under the microscope, have overlooked a very important detail. The law of heredity applies unmodified to all forms of lower life, but in the more highly developed human beings, *where spiritual laws supersede physical laws,* the law of heredity can be modified or accentuated by the conscious and determined efforts of the mother. The mother's will, thoughts, feelings, and desires, before and during pregnancy, as well as during lactation and early childhood, may reverse heredity and natural tendencies to a considerable degree.

This conscious maternal influence on the child's future is especially true in regard to his mental, emotional, intellectual, and spiritual attributes and capabilities.

By dwelling on, visualizing, desiring, and praying in faith, the mother can help to instill in a child superb qualities of character, talent, and personality necessary for potential success in life—even though these desired qualities are not possessed by the parents.[1] This is a fundamental principle of the spiritual laws superseding the physical laws, or what even the materialistic scientists finally are conceding: the power of mind over body! Indeed, it is possible and within the power of the mother to fashion the moral, intellectual, and physical fiber of her child.

What a great responsibility: not only to shape the destiny of offspring for good or ill, but also the destiny of the nation as a whole! President Herbert Hoover said: "If we could have but one generation of properly born, trained, educated and healthy children, a thousand other problems of government would vanish. We would assure ourselves of healthier minds and more vigorous bodies, to direct the energies of our nation to greater heights of achievement."

Yes, the role of a women is, indeed, magnificent and far-reaching. She is given the ability and privilege to bear children so that she might share in the glory of creation with the Source of All Life. In addition, the great personal reward of motherhood is the love which will fill her life to overflowing: the trusting love of her children, the devoted love of her husband, and the divine, infinite love of her Creator. The whole essence of her life will be that of giving and receiving an abundance of love. Woman's justifiable pride and gratification in achievements in any other field will never exceed her desire to express love and to be loved.

In order to fulfill her important roles within the Divine plan, woman is endowed with special qualities that man does not possess to the same degree. A woman is by nature more intuitive, more compassionate and caring, more spiritually aware, more gentle, warmer, kinder, more tolerant, considerate and forgiving, more altruistic and magnanimous, more aesthetically oriented, more creative and imaginative, more affectionate and romantic, more benevolent and loving. These qualities and personality attributes help her in performing the role of motherhood as well as contribute to her success in all areas where warm, personal, trusting, and caring relations are important.

Career women

But what about women who for one reason or another are not married, or cannot have children? What about the many great women in past and recent history who have attained high degrees of achievements in various fields of art, science, or statesmanship? What about a career woman—doctor, nurse, administrator, teacher? Is it not possible that they can attain great satisfaction and fulfillment in their careers or chosen fields of activity?

Yes, if the role of wife and mother, however preferred, is not possible or available, or, if a woman chooses not to perform the traditional role of motherhood, she can find fulfillment in performing other life functions for which she is prepared and inclined. There are many women who *choose* to dedicate their lives to a specific task outside of the traditional role of motherhood. No doubt there are women who are better suited to perform missions of great importance which do not include the role of motherhood. Such women make great contributions to the advancement of humanity through their specific fields of endeavor and find happiness and fulfillment in performing these roles. The woman who feels a need for the challenge and stimulation of a career outside the home in order to utilize her special talents and gifts, can do so while still exemplifying womanhood at its best. It is every woman's right and responsibility to bring her unique qualities to all facets of life. By so doing, she is being true to womanhood and to humanity. In Russia, 70 percent of all medical doctors are women, and over 90 percent of them are married. I have been associated with many brilliant and talented women who have achieved high degrees of competence in various areas of science, healing, business, arts, and management; having a career does not, however, mean that the role of motherhood *must* be relinquished. A woman can be a successful wife and mother and have a second career, as well. Although having two careers—the career of mother and wife and an outside career—is rather challenging in terms of time and energies, if the priorities are kept right, both can be successfully pursued at the same time.

Whether or not you choose the role of motherhood, you can exemplify womanhood in any career, field of endeavor, or lifestyle. By being true to yourself and developing your unique potentials, you can not only make a great contribution to the advancement of humankind, but also reach the ultimate of self-realization and attain supreme joy and fulfillment in your own life.

2

Preparing For Pregnancy

As stated in the previous chapter, bringing a new spirit into this world and raising him to be a happy and fulfilled human being is a great joy and privilege, but also a tremendous responsibility. Every prospective mother's goal should be to give her new child a good start in life by making sure that his body and mind are free from in-born illness and imperfections and that he will be equipped with built-in resistance to disease and to the constantly increasing amount of environmental stresses.

It is no secret that the chances of living a long life and enjoying excellent health in modern-day America are virtually nil. According to authoritative sources and statistics:

- 98 percent of all Americans are afflicted with dental disease.
- 70,000,000, including children, are obese.
- 25,000,000 suffer from hypoglycemia.
- 30,000,000 suffer from crippling and agonizing arthritis.
- 20,000,000 suffer from mental diseases; over 10,000,000 of them requiring medical treatment.
- 10,000,000 suffer from coronary heart disease, leading to 1,000,000 deaths a year.
- 1,000,000 new cases of cancer are diagnosed yearly and 300,000 die from it each year.

Millions of others suffer from diabetes, allergies, multiple sclerosis, muscular dystrophy, hearing and visual problems, digestive, reproductive, and glandular disorders, etc. Unbelievable as it may seem, available statistics indicate that over 2/3 of all Americans suffer from chronic diseases!

Why is there so much disease? Why, in spite of the fact that we have the most advanced medical care in the world, more doctors, more hospitals, more drugs, and better housing, higher wages, and more food to eat than in most other nations, do we have more disease than any country in the world?!

To answer this question in depth would require more space than the format and the theme of this book would allow or justify. The question is discussed extensively in several of my earlier books, especially in *Are You Confused?*, and *Health Secrets From Europe*.[1] But, the most comprehensive and scientifically documented answer to this perplexing question is given by Dr. Weston Price in his classic book, *Nutrition and Physical Degeneration*.[2] Dr. Price, with well-documented dietary records, case histories, photographs, and statistics from around the world, showed that the health of individuals and nations is determined by their *eating and living habits*. A simple, health-promoting lifestyle, and a diet of unprocessed, whole, natural foods results in the birth of beautiful, healthy babies and builds strong resistance to disease; while the diet of processed, canned, "convenience" foods with sugar and refined flour products results in sickly, malformed, defective children and adults prone to a variety of diseases.

What about our children?

In our country, there are over 400,000 miscarriages annually. In terms of infant mortality, we are in 26th place among the nations, according to U.N. statistics (1978). Each year the number of babies born with physical and mental defects increases with alarming speed. There are now 15 million American children affected in some way by one of the 1400 birth defects differentiated by medical researchers. One in ten newborn babies suffers from some birth defect; 250,000 of them serious enough to require medical attention. Over 126,000 are born severely mentally retarded. At least 1 million school-age children are hyper-kinetic to the extent of needing medical attention. In addition, more than 10 million other emotionally disturbed children need medical help. Dr. Joseph D. Noshpitz, president of the American Academy of Child Psychiatry, says that with proper screening this figure would probably double.[4]

Our medical journals, newspaper and magazine articles, and television specials sing out in hopeful tones about the newest medical advances in treatment and care of these pitiful, deformed little children. Plastic surgeons develop new ways of repairing distorted bodies. The drug industry spends millions on the testing and developing of new miracle drugs to manipulate and normalize the physical and mental functions of these retarded and deformed babies. But, *no one* teaches our young people, the future mothers and fathers, how to *prevent* all this needless suffering of both parents and children.

To be normal, healthy, and well-developed is the *birthright* of every newborn. "Primitive people in every part of the earth knew exactly how to preserve their tribal patterns of health, vitality, and beautiful, perfect bodies, and to pass this gift of radiant health to their children, throughout countless generations," writes Gena Larson, one of the American pioneers and champions for better nutrition for our children.[5] But, in our highly "civilized" country, the inherited wisdom and instincts regarding the relationship of health vs. eating and living habits is almost totally lost, and we now depend on our family doctor or pediatrician to take care of our children's health. And, many misinformed and misdirected doctors, still in a stupor from medical school indoctrination in the erroneous Pasteurian germ philosophy of disease, believe that health and nutrition are not related!

Is our sordid state of health and that of our children influenced by the way we eat and the way we live? Can the recent tremendous increase in all degenerative diseases among all ages and the epidemic growth in birth defects and childhood diseases be attributed to prenatal, natal, and infant feeding? Can breast feeding help prevent diseases in children and adults? Will the health of the parents and the kind of foods they eat have an effect on the physical and mental health of their children?

Based on the available authoritative research and a growing number of world-wide scientific studies, the answer to all these questions is an emphatic YES!

It is becoming more and more evident, supported by overwhelming research, that a child will "inherit" the quality of health that his parents have been preparing for him during their lifetime, during prenatal and infant care, and during his childhood.

Preparing for pregnancy emotionally

Parenthood, as you can see from the above, is a great responsibility. Therefore, it is important that preparation for parenthood begins as early as possible, both physically and emotionally.

Children can grow up healthy and happy only if they have loving, caring parents. The most important thing about pregnancy is that it must be *wanted.* Unwanted pregnancies rarely produce happy, healthy, and well-adjusted children. A young woman planning to become a mother must be sure that there is an unmistakable sense of desire, commitment, and responsibility on her own part as well as on the part of the father of her future child. Both prospective parents must realize that bearing and raising children is a lifetime job, and requires a total commitment.

Raising children requires patience, forbearance, and understanding. Parents must be prepared for letdowns, sacrifices, and disappointments. But, the ultimate rewards of successful parenthood far outweigh all the sacrifices. As the father of five children, I can truthfully say that of all the many joys I have experienced throughout my life—material and professional successes, wonderful friends, colleagues' and critics' praises, honors, awards and merits, world-wide travels, and international acclaim—none has given me as much true happiness, lasting joy, and sense of accomplishment, contentment, and fulfillment as the opportunity of helping to bring into this world and raise five precious, healthy, and well-adjusted children.

Preparing for conception physically

The number one requisite for healthy babies is healthy parents. Young people who get married and plan to have children should always keep this in mind.

At least for one year *before* attempting to conceive a baby, both future parents should begin making every effort to build a high level of health which will provide a suitable base for the genetic inheritance of their child.

How can you maximize your health?

Here are the essential basic factors that will add up to an optimal level of physical and mental well-being:

1. *Positive state of mind.* A health-oriented attitude, hope, faith, and reliance on your own ability as well as in a Higher Power that will give guidance, understanding, energy, and wisdom, are the most important ingredients leading to optimum health. Faith is the greatest health-building and healing power known to man. The power of faith, prayer, meditation, and positive thinking, cannot be overestimated. A positive attitude and peace of mind are two vital health factors that are missing in modern man's life. Emotional and mental stresses can tear your health down faster than can inadequate nutrition. It has been scientifically established that emotional and mental stresses—constant fears, anxieties, worries, tensions, depression, hate, jealousy, unhappiness, deprivation of love, and loneliness—can cause virtually every disease in the medical dictionary, including arthritis, ulcers, asthma, strokes, constipation, diabetes, high or low blood pressure, angina, glandular disturbances, sexual inadequacies, heart disease, hypoglycemia, and cancer. On the other hand, a positive state of mind is of inestimable value for optimal health and prevention of disease. (Read more about the health-building value of positive, health-oriented state of mind in Chapter 35.)

2. *Plenty of exercise.* Life is motion. Your body's most important nutritional requirement is not protein, vitamins, enzymes, fats, minerals—it is oxygen! You can live for months without any food, for days without water, but for only a few minutes without oxygen. Nutritionists, in their illustrative description of the body's mechanism, like to compare it to an automobile. "Just as your car runs best on pure, high quality gas, your body requires the highest quality food to run friction-free." This comparison is misleading. The automobile-gas relationship should be compared to the body-*oxygen* relationship. Oxygen is the most important nutrient for every organ and every cell of your body. How can you get enough of it?

I have often referred to the effective and optimal functioning of your body as dependent on special biorhythms or lifecycles, a kind of genetic programming which has been determined and formed as a result of man's adaptation to the historical and traditional circumstances of his environment. One of the environmental circumstances of prehistoric man was his great mobility connected with daily living. To survive and provide nourishment, man had to move a great deal. And this he had to do on his own two legs. Much walking, running, moving about, and lifting was done during most of the day. Consequently, after thousands of years of adaptation to this kind of lifestyle, man's body was genetically programmed and adjusted to function efficiently on the level of oxygen that was generated by such a mobile lifestyle.

Our present lifestyle has eliminated 90 percent of the motion and exercise our bodies used to have. We do not move on our own power any more—cars and airplanes take care of that. We do not need to exercise our muscles to get our food—we simply drive to the supermarket; and even there we use a cart to haul the food back to our car. Such a lifestyle results in a body which isn't getting much oxygen. The level of oxygen absorption is determined by the level of physical exertion. Our sedentary life has led to a chronic oxygen starvation. Our organs, muscles, brain, nerves, which were designed to function at optimum capacity on a certain level of oxygen, now are forced to cope with their tasks on a constant undersupply of this most important nutrient. The consequences are obvious: physical and mental deterioration and a growing amount of disease that has developed since man has adopted his new, sedentary, mechanized lifestyle, with its polluted air, where he is getting less and less oxygen.

The only way you can bring more oxygen into your system now is by the deliberate exercise. With exercise, I do not mean only a few calisthenics in front of your television, or some slow yoga movements—although both can be beneficial in conjunction with more strenuous activity—but vigorous daily exercise such as jogging, running, playing tennis, biking, swimming, etc., which will lead to an accelerated heartbeat and perspiration. Vigorous exercise is needed to bring the maximum amount of oxygen into tissues and organs. Vigorous exercise, and the oxygen it brings into the system, is imperative for the proper functioning of all organs, *especially the all-important lymphatic system.*

The exercise should be performed outdoors in pure, unpolluted air. There are many books on special exercises to be done during pregnancy. In the natural childbirth classes, there are usually exercises taught for mothers-to-be. However, walking, jogging, swimming, and mild calisthenics are the best forms of exercise even during pregnancy.

3. *Optimum nutrition.* See the detailed outline of the Optimum Diet for mother-to-be in the next two chapters.

4. *Fresh, pure air.* Pure air is becoming harder and harder to come by. Many live in large cities where the air is badly polluted with dangerous chemicals such as lead, mercury, carbon monoxide, cadmium, etc. Optimum health cannot be achieved if you are breathing such air. Especially if you plan to start a family and raise children, you owe it to yourself and to the future of your children to make all conceivable efforts to get out of the city smog. You may say, "It is not possible." You are fooling yourself. It *is* possible! *Everything* is possible, if there is sufficient mo-

tivation and conviction that it must be done, and a strong determination to do it. I know of hundreds of people who have done so against seemingly overwhelming odds and obstacles. If you decide to go all out for maximizing your health, spending lots of time and money for better nutrition and more exercise, your efforts will be largely wasted if you continue breathing polluted, toxic, smoggy air. Pure, unpolluted air is absolutely imperative for the health of everyone, but especially for the health of pregnant women, babies, and children.

5. *Sunlight.* Research by Dr. John Ott, director of the Environmental Health and Light Research Institute in Sarasota, Florida, shows that there is a link between light and the physical, mental, and emotional health of animals and humans.[6] Sufficient exposure to sunlight is essential for optimum health. Sunlight is the initial source of all life—without sunlight no life can exist. Until very recently, the eyes were generally thought of only as sensory organs for vision. But research during the last twenty years reveals that the eyes have other important functions. Through the eyes, light enters into the body and via an elaborate system of electro-neurotransmitters stimulates the activity of the whole body, particularly of the glandular system. Dr. Ott showed that sunlight stimulates the pituitary gland which is a regulator of the other endocrine glands. The pineal gland, located at the base of the brain, is also affected by the action of sunlight on the tissues of the eye. Both of these glands—pituitary and pineal—are major regulating glands of the endocrine system, which includes the sex glands. The proper function of the endocrine glands is essential for the health of the whole body.

The excessive use of artificial light, especially cool white fluorescent light, and specifically the use of sunglasses, has been shown to be very detrimental to the health. Dr. Ott's studies with both animals and human beings, using different forms of light, natural and artificial, showed almost unbelievable results. Here is just a few samples taken from the volumes of scientific reports:

- Calcium absorption is more efficient when patients are subjected to sunlight as compared to artificial light.
- Terminal cancer patients improved dramatically when they started to avoid artificial lighting and started being outdoors in sunlight as much as possible.
- African natives who adopt the habit of wearing sunglasses become susceptible to cancer while those who do not wear sunglasses are more resistant.
- Leukoplakia of the cervix, with complete hysterectomy recommended, disappeared when changes were made in the patients' eyeglasses and window glass, and when more time was spent in sunlight.
- Prostate cancer was also favorably affected by the same means.
- Chronic arthritis, recurrent sore throats, colds, jaundice in premature babies, tooth decay, hyperkinesis, behavioral and personality problems in classrooms and offices—all changed for the better when artificial lighting was replaced by full-spectrum lighting and/or sunlight.

One of the most dramatic studies on the relationship between light and health involved a school where for several years the leukemia incidence was five times that of the national average. All affected children attended class in two rooms where the window shades were always closed, thus preventing any sunlight from coming through the window glass, and necessitating the constant use of the fluorescent lights. After the lighting was changed to allow more sunlight through the windows, and a different type of full-spectrum lighting was installed, there were no further reported cases of leukemia among children in those two classes.

Although Dr. Ott says that his studies and the dramatic cases reported above cannot be considered "scientific proof," that more studies are needed, and although it may take a long time before his pioneering research will be approved and endorsed by medical orthodoxy, it would be wise to heed the lesson and avoid spending too much time in artificial lighting. Expose your body to real life-giving and health-building sunlight—without wearing sunglasses!

In addition to the beneficial effects of sunlight as discovered by Dr. Ott, don't forget the fact that vitamin D, which builds on the skin of your body when exposed to the sun, is of crucial importance for optimal health. Foods are very poor sources of vitamin D, and we actually depend on sun-produced vitamin D as a prime source of this important vitamin. This is especially important for pregnant women as well as young breast-fed babies, since mother's milk is a rather poor source of vitamin D. Note: do not take a bath or shower immediately after sunbathing which will wash off the vitamin D formed on the skin by the action of the sun before it is absorbed into the body.

Caution: As beneficial as sunlight is, you must avoid over-exposure! All things, even good ones, can be harmful in excess. Painful sunburns, even skin cancer, can be the result of over-exposure.

6. *Pure, natural water.* Drinking pure, uncontaminated, natural spring or well water is an important part of the Optimum Diet for optimum health. Keep in mind, however, that even well water may be contaminated with man-made chemicals if you live in an agricultural or industrial area.

Avoid prolonged use of distilled drinking water, which has become a fad recently, motivated by the universal water contamination. Distilled water is totally devoid of all minerals, and prolonged use of it may leach out the body's own mineral reserves and lead to severe mineral deficiencies and such diseases as osteoporosis, diabetes, tooth decay, and heart disease. It has been proven by extensive world-wide studies that where people drink naturally "hard" or heavily mineralized water, there is a lesser incidence of the above-mentioned diseases. Minerals, as they are naturally present in drinking water, have been an essential part of man's mineral nutrition since the beginning of his life on this planet.

Contrary to what you may have heard or read, inorganic minerals in natural waters *are* effectively absorbed and well utilized in human metabolism. And they *do not* cause hardening of the arteries, kidney stones, or other supposed diseases. Quite to the contrary! *We need* both *inorganic* and *organic* minerals for optimum health. Hunzakuts, who are considered to be the healthiest people in the world, who have never suffered from hardening of the arteries, kidney stones, tooth decay, arthritis, osteoporosis, or heart diseases, have for 2000 years been drinking mountain stream water so heavily mineralized with lime and other inorganic minerals that it is milky in appearance. This is, perhaps, better evidence than any quasi-scientific reasoning.

Unfortunately, it is becoming more and more difficult to obtain uncontaminated pure natural water in this poisoned world of ours. Most supermarkets and health food stores now sell bottled spring or purified waters. See that natural minerals are left intact in the purification process. If you must drink distilled water, add natural minerals to it, such as pure sea water—2 - 3 tsp. of sea water to 1 quart of distilled water. But, *if you can get it,* we recommend using pure, uncontaminated, naturally mineralized spring water.

7. *Sleep, rest, and relaxation.* Rest and relaxation are other factors which must not be ignored. Throughout this book, we are going to emphasize repeatedly that stress is one of the main causes of disease. A certain amount of stress is natural, cannot be avoided, and is not harmful, *if it is counteracted and balanced by sufficient rest and relaxation.*

Make a habit of having an afternoon nap or siesta. Relax with a good book or enjoyable music now and then. Don't drain yourself of all energy reserves. Conserve energy and recharge your batteries by occasional pauses and rest periods. This is of special value to the mother-to-be.

Long periods of undisturbed sleep, preferably with open windows is also imperative for optimum health.

8. *Periodic cleansing juice fasts.* Continuous over-

abundance of and overindulgence in food is a relatively recent phenomenon in man's history. Historically and traditionally, our genetic code is programmed for periodic abstinence from or drastic reduction of food, which was necessitated by the periodic unavailability of food, particularly during famines and during winter and early spring, when the storage supply of food was exhausted and the new crops were still unripe. In Hunza, and many other parts of the world, such spring starvation is a common occurrence even today. Every spring there is a period of four to six weeks when people must tighten their belts and go through a natural, unintentional partial fast because there is not much food left from winter supplies.

Although the primitive people who were forced to starve (fast) did not, of course, understand or appreciate the health benefits they derived thereby, the fact remains that periodic abstinence from food had a far-reaching beneficial effect on their health. Our ancestors' bodies used these periods to cleanse themselves from the toxic wastes accumulated during the periods of overindulgence. These periodic fasts also helped to repair and heal any health disorders, give digestive and eliminative organs a rest, and to restore and normalize the functions of all glands and organs. Because of this involuntary fast, they enjoyed better health, their resistance against disease was increased, and they lived longer. We are able to say this now, because modern scientific research has shown that systematic undereating and periodic fasting are the two most important health and longevity factors.[7, 8]

What our ancestors did against their will, forced to it by unfavorable environmental conditions and circumstances beyond their control, we must do now intentionally if we wish to enjoy the same level of health. Periodic cleansing fasts, perhaps once a year, every spring, for a couple of weeks, would help tremendously to improve our health, prevent disease, and increase life span. Because of our sedentary life and a tendency to overeat, our body mechanisms need such cleansing to keep in good working order.

Juice fasting has been shown to be the safest and most effective way to restore health and prevent disease. Periodic juice fasting will speed up the process of elimination of toxic waste matter and dead cells from the body and accelerate and stimulate the building of new cells. It will also normalize all metabolic and nervous functions and increase cell oxygenation. After fasting, the digestion of food and utilization of nutrients is greatly improved and sluggishness and further water retention are prevented.

For a mother-to-be, periodic juice fasting, at least one or two short fasts *prior* to conception, can do much to improve her chances of successful pregnancy and the delivery of a healthy offspring, with a minimum of stress on her own body. (Note: *during* pregnancy or lactation fasting is not advisable.)

(For complete instructions and detailed, hour-by-hour, day-by-day guidelines on how to fast on your own, see my book, *How To Keep Slim, Healthy, and Young with Juice Fasting.*)

If all the above-mentioned basic health-optimizing factors, including the Optimum Diet as outlined in the next two chapters, are carefully adhered to, for at least one year before conception—*by both* future parents—as well as during pregnancy and lactation, the greatest assurance for having a normal, well-formed baby, free from inborn illness and imperfections, can be potentiated, and you can expect to have the wonderful pleasure and joy of delivering and raising a happy, healthy, and well-adjusted child.

3

Optimum Nutrition
For Mother-To-Be
(and father, too)

The most important prerequisite for healthy babies is healthy parents, as it was shown in the previous chapter. Optimum nutrition is one of the most important factors in achieving an optimal level of physical and mental well-being.

Although most people agree that nutrition is a very important factor affecting one's health, almost everyone, including doctors and nutritionists—or, should I say, *especially* doctors and nutrition experts—disagree as to what kind of nutrition is good for you, or **WHAT** constitutes an Optimum Diet for optimum health.

There are those who believe that the so-called "Basic Four" food groups will assure optimum nutrition. There are those who advocate a high-animal-protein diet, with lots of meat. There are those who condemn all seeds and grains ("seeds are for the birds") and those who would eat seeds, but not grains. There are those who advocate eating only raw foods, and those who consider the discovery of fire to be the greatest boon to man's nutrition. There are those who eat only vegetables that grow above the ground, and those who consider tomatoes, garlic, and onions to be poisonous. Then there are nutritionists and health writers who wish to please everyone (just like the politicians—it's good business, you know) and advise eating anything that you like, or "what agrees with you," as long as it is natural and unprocessed. There are those who feel that you should supplement your diet with vitamins—and there are those who claim that all added vitamins are harmful and/or unnecessary and that you should get your vitamins from the foods you eat.

Lately, we seem to have more and more extreme and bizarre diets and nutritional fads. Fruitarians advise eating nothing but fruits. Raw foodists claim that cooked food is "dead" food and cannot produce anything but death—consequently, they advocate eating everything raw. Mucusless diet proponents attribute all disease to mucus-producing foods, such as milk, grains, and meats, and claim that avoidance of them can assure optimum health. Sproutarians claim that the secret of health is in eating sprouts, especially wheat sprouts and wheat grass. Even among those who adhere to vegetarian dietary philosophies there are plain vegetarians, lacto-vegetarians, lacto-ovo-vegetarians, and vegans. Then there is the macrobiotic diet with Japanese culinary flavor with emphasis on rice and soy products, all heavily salted, cooked, and fried. There are even those who suggest that we quit eating completely, and replace it with drinking, claiming that by drinking copious amounts of juices we will solve all of our health problems. Some of the newest fads put all the blame on fats and claim that by eliminating from the diet not only butter, vegetable oils, and other concentrated fats, but also all fat-containing foods such as milk, cheese, nuts, seeds, and avocados, we can eliminate all of our degenerative diseases.

The proponents of each of the above-mentioned diets claim in their books or lectures that *their's* is the diet that is the perfect one—and they have "wonderful results" to prove it! No wonder the average person is confused! The more books he reads, the more lectures he hears, the more confused and bewildered he becomes. Who is right? Whom can you believe? Why is there so much confusion and disagreement among experts?

In my book, *Are You Confused?*, I have answered these questions quite thoroughly, so I will not go into detail here, except to mention that commercialism (most nutritionists are selling the products or services that they so highly recommend), scholastic dogmatism, outdated and obsolete information (many still-popular nutrition books were written 20-30-40 years ago when many of the vitamins had not even been discovered and nutrition science was in its infancy), and personal likes and dislikes (for example, one late leading nutritionist extolled the value of eating lots of meat because he "personally liked the taste of meat"), are at the root of so much nutrition misinformation, confusion, and disagreement. Ever since *Are You Confused?* was written, I have continued to ponder about the growing number of new dietary fads and the puzzling question kept recurring: why do the seemingly intelligent creators of some of these obviously deficient diets sincerely believe that they have discovered the ultimate health-building and preventive diet? Finally, the answer dawned on me: the nutritionists, overwhelmed by the *therapeutic* effect of their diets, concluded, *erroneously,* that "what cures will prevent," that their diets can build and maintain health and *prevent* disease because they are so effective in *curing* disease. They overlooked the extremely important difference between a *therapeutic diet* and a *preventive diet.* Let me explain.

The crucial difference between therapeutic and preventive nutrition

Example: Arnold Ehret was a very sick man. After trying a long line of conventional doctors and drugs for years, his health went from bad to worse and nothing seemed to help. Finally, in desperation, he started to experiment with his own diet and he discovered that by eliminating bread, cereals, milk, cheese, meat, fowl, and fish from his diet, he miraculously became well. Since all the above-mentioned foods are mucus-producing, Ehret concluded that excess mucus is the cause of all illness, and by eliminating all mucus-forming foods from our diet, not only will we all get well, but such a diet will prevent disease if we remain on it continuously. Consequently, he wrote books, lectured, and proclaimed to his enthusiastic followers that he had discovered the optimum diet, the *mucusless* diet, and he advocated that all should adhere to such a diet to optimize their health and prevent disease.

Another example: In the past few decades, several sincere seekers of optimum health have discovered that eating nothing but fresh fruits for several months (often nothing but oranges and tomatoes) helped dramatically to restore their health. They, again, drew the erroneous conclusion that because a fruit diet made them feel so good, and because it had such a healing effect, it must be the ultimate, divinely-designed diet for man. Consequently, they recommended that all those concerned with preserving their health become fruitarians.

One more example: A man in California discovered that by eliminating all fats from the diet, even such foods as milk, cheese, butter, vegetable oils, eggs, nuts, seeds, and avocados, patients at his health center were miraculously cured from such degenerative cardiovascular disorders as angina, atherosclerosis, high blood pressure, and heart disease. After a few weeks on this diet, it was found that heart patients scheduled for by-pass surgery no longer needed surgery. Angina patients, who previously could not walk ten feet without pain, could walk miles and climb mountains. Impressed by the tremendous *therapeutic* effect of his diet, the originator of this fat-free diet concluded that the prime reason we Americans are so sick and suffer from so many degenerative diseases is that we eat too much fat. By eliminating all the fat from our diets, we can get rid of all the degenerative diseases.

What all the above-mentioned nutritionists overlooked is that although their diets, and many others, such as sproutarian, juice, grape, or other limited diets, are obviously remarkably *therapeutic,* i.e., they are able to cure disease and restore health, they are also, nutritionally speaking, far too *deficient* to *maintain health* and *prevent disease* once health has been restored. A thera-peutic diet doesn't have to be an *optimum* diet in terms of its nutritional adequacy. For the best therapeutic effect, it can be, in fact often must be, inadequate or deficient in certain nutritive elements. Eating nothing but fresh fruit for a period of time obviously has such a thorough cleansing effect on the body that many ailments, espe-cially those related to overeating, constipation, intestinal sluggishness, poor digestion and assimilation, and a slowed down metabolism, are miraculously corrected, and the functions of all organs and glands normalized. But, *if, after health has been restored on such a deficient but therapeutic diet, the patient continues to adhere to it, it will eventually create even more serious health disorders than the ones it corrected.* With an excess of mineral-binding fruit acids and the lack of suf-ficient fat and protein in an exclusive fruitarian diet, severe deficiencies and imbalances, which may lead to serious health disorders, will eventually manifest themselves.

The same applies to a fat-free diet. Because we Americans eat far too much fat (45 percent or more of the calories in our average diet come from fat), we have an epidemic of diseases related to, or caused by, excess fat in our diet, notably cardiovascular diseases, heart disease, high blood pressure, diabetes, liver and gallbladder dis-orders, and obesity. By eliminating all fats from the diet, these disorders respond dramatically and are corrected in record time, especially in combination with proper exercise. Not able to get any fat from dietary supplies, the body is forced to burn its own fatty deposits, including those in arteries, tissues, and organs—which results in a speedy recovery of all ailments related to excess dietary fat, over-eating, and lack of exercise. But, if the recovered patient stays on such a diet *after* the health has been restored, he will eventually suffer from other severe health disorders which the dietary lack of saturated and unsaturated fatty acids and fat-soluble vitamins can cause, such as multiple sclerosis, diseases of the nervous system, senility, sexual dysfunction, and mental disorders. In order to arrive at a ratio of 10 percent fat in the diet (calorie-wise), as proponents of low-fat diets recommend, many indispensable and nutritionally-superior foods, such as many grains, nuts, seeds, avocados, milk, and cheese, must be totally eliminated from the diet. Such a diet, just like a fruitarian, sproutarian, or exclusive juice diet, will have a tremendous *therapeutic* effect, but it is too deficient to be an optimum *preventive* diet, a diet that can *build* and *maintain* health and *prevent* disease.

An optimum *preventive* diet must be adequate in all the essential nutrients necessary for the maintenance of the highest level of health and prevention of disease, not only for a few weeks or months, but for a lifetime, while the *therapeutic* diet can be deficient in one or more vital nutrients and yet produce remarkable therapeutic results. The best example of this is *juice fasting*. Drinking nothing but fresh fruit and vegetable juices for several weeks is the safest, fastest, and most effective therapeutic method known. Practically every condition of ill health can be corrected by juice fasting. Yet, if you continue a juice fast indefinitely, it will eventually kill you. So it is with the various fad diets mentioned previously. They are all excellent *therapeutic diets* and are able to correct specific diseases and restore health. But as soon as health is restored, you must discontinue them, and go on an optimum *preventive* diet.

Once you understand this crucial difference between *therapeutic* diet and the *preventive* diet, it will enable you to orient yourself in the growing maze of nutrition misinformation and dietary fads and avoid confusion. Next time a persuasive and eloquent lecturer tries to convert you to his diet by the usual appeal, "If you don't believe me, just try my diet for three weeks, and see for yourself how great you feel," you respond with, "I am not interested in how I feel in *three weeks*—I would like to know what kind of diet will make me feel great and help me avoid disease for a lifetime, even for several generations." In other words, what you are looking for is not just a therapeutic diet (although therapeutic diets are valuable in the treatment of disease) but an optimal health-building, and disease-preventive diet, a diet that can assure you of the greatest potential for building and maintaining health and preventing disease.

The Optimum Diet, presented below, is not based on my subjective beliefs or wishful thinking, but on reliable empirical evidence. I have traveled around the world studying the eating and living habits of people known for their exceptional health, absence of disease, and long life, such as Abkhasians in Russia, Bulgarians, Finns, Japanese, Hunzas, Vilcabambas in Equador, Yucatan & Chihuahua Indians in Mexico, etc. The eating habits and lifestyles of these people are strikingly similar in terms of the relationship to their superior health and extended longevity.

The Optimum Diet, outlined below, is based on my above-mentioned empirical studies as well as the latest scientific discoveries in the field of nutrition and health. It is a diet that is not only optimal for a mother-to-be, but also for a lactating mother, a child, and for any man or woman of any age who is interested in optimum health and a long, disease-free life.

Here are, then, the seven basic principles of the Airola Diet of Optimum Nutrition:

1. YOUR BASIC OPTIMUM DIET SHOULD BE MADE UP OF THESE THREE FOOD GROUPS
(in this order of importance):

A. Grains, seeds, and nuts
B. Vegetables
C. Fruits

A. *GRAINS, SEEDS, AND NUTS* are the most important and potent health-building foods of all. Their nutritional value is unsurpassed. Eaten mostly raw and sprouted, but sometimes cooked, they contain all the nutrients essential for human growth, sustenance of health, and prevention of disease in the most perfect combination and balance. In addition, they contain the secret of life itself, the **germ,** the reproductive power that assures the perpetuation of the species. This reproductive power, the spark of life in all seeds, is of extreme importance for the life, health, and reproductive ability of human beings— thus, of specific importance for a mother-to-be.

All seeds and grains are beneficial, but you should eat predominantly those that are grown in your own environment. Sprouting increases the nutritive value of seeds and grains, especially their vitamin content. Wheat, mung beans, alfalfa, and soybeans make excellent sprouts.

Contrary to what you have been told about all vegetable proteins being incomplete and of poor quality soybeans, buckwheat, sesame seeds, pumpkin seeds, sunflower seeds, almonds, and peanuts all contain **complete proteins** of high biological value. But the protein in all seeds and grains, even those that do not contain **all** the essential amino acids, is extremely useful if the foods are combined and eaten together.

Seeds, grains, and nuts are not only excellent sources of protein, but also the best natural sources of essential **unsaturated fatty acids,** without which health cannot be maintained. They are also nature's best source of lecithin, a substance which is of extreme importance to the health of the brain, nerves, glands (especially sex glands), and arteries.

The **vitamin** content of grains, seeds, and nuts is unsurpassed, especially vitamin E and the B-complex vitamins. Vitamin E is extremely important for the preservation of health and prevention of premature aging. Vitamin E can also increase fertility in both man and woman, and help to prevent miscarriages and stillbirths. Thus, vitamin-E rich foods are of special value before and during pregnancy. B-complex vitamins are absolutely essential for practically all body functions, but they are particularly needed during pregnancy because they are very much involved in protecting the body against stress.

Grains, seeds, and nuts are also gold mines of

minerals and trace elements. It is becoming more and more apparent that minerals are even more important to health than the more glamorized vitamins. A balanced body chemistry, especially in terms of acidity and alkalinity, is dependent on minerals. Biochemical disorder in the system is the basic underlying cause of most disease. Grains and seeds are the best sources of such trace elements and important minerals as magnesium, manganese, iron, zinc, copper, molybdenum, selenium, chromium, fluorine, silicon, potassium, and phosphorus—all needed for mother and growing fetus during pregnancy. Sesame seeds are an excellent source of calcium, which is needed in increasing amounts during pregnancy. Molybdenum, which is still a very much ignored mineral, is present in many whole grains, especially in brown rice, millet, and buckwheat, and is involved with proper carbohydrate metabolism.

Grains, seeds, and nuts also contain *pacifarins,* an antibiotic resistance factor that increases a pregnant woman's natural resistance to disease. They also contain *auxones,* natural substances that help produce vitamins in the body and play a part in the rejuvenation of cells, preventing premature aging.

The importance of whole grains and seeds in the diet has recently been emphasized, stressing their fiber and roughage content. After several decades of eating refined and processed foods, from which the outer coating—the fiber—has been processed out, we have become a nation of people plagued by constipation, diverticulitis, colitis, and cancer of the colon and intestinal tract. Current studies show that we must go back to whole, unprocessed grains and seeds, which provide enough bulk to prevent these disorders.

The best seeds are: flax seeds, sesame seeds, chia seeds, and pumpkin seeds. Sesame seeds are an excellent source of easily digestible and assimilable calcium. Tahini and other sesame butters can also be used. Make your own, or buy them in health food stores.

Flax seeds are an excellent food, largely neglected in

the American diet. The extraordinary nutritional value of flax seeds is based on the fact that they contain a great amount of the highest quality essential fatty acids, such as linoleic and linolenic acids, or vitamin F factors. Flax seeds are also a highly mucilaginous food and are very beneficial for the healthy workings of the alimentary canal and eliminative system. They are an excellent food to prevent and/or remedy constipation, and this is very important during pregnancy. Keep in mind, however, that flax seeds and sesame seeds contain 45 - 50 percent fat; so do not overeat—they can be fattening!

The best nuts are almonds and hazelnuts (filberts). Almonds are, in terms of rancidity, the most durable of all nuts, even when they are shelled. They also supply complete high-quality proteins, as do sesame and flax seeds.

All seeds and nuts must be eaten *fresh* and *raw*. Nuts can be chewed (but well!) and seeds should be ground in your own seed grinder (available at your health food store) just before eating. Remember, ground flax seeds will turn rancid within a few days, so it is better to grind them fresh and eat them at once.

I did not mention another popular seed food, sunflower seeds, because it becomes increasingly difficult to get sunflower seeds that are not rancid. They are extremely vulnerable to rancidity and turn rancid quickly after they are shelled because the shelling process scratches and breaks the seed and exposes its oil to oxygen. How can you tell if your seeds are rancid? Spread them on a white paper and notice all the seeds that are not medium grey, but are, in whole or in part, brown, yellow, white, black—these are all rancid. Even a small quantity of rancid seeds can be extremely toxic and harmful, even carcinogenic, if consumed often. And, a pregnant woman should certainly not expose herself to carcinogens!

Nuts and seeds combine beautifully with fresh fruit for breakfast, which can also include yogurt or other cultured milk and/or cheese.

The best grains for a mother-to-be are buckwheat and millet, although most grains are beneficial. Since wheat is one of the most common allergens (foods that cause allergy in many people), be sure you are not allergic to wheat before you incorporate it as part of your diet. If eating wheat in any form (even wheat germ) gives you any trouble, such as gas, indigestion, excessive mucus, stomach pain, and increased pulse rate, leave it out of your diet completely.

Buckwheat is another excellent cereal. According to the U.S. Department of Agriculture, the proteins in buckwheat are complete and are of such high biological value that they are comparable to the proteins in meat. Buckwheat is also an excellent source of magnesium, manganese, and zinc.

B. *VEGETABLES* are the next most important food group in the Optimum Diet. Vegetables are extraordinary sources of minerals, enzymes, and vitamins. Most green leafy vegetables contain complete proteins of the highest quality. The proteins in alfalfa, parsley, and potatoes, are comparable to the protein in milk in their biological value.

Most vegetables should be eaten raw in the form of a salad. In fact, one meal of the day, lunch or dinner, should be largely made of vegetables (see next chapter). Some vegetables, such as potatoes, yams, squashes, and green beans, can be cooked, steamed, or baked. Vegetables containing an excess of oxalic acid, such as spinach, rhubarb, and the cabbage family, should be boiled in water for 3 - 5 minutes, before eating. The water in which they were cooked should be discarded, not used as a vegetable broth.

Garlic and onions are excellent health-promoting as well as medicinal foods and should form an important part of the diet. Garlic and onions contain sulfur and selenium—very important trace elements for the mother-to-be. Garlic and onions, complemented by a large assortment of natural herbs and spices, will help to improve your health as well as turn ordinary vegetable dishes into delectable gourmet foods.

C. *FRUITS* are the third most important food group in the Optimum Diet for the mother-to-be. Like vegetables, fruits are excellent sources of minerals, vitamins, and enzymes. They are easily digested and exert a cleansing effect on the blood and the digestive tract.

In addition to all available fresh fruits, in season, the Airola Optimum Diet can include dry fruits, particularly when fresh fruits are not available. Unsulfured, organically grown raisins, prunes, dried apricots, and figs are available from health food stores. Dried fruits should be pre-soaked before eating.

Fruits are best eaten for breakfast or as a snack between meals. Roughly, one food group should supply the bulk of each of the three main meals: fruits, seeds, and nuts for breakfast, cereal for lunch, and vegetables for dinner; although this order can be interchanged, of course. See the suggested *HEALTH MENU* in Chapter 4.

2. EAT MOSTLY FRESH, RAW, LIVING FOODS.

Approximately 75 to 80 percent of your diet should consist of foods in their natural uncooked state. There are numerous studies which demonstrate the superiority of raw, living foods, both for maintenance of health and prevention of disease, as well as for the healing of disease. Cooking destroys much of the nutritional value of most foods. Many vitamins are partly destroyed, minerals are leached out (if boiled in water) and all enzymes are destroyed by temperatures over 120 degrees F.

Cooking also changes the biochemical structure of amino acids (proteins) and fatty acids, and makes them only partially digestible. For example, it has been demonstrated at the world-famous Max Planck Institute for Nutritional Research that you need only one-half the amount of protein in your diet *if you eat protein foods raw* instead of cooked.[1]

Sprouting is an excellent way to eat seeds, beans, and grains in raw form. Sprouting increases nutritional value of foods; many new vitamins are created or multiplied in seeds during sprouting. Sprouting also improves the protein quality in seeds and grains. Some grains and legumes, which do not contain complete proteins, become complete

protein foods after they are sprouted. (See *Recipes &
Directions* for instructions on sprouting.)

Another excellent way to increase the amount of raw
food in your diet is to eat lots of fermented lactic acid
foods, such as homemade sauerkraut, pickles, or lactic acid
vegetables (see *Recipes & Directions*). Especially for
those who live in cold northern regions, fermenting foods
is an excellent way to preserve vegetables for winter use,
and not only preserve, but increase their nutritive value—
without cooking!

Must all foods be eaten raw?

If you have read even a minimal amount of health and
nutrition literature, you must be aware that there are
experts who recommend eating all foods in their natural,
raw state. As I've just stated, cooking destroys some of the
nutritive value of food. Also, eating fried foods, especially
if they have been fried in vegetable oils, can be hazardous,
since vegetable fats become carcinogenic if heated to high
temperatures.[2] Frying in animal fats, such as butter, is
safer, since unsaturated fatty acids are more resistant to
damage by heat. Any way you look at it, the *general* rule
of healthful eating seems to be that raw foods are preferable to cooked foods.

But there are some important exceptions to this rule,
as there are to any rule. Fanaticism in nutrition can be
dangerous. Unfortunately, some uncompromising fanatics
who are "into" raw foods, refuse to recognize that in the
science of nutrition (which is, like medicine, not an exact
science, but rather an art) there are always exceptions,
compromises, and special considerations. This is only
natural since there are great physiological, biochemical,
and structural differences between individuals, and because our present nutrition has evolved through thousands
of years of search, selection, and environmental adaptation. An example: man has long been eating a great
variety of initially wild, then cultivated, plants (vegetables). Many of these plants are excellent and edible in
their raw state. But some plants contain too many harmful

substances, such as oxalic acid, for example, and early man, therefore, avoided them. However, with the discovery of fire, he learned to use even these plants, by destroying or leaching out the harmful elements through cooking. Thus, spinach, rhubarb, asparagus, cauliflower, cabbage, and other vegetables of the cabbage family, have become a regular part of man's diet. In a raw state, especially if consumed in large quantities, they can be quite harmful.

The story of beans is somewhat similar. Many beans, especially soybeans, contain enzymes that inhibit the body's protein utilization. Man discovered very early that eating raw beans led to digestive disorders, mineral and protein deficiencies, and other discomforts. He has found that these foods become more useful if cooked. Cooking destroys the enzyme-inhibitors and makes digestion and assimilation of these foods better. Thus, cooked soybeans became an essential part of man's diet in the Orient. But soybeans can also be eaten raw after having been soaked for 24 hours in water which is changed every 6 hours. The enzyme-inhibitors are thus soaked and leached out from the beans.

There is another important factor—*the most* important in fact—that must be taken into consideration when dealing with the question of cooked or raw foods. Minerals in all dry grains and most dry beans, peas, and other legumes, are chemically bound with phytic acid, or phytin. If grains or beans are eaten very fresh, like raw corn on the cob, or raw soft peas or beans, they can be digested fairly well and the mineral content in them can be sufficiently utilized. But dry grains or beans, if eaten raw, or if just soaked overnight, cannot be digested properly and the minerals in them will be largely wasted and excreted with the phytins to which they are chemically bound. Cooking grains, as in baking bread or making porridge or cereals, helps to break down this chemical bond and releases all the vital minerals and trace elements such as zinc, iron, manganese, magnesium, molybdenum, etc., making them easily available and assimilable in the intestinal tract.

To avoid misunderstanding and confusion, let me

summarize: All seeds and nuts, and all fruits and most vegetables should preferably be eaten in their natural state—raw. Some vegetables, like those mentioned above, should be cooked, preferably boiled in water, discarding the water.But all grains should be either cooked, like in bread or cereals, or sprouted. Sprouting also breaks down the mineral-phytin bond and releases the minerals.

3. EAT ONLY 100% NATURAL FOODS

Your foods should be whole, unprocessed, unrefined, and organically grown in fertile soil. They should preferably be grown in *your own environment,* and eaten in *their season.*

That your health and longevity are in a direct relationship to the naturalness of the foods you eat is a well-established scientific fact. Where natives eat a diet of natural, whole, unprocessed, and unrefined foods, they enjoy perfect health, absence of disease, and long life. When denatured, refined, processed, man-made foods, such as white sugar and white flour, and canned and processed foods, enter into their lives, disease becomes rampant among them.

Natural foods are foods that are grown in fertile soils without chemical fertilizers and sprays and are consumed in their *natural* state with all the nutrients nature put in them intact, *nothing removed and nothing added.* White bread is, for example, a denatured food, from which most vital nutrients have been removed; the so-called "enrichment" is a hoax—over 20 vital nutrients are removed in refining the flour, while only 4 nutrients are returned. Breakfast cereals are denatured foods with some "added features"—toxic preservatives and health-destroying white sugar. Supermarket quality eggs are not natural food; they are produced by cooped-up chickens, without a rooster (thus infertile), which are fed chemicalized commercial mash. Such eggs have a lower nutritional value, less vitamins, and more cholesterol than natural eggs.

Organically grown fruits and vegetables contain more

vitamins, minerals, and enzymes than produce grown on depleted, chemically fertilized soils, as has been shown in many tests. Such foods have a greater health-building and disease-preventing potential. Researchers reported recently that anti-malignancy factors are apparently present in organically grown foods.

Synthetic, denatured, and devitalized foods will not sustain health, but will inevitably bring about a gradual degeneration of normal body functions and ultimately disease.

It is of specific importance when planning a diet for the pregnant woman to see that all her foods are natural. Only natural, whole, unprocessed and organically grown foods will assure a high level of health during pregnancy and delivery, and produce a healthy, disease-resistant baby.

4. EAT ONLY POISON-FREE FOODS

Your food should be grown without the aid of chemical fertilizers and should contain no residues of toxic insecticides, chemical additives, or preservatives. It has been demonstrated that toxic chemicals from the environment can enter the fetus through the placenta.[3,4]

Almost all food sold at supermarkets today contains some chemicals, used either in food producing or added during food processing or packing. Many of the poisons in fruits or vegetables are systemic, that is, they cannot be washed off or peeled out, as they penetrate the whole plant.

The only solution seems to be to grow your own food, or buy certified organically grown food. And, of course, to avoid eating all processed and packaged foods, which contain the most chemicals.

If, in spite of all the precautions, you are not able to avoid toxins in food and environment, use special vitamins and supplements that can minimize the harmful effects of environmental poisons, which are listed in my book, *How To Get Well,* in a special section: "How to Protect Yourself Against Common Poisons in Food, Water, Air, and Environment."[5]

5. SPECIAL COMPLEMENTARY FOODS AND FOOD SUPPLEMENTS

You can complement your three basic health-building food groups with the following special foods and supplements.

A. *MILK.* The value of milk in human nutrition has been highly disputed in the United States. Some authorities claim that milk is an excellent and indispensable food for man—others insist that milk is food for calves and poison for man, that man cannot digest milk properly, that milk causes mucus, allergies, etc.

The answer to the milk controversy is simple: both sides are right! *Milk is an excellent food for those who are milk-tolerant, and poison for those who are not.*

Who is tolerant and who is not? Simple again, as so ably explained by Dr. Robert D. McCracken, anthropologist at the University of California School of Public Health. People whose ancestors historically herded dairy animals and traditionally lived on a lactose-rich diet of milk, cheese, etc., are usually *tolerant to milk.* Their intestines contain plenty of the enzyme, *lactase,* which breaks down milk sugar, *lactose,* into a form that the body can use. Thus, milk for them is an excellent health food. Conversely, those whose ancestors never or seldom used milk as a major element of their diet, are usually *intolerant to milk,* because their intestines do not contain sufficient lactase.

So, if your ancestors come from Europe, or the Middle East, your body probably is genetically programmed to use milk and digest it effectively. If your ancestors came from Africa (except the few milk-drinking tribes), China, the Philippines, or New Guinea, or if your heritage is that of American Indians, Australian Aborigines, or Eskimos, your body may not be programmed to digest milk properly.

Thus, almost 75 percent of American Blacks have been found to be intolerant to milk, while over 95 percent of white Americans have no problem in digesting milk. As simple as that!*

Needless to say, when I recommend supplementing the diet with milk, I mean *only the highest quality, uncontaminated, raw milk from healthy animals.* Today's pasteurized supermarket-sold milk is loaded with toxic and dangerous drugs, chemicals, and residues of pesticides, herbicides, and detergents—such milk is not suitable for human consumption. If you are fortunate enough to get *real* milk, fresh, raw, "farmer's" milk from healthy cows fed organic food, then you can add milk to your diet. Note that the people we always associate with remarkable health—Scandinavians, Bulgarians, Russians—are traditionally heavy dairy food eaters.

The best way to take milk is in its soured form: as yogurt, kefir, acidophilus milk, or regular buttermilk or clabbered milk. Homemade cottage cheese can be made from any of these soured milks (see *Recipes & Directions*). Soured milks are superior to sweet milk, as they are in a *predigested* form and very easily assimilated. They also help to maintain a healthy intestinal flora and prevent intestinal putrefaction and constipation.

Goat's milk is better than cow's milk as a human food. It contains both anti-arthritic and anti-cancer factors and is recommended for these conditions. Also, after the mother has finished nursing her baby, goat's milk is much preferred to cow's milk as a part of the baby's new diet. Goat's milk is closer than cow's milk to the nutritional composition of mother's milk.

B. *COLD-PRESSED VEGETABLE OILS.* High-quality, fresh, cold-pressed, crude, unrefined, unheated, and unprocessed vegetable oil is recommended as a regular addition to the diet of the expectant mother, *but only in a very moderate quantity.* Please re-read the foregoing

---

* By the way, you *cannot* change this genetic programming in just a few generations—it would take thousands of years to accomplish this.

sentence and notice all the specifications and requirements
that I place on vegetable oil before I can recommend it for
human consumption. Such oils are almost impossible to
obtain today.

All commercially-produced, supermarket-sold oils are a
complete no-no. They are all produced either with the use
of extremely high temperatures, up to 350 degrees F, or
with the process known as chemical extraction, in which
such solvents as hexane and benzine are used. Both
methods result in a final product which has no resem-
blance to anything "natural." It is processed, filtered, refined, bleached, and deodorized. Beneficial lecithin, which
normally clouds the natural unrefined oils, has been removed. Toxic chemical antioxidants, such as BHT, have
been added. Margarines, made from such vegetable oils,
have, in addition, been saturated with hydrogen and are
even worse than the original oils from which they are
made.

But even many oils sold in health food stores are not
actually cold-pressed. Some manufacturers use a misleading term, "cold-processed," which really means that the oils
were extracted with the help of chemical solvents, such as
carcinogenic hexane. There are only a very few oils that
can be made by hydraulic pressure, and, thus, can be
truthfully labeled as cold-pressed. Sesame seed oil and
olive oil are among these few oils. Most oils are extracted
by a screw-type press. This method results in extremely
high temperatures, the oils being heated to 300 - 350 degrees F. There is evidence that exposing vegetable oils to
such high temperatures makes them carcinogenic.[2,6]
(Therefore, vegetable oils should never be used in cooking,
frying or baking.)

In addition to these hazardous manufacturing and
processing methods, there is another danger connected
with edible oils. All natural foods are extremely perishable,
and vegetable oils are no exception. Natural oils turn
rancid very rapidly. It is almost impossible to keep them
for any length of time without the use of preservatives.
Storing them in metal cans or dark bottles helps. Also,

constant refrigeration is essential. Even then, most oils will turn rancid within a few weeks or months after they are made.[7]

So, now what? Should we leave all oils completely out of the diet? How can we get truly safe edible oils?

Since my book, **Are You Confused?**, which pioneered the information on the dangers of eating rancid foods and oils, was published a few years ago, many changes have taken place in the American health-oriented segment of the edible oil industries. Spurred by my research, an effort is being made to produce better oils. There are now several brands of better quality natural oils available. Ask for these oils in your health food store. If your store does not have them, they will get them for you. Some stores sell good imported brands of virgin olive oil from France, Italy, or Spain. The best oils are olive oil and sesame seed oil. These are also the two oils most likely to be non-rancid.

Olive oil is of special interest in the pregnancy diet since it is an excellent source of the important fatty acid, arachidonic acid, which is needed for the synthesis of prostaglandins within the body. Prostaglandins are involved in balancing hormonal levels and therefore may be of importance to pregnant women, whose whole metabolism is directed by hormones.

In the beginning of this section, I said that vegetable oils (polyunsaturated fats) should be used only in strict moderation, perhaps 1 - 2 tsp. a day. This advice is based on recent research which shows that *excessive* use of polyunsaturated oils can lead to the deficiency of vitamins E, A, D, and K (by leaching them out of the body), and consequently to serious health problems, such as cancer, and cardiovascular diseases.[8] Some research also indicates that excessive consumption of polyunsaturated oils can accelerate the aging processes, causing wrinkles, crow's-feet, and other visible signs of premature aging. The best way of getting needed saturated and unsaturated fats in the diet is by eating natural fat-containing foods such as whole milk, nuts, seeds, grains, etc.

C. *HONEY*. Natural, raw, unheated, unfiltered, and unprocessed honey is the only sweetener a prospective mother should use—1 tbsp. a day is the maximum, however. Honey possesses miraculous nutritional and medicinal properties and has been used for healing purposes since early history. It has been found that most centenarians in Russia and Bulgaria use honey in their diets.[9]

Better than any other food, (with the possible exception of garlic) honey fulfills Hippocrates' requirement for an ideal food: "Our food should be our medicine—our medicine should be our food." Honey increases calcium retention in the system, which is important during pregnancy. Raw, unfiltered, pollen-rich honey also helps prevent nutritional anemia, is beneficial in kidney and liver disorders, colds, poor circulation, and complexion problems.

D. *SPECIAL PROTECTIVE FOODS* for the mother-to-be, both before and during pregnancy, are brewer's yeast, wheat germ, fish-liver-oil, and kelp. These supplementary foods are truly "wonder" foods. They are storehouses of important nutrients for the mother and the child.

Brewer's yeast is a real super-food and should form an essential part of an expectant mother's as well as a nursing mother's diet. The value of brewer's yeast as an indispensable supplement in the diet of expectant and nursing mothers is based on its following properties:

- Brewer's yeast is an excellent source of high quality proteins. Up to 40 percent of brewer's yeast is made up of protein. Especially in the vegetarian diet, brewer's yeast can be a good supplementary source of protein.
- Brewer's yeast is the best food source of B vitamins. B-complex vitamins are essential for virtually all body functions, including the growth and division of all body cells and for the production of RNA and DNA, the nucleic acids that carry the hereditary patterns. Deficiency of some of the B vitamins may cause reproductive disorders such as spontaneous abortions, difficult labor, and high infant death rate.

- Brewer's yeast is one of the best foods known to stimulate breast milk production in nursing mothers.
- Brewer's yeast is an unmatched source of the trace minerals which are specifically needed during pregnancy and nursing: selenium, zinc, iron, and chromium. Selenium is similar to vitamin E in many of its functions and is essential for the proper function of all the reproductive organs. Selenium is considered to be one of the most important factors for the prevention of breast cancer.[10] Yeast also contains the Glucose Tolerance Factor, which is vital for proper sugar metabolism—this factor is especially needed by pregnant women who also tend to be hypoglycemic (suffer from low blood sugar).[11]

The best way to take brewer's yeast is to use it as a snack food. One tablespoon of brewer's yeast powder mixed in a half glass of freshly made pineapple juice, or freshly squeezed grapefruit juice, can be taken 2 - 3 times a day, preferably one hour before meals. Taking brewer's yeast in this manner will also totally eliminate an explosive problem too often associated with the consumption of yeast—gas. Brewer's yeast should *never* be taken *with meals,* or immediately *before* or *after* meals, as is generally the case with other vitamin and mineral supplements. Yeast is a rich protein food. Protein needs lots of hydrochloric acid to be effectively digested. To assure trouble- and gas-free digestion, brewer's yeast should always be taken on an empty stomach, when there is a plentiful supply of hydrochloric acid.

Some people are allergic to yeast (even to yeast-containing B-vitamins). Thus, gas and intestinal distress may be caused not by low stomach acidity, but by allergy. If this is your problem, check with your doctor.

There are many food yeasts on the market. When I mention yeast in my lectures, I am always besieged by questions: Which of the numerous available yeasts is the best? Although all food yeasts or primary yeasts are useful in human nutrition, the true *brewer's yeast* is best. Not "brewer's type" yeast, not "primary" yeast, not "torula" yeast, not a "number so and so" yeast, but one which is labeled "brewer's yeast." True brewer's yeast is a better source of selenium and chromium and of the Glucose Tolerance Factor, than any other form of nutritional yeast. However, in all fairness, I must say that the all-important B vitamins are present in approximately the same quantities in all food yeasts.

Special important notes on yeast:

1. When taking yeast, always take 1 tablet of calcium supplement with it. Yeast is rich in phosphorus and low in calcium. An addition of calcium will achieve a better mineral balance and improve the utilization and metabolism of all the yeast's minerals. As a calcium supplement, bone meal, calcium lactate, dolomite, or calcium-magnesium tablets can be used; or you can take calcium-rich sesame seeds. Even taking the yeast with some form of calcium-rich soured milks, such as yogurt, kefir, acidophilus milk (buttermilk), etc., can be helpful.

2. Never eat *live* yeast intended for baking. Live yeast may multiply in the intestines and, instead of supplying you with B vitamins, may actually consume your body's own B-vitamin reserves.

Wheat germ is a superb food supplement loaded with complete proteins, essential fatty acids, vitamin E, and B-complex vitamins. It is important, however, that wheat germ you eat is *absolutely fresh*. Wheat germ is extremely perishable, and becomes inedible (rancid) after about 10 days.[7] Make sure, therefore, that wheat germ you eat is not rancid. Rancid foods are extremely harmful, and may cause cancer as well as damage to the fetus. There are some brands of wheat germ on the market that are dated—use them.

Wheat germ does not require cooking. It should be eaten raw, sprinkled on salads, in soups, or mixed with milk or yogurt. You can have as much as 2 - 4 tablespoons a day.

Fish liver oil is another good food supplement in the Optimum Diet. It supplies vitamins A and D in **natural** form. This is very important, since I would hesitate to recommend synthetic vitamins to pregnant women and nursing mothers. Most people, especially those living in northern regions, are deficient in vitamins A and D. Vitamin A is essential during pregnancy and lactation. Deficiency of vitamin A can cause retarded growth of the fetus as well as retarded growth in infants. Vitamin D assists in the assimilation of calcium and other minerals from the digestive tract. This is very important for proper formation of bones of the fetus during pregnancy, as well as for the formation of bones and teeth during infancy.

Make sure that the fish liver oil you get is **not fortified** with synthetic vitamins—just plain, natural, cold liver oil, or halibut liver oil. It is also available in capsule form for those who cannot tolerate the taste. Two teaspoons of oil, or 5 - 8 capsules, a day is sufficient.

There are many strict vegetarians who would object to using fish liver oil because of its being an animal product. As much as I respect conscientious objectors in any field, I would suggest making an exception in regard to fish oil, since I feel it is of extreme importance for the health of the mother and baby. Also, fish oil is not an animal tissue, and no fish is ever killed for the purpose of obtaining oil—it is a by-product of the regular fish industry. In addition to this, all the so-called vegetarian tablets of vitamin A that are available, to my knowledge, are fortified with a synthetic form of vitamin A, which should never be used by pregnant or lactating women.

However, if the vegetarian mother-to-be absolutely refuses to use fish liver oil supplement, she should make sure to expose her body to plenty of sunshine during pregnancy and lactation, since vitamin D is produced by a reaction between sunlight and skin oils, and absorbed by the body. Also, egg yolk, milk, butter, sprouted seeds, mushrooms, kelp, and sunflower seeds contain some natural vitamin D. For help with the dietary supply of vitamin A, eat plenty of brightly colored fruits and vegetables, particularly carrots,

squash, yams, melons, tomatoes, and all green leafy vegetables, as well as fertile eggs and whole milk.

Kelp is another miracle food that pregnant women
and nursing mothers can benefit from. It contains valuable
iodine and most other minerals and trace elements. It also
contains complete proteins, and vitamins C, K, A, D, E,
and B_{12} (which is otherwise seldom found in vegetable
foods). Iodine deficiency can disrupt normal function of the
thyroid gland and cause diminished hormone production.
Thyroid hormone is used for the regulation of the estrogen
in the body. Pregnant women have greater than normal
excretion of urinary iodine, which may cause iodine
deficiency. The deficiency of iodine may lead to a build-up
of excessive amounts of estrogen in the body and contribute to the development of breast cancer.[10]

It would be wise to eat some kelp, dulse, or other
seaweed, every day. Kelp is sold in tablet form, or as a
powder or granules. One-half teaspoon of granules or 2 - 3
tablets a day is sufficient. Kelp powder can be used as a
salt substitute in soups, or other dishes, or sprinkled on
vegetable salads.

E. *NATURAL VITAMIN AND MINERAL SUPPLEMENTS*

During pregnancy and lactation, I do not recommend
taking any synthetic vitamins, with one exception:
vitamin C. The reason I make an exception for vitamin C
is because (1) it is extremely important for pregnant or
lactating women, and (2) a 100 percent natural form of
vitamin C supplement in high potencies is not available.
Vitamin C sold in health food stores in potencies of 50 mg.
or more per tablet, even though it may be called "natural,"
and have some rose hips powder or acerola extract listed as
part of the content, is usually up to 95 percent ascorbic
acid.

Here are the vitamins and supplements that should be
added daily to the optimal pre-natal and post-natal diet:

C — 1,000 to 1,500 mg.

B-complex with B_{12} (must be *100% natural,* from
yeast) — 4 - 6 tablets.

A and D (from fish liver oil, 10,000 units A and 400
units D per capsule) — 1 - 2 capsules.

E — 200 - 400 I.U. of mixed tocopherols.

Brewer's yeast powder — 2 - 3 tbsp., or 10 - 15 tablets.

Kelp — ½ tsp. granules or 2 - 3 tablets.

Bone meal, preferably raw, from veal bones and
imported from the Southern Hemisphere — 3
tablets.

Calcium lactate — 1,000 to 1,200 mg.

Magnesium — 500 mg.

Multi-mineral and trace element formula with
potassium, iron (18 mg.), selenium, zinc (20 mg.),
manganese, chromium, molybdenum, etc. — 1
tablet. Or 5 - 6 tablets of "Nature's Minerals", a
100% natural mineral and trace element formula,
available in health food stores.

The reason that a phosphorus supplement is not
included in the above list is because by taking 2 - 3
tablespoons of phosphorus-rich brewer's yeast, you will get
enough phosphorus. Also, the Airola Optimum Diet, with
its heavy emphasis on grains, is rich in phosphorus.

A few tips on how to take vitamins and supplements

1. As a general rule, all vitamins and food supplements should be taken with meals, or immediately after
meals. They are better utilized when taken with foods.

2. Divide all the suggested amounts equally among 2
or 3 meals.

3. Most drugstore-sold vitamins are synthetic. This is
especially true in regard to vitamins B and E. Therefore,
you will be safer if you buy all your vitamins from health
food stores.

4. Since even health food stores sell some synthetic
vitamins, how will you know if the B vitamins you buy are
natural or synthetic? Here's a helpful hint: if a B-complex
tablet contains more than 10 mg. of most individual B's, it
is likely to be synthetic. The usual strength of 100 percent
natural B-complex vitamins does not exceed 10 mg. for B_1,

B_2, B_3, or B_6 per tablet—often it is somewhere between 3 and 7 mg. See *How To Get Well* for detailed information on the differences between natural and synthetic vitamins and how to tell which is which.[5] See also Chapter 9 in this book.

5. The above-mentioned dosages of suggested vitamins and supplements for pregnant women can be taken continuously during pregnancy and lactation if you are healthy or reasonably healthy. However, if you have some specific health problems—let's say, constipation, varicose veins, obesity, or hypoglycemia—the supplementary program can be changed and modified, even during pregnancy and lactation, to include specific therapeutic vitamins and other nutrients as suggested in my book, *How To Get Well,* as well as in some chapters on specific female health problems in Part Three of this book. When you include supplements other than those recommended above, always keep in mind, however, that I do not advise taking synthetic vitamins during pregnancy, especially in megadoses (with the exception of ascorbic acid, as mentioned before).

6. As a rule, all vitamins and food supplements should be taken together; being synergistic in action, they work best that way, complementing one another. There is, however, a notable exception to this rule: vitamin E and iron. Vitamin E and iron supplements are *antagonists.* Iron tablets have an adverse effect on the utilization of vitamin E. Therefore, when iron tablets are taken, even if the iron is an ingredient in a multi-mineral tablet, they should be taken 8 - 12 hours before or after taking vitamin E. For example, you can take the total daily dose of vitamin E for breakfast and the total iron supplement at dinnertime. Note: natural iron-rich *foods* have no adverse effect on vitamin E utilization.

7. The above doses of vitamins are only approximate doses for the average, young, healthy woman. Since there is a great difference in every person's nutritional needs, as well as in their response to vitamins and other nutritional substances, depending on age, health condition, nutri-

tional stature, the quality of the foods eaten, the ability to assimilate nutrients, the mineral content of the water used for drinking, the toxicity degree of the environment, the level of emotional stresses, etc., the suggested doses can be modified to fit any woman's individual needs. Your doctor, upon a careful examination and nutritional and metabolic evaluation of your condition, would be the person to determine the exact dosages of vitamins and supplements *FOR YOU.*

6. AVOID AN EXCESS OF PROTEIN IN YOUR DIET

The Airola Optimum Diet made of three basic food groups—seeds, nuts and grains; vegetables; and fruits—supplemented with the special super-foods and food supplements named in preceding pages, will assure you a complete supply in adequate amounts of all required nutrients for optimum health, *including sufficient amounts of complete high-quality proteins.* During pregnancy and lactation, however, the requirements for protein are increased by approximately 30 grams a day. This extra need can be filled by increasing the quantity of protein-rich foods recommended in the Optimum Diet, such as milk, natural cheese, almonds, sesame seeds, buckwheat, millet, and other grains and beans. Homemade cottage cheese, quark (see *Recipes & Directions*), is an especially good supplementary protein food during pregnancy and lactation. A moderate amount of eggs, fish, or meat may be added to this basic diet, if desired (particularly the fish in coastal areas or meat in far northern regions with long winters), *but their inclusion is not necessary.* In temperate, sub-tropical and tropical climates, the highest level of health, both that of the mother and the baby, can be best achieved and maintained without meat.

A high-animal-protein diet, as shown by recent massive research, is definitely detrimental to the health and may cause or contribute to the development of many of our most common diseases, including cancer of the colon and of the breast (see Chapter 25).

In this era of the "high-protein cult," you have been brought up to believe that a high-protein diet is a *must* if you wish to attain a high level of health and prevent disease. Health writers and "experts," who have advocated a high-protein diet, have been misled by slanted research financed by the dairy and meat industries, or by insufficient and outdated information. Most recent research, world-wide, shows more and more convincingly *that our past beliefs in regard to high requirements of protein are outdated and incorrect, and that the actual daily need for protein in human nutrition is far below that which has long been considered necessary.* Researchers, working independently in many parts of the world, arrived at the conclusion that our actual daily need of protein is only 30 - 40 grams[12] (30 grams more for pregnant and lactating women)—*even less if raw proteins from milk and vegetable sources are used* (raw protein being utilized twice as well as cooked[1]). Independent researchers, not associated with nor paid by dairy or meat industries, also point out that, contrary to past beliefs, proteins from many vegetable sources are equal or superior to animal proteins in their biological value—not inferior, as some meat cultists claim. Almonds, sesame seeds, soybeans, buckwheat, peanuts, sunflower seeds, pumpkin seeds, potatoes, and all leafy green vegetables contain **complete proteins,** which are comparable in quality to animal proteins.[13] This revealing information comes from the most reliable and respected nutrition research organization in the world, the Max Planck Institute for Nutritional Research, in Germany. This was also stressed by recent recommendations by the U.S. Senate Select Committee on Nutrition, which advised Americans to cut down on meat eating and eat more grains and vegetables[14]—actually, in verbatim, advocating the Airola Diet as expounded in all my works.

But what is even more important, the world-wide research brings almost daily confirmation of the scientific premise which I first publicly voiced in the United States ten years ago, and which then shocked high-protein-brainwashed Americans—that proteins, *essential as they are,* CAN BE EXTREMELY HARMFUL WHEN CONSUMED IN EXCESS OF ACTUAL NEED. An excess of meat in the diet, with its high content of fat, is especially likely to cause serious health disorders.

As is well documented by reliable scientific research, the metabolism of proteins consumed in excess of the actual need leaves toxic residues of metabolic wastes in tissues, causes autotoxemia, over-acidity, and nutritional deficiencies, accumulation of uric acid and purines in the tissues, intestinal putrefaction, and contributes to the development of many of our most common and serious diseases, such as arthritis,[15] kidney damage, pyorrhea,[16] schizophrenia,[11] osteoporosis,[16] atherosclerosis,[17, 18] heart disease,[17, 18] and cancer.[19, 20] A high-protein diet also causes premature aging, and lowers life expectancy.[11]

Recent American research done under the direction of Dr. Lennart Krook, shows that overindulgence in meat leads to a mineral imbalance in the system—too much phosphorus and too little calcium (meat has 22 times more phosphorus than calcium)—which in turn leads to severe calcium and magnesium deficiency and resultant loss of teeth through decay or pyorrhea.

A study made at the U.S. Army Medical Research and Nutrition Laboratory in Denver, Colorado, demonstrated that the more meat you eat, the more deficient in vitamin B_6 you become. A high protein diet can cause severe deficiencies of B_6, magnesium, calcium, and niacin (vitamin B_3). Mental illness and schizophrenia are often caused by a niacin deficiency and have been recently successfully treated with high doses of niacin. Russian researcher, Dr. Yuri Nikolayev, has been extremely successful in treating schizophrenia patients with a low-protein diet.

Extensive studies made in England showed a clear connection between a high-protein diet and osteoporosis. And doctors at the Vascular Research Laboratory in Brooklyn, New York, conducted research which indicates that excessive meat eating can be a cause of widespread arteriosclerosis and heart disease. Researchers Dr. C.D.

Langen, from Holland, and Dr. A. Hoygaard, from Denmark came to the same conclusion.

Dr. Ph. Schwarz, of Frankfort University, in Germany, and Dr. Ralph Bircher, a famous biochemist in Zurich, Switzerland, report that the aging process is triggered by *amyloid,* a by-product of protein metabolism, which is deposited in all the connective tissues and causes tissue and organ degeneration—thus leading to premature aging. This explains why people who traditionally eat low-protein diets—Hunzakuts, Pakistanians, Bulgarians, Russian Caucasians, Yucatan Indians, East Indian Todas—also have the highest average life expectancy in the world—up to 90 years! And, why the people who live on high-animal-protein diets, such as Eskimos, Greenlanders, and Lapplanders, have the lowest life expectancy in the world—30 - 40 years. Americans lead the industrialized world in per capita meat consumption—and we also are in 27th place in life expectancy among industrialized nations!

Recently, Dr. Willard J. Visek, of Cornell University, implicated high-protein diets in the development of cancer. *Ammonia,* which is produced in great amounts as a by-product of meat metabolism, is highly carcinogenic and can trigger cancer development.[19] A high-protein diet also breaks down the pancreas and lowers resistance to cancer, as well as contributes to the development of diabetes and/or hypoglycemia.[11]

These are just a few examples of recent research and overwhelming scientific evidence which show that a high-animal-protein diet is *a very dangerous course to follow.*

Not only animal proteins, but *all* proteins should be consumed in moderation. *Excessive* protein consumption, even if from such sources as milk or concentrated protein powders of vegetable origin, can be dangerous.

A good rule regarding proteins should be: *Enough, but not too much.* By eating the three basic foods of the Airola Diet—seeds, nuts, and grains; vegetables; and fruits—supplemented with milk and brewer's yeast, up to 80 percent of which are consumed in their natural uncooked state, you can be assured of obtaining *all* the vital nutrients you need for vigorous and vibrant health and prevention of disease, *including adequate amounts of complete proteins* in a natural balance and in proper combination with all the other vital nutrients. Again, during pregnancy and lactation, you must increase the quantity of protein-rich foods, as suggested earlier, but as soon as lactation is completed, it will be wise to reduce your daily protein intake to about 30 - 40 grams, or to about 10 - 15 percent of your total caloric intake.

7. CULTIVATE THE FOLLOWING HEALTH-PROMOTING EATING HABITS

1. *Eat only when really hungry.* There are all kinds of theories regarding eating and drinking—when you should or shouldn't eat or drink—*theories invented by scientists.* They tell you that you should eat a large, heavy protein breakfast with meat, eggs, etc., the first thing in the morning. They tell you when to eat heavy meals and when to eat lightly. They tell you when and how much to drink. Etc., etc. All these are unsubstantiated pseudo-scientific theories. You don't need any scientists or their theories to tell you when and how much to eat. *Nature* has provided a built-in mechanism within your brain which will tell you unmistakably *when* you should eat or drink. You should *eat when you are hungry,* and *drink when you are thirsty.* Contrarywise, you should *never* eat when you are *not* hungry (very few people are hungry in the early morning, for example, no matter what "experts" tell you) and you should never drink when you are *not* thirsty. This is the *only* sure and safe way to solve this controversial question *for you. Your* requirements for food and drink are *unique,* different from those of everybody else. But you can never go wrong if you follow your hunger and thirst signals. (Note: an uncontrollable desire to eat out of boredom or insecurity is not to be confused with the physiological feeling of hunger; see Chapter 33.)

Food eaten without appetite will do you no good. It will, in fact, harm you by overburdening the digestive organs with unwanted material and create indigestion, gas, and other disturbances. This is true even during pregnancy and lactation. A pregnant woman who forces herself to "eat for two" often only causes digestive and assimilative problems. Overeating is harmful even during pregnancy. In fact, at any time, the less you eat, the better you assimilate!

2. *Eat slowly in a relaxed, unhurried atmosphere.* Slow eating and thorough mastication (chewing) are essential for good digestion. Good chewing increases the assimilation of nutrients and makes you feel satisfied with a smaller amount of food. "Fletcherize" your food— chew every mouthful at least 40 times! Saliva contains digestive enzymes. Therefore, well chewed and generously salivated food is practically half-digested before it enters the stomach.

Also, food should be eaten in a relaxed atmosphere and *enjoyed.* Biologically, only the foods eaten with genuine pleasure will do you any good. A peaceful, unhurried and happy atmosphere around the table will pay good dividends in improved digestion and assimilation of food—and hence, in better health for you and your baby.

3. *Eat several small meals during the day in preference to a few large meals.* In my lifelong study of nutrition, I have been unable to find any scientific support for the necessity of eating a few *large* meals a day. In my travels and studies of eating habits of various natives known for their excellent health, I have found that they always eat several *small* meals a day. In addition to two or three main meals, they have some snacks in between as they go about their usual work. Watching peasants work in the fields in Russia and Ukraine, I noticed that they interrupt their work every two hours or so to eat and drink a little something: a fruit, a glass of cool sour milk, a slice of watermelon, a plate of cold summer borsch, or whole fresh vegetables, such as cucumber, tomato, carrot—or just a slice of sour bread with onions!

When a Mexican laborer goes to work he takes with him several oranges, mangoes, ever-present limes, or a large jicama, and has a snack of something every now and then.

It is better to eat four, five, or six small meals a day than two or three large meals. This is especially advisable for pregnant women and lactating mothers. Such eating habits would also solve 99 percent of all hypoglycemia, or low blood sugar, problems. Also, if you have a tendency toward obesity, you should know that while 2,000 calories eaten at two meals will result in a new fat accumulation, the same 2,000 calories eaten in six small meals, with two- or three-hour intervals, will not only fail to add weight, but may actually help to reduce.

4. *Do not mix too many foods at the same meal.* There is much evidence to the effect that the fewer foods you mix at the same meal, the better your digestion and assimilation will be. Every food requires a different digestive enzyme combination and mixing too many at one time results in less effective digestion.

5. *Do not mix raw fruits and raw vegetables at the same meal.* Raw vegetables and raw fruits require a totally different enzyme combination for their effective digestion, and, therefore, they should never be eaten at the same meal. Such combination will only result in poor digestion and gas. Neither should you ever mix fruit and vegetable juices.

It would be advisable to make one main meal of the day a *fruit meal,* where any available fruits are eaten, possibly with yogurt and raw seeds and nuts; and another meal a vegetable meal. The third main meal can be a cereal meal, with smaller meals, or snacks, in between (see the *Menu* for the mother-to-be in the next chapter).

The exceptions to the above rule: lemon and papaya. Both can be used with any foods. Avocados, although botanically a fruit, can be eaten with vegetables.

6. *When protein-rich foods are eaten with other foods—eat the protein-rich foods first!* Proteins require a generous amount of hydrochloric acid to be present in your stomach for proper digestion. When you eat carbo-

hydrate-rich foods, such as vegetables, your stomach does not secrete much hydrochloric acid, because it is not needed for the digestion of carbohydrates. If you fill your stomach first with predominantly carbohydrate foods (as you do when you start your meal with a large raw vegetable salad, as seems to be traditional in this country) and then finish your meal with a protein food, *the protein will remain largely undigested* because of an insufficient amount of hydrochloric acid in the stomach.

Therefore, it is best to eat protein foods first, on an empty stomach, when the hydrochloric acid secretion will be generous; then continue with carbohydrate foods. In practical terms this would mean: *steak first and then salad!* Or beans and tortillas first and then the salad. Or, if you wish, eat your salad *with* the protein food, but *not before.* The proof of the pudding is in the eating—it works! Try and see for yourself how your digestion will improve and how even beans will cease to be a "musical food."

NO-NO'S FOR MOTHER-TO-BE

- *Smoking.* See Chapter 28 on what smoking before, during, or after pregnancy does to the mother and the child. See also PART FOUR: Questions & Answers.
- *Alcohol.* Even a small amount of alcohol can enter the fetus and affect the baby unfavorably. Doctors now refer to this as "fetal alcohol syndrome." Studies made at the University of California at San Diego, where a follow-up was done on the pregnancies of alcoholic mothers, show that their babies are more likely to have slight facial, limb, and cardiovascular malformations. Some babies of alcoholic mothers have conical heads and are mentally retarded.[21] See "Fetal Alcohol Syndrome" in Questions & Answers.
- *Drugs.* All drugs, even "simple" aspirin, should be avoided during pregnancy and lactation because of potential harm to the fetus as well as to the mother. Despite this, American women consume, on the av-

erage, four or five different drugs during pregnancy. Drugs taken during the first trimester (first three months of pregnancy) can be especially dangerous to the developing fetus. Studies at the Georgia Center for Disease Control, in Atlanta, show that mothers who take diazepan (a tranquilizer marketed as Valium) during the first trimester are four times as likely to have babies with cleft lips or cleft palate, as mothers who do not take the tranquilizer.[22] And, I hope that the great world-wide tragedy of another sedative, Thalidomide, during the 1960's is still in the memories of women who plan to become mothers. Thousands of women who took Thalidomide during the first trimester of their pregnancies gave birth to babies whose arms and legs were nothing more than rudimentary flippers. Other drugs, especially antibiotics, may cause blindness, deafness, gross malformations, discoloration of nails and teeth, etc. Narcotic drugs, especially heroin, also affect the fetus. Babies whose mothers take heroin during pregnancy are born addicted to the drug.[22] Aspirin, if taken during the last three months of pregnancy, can cause premature labor, jaundice, and bleeding in the infant. Acetaminophen (Tylenol, Validol, and Tempra) can cause kidney problems in the infant. Antihistamines may cause seizures; sulfa drugs may cause jaundice; bronchial medication can lead to goiter; and tranquilizers may cause seizures, bleeding, and disorders in the body's temperature-regulating mechanism.[23]

- *X-rays.* Pregnant women must avoid *all* X-rays during pregnancy unless they are absolutely unavoidable according to several doctors' opinions. *That includes all dental and chiropractic X-rays.* Not only may X-rays contribute to the development of cancer in the mother, but it has been found that leukemia in children in later years is often caused by abdominal X-rays received by the mother during pregnancy.[24]
- *Excessive use of salt.* Salt (sodium chloride) is toxic in large doses. The average American diet contains 10 - 40 times as much salt as is required by the

body. Especially during pregnancy, excessive salt in the diet can be harmful and can cause, among other undesirable side effects, edema (swelling). Whole sea salt, in moderation, is the best form of salt.

- *Harmful spices.* Mustard, black and white pepper, and white vinegar, are without nutritional value, and act as strong irritants to the digestive and assimilative tract.
- *Sugar.* All refined, as well as brown, sugar must be completely excluded during pregnancy and lactation. The excess of sugar in the American diet, is, perhaps, the singularly most damaging factor to health and the major cause of our catastrophic health deterioration. Excessive sugar destroys B-vitamins in the body, leeches minerals, over-taxes pancreas, raises cholesterol, etc., etc.
- *Coffee, tea, chocolate, cola drinks, and other soft drinks.* All these stimulants (most containing large doses of caffeine) can reach the fetus through the placenta and cause health damage even before the baby is born. In a University of Washington study, Dr. Ann Streissguth and her colleagues interviewed 1,529 pregnant women regarding their use of coffee and found that the health of babies born to mothers who drank 8 or more cups of coffee a day was adversely affected by the caffeine. See "Coffee During Pregnancy", in Questions & Answers.
- *White flour,* and everything made with it: white bread, pastries, packaged cereal, pies, donuts, cookies, etc. These are nutritionless, overprocessed, and highly sugared foods that have no place in the diet of a responsible mother-to-be or nursing mother.

4

Pre-natal and Post-natal Diet

Based on the material and information in the previous chapter, the approximate daily menu and health program of an expectant or lactating mother should look something like this:

UPON ARISING

Choice 1: 1 glass of water (warm in winter) with freshly squeezed juice of ½ lime, or ¼ lemon, or 1 orange.

Choice 2: 1 large cup of warm herb tea, sweetened with honey. Choice of rose hips, peppermint, alfalfa (especially during lactation).

Choice 3: 1 glass of freshly-made fruit juice from any available fruits or berries, in season. Sweet juices should be diluted with water, half and half. No canned or frozen juices—the juice must be freshly made, just before drinking.

MORNING WALK

The best exercise during pregnancy is simple walking. An early morning walk, if possible in the company of the father-to-be, can do a lot to build the strength of the body for successful and comfortable pregnancy as well as an easy delivery. Walking is also a perfect time for reflection, relaxation, and meditation. A morning walk is a good way to eliminate the traces of so-called morning sickness, which some women experience during the first trimester.

However, if you have followed this book's recommendations so far, you are not likely to have any morning sickness.

Adjust the speed of your walk to your level of energy and comfort. If you feel tired, stop and rest, then continue. If you have the time, stop in the middle of the walk and do your favorite bending, stretching and rotating exercises. Do some deep breathing exercises, too.

If possible, get out of the city and go to the countryside for your walk. Perhaps you can drive out to the beach or to the woods. If you live in a city, and it is impossible to get out, walk on the back streets that are not heavily trafficked, to avoid smog. Remember, smog is hazardous for both you and your baby.

SHOWER AND DRY BRUSH MASSAGE

After your walk, take a shower to wash perspiration away. It is not necessary to take a cold shower; warm is alright. After the shower, dry thoroughly and then give yourself 10 to 15 minutes of dry brush massage (see Recipes & Directions) using a special natural bristle brush with a long handle. If your husband can give you the massage, so much the better. Do not press too hard over the abdominal area, especially during the last trimester of pregnancy.

BREAKFAST

Choice 1: Fresh fruit, in season: apples, bananas, grapes, grapefruit, or any other available fruit or berries—one or several fruits at the same time.

1 cup of any of the lactic acid milks: yogurt, kefir, or homemade clabbered milk, preferably made from goat's milk or raw cow's milk (see Recipes & Directions).

A small handful, or 10 - 20 raw nuts, such as almonds, cashews, peanuts, filberts or a couple of tablespoons of sunflower seeds, pumpkin seeds, or sesame seeds. Nuts and seeds can be ground in your own seed grinder (sold in health food stores) and sprinkled over yogurt. Sesame butter (Tahini) or almond butter can be used instead of whole nuts and seeds.

½ cup of cottage cheese, preferably home-made quark (see Recipes & Directions).

1 tbsp. fresh wheat germ, sprinkled over milk or cottage cheese. Use only if fresh, non-rancid wheat germ can be obtained.

Choice 2: A large bowl of fresh Fruit Salad á la Airola (see Recipes & Directions).

Choice 3: A bowl of cooked cereal, such as millet, buckwheat, oats.

1 cup of soaked or cooked unsweetened and unsulfured dried fruits: raisins, prunes, apples, peaches, apricots, etc. Or, 2 - 3 tbsp. of homemade applesauce (see Recipes & Directions).

1 glass of fresh, raw, unpasteurized milk, preferably goat's milk.

Options, if desired: ½ tsp. of honey, or 1 pat of butter, or 1 tsp. of olive or sesame oil.

Choice 4: A bowl of sprouted wheat or other sprouted seeds with a glass of yogurt or milk.

Choice 5: 2 - 3 buckwheat pancakes (see Recipes & Directions).

1 glass fresh, raw milk.

Homemade applesauce or honey or natural maple syrup.

Choice 6: 1 or 2 eggs, soft-boiled. The best (from a nu-tritional standpoint) way to prepare eggs: separate the egg yolk from the white; poach the white; then scramble eggs at the table by mixing raw egg yolk with cooked whites.

1 slice whole-grain bread made without sweeteners or fats (see Recipes & Directions).

1 pat fresh butter, if desired.

1 glass fresh, raw milk, or 1 cup of your favorite herb tea.

MID-MORNING SNACK, if desired

Choice 1: 1 apple, banana, or other fruit, or berries, in season.

1 cup kefir or yogurt, or 1 slice of natural cheese.

Choice 2: A handful (10 to 20) raw almonds or equivalent of other raw, unroasted nuts.

Choice 3: ½ avocado.

ONE HOUR BEFORE LUNCH

1 tbsp. brewer's yeast powder, fortified with B_{12}.

¼ tsp. bone meal powder (or 1 calcium lactate tablet).

½ glass freshly-squeezed grapefruit or pineapple juice.

Mix well and eat with a spoon. If the mixture is too thick, dilute with water. Make sure the yeast you use is labeled "brewer's yeast"; health food stores sell it. If fresh grapefruit or pineapple juice is not available, kefir, yogurt, or fresh lemon or lime juice, mixed with water, or apple cider vinegar (1 tsp. in ½ glass of water) can be substituted.

LUNCH

Choice 1: A bowl of cooked, whole-grain cereal, such as millet, buckwheat (kasha), or kruska (see Recipes & Directions). Any other available whole-grain cereals can be used, such as oats, barley, corn, rice, etc. Dry milk powder (non-instant type) can be added to the water in which cereals are cooked. This will raise the protein quantity as well as improve its quality. Molino cereal (see Recipes & Directions) is recommended to those who are bothered by constipation during pregnancy.

1 large glass of fresh, raw milk, preferably goat's milk.

½ tbsp. olive or sesame seed oil, or 1 pat of butter.

1 tsp. honey or 2 tbsp. of homemade apple-sauce, or dry fruit compote can be used on cereal instead of oil or butter.

Choice 2: A bowl of freshly-prepared vegetable soup, or pea or bean soup, or any other cooked or steamed vegetable course, such as potatoes, squash, yams, zucchini, green beans, fresh corn on the cob, etc.
1 - 2 slices whole-grain bread.
1 - 2 slices natural cheese.
1 - 2 pats butter.

Choice 3: Buckwheat pancakes it not eaten for breakfast.

Choice 4: For Mexican food lovers: beans and corn tortillas with fresh salsa made from toma-toes, avocado, onion, garlic, and chili.

Choice 5: Vegetable salad meal (see DINNER menu).

Choice 6: A large bowl of Fruit Salad á la Airola (if not eaten for breakfast)—or any of the break-fast choices not eaten that morning.

Choice 7: ½ cup drained, canned salmon, sardines, or tuna fish, preferably canned in water.
Small vegetable salad.
1 slice whole-grain bread.
1 pat butter.
1 cup of kefir or yogurt.

SIESTA AND AFTERNOON WALK

Important: After lunch, take ½ to 1 hour rest in bed. After the rest, go for a gentle walk, and if possible, do a few stretching, bending, and deep breathing exercises.

DINNER

Choice 1: A large bowl of fresh, green vegetable salad. Use any and all available vegetables, preferably those *in season*, including tomatoes, avocados, and all available sprouts, such as alfalfa seed sprouts, mung bean sprouts, etc. Carrots, shredded red beets, and onions should be staples in every salad. Garlic, if your social life permits. Salad should be attractively prepared and served with homemade dressing or lemon juice (or apple cider vinegar) and cold-pressed vegetable oil, such as olive or sesame seed oil, seasoned with herbs, garlic powder, a little sea salt, cayenne pepper, etc. Or, all vegetables, whole or cut, can be placed attractively on the plate without mixing them into a salad, and eaten one at a time—this is, by far, the superior way of eating vegetables.

1 or 2 middle-sized boiled or baked potatoes in jackets. Prepared cooked or steamed vegetable course, if desired: eggplant, artichoke, sweet potatoes, yams, squash, or other vegetables. Use kelp powder or sea salt sparingly for seasoning; also any or all of the usual garden herbs.

½ cup homemade cottage cheese, or 1 - 2 slices of natural cheese.

1 - 2 slices whole-grain bread, preferably sourdough rye bread (see Recipes & Directions).

1 pat fresh butter of ½ tbsp. olive or sesame seed oil (oil can be used on salad, potatoes, or vegetables).

1 glass of yogurt or other soured milk.

Choice 2: Any of the recommended LUNCH choices, if fresh vegetable salad is eaten at lunch.

Choice 3: A large bowl of green vegetable salad, as in Choice 1, plus 3 - 4 ounces broiled or poached fresh or frozen salt water fish; or an omelet, if desired. This choice no more than once or twice a week.

EVENING (BED-TIME SNACK)

Choice 1: 1 glass of fresh milk or nut and seed milk-shake (see Recipes & Directions).

Choice 2: 1 cup of yogurt or kefir with 1 tbsp. brewer's yeast powder.

Choice 3: 1 apple, eaten slowly and chewed well.

Choice 4: 1 cup of your favorite herb tea, sweetened with honey, and a slice of whole-grain bread or bran/corn muffin, with butter and a slice of natural cheese.

Vital points to remember

1. The above Menu is an outline, a skeleton, around which an individual diet of optimum nutrition during pregnancy and lactation can be built, following the guidelines in Chapter 3. Or, it can be followed as it is. The mother of my children lived on such a diet before, during, and after her pregnancies and delivered five healthy and well-developed children, who are now parents of their own healthy children. I know of thousands of people who live on the Airola Optimum Diet and enjoy extraordinary health. But my diet is very broad and, therefore, so flexible that it can be changed and adapted to your specific requirements and health conditions, your country's own

ethnic customs and climate, the availability of foods, your personal preferences, etc.

2. Whatever changes you make, keep in mind, however, that the bulk of your diet should consist of grains, seeds, and nuts (the natural, complex carbohydrates), and fresh vegetables and fruits, preferably organically grown, up to 75 - 80% of them eaten raw. Eat as great a variety of available foods as possible, but not in the same meal, of course. Do not avoid potatoes because you think they are fattening—they are not. Potatoes are supernutritious food, containing almost as much vitamin C as oranges, and proteins comparable in quality to those in eggs and meat.

3. The Optimum Diet contains all the nutrients you will need, including adequate amounts of protein, provided you make an effort to increase your protein intake during pregnancy and lactation to a total of about 70 - 75 grams by using fresh and lactic acid milks (yogurt, kefir, buttermilk)—3 - 4 glasses a day; plenty of nuts and seeds; plus such protein-rich cereals as buckwheat, millet, and oats. Natural cheese, such as Swiss, cheddar, and homemade cottage cheese (quark), are good protein sources. A small quantity of eggs, fish, or meat may be added to this diet, if desired, *but their inclusion is not necessary.* An adequate amount of protein can be obtained without eggs, meat or fish, on a pure lacto-vegetarian diet.

4. Remember, however, that even though there is an increased need for high-quality protein during pregnancy and lactation, of even more importance is the need for perfect digestion and assimilation of the proteins consumed. Overeating—eating a large quantity of food at one meal—hinders the digestion and assimilation of nutrients, even protein. Therefore, it is better to eat several small meals a day rather than two or three large meals.

5. The menu lunch and dinner is interchangeable. Ideally, a fruit meal should be eaten for breakfast, a cereal meal for lunch, and a vegetable meal for dinner.

6. Do not drink liquids with meals, unless you are very thirsty. Milk, yogurt, and vegetable and fruit juices are foods, and can be used with meals.

7. Divide all vitamins and supplements into three equal parts and take them with breakfast, lunch, and dinner. See other instructions regarding vitamins in Chapters 3 and 9.

Conclusion

The Optimal pre-natal and post-natal diet, as described in Chapters 3 and 4, will help you retain your own health during pregnancy and to nurture, deliver, and nurse a well-formed and healthy baby. Once it was thought that if the mother was malnourished and didn't have enough nutritional resources to supply the growing fetus, the fetus would take from the mother's own tissues and reserves whatever it needed for its own growth and optimal development and leave the mother suffering from severe pregnancy-caused deficiencies. It was believed that the mother would lose "one tooth with every child" she had. Now we know that if the mother is undernourished by an inadequate diet during pregnancy, not only will she suffer, but the baby will suffer severe deficiencies and potential health damage as well. Although most babies may appear to be healthy at birth and may be growing and doing well during infancy, their full potential for physical, mental, and intellectual development may never be reached if the mother was malnourished during pregnancy. There are many studies which show that both the fetus and the mother benefit from optimum nutrition during pregnancy. The Optimum Diet, as described in this and the foregoing chapters, can help prevent such pregnancy complications as miscarriage, premature birth, stillbirth, infant death, congenital malformations, convulsions, and epilepsy. Dr. E. Thurston, author of an excellent book, **Nutrition for Tots and Teens**, says that optimum nutrition "can also favorably affect such elusive attributes as brain development and nerve stability as well as resistance to infections, anemia, diabetes, and other degenerative diseases." Studies also show that optimal pre-natal and infant nutrition can help produce an excellent set of teeth and prevent tooth decay.

The magnificent rewards for adhering to an optimum nutrition program during your pre-conception period, pregnancy, and lactation will be not only that you will give life to a healthy, wellformed child, but also that you, too, will enjoy the highest level of physical and mental well-being.

5

Understanding Your Pregnancy

The Miracle of Creation

The miracle of pregnancy is that within a woman's uterus a human being grows and develops from a single fertilized egg, which, although so small that it can be seen only under a microscope, carries the genetic programming for an individual with unique physical and mental attributes, abilities and characteristics. This is rather difficult to comprehend if we view pregnancy only from the de-spiritualized, materialistic medical science's viewpoint. But, if we look at pregnancy from the viewpoint as expressed in Chapter 1 of this book, then the miracle of creation will be easier to grasp. The position I take in this regard is that although most of the physical attributes are hereditary, and genetically transferred from the parents to the newborn, most mental, emotional, moral, and spiritual attributes and capabilities of the child are influenced, modified, and affected by the parents' conscious and willful thoughts, desired wishes, and hopes, as well as their stands and actions in mental, moral and spiritual spheres, before and during conception and pregnancy, and during the early life of the infant. Researchers who studied this relationship believe that the "genetic component of personality" is influenced by the hormonal and biochemical changes in expectant mother's body effected by her thoughts and emotions.[12, 13]

89

For the total success of your pregnancy, which will culminate in the birth of a new human being, you must understand the spiritual significance of pregnancy as well as the nature of the physiological and biological processes and the profound physical and emotional changes you undergo during pregnancy.

Ideally, of course, you shouldn't need to read books or manuals on pregnancy and childbirth. Every woman possesses powerful instincts that can guide her in all phases of this perfectly natural process. The human race has been perpetuated for thousands, perhaps millions, of years by parents equipped with intuition and common sense, without the help of pediatricians and/or books on childbirth and infant care. Unfortunately, recent generations of women seem to have lost confidence in these instincts (or rather, were taught by their doctors not to rely on them) and, consequently, do not feel safe unless they are guided through pregnancy by experts. So, if you are one of those who feels that you want to know what is going on within your body, as well as what's happening to your emotions during this important phase of your life, read on.

How conception takes place

Conception takes place when the male's sperm (spermatozoa), which is manufactured in the testicles, and the female's egg (ovum) unite. This normally happens a few minutes or hours after sexual intercourse. Fertilization of the ovum occurs in the fallopian tube, a tube leading from the ovary to the uterus. The fertilized egg then travels to the uterus, where it attaches (implants) itself to the uterine wall and begins to grow and develop into a fetus.

During one ejaculation, the male releases as many as 400 million sperm. Upon entering the vagina, the sperm travel at a speed of about ¼ inch per minute, heading for the uterus and then the fallopian tubes. With the aid of muscular contractions as well as natural chemical and hormonal assistance, the sperm may reach the fallopian tubes and fertilize an egg within a few minutes after intercourse. A woman's orgasm may speed up the movement of the sperm. During the orgasm, the cervix descends and enlarges, increasing the size of the passageway to the uterus. This makes it easier for the sperm to travel and meet the egg.[1] Also, the sperm travel more easily in an alkaline environment, and orgasm changes the normally acid vaginal secretions into more alkaline. The uterus, too, is trying to speed up the movement of the sperm. It expands and contracts intermittently, creating a suction-like effect.

How soon or how long after intercourse is there a possibility of conception? The egg, after it is released from the ovary, may survive as long as 72 hours, so there is always a possibility that conception can occur during the three days following ovulation (see Chapter 22, "Birth Control: Natural and Unnatural"), although during the first 24 hours the chance (or the risk) of fertilization is greatest. The male sperm, on the other hand, may survive within the woman's body for as long as seven days, although it is generally considered that after the first two days they are not able to penetrate and fertilize the egg.

From the above, it is obvious that the best chances to conceive are if intercourse is performed at the exact time of ovulation, which is normally fourteen days before the next menstrual period. It is also possible to get pregnant by making love up to 72 hours before or 24 hours after ovulation.

Boy or girl

According to some experts on conception and pregnancy, the baby's sex may be determined by carefully planning the time of intercourse in relationship to the time of ovulation.

The baby's sex is determined by the chromosome type of the sperm. About half of the sperm released during intercourse carry an *X chromosome,* which will produce a girl. The other half carries a *Y chromosome,* which will produce a boy. For reasons unknown, the boy-producing sperm are smaller, lighter, and faster, but they die sooner than the sperm that produce girls. The male sperm (andro-sperm) lives only about 24 hours, while the female sperm (gynosperm) lives two to three days.

So, here's how you can help to choose the baby's sex. Intercourse at the exact time of ovulation favors the conception of a boy. Intercourse two to three days before ovulation increases the chances of conceiving a girl, because most of the male-producing, quick-dying sperm, will be dead by the time the female's egg is released during ovulation.

Dr. Landrum B. Shettles, M.D., who discovered this method of pre-determining the sex of the baby, claims that it is eighty percent accurate. The method also includes douching with mild alkaline or acidic solutions before intercourse to alter the pH of the vaginal tract (alkaline for boy and acidic for girl), as well as the presence or absence of female orgasm. The female orgasm favors the birth of a baby boy, since it opens the entrance to the uterus, produces alkaline lubrication, and facilitates the speedier movement of the fast-traveling male-producing sperm.[15] Of course, the success of this approach to choosing the sex of your baby depends largely on the ability to know the exact time of ovulation—which is not always easy. (See Chapter 22 for the most effective ways to determine the time of ovulation.)

New studies made in France and Canada show strong evidence that by manipulating her nutrition before conception, a mother can dictate the sex of her future child. The nutritional principle of sex pre-determination was discovered by Dr. Joseph Stolkowski, professor of physiology at the University of Pierre and Marie Curie in Paris. In a nutshell: if a woman eats lots of dairy products, she will probably conceive a girl, but if she eats lots of salty foods, she most likely will conceive a boy. The diet changes the body chemistry in such a way that a woman's egg is more receptive to a certain type of sperm. Following such dietary changes, 81 percent of the women in the Canadian study, and 87 percent of those in the French study had the infant of the sex that they selected. Dr. Stolkowski explained that if you want a girl, make your diet rich in calcium and magnesium (dairy products) and if you want a boy, your diet should be rich in potassium and sodium. Of course these minerals can be also added to the diet in supplementary form. The dietary changes should be made at least six weeks before conception.

Additional research on this dietary approach to determine the sex of the child is underway in Paris. In the meantime, if the principle is correct, it would seem that the lacto-vegetarian diet, as advocated in this book, would favor the birth of a girl, unless, of course, you add more salt to your diet than is normally advisable.

First trimester

During the first three months following conception, the fetus develops almost all of its physical human characteristics: all vital organs—brain, sexual organs, endocrine glands, and digestive organs. Its heart pumps blood through well-developed arteries and veins. The stomach produces digestive juices, the liver produces blood cells, the kidneys function and produce urine. The fetus can move, turn its head, and can swallow, and the testes of the male fetus already produce androgens (male hormones). And all this while the fetus is only three inches long and weighs about half an ounce!

The first trimester is the most critical for the child's future development. The fetus depends on its mother for all the nutrients it needs for growth and development: proteins, vitamins, minerals, etc. Extensive animal studies as well as human studies made during times of severe deprivation, such as during World War II, when diets were deficient in vital nutrients, showed an increased amount of fetal brain damage, premature births, and stillbirths.

In addition, during the first trimester, the developing fetus is most sensitive to toxic influences to which the mother-to-be is subjected, such as drugs, tobacco, alcohol, and X-rays.[1, 2, 3] For example, women who take Valium (a common tranquilizer) during the first trimester are four times as likely to have babies with cleft lips or cleft palates as mothers who do not take tranquilizers.[1]

Three phases of growth

The current medical understanding of the growth of the fetus seems to be that there are three distinct phases of growth. The first phase is *hyperplasia,* or cellular proliferation. During this phase, the growth occurs through rapid multiplication of the *number* of cells. Thus, it is a quantitative growth. During the second phase, although the cells still multiply, they also begin to *enlarge*. This process of qualitative growth, or enlargement of the cells, is called *cellular hypertrophy*. The third and final growth phase is virtually exclusive cellular hypertrophy.[4]

The understanding of this growth process is very crucial. It appears that the brain, for example, reaches its full cellular proliferation during early stages, perhaps exclusively during the first trimester. If the mother's nutrition is inadequate during the first 13 weeks of pregnancy, the development of the fetus' brain, nervous system, and vital organs may be curtailed. And, even though during the later two trimesters the nutrition is optimized, the brain may never grow to its full potential. The final number of brain cells may be significantly less than the total number of brain cells in an adequately nourished fetus' brain. Thus, brain function may be permanently impaired.

Studies show that different organs attain their full cell number at different stages, the lungs and brain being among the first to reach full cell count.[5]

Second trimester

During the first trimester, some mothers feel sick: "classic" morning sickness with nausea and vomiting are common, especially if the mother is inadequately nourished. In addition, the mother's emotions and feelings about pregnancy are crucial for her level of well-being. If the baby is really wanted, and the attitude of both parents is nothing but joy and gratitude, the mother is likely to feel wonderful through all three trimesters. Furthermore, studies show that women who wanted to become pregnant have much fewer complications during labor and delivery than women not consciously desiring pregnancy. Therefore, the attitude, or the state of mind, is of paramount importance not only in regard to how the mother feels during pregnancy, but also for the successful completion of the delivery.

As the second trimester progresses, the mother begins to feel better and better. Indeed, often she feels better than she did when not pregnant.

The mother now feels the presence of the living human being within her body. The baby's movements are felt periodically. The mother's appetite improves. Her breasts begin to increase in size and she is beginning to gain weight.

Proper weight gain

Every adequately nourished woman will gain weight during pregnancy. The question, so often asked by pregnant women, is, how much weight gain is appropriate? In our weight-conscious culture, women often worry more about their appearance, even while they are pregnant, than what is best for the baby. And, many obstetricians urge mothers to restrict weight gain during pregnancy—in fact, often they put mothers-to-be on strict diets at a time when both the mother and the growing fetus need more nutrients.

Since each pregnant woman differs in regard to weight, body build, pre-pregnancy weight (degree of underweight or overweight at the time of conception), physical activity, and basal metabolism, an exact desirable weight gain cannot be specified for all women. But, in general terms, the pre-natal weight gain, as recommended by the Committee on Maternal Nutrition, Food and Nutrition Board of the National Research Council, is 24 pounds.

There usually is little or no change in the weight of the mother-to-be during the few weeks following conception. The steady weight gain commences near the end of the first trimester and continues through the second and third trimesters at a rate of about 400 grams (a little less than a pound) per week. According to this pattern, the total weight gain during the whole pregnancy would be around 11 kg. (kilograms), or approximately 24 pounds.

Some women ask, why such an increase when the average baby weighs only 3.5 kg. (8 pounds)? The break-down is as follows: approximately 3.4 kg. (7¾ pounds) are in the fetus, about 0.6 kg. (1½ pounds) are in the placenta, and about 1.0 kg. (2¼ pounds) is in the amniotic fluid. This leaves about 6 kg., or roughly 13½ pounds gained by the mother. Don't forget that the size of the uterus and the breasts are increased considerably during pregnancy. There is also an increase in maternal blood volume. During the third trimester, there also is weight gain for the mother through accumulation of extra cellular fluid. In addition, about 3½ pounds are stored by the mother as fat and extra protein to act as a reserve to meet the demands of stress during the immediate post-natal period.

Third trimester

By the time the fetus is six months old, it is in many ways a fully-developed human being. It is about thirteen inches long and weighs about one and a half pounds. This miniature being is very active and the mother can identify various parts of his body—an elbow, a knee, a tiny bottom —as it moves and squirms within the uterus.

During the third trimester, the demands of nutrients are especially heavy. The baby will absorb up to 84 percent of all the calcium the mother gets in her diet, and 85 percent of the iron. The calcium is needed for the rapid skeletal growth of the fetus. The extra iron is needed for two purposes: (1) to supply it to the fetus and the placenta; (2) to meet the demand created by the significant increase in maternal blood volume and in total erythrocyte quantity during pregnancy. Peak blood volume prior to delivery is about 50 percent greater than non-pregnant volume.

The average pregnant woman needs 870 mg. of iron during the course of a normal pregnancy, in addition to her normal needs, to meet both the fetus' and her own body's increased demands. This divides out to about 4 to 5 mg. of absorbable iron per day, at least during the latter half of pregnancy. Since only about ten to twenty percent of dietary iron is absorbed (even less of supplementary iron) it is important to eat plenty of natural iron-containing foods and take iron supplements during that time. The best natural sources of iron are: apricots, peaches, bananas, prunes, raisins, brewer's yeast, blackstrap molasses, whole grain cereals, beets, beet tops, turnip greens, alfalfa, spinach, sunflower seeds, walnuts, sesame seeds, dried beans, lentils, kelp, liver and egg yolks. (See Chapter 13 and 30 regarding iron-deficiency anemia in infants and women.)

A sufficient amount of gastric enzymes, especially of hydrochloric acid, is needed for proper assimilation of iron. So, if your digestion is not too good, one tablet of HCl, taken with meals, can be helpful. For these reasons, the iron-containing fruits, which contain their own enzymes and acids that aid in the digestion and assimilation, are the most reliable sources of dietary iron. Vitamin C also aids in the absorption of dietary and supplementary iron. Note: coffee and tea interfere with iron absorption. Also, remember what we said in Chapter 3: supplementary iron is antagonistic to vitamin E. Therefore, it should be taken ten to twelve hours after Vitamin E supplement is taken. For example: you can take a full daily dose of vitamin E in the morning, and iron supplement with dinner.

One of the most common iron supplements prescribed by obstetricians is ferrous sulfate. This form of iron supplement is definitely not advisable. Its toxicity is well known. It increases tremendously the need for oxygen, pantothenic acid, and several other nutrients as well as destroys vitamins, E, A, and C.[7] It also can cause liver damage and can even bring about miscarriages and premature or delayed births.[8]

If an iron supplement is taken, get it from health food stores, where it most likely would be from natural sources.

Folic acid, or folate, is another specific supplement that may be needed during pregnancy. The usual dosage is 1 to 2 mg. Dosages up to 5 mg. can be taken if recommended by a doctor.

Regarding extra protein need during pregnancy, the opinion of experts varies considerably. For example, the official RDA (Recommended Daily Allowance) by the Food and Nutrition Board, 1968 edition, was 10 grams additional protein per day during pregnancy.[9] However, in the 1974 edition, the RDA is an additional 30 grams protein for pregnant women—they tripled the protein requirement!

Based on the calculation of actual additional protein needs (amounts of protein in the uterus, amniotic fluid, and fetus), 10 grams per day would be sufficient additional protein during pregnancy, assuming complete utilization.

However, based on the nitrogen balance studies (which are rather inaccurate) the need may be in the neighborhood of 30 grams.[11]

Since proteins in their raw forms are utilized twice as effectively as when cooked, the amount of high-quality raw protein in the Airola Optimum Diet, derived from raw milk and natural cheese, plus sprouted grains, seeds, nuts, cereals, and vegetables, will supply plenty of high-quality proteins. With an added supplement of approximately twenty to thirty grams a day (through increased use of natural milk products, brewer's yeast, nuts, soybeans, and other protein-rich foods), all the protein needs during pregnancy can be adequately met.

Immunity transferred

If the mother is healthy and well-nourished during pregnancy, she will pass on to her baby immunity to a number of diseases, which she herself may have contracted in the past. The antibodies that her body produced when she was subjected to certain infectious diseases are still present in her body and they can be transferred through the placenta to her new baby. Thus, her baby will have a certain resistance to such diseases as mumps, measles, whooping cough, influenza, etc. This transference of protective antibodies is continued through the mother's milk if the baby is breastfed. (See Chapter 20, *Immunization: A New Look.*)

Pregnancy complications

Pregnancy is not a sickness or any kind of abnormal condition. It is a perfectly natural, healthy state. Normally, a woman feels just great, "better than ever," during pregnancy. Many of the minor health problems, aches and pains, and even some of the more serious health disorders, such as arthritis, for example, tend to disappear completely during pregnancy.

But, occasionally, some women may experience discomforts. Some suffer from constipation or heart burn. If you follow the Optimum Diet as described in Chapters 3 and 4, you won't have problems with constipation. Some women experience cravings for certain, often exotic, foods. This is usually a sign of nutritional deficiencies. Many women who lived on my Optimum Diet during pregnancy have reported to me that they never felt the cravings for unusual foods. When the body is adequately nourished and the fetus receives all the nutrients it needs, there isn't any unusual desires or cravings for food.

Some women complain of swollen legs and varicose veins during the last trimester. One of the reasons for this is a high sodium (salt) intake; another reason: increased need for potassium, calcium and magnesium. Also, the increased weight of the abdomen causes extra stress on the legs. This can be alleviated if you take the time for a daily rest in bed, elevating your legs slightly. Also, exercises, and other suggestion for varicose veins, as mentioned in Chapter 26, can be beneficial.

If there are no unusual symptoms or any kind of abnormality, there is no need to worry about your health during pregnancy. Neither is there a need to constantly check with your doctor (beyond regular checkups) to see if everything is OK. If you feel OK, everthing *is* OK! If it is not, you will know it.

The danger symptoms, however, should not be overlooked. If there is a heavy vaginal discharge of any kind, bleeding, irritation in the genital organs, swelling of the ankles, or the stopping of the movements of the child in the womb, the doctor should be contacted at the earliest possible moment.

Preparation of the nipples

Preparation for breast feeding should begin not later than in the beginning of the third trimester. Small breasts can be just as good milk producers as big ones, but small nipples are not very convenient for the baby to hold and suck effectively. Nipples should be well shaped and protruding.

Therefore, if your nipples are small, and especially if they are retracted, they should be gently pulled out each day and massaged. This preparation is to accustom the nipples to being handled, sometimes rather roughly by a hungry baby, and prevent cracking and soreness during breast feeding.

Most women, even though they never give any special care to their breasts during pregnancy, do not run into any difficulty. However, some women, especially redheads and those with very fair complexions, do have occasional difficulty with tenderness or soreness.

Here are a few things you can do to prepare your breasts for nursing:

1. Do not use too much soap on your breasts or nipples during bathing. Soaps dry out the skin, removing natural protective oils, and dryness encourages both cracked nipples and stretch marks. Breasts and nipples should be washed only with plain warm water, or you may add ¼ teaspoon sea salt to one cup of water. This will strengthen them for nursing.

2. Massage your nipples gently with fingers during your bath and several times during the day. Also, pull your nipples out with your fingers, quite firmly, but not to the point of pain.

3. Going without a bra, even if only for a part of the day, is also helpful. It exposes nipples to the air and the gentle stimulation by friction of your outer clothing.

4. If your nipples are inverted (depressed, and not protruding—and many women do have this problem) you can

help by gently pulling the nipples out and stretching them several times a day. If nipples are so small that you cannot grasp them with your fingers, try to take the whole areola (the dark area around the nipple) between your thumb and forefinger and gently squeezing outward, like milking, push the nipple out. Do this a couple of times a day. Even if you cannot get the nipple out too much now, it helps, and the baby will do the rest later on. Not wearing a bra will also help those with depressed nipples.

Some natural birth advocates recommend hand-expressing a few drops of colostrum from each breast every day during the last six weeks of pregnancy. Colostrum is the fluid secreted by the breasts before milk comes in and is a very important first nutrient for the newly born baby. The suggested reason for this pre-delivery expression of the colostrum is that it supposedly helps open milk ducts and prevents engorgement later when nursing begins. Personally, I do not feel this routine is necessary; possibly it is even harmful. It doesn't impress me as being natural, either. If a few drops of colostrum come out on their own a few days before birth, it's OK, but I don't think a deliberate expression is necessary.

Stretch marks

One area of much concern to many women is stretch marks. Many women think that stretch marks are an undesirable but unavoidable side effect of pregnancy.

This may not need to be so. If the mother is well nourished for a year before the pregnancy and during the pregnancy, adheres to the Optimum Nutrition Diet, and takes all the vitamins and supplements as recommended in this book, she will, most likely, not have any problem with stretch marks at all. I have seen many women who have followed my nutritional program and special preventative routines, and you would never know by looking at their bodies that they have ever been pregnant.

Stretch marks are the result of the body's weakened cellular and collagen integrity and inability to meet the demands of stress. This skin is not elastic enough to shrink back to its original size without leaving marks. The deficiencies of vitamins and minerals are definitely involved, particularly deficiencies of vitamins E and C-complex, zinc, silicon, and pantothenic acid. The deficiency of mucopolysaccharides may also be involved.

To prevent stretch marks, here is what you can do:

1. Build your body's nutritional integrity to the optimal level by eating the Optimum Diet for one year before, and throughout the pregnancy. See Chapters 3 and 4.

2. Take all the vitamins and supplements as suggested in Chapter 3, especially vitamins E and C, the minerals including zinc and silicon, and bioflavonoids. Sunflower seeds and pumpkin seeds are good sources of natural zinc. Take horsetail tea for silicon.

3. As soon as you know you are pregnant, start a daily routine of gently massaging your body, especially the breasts, abdomen, and buttocks, with a few drops of my special "Formula S." Morning and/or evening, after a bath or shower, are the best times. Here is the

Formula S

4 tbsp. virgin olive oil, cold-pressed
4 capsules vitamin E, 1000 I.U. each
   capsule, mixed tocopherols
2 capsules of vitamin A, 25,000 units
   each capsule.

Mix the ingredients in a little jar and keep refrigerated, tightly closed. Make a new batch when the first one is gone. Add a few drops of a pure, natural perfume (essence of flowers) if you and/or your husband prefer.

4. Aloe Vera gel, internally and externally, is also helpful.

Mother's emotions during pregnancy

Both prospective mother's and father's attitudes during pregnancy are of paramount importance. The father must support his wife each day in her objective to produce a perfect, healthy, and beautiful baby and provide not only the best of food, clothing and shelter, but also an atmosphere of joy and love in which this can best be accomplished. He must provide an atmosphere as safe and as peaceful as possible.

You are now approaching your expected date of delivery. Your excitement and anticipation are slowly building up. Each day you are growing more and more enormous. And, occasionally, you are just a little apprehensive and worried. Will the delivery be easy? Will the baby be without defects? Will it be a boy or a girl; a small or large baby? A small baby does not necessarily mean a swift, easy labor, nor a large baby a long and painful one. The proper preparation, exercises, and foremostly, the emotional attitude, relaxation, and peace of mind, are much more relevant factors.

Apprehensions and worries are natural during the last few weeks before delivery, especially if it is the first pregnancy. But with conscious effort you must try to develop a relaxed, confident, peaceful attitude. And, avoid or minimize all emotional conflicts and stresses, if possible. The unborn baby is very sensitive and responsive to what's happening "outside" at this stage. For example, it responds negatively (with violent motions) to loud noises. Some of the young people today don't seem to be able to listen to music unless it is unbearably loud. Turn the sounds down—a baby likes soft, gentle, mellow sounds. Dr. Lester Sontag experimented with various loud sounds and found that not only do babies react with kicking and violent movements, but their heart rate increases, indicating raised blood pressure.[12] Researchers believe that there is a genetic component of personality influenced by the uterine environment. When the mother-to-be is emotionally upset, the excessive amount of adrenalin and other hormones cause physical and biochemical changes in her body which also affect the unborn baby.[13]

In one study, several women were observed during the last trimester of their pregnancies and their babies followed up after delivery. The babies of those women who suffered severe emotional crises, grief, fear or anxiety during pregnancy, were irritable and hyperactive, and several had severe feeding problems.[12] Thus, the importance of avoiding emotional upsets and stresses during pregnancy cannot be overemphasized.

If you are easily upset, apprehensive, and worried, herbs and herbal remedies, especially Bach Flower Remedies, can help to stabilize your emotions. During the last trimester, a mild tea of one or several of the following herbs can be helpful: valerian, scullcap, lady slipper, rosemary, camomile, garden sage, hops, and licorice root. One combination of five flower essences, known in the Bach Flower Remedy system as Rescue Remedy, can be of great help during the last trimester.*

Television viewing during pregnancy should be severely curtailed, preferably avoided. There is a danger from radiation, especially from color T.V. There is growing evidence that long hours of television viewing by the mother may result in the child being particularly susceptible to leukemia.[14] I would suggest avoiding air travel during the third trimester, as well.

Gentle walks, plenty of mild and medium-vigorous exercise, good nutritious foods and supplements as outlined in this book, plus a confident, relaxed, peaceful attitude can make the nine months of your pregnancy the most unforgettable and joyous time of your life. You are now approaching the final phase and the culmination of pregnancy—bringing a new human being into the world— the most fulfilling and blessed event that any human being can experience. In co-partnership with God, you will perform the wonder of wonders: the Miracle of Creation!

During the last few weeks of pregnancy, your thoughts, as well as much of your attention and feelings should be directed towards your baby who is about to be born. Meditate and dwell on how pleasant and easy your delivery will be. Visualize your baby as a sweet, beautiful, defect-free, healthy, intelligent, talented, and lovable new spirit which will enrich your life and fill it with joy, love, and purpose.

---

*A list of Bach Practitioners can be obtained from: Dr. Edward Bach Healing Center, Mount Vernon, Sotwell, Wallingford, Berks., England.

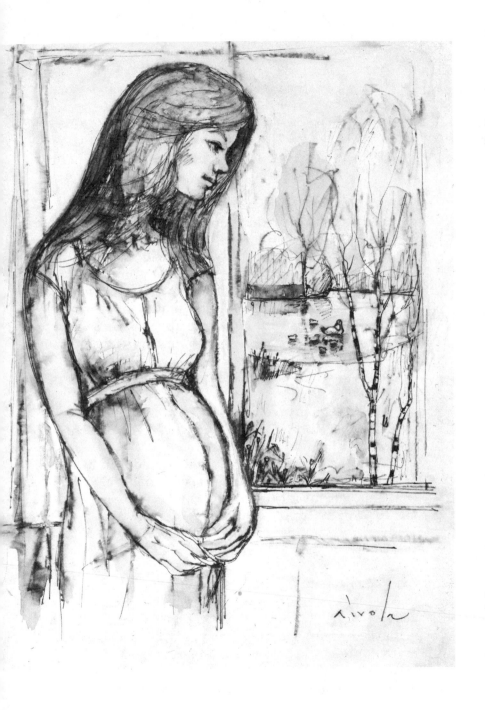

Natural Childbirth

You have been preparing for this big event for at least a year or more. Your preparation began long before conception. When you and your husband decided to have a child, you prepared your body by periodic cleansing fasts and by optimizing your nutrition so that your physical and mental health would be at the optimum level when conception occurred. Then, for nine months, you carefully nurtured your baby within your womb, preparing the physical body as well as the mind of a new spirit to enter into this world.

And now, the supreme and marvelous event is dawning!

You are finally going to have a baby!

And, of course, you are going to have your baby by *natural* birth.

If you have been reading natural childbirth literature, or attending classes or workshops where natural childbirth is taught, you must be aware by now that there are several methods of natural childbirth. There is the "Lamaze Method," the "Bradley Method," the "Dick-Read Method," the "Spiritual Midwifery Method," etc. Which "method" are you going to use?

You might as well admit to yourself right at the outset that what you really want, the way you really wish to deliver your baby is by the "original" divinely-designed method, the way babies are supposed to be delivered, and the way they have been delivered for millions of years. Not by any methods devised or developed by this or that man, doctor, or "expert," but by the method developed by the

Master himself, the One who designed and created the "original."

During the past century, with the advance of modern medical science, the responsibility for man's health has been gradually taken away from whom it belongs—man himself—and usurped by the doctors. This remunerative seizure of control over what should have been man's birth-right and responsibility has had disastrous effects on the health of the human race. The area where this usurpation of control brought the most disastrous consequences was in the birth of babies. What was once a perfectly natural, simple, common, and joyous family event, attended and aided by husband, children, and older relatives with experience in childbirth, became a medical case, handled by total strangers in white, within sterile cement walls of the huge impersonal hospital complex. The mother was taken away from the family and all the relatives, including her husband, sedated by strong anesthetics, drugged, cut, and manipulated. Being unconscious and not having control over her muscles, and thus, not being able to participate in the labor, the baby often had to be pulled out with steel instruments. Then, while the mother was recuperating from the heavy stress of drugs and sedatives, the baby was taken into the nursery, given drugs, and forcefully fed glucose (sugar) water. Finally, when the baby was brought to the mother, sometimes after the lapse of several days, and the mother, still in possession of some degree of instincts, wanted to breast-feed her baby, she was told by the omniscient doctor that breast feeding was a superstitious custom of the unenlightened past, that the formula he prescribed was far superior nutritionally to her own milk, and that modern bottle feeding would be less bothersome both for her and the baby, would not cause sagging breasts, and would produce a super-healthy and smart baby. Then, he gave the mother powerful drugs to suppress her own milk production, and handed her a sheet with feeding instructions which included giving the newborn baby canned baby foods, with meat and cereals beginning in the second or third week after birth!

In case you think I am exaggerating, I can assure you that this is an exact re-enactment of the standard procedure of the hospital delivery years ago—and similar experiences happen even today! No wonder this medical practice of scientific childbirth produced several generations of people with the lowest health level in human history—both mentally and physically!

Many experts believe that not only are our physical and mental ills related to the unnatural ways in which our children are conceived, nurtured, delivered, and fed, but many of our social ills, especially family breakdown and a discernible alienation between parents and children, may be linked to the lack of natural "bonding" which occurs between parents and infant in the very first few minutes after the birth; which, of course, is not possible in the above-described hospital-type medical delivery.

But, as with all fashions, social and medical customs change with the times. There has been, during the past few years, a rapidly-growing movement towards living a more natural life, eating more natural foods, even delivering babies in a more natural way. Doctors are slowly and quietly changing too, and, forced by the growing consumer (patient) interest and demand, moving gradually, albeit sometimes reluctantly, towards supporting the more natural approach both to living and healing. The dark age of medicine—the Pasteurian era of relentless hunting for vicious germs and reliance on deadly drugs and the surgical knife in an unsuccessful attempt to keep people healthy—is coming to an end. We are moving towards a more natural, holistic approach to health where the well-being of the total person—even the whole family—is taken into consideration. A *new look* at the old ways of delivery is a logical consequence of such a development.

The key word—NATURAL

When you look at the growing number of new natural childbirth "methods" that are becoming increasingly popular, you will discover that they really do not offer anything *new*. They have been developed as an inevitable reaction to the de-humanized and outright dangerous orthodox hospital-type medical delivery. All the natural childbirth methods mentioned earlier have one thing in common: they all advocate the return to the old-fashioned, natural, drugless, family-oriented deliveries; away from hospitals, anesthetics, and strange, unfriendly environments; bringing the important event of the birth of a new baby back home where it belongs.

What do we mean by *natural* childbirth?

Here are the basic principles behind the philosophy of natural childbirth:

1. The pregnancy and the consequent birth are perfectly natural, healthy, normal functions of the human female body, as normal and natural as the processes of eating, eliminating, or performing any other bodily function.

2. Pregnancy is not a disease; not a pathological condition which requires diagnosing or treatment by medical experts, except where there is a pathological involvement connected with it. Analogy: the normal, natural, and very involved and complex process of feeding, digestion, and assimilation of food is performed by individuals on their own, using the hunger instinct and taste as their guiding lights for the proper selection of food. Only when there are malfunctions and disorders in the digestive and eliminative process is the involvement of the professional practitioner justified. Drugs, X-rays, anesthetics, sedatives, painkillers, and tranquilizers have no place during pregnancy or childbirth. Medical intervention is justified only if there are medical complications.

3. The birth of a baby is a very important family happening. It is, perhaps, the most important event in a woman's life. It is a marital experience. Mothering is an inadequate term to describe such a complex, physical, emotional, psychological, and spiritual event as childbirth. Parenting is a more suitable term. Both parents are vitally involved in this pivotal experience of their lives. Their closeness, love, and caring for each other are strengthened by sharing the joys as well as responsibilities of parent-

hood. It is, therefore, unnatural to keep them apart during such an important and joyous experience. Natural childbirth means that the father joins the mother during this all-important and thrilling event, supporting, encouraging, and helping her, sharing the joy, wonderment, and excitement with her.

Is natural birth painless?

The concept of pain associated with childbirth is deeply engraved in the collective memories of most civilized women. The Biblical account of the creation and the decree, "In sorrow or suffering thou shalt bring forth children," may have been adulterated by the translations, according to some scholars. It could have been translated to "with labor," or "with hard work," which does not necessarily involve pain.[19] In primitive cultures, where women are unfamiliar with the Biblical account of childbirth and consequently have no negative feelings or fear associated with it, they deliver babies in an easy, natural, matter-of-fact way, without suffering or pain. In our culture, especially since the moving of childbirth from the home to the hospital, with its sedative drugs and anesthetics, the mother-to-be *expects*, in fact *fears*, that the childbirth will be associated with pain. Emphasis on pain is pronounced throughout the whole experience. The phrase, "labor pains," is the basic textbook designation for the contractions during childbirth. The mother-to-be is conditioned to think that pain in childbirth is inevitable. But is it?

The Grantly Dick-Read Method

Some doctors didn't think so, and started to question the inevitability of pain. English doctor Grantly Dick-Read was one of the first to develop a natural-birth technique that virtually eliminated all pain during childbirth. His first book, *Natural Childbirth*, was published in 1933. His second book, *Childbirth Without Fear*, was published in the United States in 1944.[1] Today, Read's method, with some variations, is one of the two most widely used natural childbirth techniques in this country. It is based on the fundamental belief that *fear and tension*, learned through cultural conditioning and transmitted from mother to daughter over the generations, is responsible for pain. "Superstition, civilization, and culture," he wrote, "have brought influences to bear upon the minds of women which have introduced fears and anxieties concerning labor. The more cultural the races of the earth have become, so much the more positive they have been in pronouncing childbirth to be a painful and dangerous ordeal."

Fear, through the sympathetic nervous system, generates tension, and that tension, in turn, produces pain. By removing fear from childbirth, tension is reduced and pain is minimized or eliminated. Dr. Read's method of removing pain and achieving painless childbirth is based on:

a. education
b. correct breathing
c. relaxation, and
d. special exercises.

Education is extremely important. The more completely the mother- and father-to-be understand all the aspects and phases of pregnancy and childbirth, the female anatomy and physiology, the process of labor and delivery, the easier it becomes for them to avoid anxiety and fear.

The Russian methods

Russian doctors have developed the so-called psychoprophylactic method (PPM), which is largely based on conditioning techniques developed from Pavlovian physiology. The main goal of this method is the substitution of new or conditioned responses for what was previously felt as pain.

Dr. Platanov was the first to advocate hypnosis as an anesthesia for pain relief. He performed hundreds of hypnotic deliveries and claimed that women who deliver in this way "fulfill a normal and magnificent act with a quiet smile on their lips, rather than tears in their eyes, writhing and sobbing in useless pain."[2] He believed that both mother and baby benefited from childbirth with hypnosis, since harmful drugs were avoided and pain was reduced.

Another Russian pioneer was Dr. I. Velvovsky, who studied painless childbirth as early as 1920. He wrote: "The teachings of Pavlov have strengthened the conviction that childbirth, in so far as it is a natural act, need not be accomplished by painful manifestations."[3]

The other major Russian pioneer in the Pavlovian concept of painless childbirth was Professor A. Nicolaiev. It was he who coined the name "psychoprophylaxis" in 1949, the term now used universally to describe natural childbirth without pain, based on conditioning techniques derived from Pavlovian research. Dr. Nicolaiev made the very first physiological analysis of pain in childbirth. Nicolaiev used post-hypnotic suggestion, rather than hypnosis, during pregnancy. The woman was hypnotized *before* the birth, instructed not to feel pain during the birth, and then was awakened for the birth itself. She was able, thus, to participate actively in the birth process, yet feel no pain.

Now, PPM, or psychoprophylaxis, is a commonly-used method of childbirth in Russia. In fact, since 1951, PPM is the official method of childbirth in the entire country. Based on Pavlov's concept that fear is a conditioned response, PPM asserts that it can be eliminated by deconditioning or unlearning by proper education. When a woman feels the sensation of uterine contraction stimulated by labor, she responds with fear and pain, being so conditioned by tradition and social factors. The PPM method is based on forming new positive conditioned reflexes such as deep-breathing exercises and relaxation when the uterine contractions occur, and replacing with them the old ones of pain and fear.

Lamaze method

The Lamaze method is actually the Russian PPM method with a few minor modifications.[4] Dr. Fernand Lamaze, a French obstetrician, heard Dr. Nicolaiev speak in Paris, visited the Soviet Union for firsthand observation, was impressed by what he saw, and then introduced the method in France. Although he humbly gives all the credit for "his" method to Russian pioneers, in the United States the original Russian work is hardly known and the PPM method is, therefore, commonly-referred to as the Lamaze method.

According to Lamaze (and PPM), peripheral uterine sensations (contractions), upon reaching the brain, are translated into consciousness. Such contractions are painless, and yet, most women today experience pain during labor. Why? Because, in the minds of the women, pain and childbirth have for so long been associated, that their emotions and conditioned reflexes interfere with the contractions to make them painful. The Lamaze method uses various devices and techniques to recondition the thinking and develop a new, painless, positive conditioned response to contractions. Like Dr. Read said, fear of pain results in pain. The Lamaze method shows how to suppress the painful conditioned reflexes, and, by reshaping nervous function and positive conditioning of consciousness, teaches a woman to deliver her baby without pain.

Most cities in the United States now conduct classes in natural childbirth. Some use Dr. Read's method, some Dr. Lamaze's method. Some classes use a combination of both. If you are interested in natural childbirth without fear and without pain, you should join such a class. Your doctor or the local La Leche League, or one of the hospitals, can give you the addresses of such classes.

A recent study by Dr. Michael Hughey, of Evanston Hospital in Illinois, in which 500 Lamaze-prepared pregnant women were compared with a control group of 500, matched for age, race, number of children, and educational level, showed that the group trained in the Lamaze method of natural birth, without anesthetics, had 75 percent fewer deaths during delivery, 33 percent less post-partum infections, and fewer lacerations. The control group, which was not prepared with the Lamaze techniques, had 3 times the frequency of toxemia and twice the number of premature infants.

Father's participation in childbirth

All natural childbirth methods include having the father at the mother's side during their most momentous experience—the birth of *their* child. The courses in natural childbirth encourage both parents to be in attendance. The husband is trained to coach and assist his wife during delivery. The father, who actively participates in the birth, performs a variety of important functions: he renders physical assistance by coaching his wife on breathing procedures, massaging her back or abdomen, and keeping track of the progress of labor; he also provides essential emotional support for his wife and adds to her feeling of safety, security, and confidence. Most theorists on natural childbirth feel that such active sharing of a family's most important event adds strength to the marriage and to the total family relationship. Dr. Irwin Chabon said: "His help, sympathy, and understanding are of incalculable value in sustaining the emotional health of his pregnant wife."[5]

Dr. Deborah Tanzer, author of *Why Natural Childbirth?*, conducted a pioneering scientific study on the psychological impact of childbirth. One of the primary objects of the study was to evaluate the conflicting claims for and against the husband's participation in labor and delivery. Her controlled study showed conclusively that the husband's presence and active participation during childbirth contributes "strongly and positively" to the welfare of the mother and makes the experience more "rapturous and joyous," and the husband's participation added a new dimension to their marriage. Dr. Tanzer writes: "As far as marital relationship is concerned, there seems little doubt that it has been enhanced as a result of their mutual experience of birth. The couple has moved *together* from the status of a twosome to that of a family ... In terms of the effect on the wife and on the marriage itself, my research indicates that the father belongs at his wife's side through labor, delivery, and on to the unforgettable early moments when a new life has been created."[2]

Dr. Robert A. Bradley, author of the book, *Husband-Coached Childbirth*, is one of the pioneer advocates of childbirth as a husband-wife joint venture. As a prerequisite for the husband's participation, however, he stipulates that both parents are well-trained in all the details of labor and birth: the wife has been shown how to perform in labor and has prepared her birth-giving muscles by special exercises; and "the husband has been prepared so that he understands how, why, and what his wife is doing, enabling him to coach, guide, and encourage her in her ennobling work. He should be well-acquainted in advance with her appearance in the various states of labor. By being prepared for her objective appearance, he not only feels serene and self-confident through familiarity, but can apply his knowledge by acting as a coach to actually see to it that she performs properly. She, in turn, feels secure knowing that her ever-present coach not only loves her, but knows what she is about to do and how to guide her."[6]

Dr. Bradley has delivered babies by natural birth for over twenty years and has experience of more than seven thousand cases of the husband in the delivery room. His work has influenced the attitude of many obstetricians and hospitals across the country, and now husbands are welcome in many delivery rooms for active participation during the childbirth. When the state of California ruled that husbands must be allowed in the delivery rooms, the ruling was based on a survey of 45,000 cases of husbands in attendance, which concluded: "there was not one infection traceable to this practice, and not one malpractice suit."[2]

Bonding: what the newborn baby needs most

When a baby is born, the strongest natural instinct of most parents is to hold their child. Not after a few hours, or even minutes, but right away! In those first moments of contact, the powerful ties that bind mother and father to the child are formed. Scientists call this process *bonding*.

Studies show that the amount of bonding that takes place after birth can have a permanent effect on the future development of the child's personality and character, as well as on the quality of the relationship between parents and child.

Yet, according to a recent study by the American Hospital Association, 75 to 80 percent of U.S. hospitals not only do not permit fathers in the delivery rooms, but interfere with the bonding process by separating parents and children immediately after the birth. The baby is handed not to the mother, but to the nurse, checked by a medical team, and whisked straight to the hospital nursery. Many mothers are not able to see or hold their babies until several hours later. And for the rest of the hospital stay, most parents only see and hold their newborns at specified times.

Luckily, the American Medical Association is finally recognizing the importance of bonding and recently adopted a resolution urging hospital medical staffs to review and humanize their delivery practices and develop policies that promote bonding.

The importance of bonding has been recognized by many professionals for a long time. Dr. Joost Meerlo stated in 1968:

"The psychological impact of the father on the emotional development of the child has long been overlooked... The example set by the father is vital for shaping the destiny and eventual emotional independence of the adult-to-be. The joint relationship of parents with the child begins at birth."[7]

It is important that the baby is given to the mother to hold as soon as possible, right after the placenta is expelled. A newborn baby should come in close contact with his mother's body, preferably lying on her stomach, where he can hear the mother's familiar heartbeat and feel the warmth to which he was so accustomed while in the womb. The baby should hear his mother's and father's soft, gentle voices, and experience their touch.

It is also important that the baby is put to his mother's breast as soon as possible after his birth. Although the mother's breasts do not have milk for three or four days following the birth, they do have a fluid called *colostrum*, which has an exceptionally important nutritive value for a newborn baby and also contains immunizing substances for the baby's protection in the new environment.

Home birth vs. hospital birth

More and more women are choosing childbirth at home over hospital delivery. Between 1972 and 1975, a period during which total births actually declined, the number of out-of-hospital births in the United States increased by 60 percent. Many obstetricians enthusiastically support the home-birth idea. In Chicago, a group of physicians has organized the American College of Home Obstetrics to support families and doctors interested in home birth. Home-birth societies and centers are springing up everywhere. I will list several national home-birth organizations later in this chapter so that women who want to know more about home birth may write for information.

The AMA, concerned about the growing number of women who have chosen to give birth at home rather than accept traditional maternity procedures, prepared a statement urging hospitals to "humanize delivery practices." "There is no question that we are responding to a rising consumer interest in the lifelong importance of childbirth." One reason why hospitals have been reluctant to change their methods is the fear that relaxation of their rigid rules might lead to an increased risk of infections in the newborn. Now the AMA admits that this is not the case. Family-centered procedures, such as allowing the father in the delivery room and letting both parents hold the newborn baby right away, have not resulted either in increased infections in the baby, or increased mortality.

Actually, a recent remarkable study by Dr. Lewis Mehl and his associates at the Institute for Childbirth and Family Research, Berkeley, California, showed that home births are much safer than hospital births. The massive study of more than 2,000 births from 1971 to 1976, of which roughly half were home births, showed that women in the

hospital group had
- 30 times more forceps deliveries;
- 30 times more birth injuries;
- 6 times greater incidence of distress in labor;
- 8 times greater frequency of babies being caught in the birth canal.
- 4 times as many babies in the hospital needed resuscitation.
- Infection rates were 4 times higher in the hospital.
- Mothers were 3 times more likely to hemorrhage in the hospital than in the home.

This was a scientifically-executed study, where home births were carefully compared with the same number of equivalent hospital births, matching pair for pair, mothers of the same age, number of previous children, income, education, state of health, and medical history.[8]

Dr. Mehl explained that the greater risk for hospital births is because of the greater number of procedures done in the hospital. Excessive use of forceps leads to a greater number of permanent birth injuries such as facial nerve injuries, fractured skulls, and facial nerve paralysis. "There is also a higher incidence of Caesarean sections in hospitals because doctors are more likely to intervene, instead of letting labor pains progress and seeing what happens," said Dr. Mehl. The key problem of hospital births, he said, is that most doctors in the delivery room, "tend to regard birth as a disease, rather than a normal process. Consequently, there is also a greater use of pain-killing medication."

Dr. David Stewart, Executive Director of the National Association for Parents and Professionals for Safe Alternatives in Childbirth (NAPSAC), a leading national organization supporting a family-centered childbirth program, both in and out of the hospital, says that other studies have yielded similar results as the studies by Dr. Mehl. " The conclusion that we draw is that hospitals pose hazards to mothers and babies unique to the hospital."

NAPSAC does not advocate home birth for every woman. It recognizes that hospitals are necessary for some mothers who have true medical problems, and one of NAPSAC's main goals is to implement a human, family-centered hospital maternity program. "But," says Dr. Stewart, "current scientific studies, as well as a number of working out-of-hospital childbearing centers and home-birth programs, show that out-of-hospital births can be a safe, viable alternative for many and are actually safer than hospitals for the normal healthy mother and baby."[8]

Mothers choosing home birth must be aware that there are certain risks. In medical emergencies, sophisticated hospital equipment may save lives. On the other hand, the very availability of such equipment tempts hospital personnel to intervene unnecessarily, perhaps even danger-ously, in normal births. Artificial induction of labor with drugs carries a certain risk to mother and child. Drugs used to stimulate labor may produce contractions so strong that they can interfere with the baby's oxygen supply. Despite this, Dr. Robert Caldeyro-Barcia, president of the International Federation of Gynecologists and Obstetri-cians, estimates that 90 percent of hospital inductions are unnecessary and are performed to speed up a normal birth.[9]

Dr. Robert S. Mendelsohn, nationally syndicated columnist and an associate professor of Preventive Medi-cine and Community Health at the University of Illinois, feels that hospitals are dangerous places for newborn babies because they "are always exposed to the people in the next bed, and there are resistant germs in the hospital that you can't get anywhere else in town. In the nurseries, there are unnecessary tests, unnecessary injections, like routine vitamin K (given in some places), bilirubin lights (special treatment for skin yellowing) used too frequently when you don't need them." And, finally, Dr. Mendelsohn said, "there is psychological damage resulting from sepa-ration from the mother."

One mother-to-be I know, who plans to have home births, sums up her attitude thus: "Sure, there are risks, but not as great as at the hospital. In the end, I think the benefits of home birth are well worth the risks."

And what are the benefits of home birth, other than the avoidance of increased health hazards to mother and baby in hospital births as cited above?

Here are some of the other benefits:

- At home, parents retain complete control.
- Labor and delivery in one room, in a familiar, serene home environment.
- Husband coaching and supporting his wife throughout.
- Infant can be nursed immediately after birth, and remains with his mother.
- No routine pubic shave (Michael L. Gerber, M.D. reports that shaving of pubic hair results in twenty-fold increase in superficial post-partum infections in the perineum), enema, or episiotomy (cut in the vagina to enlarge the birth canal).
- No drugs or anesthetics. Although most physicians admit that an unmedicated birth is the safest for both mother and baby, many hospitals still administer massive doses of drugs whether the mother wants them or not.
- The absence of harassment. As one doctor, whose wife recently had home birth says, "In the hospital, there is always a nurse who thinks she knows better than the mother."
- The comforts of home: comfortable bed, mountains of pillows, favorite foods, complete privacy if desired, favorite music, soft lights, comfortable temperature, the company and devoted care of people she knows and trusts.
- Sympathetic doctor or midwife giving full-time attention and supervision. The assurance that in case of a complication, mother will be driven to the hospital by experienced professionals.
- The physician's bill for a home delivery is now covered by many insurance plans.

Where can you get the names of doctors who are willing to attend home births? Most child-birth education centers can provide one or two names of doctors in your town.

Can any woman give birth successfully at home?

Definitely not. A woman who suffers from heart disease, diabetes, kidney disease, epilepsy, anemia, or hypertension should not consider home birth. Home birth is generally not advisable for a woman giving birth for the first time at age 35 or older. Neither is a woman who carries more than one child, or one whose medical history includes Caesarean section, a candidate for home delivery.

A careful preparation for natural childbirth is essential for all those who choose home birth. If any of the natural childbirth methods mentioned in this chapter are chosen, both parents-to-be should attend a training and education workshop or class. You can find them in most cities. In classes, the breathing and relaxation techniques that can ease the labor and delivery are taught. Most classes also provide information about preparation for breast feeding, possible complications, and special exercises to help the mother during pregnancy, during labor, as well as after the delivery.

Early in the pregnancy, a physician or a nurse with midwife training who is willing to attend a home birth, should be chosen. Regular checkups of blood pressure, weight gain, urinary sugar and protein levels, fetal position, heart sounds, etc., are important. Blood tests and pelvic measurements should also be made.

The parents-to-be should maintain a reasonably clean house, live preferably not more than 20 minutes from the hospital (in case of complications), and have a competent birth attendant available on short notice.

If you wish more information on home birth, you may write to:

National Association of Parents and Professionals for Safe Alternatives in Childbirth (NAPSAC), Box 1307, Chapel Hill, N.C., 27514

Association for Childbirth at Home International, Box 1219, Cerrito, California, 90701

HOME, 511 New York Ave., Takoma Park, Md., 20012

Gentle Birth Foundation, 142 Calumet, San Anselmo,

CA, 94960

International Childbirth Education Association, Box 20852, Milwaukee, Wisc., 53201

La Leche League, International, Inc., 9616 Minneapolis Ave., Franklin Park, Illinois, 60131

All the above-mentioned organizations have available a great amount of literature on natural childbirth, home birth, alternative birthing, breast feeding, and related subjects.

Alternatives to home delivery

Attractive compromises to home deliveries are now available in some hospitals or in special centers in many larger cities—*family-oriented maternity centers.* In New York City's Childbearing Center, parents can stay in a comfortable and cheerful townhouse where the birth takes place. Relatives and friends can visit, food can be prepared in the Center's kitchen, where parents' wishes are respected, and the baby can be taken home the same day if there are no complications. Such centers are available in several cities.

A number of hospitals around the country are developing rooming-in facilities, in an effort to combine the warmth and comfort of home with the safety of a major medical facility. Looking at it realistically: since for most women it is not yet possible to have babies at home, the next best thing is to bring home into the hospital.

Danger of drugs used during childbirth

Although there is a strong move away from the use of drugs during childbirth, many doctors attending delivery in most hospitals are still using drugs on a massive scale, often against the wishes, or even the knowledge of the mother.

Drugs can be extremely harmful, not only to the mother, but also to the baby. A long-held belief that the placenta provides an almost impenetrable barrier and guards the fetus from harmful substances, has finally been discarded. We now know that almost every substance injected into, or ingested by the mother, can reach the fetus within minutes. Alcohol, nicotine, antibiotics, barbiturates, tranquilizers, aspirin—all get through the placenta and affect the fetus. (See also Chapter 3 on the danger of taking drugs during pregnancy.)

Dr. Virginia Apgar, a world-renowned authority on birth defects, and Dr. Sydney S. Gellis, Chairman of the Department of Pediatrics at Tuff's University School of Medicine, warn that almost all commonly-used drugs can produce abnormalities and birth defects in infants if taken during pregnancy.[10] Barbiturates and aspirin have been shown to cause excessive bleeding in newborn infants. Sulfa drugs increase the risk of brain damage. Antihistamines and antidepressants can produce abnormalities. Phenacetin, which is present in a number of over-the-counter preparations for reduction of fever and achiness, may induce excessive breakdown of red blood cells in the fetus or liveborn infant. Tranquilizers, taken during pregnancy, can adversely affect the baby's response to stress and lower his learning performance.[11] Even cyclamates, a common artificial sweetener, which is now suspected to be carcinogenic, if taken during pregnancy, can pass into the developing fetus.[12]

Anesthetics commonly given to the mothers during childbirth are dangerous both to the mother and the child. One authority refers to anesthesia as a "killer in obstetrics."[13] Another authority says that "Anesthesia as a cause of maternal mortality has reached fifth place in New York City, behind hemorrhage, infection, toxemia, and heart disease."[14] *Williams Obstetrics*, an authoritative textbook, has this to say about anesthetics. "Anesthesia is playing an increasing role in maternal mortality. It is a decisive factor in 5 percent of such deaths and a contributing cause in another 5 percent."[15] Inhalation and spinal anesthesias are called the prime offenders. If you *must* have pain relief during a hospital delivery, Dr. Abram Ber, a certified anesthesiologist who now practices holistic medicine, recommends epidural analgesia, administered by a competent M.D. anesthesiologist.

Although very few reports of severe harm or death caused by sleep-inducing drugs used during delivery reach the press, most responsible doctors seem to agree that there is a serious element of risk for the safety and life of the mother as well as of the baby.

Anesthetics given during labor and delivery rapidly cross the placenta and enter the baby's bloodstream. The greatest danger to the baby is fetal anoxia, or severe oxygen deficiency caused by the drugs' depressant effects on the respiratory center. Suffering from lack of oxygen, babies of medicated mothers are frequently born limp, bluish, unable to breathe spontaneously, and may need oxygen or other resuscitative measures. From 15 to 65 percent of babies of medicated mothers show symptoms of anoxia. Severe cases of anoxia (also called asphyxia, or hypoxia) can cause brain damage in the baby, or even death.[16] In contrast, babies of unmedicated mothers are usually healthily pink, active, and able to breathe spontaneously in up to 98 percent of cases.

Brain damage can also be caused by analgesics (pain-killing drugs) given to mother during labor and delivery. Demerol, a commonly-used drug for this purpose, has been known to cause brain damage.[2]

The American Journal of Disease in Children reported on comparative studies of babies of medicated and non-medicated mothers. It found that standard delivery room medications such as meperidine and promethazine impaired behavioral functioning of most babies for several days, and even changed their brain wave patterns.[17] The baby's sucking ability after birth is weakened by administration of drugs during delivery. Drugs may also adversely affect the mother's milk production.

Prompted by the mounting evidence of extreme danger from drugs during pregnancy and delivery, an editorial in the prestigious *New England Journal of Medicine* declared: "Physicians must think more seriously before administering any drug to a pregnant woman."[18]

Or, as famous authority on birth defects, Dr. Apgar, stated, "Don't ever use drugs unless you have to!"

The current sharply stepped-up interest in natural childbirth and home birth is spurred by a growing reaction by parents against drugs in pregnancy and at delivery. Natural childbirth mothers and babies need not be subjected to the harmful effects of medication.

Possible complications at birth

First, let me assure you that complications at birth are rare. About 95 percent of all births to healthy mothers happen *without* complications.[19]

However, it is good to be informed of even rare possibilities. It is much easier to decide on choices and courses of action if the parents-to-be are prepared and educated in all phases of labor and delivery.

Premature delivery is the most common complication of pregnancy. In the United States, about 5 percent of all babies are born prematurely, some deliberately. Doctors may induce premature labor in conditions such as diabetes, toxemia, or the Rh-negative problem, to forestall death of the fetus in the last few weeks of pregnancy. Sometimes this is also done with multiple births. It is common that women with the above-mentioned conditions have premature births even without inducement.

However, in most cases of spontaneous prematurity, the causes are unknown. If the fetus is expelled before it reaches 500 grams (1 lb.), it is considered a miscarriage. By the time it weighs 3 pounds, it is already considered a premature infant. If the infant is over 5½ pounds, he is considered a full-term baby.

Premature babies always have to be kept under special observation until they reach their full-maturity potential. If the infant survives the first week, chances are good that he is strong enough to carry on.

Premature rupture of the membranes, i.e., the spontaneous rupture of membranes before the onset of labor, is another possible complication to watch for. The delicate fetal membranes (the amniotic sac) are like a plastic bag in which the placenta is encased. The fetus is suspended in the amniotic fluid inside. This membrane protects the baby from bacterial infections. If membranes rupture within a few hours before the onset of labor, this is no problem. If after the rupture, labor does not ensue, especially for several days, there is always the possibility of an infection—although even then the infection is the exception rather than the rule. However, when this happens, it is good to have capable professional supervision since intrauterine infections can have serious consequences for both the baby and the mother.

Breech presentation is another birth complication which occurs when the baby is mislocated in the mother's abdomen. The baby usually comes through the birth canal head first with his chin bent down on his chest. When the baby is turned around and the buttocks or feet appear first, the delivery is called a breech presentation. For every one hundred deliveries, about three present with the bottom or the feet first.

If the pelvis is large enough, breech delivery can be made without complications. A doctor noticing the likelihood of a breech presentation in the last month's examination, may attempt to "turn the baby around" by external manipulation—a procedure called external version. Sometimes the baby will turn on his own accord within a week or two of delivery. But if the pelvis is known to be small, and the baby's head large, the breech birth can be risky and doctors often consider a Caesarean section to assure safe delivery.

Umbilical cord accidents happen when the cord forms knots or entanglements about the baby and causes impaired circulation in the cord. The umbilical cord is usually about two feet long, but can be much longer or shorter. Constriction is likely if the cord is short and if the baby moves around a lot, especially in the last days before birth. Constriction is most common during labor as the baby moves down the birth canal and stretches the cord. If circulation is completely shut off, for even a few minutes, a stillbirth will result.

Sometimes, especially in breech position, and after the rupture of the membranes, the cord can slip into the vagina ahead of the baby. This condition is called **_prolapse of cord._** Then, as the baby moves down, the cord could be pinched between the baby and the sides of the birth canal. Again, constriction can be severe enough to cause complications.

A **_Caesarean section_** is an obstetrical operation in which delivery of the fetus is made through an incision in the abdominal and uterine walls. Naturally, several legends connect Caesarean delivery to Emperor Julius Caesar. One is that Caesar was born in this manner. Another is that Caesar passed a law ordering the operation to be performed upon dying women during the last two weeks of pregnancy to save the child.

Caesarean sections are now performed in most hospitals in increasing numbers. It is estimated that from 10 to 20 percent of all hospital deliveries today are by Caesarean. Although a Caesarean section can be life-saving, both for the mother and the child, especially in cases of birth complications mentioned above, such as umbilical cord accidents, severe toxemia, complicated breech presentation, premature rupture of membranes, uterine inertia, or when pelvic bones are too narrow, or the baby is too large, the growing concern among doctors is that Caesarean sections are now performed even in cases that do not require it. A Caesarean section, although now perfected to the point that it is relatively easy and safe, still carries with it the risk of any surgery, especially in that it always involves the use of drugs and anesthetics. It should be performed only in cases when there is absolutely no alternative. In addition, some doctors now schedule the operation ahead of time, not waiting for the labor signs. This is definitely ill-advised. Some doctors claim that a Caesarean cannot be performed once labor begins. This is not so. Not only can it be, but, in some respects, a few hours of labor makes the Caesarean operation easier.[20] Also, if a Caesarean is performed after the contractions of real labor have begun, it can prevent hyaline membrane formation in the baby's lungs.[6] Hyaline membrane disease occurs more often in babies delivered early and by Caesarean section.

Labor and delivery

If this is your first pregnancy, you have been wondering through the last several months how it will feel when the time for the birth finally arrives. If you have been preparing for natural childbirth, especially home birth, and have attended special childbirth classes, you are "an expert" by now and well prepared for what signs to expect. Many months of mental and physical preparation have taken place, and now the much-awaited baby is going to be born!

"How do I know when labor begins? What if I find out too late to call the doctor or get to the hospital on time?", many a young mother-to-be wonders. Don't worry! You *will* know in time. You read stories in papers of babies appearing suddenly without warning and of the father having to tie the cord with his shoe string! Such happenings are as exceptional as they are rare, and that's why they make the news. Over years of practice and thousands of deliveries, obstetricians usually can count on the fingers of one hand the cases when the mother didn't get to the hospital on time.

Towards the end of the ninth month, even before the actual contractions are felt, you may have a few definite signs. One is known as "lightening," when the baby moves down with its head settling in the pelvis, thus relieving the pressure on the diaphragm. You may feel that you can breathe easier. This can happen weeks before the birth. You may also urinate more frequently since now the pressure on the bladder is increased.

When actual labor begins, you will have definite contractions at even intervals of 15 to 30 minutes. The contractions last 15 to 20 seconds and feel somewhat like menstrual cramps. The discomfort can be in front or back of the abdomen, but always in the middle.

Once true labor begins, nothing stops it until the baby is born. Usually, the first baby takes 10 to 12 hours of labor—so you have plenty of time to prepare for home birth or to get to the hospital. The intervals between contractions will become shorter and shorter, while the contractions last longer and longer. Most doctors advise waiting until the contractions are coming every 10 minutes before calling them or driving to the hospital. You still get there in time!

Sometimes during labor you will notice a rapid flow of liquid from the vagina. This means the membranes have ruptured and fluids are running out. Often there is no gush of water, just a few tablespoonfuls, just a constant dribbling, enough to saturate a few sanitary napkins. Sometimes the membranes may rupture before labor begins. If so, let your doctor know. Sometimes there is a "show," a slight discharge of blood. This may happen even several days before the rhythmic labor contractions begin. Again, don't worry, but let your doctor know. Most likely it is blood from little broken vessels of the cervix as it begins to dilate.

Labor is divided into *three stages.*

The *first stage* is the longest one and takes from 8 to 12 hours for most women having their first baby; usually, it is much shorter in subsequent deliveries. The first stage is the dilating stage and it is considered completed when the cervix, or neck of the womb, is completely dilated. At the end of the first stage, the contractions are coming every 2 to 3 minutes and are 40 to 50 seconds in duration. Now is the time to practice everything you have learned about the painless childbirth in your classes: deep breathing, gentle massage, preferably by your husband, and other techniques such as relaxation and mental concentration that eliminate or greatly minimize the labor pains.

The *second stage* of labor is the actual delivery or expulsion of the baby. It is also called the *transition* stage—transition between the uterus and outside world. It extends from the time the baby's head gets to the floor of the pelvis and starts to distend the vaginal opening, through the actual birth. With the first delivery, this stage usually last 50 minutes to 1 or 2 hours. In subsequent births, it may last just a few contractions and be as short as 1 to 10 minutes.

Again, remember the exercises, deep breathing, relaxation, and other techniques of painless childbirth. These exercises you must do now if you are having a natural childbirth without anesthetics. Actually, you are over the most difficult part of labor, the first stage. The second stage—the actual birth—is much easier and faster. The baby's head will appear through the vulvar opening and it is pushed out by each successive contraction. Then the most important moment, the "crowning," occurs, when the vulva has encircled the largest diameter of the baby's head. It is smooth sailing after that. The following contractions will help to deliver the shoulders, and then the rest of the body slides out along with the umbilical cord. The doctor may hold the baby by the feet, head down, to help drain mucus from the respiratory passages. But don't expect that. This is what you usually see in the movies. In reality, very few doctors lift the baby by the feet, since the baby usually begins breathing right away on his own, and gives a welcome cry. A drop of silver nitrate is put into each eye in order to prevent eye infections from the germ that causes gonorrhea, which may have been picked up during the passage through the birth canal; this is required by law in most states, and prevents what used to be a leading cause of blindness in infants.

At this point, the baby is still attached to the mother by the cord. When the blood has stopped pulsating through the cord, it is clamped or tied off in two places: one close to the baby's abdomen, and the other a little bit further up. It is then severed with a sterile surgical scissors in between the two ties. Your child is now born! This is probably the most incredible and joyous moment of the whole experience!

The *third stage* of labor lasts from the birth of the baby until the delivery of the placenta, or afterbirth. This usually takes only 5 to 15 minutes and there is just a minimal amount of discomfort. Once the placenta is delivered, all in one piece, labor is over, and the childbirth is completed.

Episiotomy

What about the episiotomy? A worried, first-time mother often wonders: "Do I have to be cut?" Episiotomy is a small surgical incision made betwcen the vaginal and rectal openings, in the perineum, and its purpose, supposedly, is to prevent tearing of the tissues. Doctors claim that in most deliveries, episiotomy is necessary to enlarge the vaginal opening. You mean, the creator made a mistake and didn't design the opening big enough for the baby to come out? He did design all the animals correctly— none of them need to be cut! For millions of years, before the advance of modern surgery, women delivered their babies without episiotomies. Somehow, in my logical mind, this doesn't quite compute. Could it be possible that the doctors made the mistake, not the Creator? The truth is that the supposed tearing of the vaginal opening is a very rare occurrence. If the attending doctor would only wait long enough, and if he would not drug the mother to the state where she loses all her reflexes, he would find out that there is actually nothing wrong with the original design, and that the opening *is* big enough, after all, even in first deliveries. Personally, I feel that in most cases, episiotomies are unnecessary and that they have no place in what I call a natural childbirth.

First few moments of baby's life

In the past, the general obstetrical practice was to cut the umbilical cord immediately after the birth of the child, Now, most doctors wait until after the pulsation of the cord has stopped. Both practices are undesirable.

The umbilical cord contains a large amount of oxygenated blood, and the child needs all the blood he can get to function at his best during the first moments of his life. Anoxia, or oxygen deficiency, is one of the most common birth complications. Many doctors, especially in Europe, have recommended to wait with the cord cutting at least until the placenta is expelled, which may be 5 - 10 - 20 minutes. This way, the baby will receive most of the oxygenated blood that is stored in the cord and placenta, which can help prevent anoxia.[21] You may like to discuss this with your doctor and show him the report on studies mentioned in the above reference.

How soon should the mother hold her baby? As soon as possible. Preferably right after the third stage of labor, or after the placenta is expelled, even before the cord is severed, but certainly as soon as the cord is cut. The infant can be put on his mother's abdomen, covered with a warm blanket, and both mother and father should gently hold and touch him. The baby's mouth should be put to the breast and if he has the desire to suckle, all the better. It is important that the infant take some of the colostrum from the breasts as soon as possible. Although the breasts will not have "real" milk for 2 - 3 days, they do contain colostrum, a substance, as mentioned earlier, which is extremely important to the health of the baby. It contains antibodies, particularly secretory IgA, vitamins, and proteins, which are specially formulated to nourish a newborn and to give an early protection against the germs and other hazards of the infant's new environment. Although antibodies are not always easily absorbed into the infant's bloodstream, they work locally, offering protection against allergy and pathogenic bacteria and other harmful substances that enter through the gastrointestinal tract.

Most authorities recommend that if the mother and baby are healthy, and if the baby is not premature and the birth was not medicated, the baby should be put to the breast and nursed as soon after delivery as possible, often on the delivery table. Pediatricians seem to agree that there are certain benefits attached to this practice. Some believe that the early physiological loss of weight is prevented by very early breast feeding, since the suckling reflex is at its height 20 - 30 minutes after birth, then diminishes rapidly.[22] Dr. Robert Bradley says that immediate breast feeding after delivery can help the uterine contractions needed to separate the placenta from the uterus, since the uterus contracts by reflex from breast stimulation.[6]

Some doctors in hospitals have told mothers that they may not nurse their babies because the babies must be immediately placed under a heat lamp, wrapped in aluminum foil, or put in a heated bassinet. Many obstetricians disagree with this practice, and do not feel that a full-term baby needs artificial heat.[23] And, certainly, no baby is going to get too chilled wrapped in a blanket and placed in the loving arms and on the warm body of his waiting mother.

To hold the baby as soon as possible after the birth has another important function. As I mentioned before, **bonding**, the powerful psychological, emotional, and spiritual tie, is formed between mother, father, and child **right after the birth**, during the very first moments of his life, by immediate close physical contact. In natural childbirth it is important, therefore, that the baby be given to the mother and father to hold as soon as possible, so he can feel the warmth and security of his mother's body, hear her heart beat and the gentle soft voices, and experience the touches of his parents. This establishes a solid bonding between them and leads to a physical and emotional closeness that will last for a lifetime.

One more thing. In hospitals, the baby is cleaned and washed right after he is born, which removes the *vernix*, the buttery coating covering the baby's skin. It is believed that the vernix is important for the health of the baby and should not be removed or washed away too soon. Among other purposes, it may guard the body against heat loss.[2] Therefore, if yours is a home birth, do not remove the vernix, but spread it gently around the baby's body with your hands. The vernix will sink into the skin within the next 24 hours.

Finally, the baby is happy and falls asleep. Now he can be gently moved from his mother to rest close by, in an area where it is warm, quiet, and the light is not too bright. The mother can rest now, too. And, just rejoice and celebrate the most unforgettable and fulfilling experience of her life—giving birth to a new human being and bringing a new member into the family!

SUGGESTED READING ON NATURAL CHILDBIRTH

1. *Painless Childbirth*, by Fernand Lamaze, Pocket Books, Simon & Schuster, N.Y. N.Y., 1976.

2. *Preparation for Childbirth*, by Donna and Roger Ewy, New American Library, N.Y., N.Y., 1972.

3. *Thank you, Dr. Lamaze*, by Marjorie Karmel, Dolphin Books, Doubleday, Garden City, N.Y., 1965.

4. *Maternal Emotions*, by Niles Newton, Harper & Brothers, N.Y., N.Y., 1973.

5. *Mother Love*, by Alice Bricklin, Running Press, Philadelphia, PA., 1975.

6. *Husband-Coached Childbirth*, by Robert A. Bradley, M.D., Harper & Row, N.Y., N.Y., 1965.

7. *Why Natural Childbirth*, by Deborah Tanzer, Doubleday & Co., Garden City, N.Y., 1972.

8. *Childbirth Without Fear*, by Grantly Dick-Read, M.D., Harper & Row, N.Y., N.Y., 1970.

9. *Life Before Birth*, by Ashley Montagu, New American Library, N.Y., N.Y., 1965.

10. *Awake & Aware*, by Irwin Chabon, M.D., Dell Publishing Co., N.Y., N.Y., 1970.

11. *Birth, Facts & Legends*, by Caterine Milinaire, Harmony Books, N.Y., N.Y., 1974.

12. *Natural Childbirth and the Christian Family*, by Helen Wessel, Harper & Row, N.Y., N.Y., 1973.

13. *Safe Alternatives in Childbirth*, by David & Lee Stewart, NAPSAC, Box 1307, Chapel Hill, N.C., 27514.

14. *A Practical Training Course in the Psychoprophylactic Preparation For Labor*, by E.D. Bing, M. Karmel, and A. Tanz, N.Y., 1961.

15. *Childbirth. A Manual For Pregnancy and Delivery*, by John S. Miller, Atheneum, N.Y., N.Y., 1963.

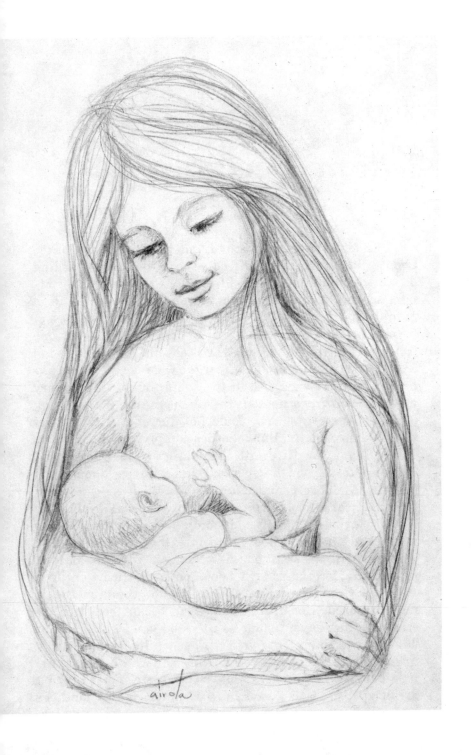

7

Infant Feeding

I have never been able to fathom how people can argue about which mode of baby feeding is better: breast feeding or bottle feeding of artificial formula. It is just plain common sense (an ingredient which apparently is missing in many a pediatrician) that the young of any species of mammals are best nourished by milk from the same species. There must be some valid reasons why females are equipped with milk-producing organs. Of course, it is easy for *me* to see: I was born at the beginning of this century when *all mothers* nursed their babies. And, if the young mother, for some reason, could not nurse, a suitable "wet nurse" was sought. Baby bottles simply did not exist.

Today it is different. A young mother has been educated to rely on her pediatrician's advice about baby feeding. And her pediatrician, especially if he graduated from medical school during the first two decades following World War II, probably had only heard breast feeding mentioned in his school as something from a distant, ignorant, and superstitious past. He was educated only in prescribing formulas. Text books on pediatrics from that era scarely mention breast feeding. So the young mother is now confused. Her grandma says to breast-feed. Her liberated mother says, "Don't be silly—do you want to be tied down to your baby for a year?" Her own instinct says that nursing is the right thing to do, and she wants to hold her new baby to her breasts. But, her pediatrician says that artificial formula is easier, just as nutritious as mother's milk, more convenient, less bothersome, will not cause her breasts to sag, and will produce a healthier baby. So, whom to believe?

In the beginning of this century, 99 percent of all babies were breast-fed. By 1956, only 38 percent were breast-fed. And, by 1966, only 18 percent were breast-fed. This rapid decline was due to many reasons:

- The "emancipation" movement among women after World War I.
- Fast-growing industrialization and urbanization, which resulted in many mothers working outside the home.
- The inadequate and misguided pediatric education in medical schools influenced by the biased research funded by baby food manufacturers.
- The new women's "liberation" movement since World War II, which depicts breast feeding as demeaning and confining.
- The great pressure on the new mother to bottle-feed her baby from massive advertising in all media by baby food manufacturers and drug companies. Just open any women's magazine or baby-care magazine! Millions of dollars are spent on advertising artificial baby-feeding compounds and baby food, and not a penny on advertising breast feeding.

Fortunately, there is now a definite trend back towards breast feeding. The unexpected benefit from the liberation movement was that enlightened women who want to be truly liberated all the way, want also to free themselves of the dehumanizing, synthetic, chemicalized threat of misdirected science and "return to nature." And, breast feeding seems to be the most natural thing in the world. Young, educated, new-age women of today are much more health oriented than the women of a generation ago, and they recognize that breast feeding will produce healthier babies. A survey taken in 1977 showed that only 8 percent of grade-school educated women breast-fed their babies, as compared to 32 percent of college educated women. And, there is a growing number of unorthodox, enlightened doctors, even pediatricians, who realize the mistake made by the medical profession regarding breast feeding in the past, and now are actively supporting the movement back towards nursing.

But, more than anyone else, the lay women's organization, La Leche League International, can be credited for the fast-growing trend towards breast feeding. They are doing great work in advising women, have branches in all major cities, print books, pamphlets, hold educational meetings, and give counsel by correspondence and telephone. Their excellent book, *The Womanly Art of Breast Feeding*, should be read by every woman who is interested in having a healthy baby. It is available from their headquarters: La Leche League International, 9616 Minneapolis Ave., Franklin Park, Ill. 60131.

Why breast feeding is better

There are many reasons why breast feeding is superior to artificial bottle feeding or feeding with baby foods.

1. Breast milk is better digested and assimilated than formulas based on cow's milk. Breast-fed babies have much less digestive upsets and disorders.[1, 2]
2. Breast feeding encourages good facial and dental development. Bottle-fed babies are more likely to have poorly developed dental arches, palates, and other facial structures in adulthood.[2]
3. Breast feeding prevents anemia in both mother and baby.[3, 4, 5] Iron is almost totally lacking in cow's milk (see Chapter 13).
4. Breast-fed babies are less likely to suffer from skin disorders such as eczema.[6, 7] (See Chapter 21.)
5. Breast-fed babies are less likely to develop allergies later in life, which are common in bottle-fed and baby food-fed babies (see Chapter 12 on Allergies).[8, 9,10]
6. Breast-fed babies have decreased susceptibility to infections of all kinds. Mother's milk supplies antibodies which help to fight infections.[11, 12]
7. Breast feeding can help prevent the possibility of breast cancer in the mother. Statistics show that

women who have never breast-fed, are more likely to get breast cancer (see Chapter 25 on Breast Cancer). [12, 13, 14]

8. Breast feeding is a natural method of spacing babies. An extensive study shows that mothers who fed their babies artificially were about twice as likely to get pregnant again before the baby was nine months old. [2]

9. Breast feeding prevents overfeeding and consequent infant obesity, the cause of a constant obesity problem as the child grows up, as well as many other health problems. Artificial feeding is the main cause of infant obesity (see Chapter 15). [15, 16]

10. Breast feeding reduces infant mortality. The World Health Organization claims that the new vogue of artificial feeding is one of the reasons for such a high infant mortality rate in the developing world. [17]

11. Babies who are fed entirely on breast milk don't get constipated, as formula-fed babies frequently do. [2] Breast milk does not solidify in the intestinal tract as does cow's milk.

12. Breast milk encourages the growth of desirable, beneficial bacteria in the baby's digestive tract. Formula promotes the growth of less desirable, putrefactive bacteria. [11, 18]

There are other obvious and common-sense reasons why breast feeding is preferable: it is available immediately—the crying baby doesn't have to wait for formula to be warmed; breast milk is always the right temperature; night feedings are much easier; breast milk digests more rapidly because it is raw, natural, and contains its own digestive enzymes; travel is safer and less bothersome if baby is breast-fed.

Breast feeding also helps to build a secure, loving relationship between a child and its mother, which can last throughout the child's entire life. A baby needs the feeling of warmth and security of the mother's body. Both mother and baby feel better physically as well as emotionally if the baby is breast-fed. Because of the inherent, deep-seated instinct, the mother who feeds her baby artificially may feel a certain degree of guilt for abandonment of her obligation and responsibility towards her baby, which may develop into even stronger feelings of guilt and remorse if the child later suffers from health problems and/or is mentally or physically handicapped.

Why formulas and baby foods are harmful

In order to understand why feeding a newborn baby artificial formulas, based on cow's milk, is harmful, you must know a little about the physiology and the chemistry of the infant digestive system.

When the baby is born, the little gastrointestinal tract and digestive system are still in the process of development and are not yet ready to undertake the difficult and complex task of liquifying and digesting foods. The salivary secretion in the mouth will not begin for a number of weeks. The starch-digesting enzyme, *ptyalin*, is found in salivary secretions. This enzyme will not be present in a newborn child in any appreciable quantities for at least six months. Another starch-digesting enzyme, which is secreted by the pancreas, is also not present in sufficient amounts of digest starch. Amylase generally does not appear until the eruption of the molar teeth, possibly not before 28 to 36 months.[19] The first teeth appear at the age of five to six months.

All the above facts suggest that: 1) the baby is not physiologically prepared for mastication and consequently should not be fed any solid foods for at least six months; 2) that the baby's digestive system is not equipped to efficiently digest foods rich in starch, such as cereals, until maybe one year or even longer, and, therefore, he should not be fed starchy foods for at least that long.

Despite these physiological facts, cereals are the first food usually prescribed by the pediatrician, and as early as four to six weeks after birth. Feeding young infants foods that they cannot digest is a main cause of allergies.[10] The arguments that feeding the young baby cereals, strained vegetables, ground meats, pureed fruits, and other solid, or semi-solid cooked and canned foods will enhance their growth and accelerate the anatomical and physiological development of the infant's digestive tract, are not supported by any valid evidence or studies.[20] In the opinion of Dr. L.F. Hill, a leading expert on infant nutrition, the early introduction of solid foods into the infant diet "is the result of empiricism and competition, not of sound nutritional principles. It is attended by certain dangers, which are not compensated for by any discernible advantages."[21]

Not only is the baby unable to digest the starches and proteins in all these cereals and baby foods, but they contain salt, sugar, fillers, and other chemicals that young babies do not need and which are detrimental to them.

Besides that, the early feeding of solid or semi-solid foods and concentrated formulas contribute to the development of obesity in infants.[22] Bottled formulas supply much more calcium, protein, and calories than the beast-fed baby receives. There is evidence that the number of fat cells in children is determined very early in life and that the tendency towards obesity can persist from infancy and childhood into adult life.[23] Infant obesity also may be linked to the greater incidence of degenerative diseases later in life.[24] (See Chapter 15 on Infant Obesity.)

Milk, fat, and milk-sugar digestants

By studying the infant digestive system, we find that during the first year of the baby's life, he can only efficiently digest proteins, fats, minerals, and lactose—the food elements present in mother's milk.

The baby's stomach secretions contain **pepsin**, a proteolytic enzyme, and **hydrochloric acid**, both of which are effective protein and mineral digestants. In the baby's pancreatic secretions, there are other enzymes: protein-digesting **trypsin**, and the fat-digesting enzyme, **steapsin**. The only carbohydrate that baby can digest easily is the milk sugar, or lactose, with the help of the enzyme **lactase**, which is present in the baby's small intestine.

Apparently nature intended the young humans to subsist primarily on the milk protein, minerals, sugars, and fat, since all the enzymes necessary to facilitate their digestion are found in considerable amounts in the stomach of the newborn infant. And so, our ancestors, as far back as records or indications exist, fed their babies nothing but breast milk for as long as one or two years, sometimes even longer. These "primitive" mothers displayed an incredible degree of instinctual wisdom (and do so now in some cultures) when they wished to feed their babies other food than breast milk: they first masticated and salivated it thoroughly in their own mouths (and saturated it with their own digestive enzymes!) and then passed it directly to their infant!

But, you may now wonder, if a baby can digest milk so well, why not feed him cow's milk? Here's why.

Mother's milk vs. cow's milk

The main ingredient in most baby formulas is cow's milk. Although in appearance mother's milk and cow's milk are much alike, their nutritional composition is very different.

Let's take the *protein* first. Cow's milk contains almost three times as much protein as mother's milk. This is, of course, motivated by the physiological need: the calf is much larger, and it doubles its birth weight in fifty days, while the human baby does so in one hundred days.

The difference in protein quality

Also, there is a significant difference in the *quality* of protein. The protein of cow's milk is 85 percent casein, and 15 percent whey protein (lactalbumin and lactoglobulin). In human milk, casein constitutes only 40 percent, 60 percent being the whey fraction. Whey proteins are water soluble and are easier to digest than casein protein. Casein forms hard, rubbery curds in the stomach, which are poorly digested,[1] since it is not readily attacked by digestive enzymes. The undigested protein may be the cause of malnutrition, diarrhea, or hard stools for the infant. We must remember that the infant calf, for whom nature has designed cow's milk, has four stomachs which contain the powerful digestive bacteria and the casein-curdling enzyme, rennin, neither of which are found in the human stomach.[25]

The amino acid composition of cow's milk and human milk is different. Human milk provides more cystine, a sulfur-containing amino acid. This is significant because sulfur and nitrogen retention are vital for effective protein assimilation. Perhaps this is one of the reasons why almost 100 percent of the protein in breast milk is effectively used by the infant, but only 50 percent of the protein in cow's milk is used. Of the remaining 50 percent, some is digested, but not utilized, and is excreted in urine. This causes undue stress on the little kidneys.

The difference in fat quality

The *fat* differences between human and cow's milk are significant. Although both milks contain about 4 percent fat, the cow's milk contains much more (10 percent against 1.4 percent in human milk) of the short-chain fatty acids and relatively few of the long-chain fatty acids, which are more easily digested.[26] While the calf's digestive system is equipped with the ability to alter these coarser short-chain fatty acids, the baby's digestive system is not. And the excess of poorly-digested fats may be responsible for some infant diarrhea and other digestive problems.[27]

Mother's milk contains approximately 7 percent linoleic acid, one of the most important of the unsaturated fatty acids, while cow's milk contains only 3 percent. Studies have shown that infants receiving linoleic acid need fewer calories to maintain the same weight gains as infants who do not get linoleic acid. Also, such conditions as eczema, diarrhea, diaper rash, and high blood cholesterol have been corrected when sufficient unsaturated acids were given.[19] The commercial baby formulas often contain coconut oil, which is 70 percent *saturated* fatty acid!

Extensive studies have shown that fats in human milk

are absorbed very easily by the baby, while fats in cow's milk, even when it is homogenized to break down the large fat globules, are digested only with great difficulty.[28] Goat's milk is more like human milk in this regard, since it contains smaller, more easily-emulsified fat globules.

The difference in carbohydrates

The *carbohydrate* difference between cow's milk and human milk is just as great. Mother's milk contains almost twice as much lactose (milk sugar) as cow's milk. Not only is the proportion larger, but the property of the lactose is different. Cow's milk lactose, which is largely alpha-lactose, is unable to maintain or support the life of *Bacillus bifidus* flora. The presence and support of this bacteria population in the intestines of the baby is very important as these friendly bacteria not only inhibit the presence of less desirable, pathogenic (disease-producing) bacteria, but also help to produce B-vitamins and important lactic acid.

During the process of digestion, lactose breaks up into two other forms of sugar: *glucose* and *galactose.* Galactose is vital, among its other functions, for the development of the myelin sheaths, or the coating around the nerves. Keep in mind what I said earlier: many of the baby's vital organs are not fully developed at birth—they continue to grow and develop in early infancy. The myelination of the nerves begins as soon as the child obtains lactose from the mother's milk and the process continues for several months after birth.

Therefore, feeding the young infant sucrose, dextrose, maltose, honey, molasses, or any other form of sugar during early infancy is one of the most harmful nutritional practices I can think of. Yet, many commercial baby formulas and baby foods contain these various forms of sugar. I have a strong suspicion that this perverted practice—feeding baby the forms of sugar other than lactose—is a contributing factor in the catastrophic increase in mental and nervous breakdowns in adults, as well as multiple sclerosis.

The difference in vitamins

Human milk has ten to twenty times more vitamin E than cow's milk. Artificial formulas are, therefore, fortified with some additional vitamin E, but it is usually totally destroyed by iron, which is also added to the formula. Supplementary iron, as we have seen before, is a vitamin E antagonist, and destroys it if consumed at the same time. The matter is aggravated by the vegetable oils which are also a usual ingredient in baby formulas. Unsaturated fats in oil increase the need for vitamin E, while iron destroys it. What a vicious cycle! A perfect example that it doesn't matter how ingenious the chemists are who design baby formulas, they cannot duplicate mother's milk! Only 0.3 to 0.7 units of vitamin E is supplied in 24 ounces of formula— just a fraction of the amount furnished by breast milk.[29]

Vitamin C, although present in cow's milk in good quantity, is largely destroyed during pasteurization and storage. And since milk in formulas is always old as well as pasteurized, it has very little vitamin C left. B vitamins, as well as enzymes, are also destroyed in the process of pasteurization. Human milk has twice as much vitamin A as cow's milk.

The difference in minerals

Cow's milk contains three to four times more minerals than human milk. This is, of course, nature's provision for the rapid growth of calves, which reach the weight of 400 pounds in six months. Even if cow's milk is diluted with water, its mineral content would still be too high for the trouble-free metabolism of a young human infant.

Intestinal flora

Normally, our intestines contain many kinds of bacteria which help in breaking down of foods and also manufacture many of the vitamins of the B-complex. As soon as the baby is born, through exposure to a diversity of bacteria in the environment, a rapid colonization of the intestines begins. The kinds of bacteria that establish themselves there will have a tremendous importance on the infant's immediate health, as well as on his life-time health. The difference in the intestinal flora in breast-fed and bottle-fed infants is enormous. With breast feeding, most of the intestinal bacteria (99 percent) consist of beneficial *Lactobacillus bifidus*. The number of undesirable, putrefactive bacteria is very low, or even absent in these infants. Their stools have a low pH, high redox value, and an unoffensive odor. Bottle-fed infants, in contrast, have mostly undesirable intestinal flora composed of many Gram-negative anaerobes such as *Bacteroides*. The number of putrefactive bacteria is much larger, the pH is high, and the odor of the stool offensive.[30]

The most remarkable thing is that the difference in intestinal flora, established in early infancy by the mode of feeding, can persist for as long as thirty years. One can examine the stool of any person up to the age of thirty years and tell, by the presence or absence of certain essential bacteria, whether or not that person was breast-fed as an infant.

Protection against infections

Breast-fed babies have an increased protection against infections of all kinds. There are many factors related to that, one being the more favorable intestinal flora just mentioned. A large quantity of the beneficial *Lactobacillus bifidus* in the alimentary canal in combination with lowered pH, provide unfavorable conditions for the growth of *E.coli.*

However, the most important factor is that mother's milk contains antibodies and immunity factors, that are transferred to the infant through breast feeding. First, the fetus receives through the placenta IgG antibodies before birth. Then IgA antibodies are obtained from the ingested colostrum. IgA antibodies are eventually produced within the human body by the cells of *lamina propria*, but before this is possible, the infant is protected by antibodies received through colostrum and mother's milk. The amount of IgA antibodies in colostrum is highest immediately after delivery and gradually decreases for the next five days.

This is one of the reasons why the baby should be given colostrum as soon as possible after birth and nursed with it all the time until milk appears.

Staphylococcus infections are responsible for up to 80 percent of gastroenteritis in children before the age of four months. *E. coli* infections are other common causes. Colostrum contains specific IgA antibodies and bactericidal factors against *Staphylococcus* as well as against pathogenic strains of *E. coli*.[11]

The other factor thought to have an anti-microbial effect upon E. coli bacteria is *lactoferrin*, a protein-bound iron which is also found in mother's milk. Cow's milk contains less lactoferrin than human milk.[31]

The choice is clear

In the light of the scientific evidence presented above, and a huge amount of individual experiences that are available in massive literature on the subject, it can be logically concluded that anyone who believes or claims that artificial formula is as good as breast milk for baby feeding has not studied the facts.

Breast feeding is a simple, natural, normal function and assures optimal infant nutrition. Mothers have happily nursed their babies through the ages. It is not more complicated, and is just as right, today. All that is needed is a little common sense and letting your instincts and e-motions override the sales pitch by the baby-food and baby-formula manufacturers.

A mother's emotional attachment to her baby is strengthened through breast feeding and this helps build a base for a long and loving relationship. The baby needs the feel of warmth and security of his mother's bosom. Especially in the first few hours after the birth, when the mother can hold her baby, breast feeding is a powerful, pleasant process of mutual interaction between mother and child. When the baby sucks at the breast, sensory impulses cause the release of the pituitary hormone, *oxytocin*, which helps the uterus contract and return to normal.

Finally, if nothing else is convincing enough so far,

perhaps the final argument—the pocketbook—will tip the scales. Medical costs are usually ten times greater for bottle-fed babies than for those who are breast-fed.[32] Not to mention the fact that breast milk is free, while artificial formulas can be rather expensive.

Any way you look at it: *breast feeding is better for the baby, better for the mother, and better for the entire family!*

How long to nurse?

If breast milk is plentiful, nurse for at least one year, preferably eighteen months. In some cultures, babies are breast-fed even longer. Obviously, this is *in addition* to solid foods, which are usually given as soon as the baby can chew. If the mother is well-nourished, her milk will be both plentiful and adequately nutritious to sustain the baby for at least a year. If, for any reason, she does not have enough milk, or if she is not able to continue breast feeding for some other reason, *she should breast feed her baby for as long as humanly possible*. One week is better than none; one month is better than one week; three months is better still.

If milk supply is low

Optimum nutrition, as described in Chapters 3 and 4, plus special supplements which help increase milk production—brewer's yeast, green vegetable juices, alfalfa tablets, vitamins, and minerals—will help produce all the milk your baby needs. Even so, almost every mother will occasionally feel that she is emptied by a hungry baby. The main causes for this are too much stress, lack of sleep, and excessive worries. Adequate rest and sleep are necessary for the manufacture of B vitamins in the system, and B vitamins control milk production to a great extent. If the milk supply lessens temporarily, do not become alarmed and rush for a bottle to supplement your own milk. Listening to your hungry baby cry is the most effective milk-production stimulant known! Brewer's yeast is the next best! Also, drinking plenty of liquids is very important.

You should drink at least eight to twelve glasses of various liquids a day: water, juices, vegetable broths, herb teas, etc., especially during the hot weather.

Most mothers are aware of the importance of the prenatal diet. They feel their baby growing in their bosom and are lovingly conscientious about the extra nutrients the growing fetus needs. However, once the baby is born, mothers often forget that after his birth, the infant's growth is still, if not more so, dependent on *her* nutrition. The breast milk production requires about 1,000 to 1,500 extra calories per day. Thus, for the mother's own maintenance and the adequate milk supply for her baby, she has to almost double her caloric intake.

Furthermore, it is now more important than ever to see that the diet does not contain empty calories from such nutritionless foods as white sugar and white flour products and an excess of fats and fatty foods. A lactating mother needs about 70 - 80 grams of high-quality proteins a day. This can easily be obtained from the Optimum Diet as recommended for the mother-to-be in Chapters 3 and 4. Brewer's yeast, of course, is an excellent milk-producing food, and also a superior source of high-quality protein. Cottage cheese, especially homemade (see Recipes & Directions), is a good way to make sure you get enough protein. One half cup of uncreamed cottage cheese will supply almost 20 grams of protein. Cheese and fresh milk are also excellent sources of calcium, which a lactating mother needs in abundance. Almonds and sesame seeds are other excellent sources of calcium. So is carrot juice. Many nursing mothers have a negative calcium balance, but only 1 quart of raw, certified milk, fortified with 1 tsp. of calcium lactate powder, taken daily, will give all the calcium a lactating mother may need—this is, of course, in addition to the Optimum Diet. Lots of calcium-rich vegetables also should be eaten each day: dark leafy vegetables, such as turnip, dandelion, and collard greens, endive, watercress, broccoli, brussel sprouts. (Note that onions, garlic, and vegetables from the cabbage family, eaten by the nursing mother, may cause gas in some babies.)

And, don't forget vitamin D. It is needed so that calcium can be effectively assimilated from the foods and also to have an adequate amount of this important vitamin in breast milk. Frequent sunbathing is the best source of vitamin D; also take cod liver oil regularly.

The herbs that help to promote the flow of milk are: oat straw, alfalfa, fennel seed, caraway, borage seed and leaves, rosemary, milkworth, and blessed thistle. Use them as herb teas. (See more on herbs during pregnancy and lactation in Questions & Answers.)

Even if you are temporarily ill (unless the illness has directly involved the mammary glands) do not deprive the baby of breast milk. The baby will not be infected by your milk, but could possibly be infected by an airborn bacteria or virus—wear a mask if you wish.

When not to breast-feed

There may be times when it might be inadvisable to nurse. A mother's serious illness or grossly inadequate diet, could affect the quantity and quality of her milk. Obviously, an experienced doctor, that has a positive attitude towards breastfeeding, must be consulted in such cases, and his advise followed.

How often to nurse

There are many theories about how often to nurse a baby, and each pediatrician adheres to his own. Some advise to feed the baby at certain intervals, and, even if the baby seems to be hungry and cries for food, he must wait until the scheduled time.

The only method of feeding a baby that makes sense to me is *demand feeding*, that is nursing the baby when he cries to be fed, or shows other signs of being hungry. Between meals, a baby should be allowed to sleep or play as long as he wishes. During the feeding, let him take as much milk as he wants, but do not urge him to take one more swallow than he wants. The meal should last about twenty minutes, ten minutes at each breast, and if the mother's milk supply is plentiful and the baby is healthy, this should be sufficient to satisfy him.

Usually, breast-fed babies prefer a 2 to 3 hour span between feedings. Bottle-fed babies can have longer intervals, but this is because mother's milk is digested more rapidly and easily than cow's milk (formula).

This type of demand feeding is based on the belief that the baby knows best how much and when he needs food, and will satisfy his own needs. Demand feeding will make life easier and more comfortable both for mother and baby than will a rigid schedule. Also, if a nursing baby receives a feeding when he cries for it, he will soon establish in his mind the assurance that he is in the hands of someone who loves him and cares about his needs.

Problem of oversupply

What if your baby is satisfied but there is plenty of milk left? If your breasts are consistently incompletely emptied it may cause an early decline in milk production. If you are one of those who consistently has too much milk, it may be necessary to express the excess milk by hand by gently compressing breasts toward the nipple. A breast pump may be considered. This extra milk should be frozen for later use if the necessity should arise.

What if nursing is impossible?

If, for some unavoidable reason, the baby cannot be nursed, the only recourse will be substitute nursing. By far the best substitute is a "wet nurse." A wet nurse is a woman who has given birth and has a plentiful supply of milk, but for some reason or another, has no baby to nurse. In "less developed" cultures, wet nurses are almost always available, and mothers who cannot nurse their babies themselves make heroic efforts to acquire a wet nurse— often bringing her from long distances. Here's a new area of activity for the La Leche League: contact service for available wet nurses!

If a wet nurse cannot be found, the only recourse left is

bottle feeding. Do not use any of the available commercially-sold, ready-made, powdered or canned formulas. They are all undesirable for one reason or another. They are all cooked, pasteurized, or heated; they contain the wrong type of sugar; they contain synthetic types of vitamins or the wrong type of iron; they contain too much vegetable oil; metal or plastic containers may leave toxic residues in the formula; etc., etc.

Here are a few simple homemade formulas for bottle feeding.

Formula Number One

Find a safe source of certified raw goat's milk. Dilute with pure bottled spring water in the amount specified by your doctor, depending on the age of your baby. Usually, goat's milk is diluted 2/3 milk to 1/3 water. Add milk sugar (lactose) to sweeten to about the same taste as mother's milk—about 3 tbsp. to each quart of formula. Milk sugar is sold in drug stores without a prescription. If the baby is over three months of age, a small amount of black strap molasses and brewer's yeast powder may be added to the above (½ tsp. each per quart).

Formula Number Two

The same as Formula Number One, but made with **certified raw cow's milk**, if safe goat's milk is not available. Dilute cow's milk with bottled spring water, half and half. Sweeten with 3 tbsp. milk sugar per quart of formula. Never use pasteurized and/or homogenized milk for baby formula. Homogenization breaks up the cream globules into tiny particles which then permits an enzyme in the cream, xanthine oxidase (XO), to enter the blood stream through the intestinal wall instead of being excreted from the body. XO damages the tissues of the arteries and heart, and the body reacts by raising the cholesterol level of the blood. Pasteurization damages the quality of proteins, fat, and minerals in milk, and destroys vitamins. Calves thrive on raw cow's milk, but get very sickly if fed pasteurized milk from their own mother. This should tell us something.

Formula Number Three

This is a milk-free formula. Frequently, infants are allergic to milk or cannot do well on it for some reason. This is a vegetable broth formula, which is nutritious and satisfying. However, it is not recommended for long-term bottle feeding, but rather for an occasional or supplementary use.

Take 1 medium carrot, 2 medium potatoes, ½ small beet, 2 stalks celery, 1 medium zucchini, 3 large stems parsley (or other greens, such as comfrey).

Chop and place in a large pot with about 4 cups of bottled spring water. Cover and bring to a boil. Lower heat, and simmer for 20 - 30 minutes. Strain vegetables out, add three tablespoons milk sugar (lactose). Take 1 oz. raw almonds and 1 oz. sesame seeds. Grind them fine in a seed grinder. Then pour vegetable broth in a blender and add the ground seeds. Blend at high speed for 1 - 3 minutes and liquify well. Strain through fine cloth. Refrigerate immediately. Shake well and heat to body temperature before feeding. This recipe will yield approximately 18 - 20 ounces, enough for a day's feeding.

Formula Number Four

1 cup full-fat soy flour or powder

4 cups water (pure bottled spring water)

3 tbsp. lactose

1 tbsp. vegetable oil (preferably virgin cold-pressed olive oil)

1 tbsp. brewer's yeast; or nutritional yeast, if baby prefers the taste

¼ tsp. calcium lactate powder

⅛ tsp. magnesium oxide powder

½ tablet of kelp or equivalent in powder

Mix soy flour in 4 cups of water and boil for 20 minutes. Cool and mix with other ingredients in blender. Bottle and store in refrigerator.

When soy formula is given, the infant should receive these additional supplements daily:

ascorbic acid—50 mg., in liquid form

cod liver oil—¼ to 1 tsp., depending on age
vitamin E—30 I.U.

If the baby is given goat's or cow's milk formulas
(Formula Number One or Formula Number Two), he
should receive 1 tsp. of vegetable oil a day, such as sesame
oil or olive oil, in addition to the regular infant supplements recommended in Chapter 9.

OTHER HELPFUL HINTS ON BABY FEEDING

Formula between breast feedings

Some pediatricians offer a "compromise" advice to
mothers who express a desire to nurse: formula feeding
intermittent with breast feedings. This is not only unnecessary, but will invariably lead to an early decline in
milk production. Breast milk contains *all* the nutrition
your baby may need, and, with frequent nursing, *on demand*, your milk will take care of the baby's needs. Also,
easier sucking from the bottle may make the baby lose
interest in breast feeding.

One or two breasts?

Each time you nurse your baby, do so from both
breasts. The average length of time is five to ten minutes
on each side. Some mothers let one breast be emptied
completely first, then move the baby to the other breast,
which often will be left half full if milk is plentiful. In such
a case, begin next feeding from the last-used side first, and
so on.

Getting started

Sometimes, a big breast presses against the baby's
nose and interferes with his breathing. With your hand,
gently press the breast away from the nipple. This will
help the baby to suck on it without disturbance. Just place
the nipple next to the baby's mouth and he will do the rest.

Breast engorgement

Shorter, more frequent feedings will help relieve engorgement and will also be easier on the nipples, which are sometimes sore during the early weeks of nursing.

Burping

Both bottle-fed and breast-fed babies usually need burping, although some breast-fed babies need burping only in the early months. When you switch from one breast to the other, or when the baby is through with nursing, try a little gentle patting on his back, holding him in upright position leaning over your shoulder. If the baby falls a-sleep at the breast, don't bother burping him, just lay him down on his side or tummy.

Does baby need water?

A baby who is fed exclusively with breast milk does usually not need extra water, not even in hot weather. If there are plenty of wet diapers, your baby is getting enough fluids. If the weather is extremely hot and diapers remain dry for too long, you may give, by spoon, pure bottled spring water, warmed to body temperature and sweetened a little with milk sugar.

Is baby getting enough?

Mothers constantly worry if their baby is getting enough food. Don't worry. Again, if there are plenty of wet diapers, your baby is getting enough food. But your friend's baby the same age is bigger! So what? Babies come in different sizes, and grow at different speeds. Weight loss after birth is different, and some babies take three weeks to regain their birth weight, while others only one, or not even that. If your baby is gaining about a pound a month, it is an acceptable gain. So, don't worry! Besides, bigger, fatter babies are not necessarily health-ier—quite the contrary! Overfeeding may lead to the development of a tendency to be obese throughout adult life. The fat cells that we build during the first few months will be there, waiting to be filled, throughout life. Your friend's pudgy baby may be a candidate for a life-long weight problem.

Is your baby constipated?

Breast-fed babies do not get constipated, as bottle-fed babies usually do. Some babies may have as many as five or six bowel movements a day; some only one every three, four, or even six days. This is all normal, and no cause for worry. The stool can vary in color, and is usually quite loose. (See Chapter 21 regarding infant diarrhea and constipation.)

Can you diet or fast while nursing?

The answer is an emphatic "NO". Not only the milk supply may drastically decline during the diet, but—what is worse—during dieting or fasting poisons stored in the fatty tissues of the body, such as DDT, for example, as well as other systemic and metabolic toxins, may be released into the blood stream and then excreted from the mother's system via the breast milk, poisoning the infant. Therefore, if you are overweight and wish to go on a reducing diet, you must wait until you finish nursing your baby.

Can you spoil your baby?

No. Little babies of nursing age cannot be spoiled by over-attention and "over-babying." Little babies *need* all the loving, "babying," fussing over, cuddling, and comforting they can get, especially during the early weeks of their life. Tender Loving Care (TLC) is your baby's most important need. Your warmth and closeness which the baby experienced before birth must not be cut off abruptly, but continued for as long as possible after the birth.

You can never pay too much attention to an infant. Someone said: "If you baby babies when they are babies, you won't have to baby them when they are adults." A baby who gets lots of attention will grow into a self-reliant and independent adult. "Babying"—a maximum of loving, attention, cuddling, playing, etc.—will be helping the baby to develop a strong image of himself and gives a sense of security at the age when a sense of selfhood is too tender and immature.

Should a baby's cries be ignored?

Again, some infant-care books advise to leave your baby alone in a closed room and let him cry, until his scheduled feeding time has come, or until he wears himself out and falls asleep. Sometimes a compassionate mother is in another room, crying herself, wanting desperately to put her crying baby to her bosom and comfort him, but she is afraid to act against the advice of the "baby-care expert." I would not be surprised if much of children's and adolescents' problems today—drug abuse, crime, irresponsibility, sexual promiscuity, extreme sense of insecurity as expressed in disregard of authorities, whether it is parents, teachers, or police—are caused by the de-humanized scientific raising of children according to the child-rearing experts' books that advised not to spoil babies.

No, baby's cries should *not* be ignored. Crying is the only way your baby can communicate. A crying baby is trying to tell you something: "I'm hungry," "I'm lonely," "I'm wet, or hot, or cold," "I'm sad," "I'm tired and I want to sleep, but I won't because I'm angry because I'm ignored!"

Don't let babies cry so they can "develop their lungs." They can develop their lungs later when they take up running. Find out why the baby is crying, change his diaper, nurse him even though he was nursed recently, cuddle and pet him, comfort him, speak to him and look at him lovingly, assure him of your love and concern, rock him gently. And, see, a miracle has happened—your baby has stopped crying! He is happy!

What: rocking a baby?

Yes, why not? Babies have experienced constant motion in the womb, and it will take awhile before they become accustomed to the still, motionless existence outside. Most mothers have a natural, instinctive desire to rock a crying baby and they have found that the baby feels happy and comforted by such treatment. Gentle rocking has a calming, reassuring effect on the baby. Mothers who

have read baby-care books and were convinced that rocking is a no-no, still have found that the best way to comfort
a crying baby is to hold him right to the bosom and walk,
briskly pacing the room, which, of course, gives the baby
the reassuring, rocking motion.

Naturally, violent, quick swinging or shaking should
be avoided; it may scare the baby. But gentle rocking,
either in mother's or father's arms, in the baby's cradle, or
in a rocking chair, is perfectly alright. Ask your grandmother! She will know. And, believe me, she is a much
more reliable and experienced expert on baby rearing than
most writers of child-care manuals are.

Family sleeping

Should your baby sleep in a separate bed or crib in a
separate room? Should the newborn sleep in the same bed
with his mother?

Although in our society co-family sleeping is taboo, in
other cultures it was always practiced, and is practiced
now. It is true that in most primitive countries, they don't
have "another room," or even another bed. Then again,
maybe this was a more natural way to raise contented,
serene children. Young children have a strong need to be
close to their parents. Shoving them away to a separate,
closed room can damage them emotionally and lead to
insecurities and phobias. Babies are not little mechanisms
that can grow and function on their own as long as they
recieve adequate nutrition. When grown to adulthood, their
total personality will have been greatly affected by the
amount of love, warmth, and security they received while
babies.

There is nothing wrong in letting a little baby sleep in
your bed, provided it is spacious enough. The baby will
appreciate such closeness and warmth. It is also so much
easier on a nursing mother—no need to get up at night—
just move the baby to her breast and feed him.

If sleeping in the same bed is impractical, or just too
contrary to your present beliefs, a baby crib should be kept
in the same bedroom, close to your own bed, so that you

can look, talk, smile, or reach out and comfort the baby, if needed, right from your own bed.

Finally...

The most important thing for successful breast feeding is having confidence in yourself. Don't be surprised if somewhere along the line you will make a few mistakes. Most mothers do, no matter how many baby-care books they read. Trust your motherly instincts more than anything else. If you show lots of love to your baby, he'll forgive your mistakes! As time goes by, your knowledge and confidence will grow, you'll feel more competent and efficient, and you will take more and more pride and pleasure in nursing your baby—realizing that by breast feeding him you are building a bond of security and loving relationship between you and your child which can last for his entire life.

SUGGESTED READING ON INFANT FEEDING

1. *The Womanly Art of Breastfeeding*, La Leche League International, 23rd edition, 1977, Franklin Park, Illinois.

2. *Breastfeeding and Natural Child Spacing*, by Sheila K. Kippley, P.O. Box 11084, Cincinnati, Ohio.

3. *Please Breast-Feed Your Baby*, by Alice Gerard, New American Library, 1970, New York, N.Y.

4. *Management of Successful Lactation*, Child and Family Booklet, Box 508, Oak Park, Ill., 1972.

5. *The Family Book of Child Care*, by Niles Newton, Harper & Row, New York, N.Y., 1957.

6. *Nursing Your Baby*, by Karen Pryor, Pocket Books, Simon & Schuster, New York, N.Y., 6th Printing, 1974.

7. *White Paper on Infant Feeding Practices*, Center for Science in the Public Interest, Washington, D.C., 1974.

8. *The Grandmother Conspiracy Exposed*, by Lewis A. Coffin, M.D., Capra Press, Santa Barbara, 1974.

9. *The Tender Gift:* Breastfeeding, by Dana Raphael, Schocken Books, New York, N.Y., 1976.

10. *Abreast of the Times*, by R.M. Applebaum, M.D., LLL, Franklin Park, Ill., 1969.

11. *Breast Feeding*, by M.P. Warner, M.D., Budlong Press Co., Chicago, Ill., 1975.

12. *Natural Rearing of Children,* by Juliette de Bairaéli-Levy, Arco Publishing Co., New York, N.Y.

An excellent source of reliable, authoritative information on breast feeding is:

La Leche League, International, Inc., P.O. Box 1209 Franklin Park, Ill. 60131-8209.

Write for their catalogs and reprints.

8

Solid Foods: When, What Kind, How Much

As you have seen from the massive scientific evidence presented in the previous chapter, human milk is, unquestionably, the best nutrition for infants. Mother's milk is superior to any of the "scientifically"-concocted artificial formulas ever devised. Mother's milk provides *optimal* infant nutrition. It contains *everything* that the infant needs for its sustenance, growth, and development.

But, mother's milk was meant to be the ideal food only until the infant matures to the point where he should begin to eat solid foods. The question is: when *is* the proper time to begin introducing solid foods to an infant?

During the last fifty years, there has been a growing tendency to give babies solid foods at an increasingly earlier age, even as early as during the first two weeks of life. Efforts have been made to scientifically justify the early introduction of solid foods in infant nutrition, but no one has been able to prove that this practice has any nutritional or medical advantages. Quite the contrary! More and more pediatric experts are beginning to realize that an early introduction of solid or semi-solid foods is extremely dangerous and can lead to a host of health problems for the child, even for a lifetime.

One of the most obvious consequences of early feeding of solid foods, or any kind of foods—even liquid or semi-solid foods—other than mother's milk, is the development of allergies.[1] (see Chapter 12). A baby's digestive system lacks the necessary digestive enzymes for him to properly digest any foods other than mother's milk. He cannot even digest cow's milk effectively. Thus, if fed foods he cannot digest efficiently, the infant's body reacts to them as toxic matter and develops an immunological rejection response. The usual symptoms of such a rejection are gastrointestinal disorders such as colic, or diarrhea, skin rashes or eczema. All foods other than mother's milk can bring mild to severe allergic reactions, but the most common allergens are cow's milk and milk products, eggs, chicken, citrus fruit or juices, tomatoes, soya products, corn, rye, oats, and wheat in all forms. Studies show that most cases of infant allergy develop in the early months of life. If babies are breast-fed exclusively for at least 6 months, the incidence of allergy is reduced to zero percent.[2]

As mentioned earlier, the first baby teeth appear at the age of 5-6 months—a clear indication that the infant was not intended to eat solid food before that age.[3] The molars do not appear until the second year.

The early introduction of solid foods will also inevitably decrease the mother's milk supply by decreasing the need. It has been shown consistently that the oftener the breast is emptied, the more milk is produced.[4]

The supposed purpose of an early introduction of solids is to improve the quality of the infant's nutrition. Actually, it accomplishes just the opposite. One of the country's leading pediatric specialists, Dr. L. F. Hill, says that "The addition of solid food in the first few weeks of life may well have the effect, through satiety, of lessening the volume intake of milk. Although the total caloric requirements might be adequately met, the feeding of solid foods nutritionally inferior to milk, at the expense of milk, could result in worsening of the nutritional state of the infant rather than bettering it."[5]

One of the underlying reasons for the current fad of feeding baby solid foods at a very early age is our culturally-motivated desire to have bigger babies. Bigger babies are better babies in the minds of many parents. Overeating and consequent obesity may be characteristic of the parents, and they, perhaps subconsciously, want their babies to be like themselves. They also want their babies to grow "big and strong." A six-feet tall, 200 pound athlete is many mother's dream. Consequently, they try to give a young baby "super-nutrition," as much food as he can take. Such overeating not only results in pudgy, obese babies, but will also damage their health and shorten their life span. The trend towards forcing children to grow bigger and faster may be linked to the increased incidence of degenerative diseases later in life.[6]

Although plump babies may look "cute," especially to their parents and grandparents, infant obesity can have very serious consequences. Not only does it almost always lead to a life-long struggle against excess weight, but also the chances of developing cardiovascular disorders, high blood pressure, diabetes, and heart problems are greatly increased.[6,7]

First three months

During the first 3 months of an infant's life, mother's milk alone is sufficient for optimal infant nutrition. If the mother eats an adequate diet as described in Chapters 3 and 4, her milk will contain all the nutrients the baby needs. No solid or semi-solid foods or juices, canned or fresh, are recommended during the first 3 months.

Three months to six months

Still no solid foods. But, during this period, two vitamin supplements can be added to the infant's breast-milk diet:

1. *Cod liver oil*. When your baby reaches the age of 4 months, give him a few drops of cod liver oil daily. Make sure it is *plain* cod liver oil, not fortified with synthetic vitamins. Start with 1 drop and increase the dosage very gradually, until the baby is getting 5 drops daily by the age of 6 months, ½ teaspoon by the age of 8 months, and 1 teaspoon at 12 months. Cod liver oil will supply your baby with natural vitamins A and D. The best time to give cod liver oil to a breast-fed baby is right after feeding and burping. After weaning, give cod liver oil after breakfast. Make sure the cod liver oil you buy is fresh and not rancid. Buy in small bottles and store in the refrigerator.

2. *Vitamin C*. Even the breast-fed baby can be deficient in vitamin C if the mother's diet doesn't contain sufficient amounts, or if excessive stresses or biochemical and metabolic derangements deplete her regular "allotment" of vitamin C for baby's milk. Therefore, it will be wise to give your baby a small amount of supplemental vitamin C to prevent such a possible deficiency. Vitamin C in small doses is totally harmless, even for little babies.

When your baby is 3 or 4 months old, start giving him about ¼ teaspoon freshly made, strained orange juice, diluted with a spoonful of pure water. You can give it from the tip of a teaspoon, or mixed with water in the bottle. Try to get organically-grown oranges, if possible. They are often sold in natural food stores (see listings in the yellow pages).

If your baby shows an allergic reaction to orange juice (some babies do) you may replace it with a few drops of vitamin C solution for a few weeks, then try juice again, to confirm possible allergy. Since vitamin C in liquid form loses its biological activity rapidly, make your own, fresh vitamin C solution, small quantity at a time. Buy powdered or crystalized vitamin C (ascorbic acid) in your health food store or drug store, or you can use vitamin C tablets, if you can't get it in powdered form. In ¼ cup of warm water, dissolve ½ ounce of powder, or 25 500-milligram tablets. Keep in a brown glass jar (to avoid light) or in a drip bottle, in the refrigerator. This solution will supply approximately 1000 milligrams (1 gram) per teaspoonful, or about 20 milligrams per drop. One or two drops a day is sufficient. In case of any kind of illness, especially infection or colds, you may double or triple the vitamin C dosage.

Remember, orange juice must be freshly made, squeezed from fresh oranges, preferably organically-grown. Never use canned or frozen orange juice. Your baby deserves the best. And fresh orange juice is actually also less expensive.

The best time to give orange juice or vitamin C is *between* nursings—1½ hours before or after breast feeding.

Six months to eight months

Most babies can continue on mother's milk alone during this period and will still get all the nutrition they need. If for some reason you feel—but most importantly, if your baby feels—that an introduction to solid foods should begin, you may do so. Six months is the *earliest* age that foods other than mother's milk should be introduced into the infant's diet. But, always remember that all babies are different. They are individual in their nutritional needs. Only your baby knows which food and how much he wants. When infants are no longer satisfied with breast milk or formula, or demand to be fed with increasing frequency, then they are probably ready for other foods. However, if your baby is happy, growing normally, and seems to be satisfied, it would be wise to postpone introduction of other foods at least until the age of 8 months.

The *number one rule* for introducing new foods to the baby's diet is: start with only *one* food at a time and continue with it for at least 5 days to 1 week. In this way, if the baby cannot handle that particular food well and develops a sore bottom or other negative reaction, you can eliminate this particular food and try another one.

The *number two rule* is to start with juices rather than whole mashed vegetables or fruits. Juices are easier assimilated and better tolerated by the baby—also are more like mother's milk in consistency. At first, give 1 teaspoon of juice diluted with pure bottled water. Increase amounts gradually. Warm both water and juice to room temperature and feed from the tip of a spoon, or from the bottle.

The best juices to start with are carrot, apple, or orange juice. Do not mix fruit and vegetable juices at the same feeding.

After a few weeks of juices, you can begin giving the baby some fruits and vegetables in finely mashed or liquified form. Use your blender to liquify vegetables and fruits, or mash them by hand. Mashed ripe bananas are an excellent food at this time.

As the weeks pass by and the baby's appetite increases

and the digestive system develops and is ready for more solid foods, increase the assortment and quantity of foods. Ripe fruits, berries, and vegetables in season, such as apples, avocados, apricots, peaches, pineapple, pears, blueberries, raspberries, carrots, beets, rutabaga, papaya, melon—anything available. Some foods like avocado, papaya, and melons are spoon-ready—just scrape with a spoon and give to the baby. Others can be mashed, blended, or grated.

However, remember two things: 1) proceed gradually and cautiously, watching for possible negative reactions; 2) if you are still nursing your baby, do not stop! Your own milk is still your baby's most important food. Fruits and vegetables are an *addition to the main diet,* not the other way around.

During this period, continue with vitamin C and cod liver oil supplements. And, please do not use any canned fruit and vegetable purees. They are more expensive, contain sugar, salt, and other additives, and are not even half as nutritious as fresh baby foods you can make so easily in your own kitchen.

Eight months to twelve months

If your own milk production is plentiful, continue nursing as before, with supplements as outlined earlier.

Now you can begin giving your baby lactic acid milks, such as yogurt, or kefir, but only in very small amounts. All milk products must be of the highest quality, preferably made by you from raw, unpasteurized and unhomogenized milk (see Recipes & Directions).

Another important addition to your baby's diet now is brewer's yeast (which, of course, you are taking every day yourself). Start with ¼ teaspoon, added to fruit juice, papaya mash, or yogurt. Increase gradually to 1-2 teaspoons a day by the 12th month. Brewer's yeast is an excellent source of iron, zinc, selenium, chromium, B-complex vitamins, and high-quality proteins [8] —all very important for your baby. Watch for baby's reaction when you start giving him brewer's yeast, since some babies are allergic to it. Do not be tempted to give him large quantities knowing how nutritious it is.

You can also give one tablet of Nature's Minerals. It is a 100 percent natural mineral tablet, providing all of the known minerals and trace elements (see next chapter).

As your infant grows, use less and less water to dilute his food and his juices. You can now give him more orange juice with added vitamin C, and more cod liver oil, reaching 1 teaspoon by the age of 1 year.

Your baby's first birthday

You see, you made it with flying colors—and you were so worried!

If you are not pregnant again, you may continue nursing as long as you have milk and as long as your baby wants it. Many mothers I know have continued nursing until their baby is 18 or more months, then stop by weaning gradually. How do you wean? Simply by feeding the child more and more other foods, cutting back gradually on the number of breast-feedings, until, finally, you are giving him only one feeding a day (before putting him to bed at night); then one every second day—and then stop completely. Give your baby raw, certified goat's milk as a "substitute." Goat's milk should become a part of the child's diet from now on, anyway.

Now you can begin giving some raw seeds and nuts. Grind almonds, sesame seeds, sunflower seeds, or filberts (one kind at a time) in your seed grinder. Mix a little with yogurt or fruit mash. As your child grows, seed or nut butter may be used on slices of banana or apple, or celery stalks, rolled in lettuce leaves, or spread on whole grain bread. Health food stores sell ready-made almond and sesame seed butters (tahini).

When you buy nuts and seeds, as well as oils, make sure they are fresh, not rancid. Rancid seeds or oils can be extremely harmful, especially for very young children.[9] Buy nuts in their shells and crack them. Buy small quantities and store in the refrigerator. When you use shelled sunflower seeds, seperate and throw away all seeds that are dark, black, brown, yellow, or white before you grind them. Rancid seeds and nuts can usually be distinguished by their color, odor, and taste.

After his first birthday, you can introduce some cooked or steamed vegetables, in addition to raw vegetables, into your child's diet. Potatoes, boiled and mashed, are loved by children. They are a very good food, containing large amounts of vitamin C as well as high quality protein which is equal to the protein of milk or eggs in its biological value.

Somewhere between 1½ and 2 years of age, your child can begin eating grains and cereals. Start with oatmeal or millet cereals (see Recipes & Directions). Cook them in a 50-50 mixture of whole milk and water. Begin with small amounts and increase gradually. Use only one cereal at a time, waiting for at least a week before introducing another. This way you can discover any possible allergic reaction.

Other good cereals are buckwheat (see Recipes & Directions), whole rice, and corn mash. You can also start introducing beans, peas, and lentils, in soups or any other favorite manner.

Whole grain breads can also be started at this time. But again, very carefully. Do not overfeed, especially on wheat bread. Wheat is one of the most common allergens and usually the first grain to cause any digestive problem. Of course, if you have followed my program so far, your child most likely will not have any problems with allergies. Buy locally baked whole-grain bread made without oil from freshly-ground flour. It would be even better if you could bake your own. It's not difficult to bake homemade bread. It's even easier with the convenient appliances available today. See recipes and instructions for bread-making in Recipes & Directions.

Feeding pre-schoolers

As soon as your child is able to chew foods effectively, he can begin eating the regular Airola Optimum Diet as described in Chapters 3 and 4, with some special modifications at first.

Do not get discouraged if your child refuses to eat some of the good foods you want him to eat. Be patient.

Children must learn good eating habits. Remember how long it took *you* to learn to eat nutritious foods. The worst thing you can do is to *try to force* him to eat something he doesn't want to eat, or doesn't understand the reasons why he should eat. This is a sure way for your child to develop a dislike for a certain food that can last for his lifetime. Let him *discover* the value and the better taste of nutritious foods on his own. During the meal, when the whole family is seated at the table, let all members, especially children, choose what they like best *from the foods served*. If, of the whole large vegetable salad your child picks only carrot pieces and refuses to eat anything else, that's alright. The next meal maybe it will be celery or zucchini instead of carrot. A child's taste must be developed gradually—and only he knows how and at what speed. You may ask, "If I leave it to him, what if he wants nothing but ice cream?" What ice cream? The secret is: do not have on the table, or in the refrigerator, or in the house, anything that isn't good for your child, or for yourself, for that matter! Also, try to offer a variety of choices. Look at the proposed menu in Chapter 4—there is a great variety to choose from. If your child doesn't seem to like one cereal, try another. Or make buckwheat pancakes, they are just as good as any of the cereals. And, I have never yet seen a child who refused to eat buckwheat or oatmeal pancakes with some honey or homemade applesauce!

When our five children were growing up, I remember that we never had any problems getting them to eat fruits or cereals. As a rule, most children love fresh fruits and berries—any kind, any time. They also love soups, breads, homemade muffins, milk shakes, yogurt, seeds, and nuts. However, one group of foods that we knew was very important for them—fresh vegetables—was received with something less than enthusiasm. A vegetable salad doesn't seem to appeal to kids until they are older, sometimes not until high school age. So, here's what we did. We placed the whole salad, homemade dressing and all, in the blender, added some homemade yogurt or kefir, and blended for 15-30 seconds, beginning with low speed and finishing on high. Then we poured the mixture into a cup or glass and served as a "salad shake." Our children all seemed to prefer their salad in such a semi-liquified form.

If your child is a picky eater, he is not unique—most children are. Your child may not want to eat anything but bread and milk. It's okay; let him enjoy it! Homemade whole grain bread with high-quality raw milk provides excellent nourishment. If not reprimanded or forced, children soon find another favorite—always keep alternatives or choices in sight and available.

Now, here's the ultimate secret of feeding children nutritious foods: set a good example! If children see that their parents and siblings enjoy eating a certain food, they will try it, too—much more readily than if they are just *told* to eat it.

Again, always have good nutritious foods available for your children and let them decide which ones they want to try first. They have instincts, too, you know; don't kill their natural instincts!

Snacks

Children seem to like between-meal snacks. Perhaps snacks—"goodies"—reinforce the sense of love and security between them and their parents. And, of course, they see other children in the neighborhood eating snacks or candies! Don't let this be a problem. Just make your own high-quality, wholesome snacks and consider them to be a part of your child's total daily nutrition.

Here are just a few ideas—but let your creative imagination guide you.

- Halvah (see Recipes & Directions). Make small balls and roll them in raw, hulled sesame seeds.
- Homemade ice cream (see Recipes & Directions).
- Fruit juice popsicle. Make your own juice and freeze on a stick. Wooden sticks are available in the paper goods section in your department store.
- Frozen banana. Cut banana in half and freeze on a stick.
- Popcorn. Pop without any fat, then serve with a little raw butter.

- Homemade oatmeal cookies or corn muffins, sweetened with honey (see Recipes & Directions).
- Dried bananas, apricots, or apples.
- Carob candy, a chocolate-like product (you can make your own or buy it at a health food store).

Health food stores also sell small yogurt cups with natural fruit flavorings, and natural ice cream, sweetened with honey.

Again, if you give your child a good start in life, by nourishing yourself well during pregnancy and feeding him after he is born as I have recommended so far, he will not develop a sweet tooth or be overly interested in "goodies." It is more of a psychological than physiological need.

Warning regarding snacks: Do not reward children's good behavior with sweets or goodies, nor offer them as a solace when they are unhappy—it will create a bad habit which will easily carry over into adulthood.

Forbidden foods

1. *Sugar*. You should never have white sugar in your house. Establishing a taste for sugar in the young child is doing him a great disservice, as this can contribute to the development of serious degenerative diseases not only during childhood, but also in later life.

2. *Supermarket-sold, prepackaged cereals*. Some of them are almost 50 percent sugar. How much better to give your children home-cooked, wholesome, whole-grain cereals!

3. *Carbonated beverages, especially cola drinks*. Not only do they contain large amounts of caffeine, but also sugar, phosphoric acid, and other harmful ingredients.

4. *Coffee or regular tea*. Use wholesome herb teas, instead.

5. *Chocolate*. It prevents absorption of minerals, interferes with calcium metabolism and damages the liver. It also contains too much copper which can contribute to the development of schizophrenia and/or diabetes. Use natural chocolate-like candy made from carob. It tastes just like regular chocolate and is good for your children.

6. *"Regular" candies, cookies, donuts, cakes,*

ice-creams, etc. These are all loaded with sugar and also artificial flavorings and colorings—a sure way to create hyperactive children (see Chapter 14).

7. *Strong seasonings and spices*: salt, white and black pepper, white vinegar, mustard—especially in the diet of very young children, whose tastebuds are sensitive. Anyway, they prefer and enjoy the natural taste of un-seasoned foods. White or black pepper and mustard have no nutritional value and they are very harsh irritants to the delicate linings of the gastrointestinal tract. Salt should be used very sparingly, if at all. Natural, unpro-cessed foods contain all the sodium children may need.

When not to feed

It would be unrealistic to think that your child will always enjoy the best of health and disposition. Little children do get "out of sorts" occasionally: a slight fever, a runny nose, or one of the so-called childhood diseases. These illnesses are not a reflection on the care you give your child, but are due to their first encounters with germs and viruses. In Part II of this book we will deal with some of the most common childhood diseases.

You will notice that among the very first signs that your child is not well is the refusal to eat. *Under no circumstances should you force a sick child to eat if he refuses to*. His natural healing instinct tells him that his body prefers not to have any food at that time. This gives his body a chance to mobilize all its resources and energies for the healing process. Digesting and assimila-ting food requires lots of energy. When health is restored, his appetite will return, and then your child will ask for food. If he has a fever, even a slight one, keep him in bed. If his temperature is 101 degrees (Fahrenheit) or more, and persists, call your doctor to make sure that no serious illness is involved. In the meantime, keep your child in bed, show him lots of love and attention, give him plenty of liquids such as juices, and possibly vegetable broth. Also, give extra vitamin C dissolved in orange juice—the older the child, the more vitamin C (see next Chapter for suggested dosages).

Final words of advice ...

When it comes to infant and child feeding, the most important thing for you, as a mother, is to relax and enjoy your precious child. Don't worry excessively or take things too seriously. Have a sense of humor. Don't become a rigid fanatic! Trust your motherly instincts when you don't know what to do or "the book doesn't mention it." Do the best you know how, and with time you will learn to do better. Strive for a pleasant, enjoyable, happy atmosphere at meal time. Food prepared and served with love is *more* nutritious. I'm serious! Because, it is not what you *eat*, but what you *assimilate* that counts. And your assimilation, as well as your child's, is enhanced if you all *enjoy* the meal, knowing that it is your great love and care for him that moved and motivated you to create it.

Vitamins And Supplements For All Ages

All nutrition experts are in complete agreement that vitamins, minerals, high-quality proteins, carbohydrates, essential fatty acids, enzymes, and trace elements are essential both for the maintenance of good health and the prevention of disease. The disagreement and confusion starts when these experts try to determine how you should obtain all these necessary nutrients and guard yourself against nutritional deficiencies.

The official medical thinking is that a "well-balanced" diet of the four basic food groups will take care of all your nutritional needs. That is, you should get your vitamins "with a knife and fork." The usual story you hear from the average doctor is that vitamin and mineral supplements are a waste of money and absolutely unnecessary, except in cases of indicated deficiencies—and then, of course, the condition must be determined by the doctor and the vitamins prescribed by him.

Unfortunately, even many health writers and lecturers, particularly those who represent some of the strict dietary fads that are so popular today, agree with this official no-vitamin-or-supplement view. They insist that taking vitamins and food supplements is unnatural, and that you can obtain all the vitamins and other nutrients you need from a well-chosen and well-balanced diet of nutritionally sound natural foods. They also claim that the addition of concentrated vitamins and supplements can be detrimental to your health.

But there is another point of view to which an increasing number of the world's most prominent nutritionists and progressive medical researchers are turning. Their contention is that, while under ideal conditions—100 percent natural, poison-free foods and a poison-free environment—you would not need any food supplements at all, under the present conditions, when the available foods are devitalized by unnatural growing methods, refining, processing, and storage, and our environment is polluted, *food supplements are imperative*, if health and vitality are to be maintained.

The poor mother is caught between these contradictory opinions by the experts and is thoroughly confused. Should you and your husband, or should you not, take vitamins and food supplements? Can you get your vitamins with a knife and fork? And isn't this the most natural and sound way to acquire proper nutrition? Also, should you give vitamins and supplements to your children? If so, when, how much, and what kind?

Changed foods and environment

Ideally, you should obtain all your nutrients in needed amounts from the foods you eat, without the addition of any food supplements. A hundred, or even fifty years ago, such advice would have been both sound and workable. Your grandparents ate wholesome foods which were organically grown on their own farms, without the aid of chemical fertilizers. They ate fresh fruits and vegetables from their own gardens, grown without poisonous sprays. They obtained meat, eggs, and dairy products from their own healthy farm animals. They ate no processed or refined foods. The natural unrefined foods your grandparents ate contained more protein, more vitamins, and more minerals than the foods of today, grown on depleted soils and denatured and devitalized by processing and refining. The eggs they ate were fertile eggs, produced by hens that ate worms, bugs, grass, etc. Such eggs had more vitamins, more lecithin, and twice as much unsaturated fatty acids as today's eggs, produced in "egg factories" by chicks that never see the sunlight—or the rooster!—and eat only chemicalized and medicated mash. The grains, the vegetables, the meat, and the dairy products your grandparents ate had a higher protein content, and a higher vitamin and mineral content, and they were free from DDT, hormones, preservatives, insecticides, and other chemicals and drugs, unknown fifty years ago. For example: American wheat grown one hundred years ago contained 18 - 20 percent protein. Today's wheat, grown on depleted soils with the help of powerful artificial fertilizers, contains only 9 - 14 percent protein—only *half* of what it should be! This is true in regard to minerals as well.

Those who today advocate eating regular natural foods as the only source of vitamins and other nutrients, live in a dream world of yesterday. What was yesterday's law is today's folly. It is a sad fact that due to vitamin-, protein-, and enzyme-destroying practices of the food-producing and food-processing industries our *modern-day foods, not only those you buy at your supermarket, but also in your health food store, are nutritionally inferior to the food your grandparents ate two or three generations ago.* Even those so-called organically grown foods are grown in a polluted atmosphere, are watered by polluted water, and contain residues of toxins from fallout, etc. Also, if you buy your organic foods from your health food store, they are probably delivered there from California or Florida, are many days old, and their vitamin content thus dangerously reduced. So it really doesn't matter how well you balance your meals, or if you are a meat-eater, a vegetarian, or a raw-foodist, *you still run a risk of malnutrition if you try to get all your vitamins exclusively from the foods you eat.*

It is medically a well-known fact that even minor deficiencies of one or more of the vital nutritive factors will result in deranged chemistry in the human system, and lower the body's resistance to disease.

Thus, food supplements are necessary as nutritional insurance against disease. Well chosen food supplements are an easy, inexpensive way to improve your diet and assure optimum health for you and your family.

The prime purpose of food supplements is to fill in the nutritional gaps produced by faulty eating habits and by nutritionally-inferior foods. Food supplements will replace in your diet the nutrients missing in food grown on depleted soils, lost in storage, or removed by food processing.

Protective and healing property of vitamins and supplements

There is another good reason to supplement your and your children's diet with an extra supply of vitamins, minerals, and other nutrients. Many of these substances have protective properties against some of today's most toxic environmental factors. They can protect you from the harmful effects of poisonous additives and residues in your food, water, and air. They can also be used as powerful healing agents in the prevention and treatment of most conditions of ill health.

Here are a few examples:

Vitamin C. You need 100 mg. to 200 mg. of vitamin C a day for the maintenance of normal, healthy functions of your body. But when you take the same vitamin in huge doses, we'll say 5,000 to 10,000 mg. a day, it will assume totally different functions and can perform such miracles as:

- Killing pathogenic bacteria, acting as a harmless antibiotic.
- Preventing and curing colds and infections, having a natural anti-histamine activity.
- Effectively neutralizing various toxins and poisons in the system, being a most potent detoxifier.
- Speeding healing processes in virtually every case of ill health.
- Increasing sexual virility.
- Preventing premature aging by strengthening the collagen, and slowing down the degenerative processes.

Vitamin E. For normal, healthy functions of all your organs and glands, you need, perhaps, 100 I.U. of vitamin E a day (the official estimation is only 15 I.U.). But when you take large doses of vitamin E, such as 600 to 1,600 I.U., or even more, it assumes a drug-like role and can perform the following activity:

- It markedly decreases the body's need for oxygen by increasing cell oxygenation.
- It protects against the damaging effects of many environmental poisons in air, water, and food.
- It saves lives in cases of atherosclerotic heart disease by dilating blood vessels and acting as an effective anti-thrombin.
- It prevents scar tissue formation in burns, sores, and post-operative healing.
- It has a dramatic effect on the reproductive organs: prevents miscarriage, increases male and female fertility, and helps to restore male potency.

Vitamin A. The official recommended daily allowance is set at 4,000 U.S.P. Units. But when taken in such large doses as 50,000 U.S.P. Units per day, or even more under doctor's supervision, vitamin A has been known to:

- Cure many stubborn skin disorders.
- Cure chronic infections and eye diseases.
- Increase the body's tolerance to poisons and infections.
- Prevent premature aging, particularly the aging processes of the skin.

Niacin. The official recommended allowance is set at 10 mg. but many doctors around the world have been using large doses of niacin (up to 25,000 mg.) to treat schizophrenia, actually achieving dramatic cures with mega-vitamin therapy.

Vitamins E and B_{15} will protect you against harmful effects of air pollution. As you know, the most injurious substance in polluted air is carbon monoxide. Carbon monoxide induces hypoxia by preventing oxygen from being absorbed by the lungs. Insufficient supply of oxygen to the tissues is considered to be a major cause of our worst diseases. Many scientists (O. Warburg, H. Goldbratt, et al.) believe that a chronic lack of oxygen is responsible for the formation of cancer cells, thus being one of the causes of cancer. Vitamin B_{15}, or pangamic acid, increases the body's resistance to hypoxia, or lack of oxygen, by reducing the body's need for oxygen. And vitamin E increases cell oxygenation by as much as 60 percent. Thus, both vitamins, E and B_{15}, can help to protect you from slow poisoning by carbon monoxide, to which everyone is subjected.

One of the gravest environmental dangers to our health today is universal lead poisoning. Lead is one of the most toxic metals, and even small amounts of it can be fatal. Lead poisoning can cause damaged kidneys and liver; it can affect the nervous system, and even cause insanity. Some researchers believe that lead also can cause multiple sclerosis, interfere with fertility, and cause miscarriages and sexual impotence.

Lead comes into the atmosphere mostly from automobiles which burn gasolines treated with lead. It pollutes the air, settles on soils and on the crops, and is absorbed by vegetables and fruits. In the United States, over 200 million pounds of lead enter the atmosphere from automobile exhaust pipes each year—that's almost one pound per capita! It has been shown that vegetables grown in gardens in a little town in New York State contained over 100 parts per million of lead—this is over 30 times the maximum permitted dose in canned foods. Even organic gardens can not escape this contamination.

It has been demonstrated that such supplements as calcium, vitamin D, vitamin C, thiamin (B_1) vitamin A, potassium, garlic tablets (Kyolic) and algin have a preventive and corrective effect in lead poisoning. These substances can protect you against the toxic effects of lead.

Calcium has also been shown to have a protective property against other toxic substances, for example, mercury and strontium 90, to which we are all subjected in this age of atomic tests. Inexpensive food supplements, such as calcium lactate or bone meal, are good sources of easily assimilable calcium.

In this polluted world of ours, where lethal poisons are lurking everywhere—the air, water, food, clothing, cosmetics, household items, etc.—food supplements are virtually your only available protection against their harmful effects.

Natural vs. synthetic vitamins

Assuming that after reading the presentation in this chapter so far you have become convinced that supplementing your diet with vitamins and food supplements is imperative in this age of a universally toxic environment and nutritionally inferior foods, the next step would be to find out which supplements to take.

There is great controversy in regard to the usefulness of synthetic vitamins. Most drugstore-quality vitamins are made of synthetic chemicals—they are not derivatives of natural food substances. Most vitamins sold in health food stores are concentrations of vitamins extracted from such natural sources as rose hips, green peppers, and acerola (C), brewer's yeast and liver (B), fish liver oil (A and D), kelp (iodine), bone meal (minerals), etc. Most health authorities claim that synthetic vitamins are useless, ineffective, and may be harmful. Most medical doctors and spokesmen for the chemical drug industry claim that "a vitamin is a vitamin is a vitamin," that synthetic vitamins have a molecular chemical structure identical to the so-called natural vitamins, and that they are just as effective in therapeutics. Who is right?

Actually, both sides are partially wrong in their mutual accusations. Some synthetic vitamins, such as a-scorbic acid (vitamin C), irradiated ergosterol (vitamin D), and many synthetic B-vitamins have been successfully used in therapeutic practice, particularly when large doses are required. Of course, there is much research which shows that vitamin C complex *is* more effective than plain ascorbic acid. Bioflavonoids—rutin, citrin, and hesperidin, which always accompany vitamin C in natural foods— being *synergists*, increase the therapeutic effect of vitamin C. But this does not mean that synthetic ascorbic acid is useless. In acute conditions of poisoning or in-fection, ascorbic acid in large doses can be useful, preferably in combination with fresh citrus juices that contain natural bioflavonoids.

Vitamin E is another vitamin that is controversial in this respect. Proponents of natural vitamins advise taking vitamin E rich vegetable oils, particularly wheat germ oil, because natural vitamin E occurs in the form of mixed tocopherols (Alpha, Beta, Gamma, Delta). But Drs. Evan and Wilfred E. Shute, the world's foremost authorities on vitamin E, used only isolated alpha-tocopherol in their large practice and research work. They contend that alpha-tocopherol is *the* active part of the vitamin E complex, and that the other tocopherols are not necessary.

The solution to the controversy, *synthetic vs. natural vitamins*, seems to be that isolated and synthetic vitamins and minerals in large doses have their rightful and indispensable place in the short-term treatment of acute disease and severe deficiency conditions, but those who do not suffer from any specific disease or deficiency, but are interested in food supplements for prophylactic reasons—that is, to protect their health and to prevent disease and premature aging—should use natural vitamins and natural food supplements, such as brewer's yeast, rose hips, fish liver oils, lecithin, wheat germ, bone meal, and kelp, because in these supplements all the nutritive factors are present in their natural, balanced combinations, which is essential for better assimilation and maximum bio-logical effect.

When, what kind, and how much to take

First, you must remember, as stated in Chapter 3, that every individual's nutritional needs are different. We are, biochemically speaking, unique, and our requirements for most nutrients vary considerably. Some persons need up to 4 - 5 times more of certain vitamins than do other people. Also, there is a great difference in every individual's re-sponse to vitamins and other supplementary nutrients, depending on such factors as his or her health condition, age, nutritional stature, special personal needs, the ability to assimilate nutrients, the mineral content of the water one drinks, the degree of the toxicity in the air and environment, and the level of emotional stresses. Due to many physical and mental disorders, vitamins may not be utilized properly. Poor health, diarrhea, the lack of sufficient digestive enzymes, intestinal parasites, infections, gall bladder and liver disorders, mental stresses—these are just a few conditions which interfere with vitamin utilization.

Then, there are countless vitamin antagonists which destroy or interfere with ingested vitamins, such as smoking destroying vitamin C; aspirin and other drugs destroying and increasing the need for vitamin C; alcohol destroying vitamin B; rancid foods destroying vitamin E; chlorinated water destroying vitamin E; laxatives causing deficiencies of vitamins C and B; etc., etc.

Therefore, the following recommendations must be considered only as a very general suggestion of what the "average" person may need in terms of vitamin and food supplements. And, since there are no "average" people, you and your doctor must adjust the suggested doses to fit your or your child's individual and personal needs.

INFANTS AGE 1 to 3 MONTHS

No supplements, if baby is breast-fed exclusively and the nursing mother is healthy.

If the baby is formula-fed with homemade formulas, similar to those described in Chapter 7:

Cod liver oil, plain—¼ tsp. Make sure oil is fresh, not rancid. Buy in small bottles and store in refrigerator.

Fresh orange juice, strained—¼ tsp., or 50 - 100 mg. of vitamin C in liquid form. See Chapter 8 for instructions on how to make vitamin C solution.

INFANTS AGE 3 to 6 MONTHS

If baby is breast-fed:

Cod liver oil, plain—¼ tsp.

Orange juice, strained—¼ tsp. If baby is allergic to

orange juice, as some babies are, give vitamin C
solution, 2 or 3 drops a day.
If baby is formula-fed:
Cod liver oil, plain—½ tsp.
Orange juice, strained—½ tsp., or equivalent in liquid
vitamin C solution.

INFANTS AGE 6 to 12 MONTHS

Cod liver oil—1 tsp.
Orange juice, strained—1 - 2 tsp., or equivalent in
liquid vitamin C.
Brewer's yeast powder with B_{12}—½ - 1 tsp.
Vitamin E, 30 I.U. capsule, mixed tocopherols—1 capsule every second day. Puncture the gelatin capsule
with a pin, and squeeze the content directly into the
baby's mouth.
If the baby is formula-fed, add:
"Nature's Minerals"—1 tablet. Crush tablet and mix
with juice or formula.

CHILDREN AGE 1 to 3 YEARS

Cod liver oil—1 tsp.
Fresh orange juice or grapefruit juice—3 - 4 tbsp.
Vitamin C—100 mg.
Brewer's yeast powder with B_{12}—1 tsp. or 3 tablets.
Vitamin E, mixed tocopherols—30 I.U.
"Nature's Minerals"—2 tablets.

CHILDREN AGE 3 to 6 YEARS

Cod liver oil—2 tsp.
Vitamin C—100 mg.
Vitamin E, mixed tocopherols—30 I.U.
Brewer's yeast powder with B_{12}—2 tsp. or 5 tablets.
"Nature's Minerals"—3 tablets.
Bone meal, raw, unheated—1 tablet.

CHILDREN AGE 6 to 12 YEARS

Cod liver oil—2 tsp.
Vitamin C—200 mg.
Vitamin E, mixed tocopherols—30 I.U.

Brewer's yeast powder, with B_{12}—1 tbsp. or 6 tablets.
"Nature's Minerals"—5 tablets.
Bone meal, raw, unheated—2 tablets.

CHILDREN AGE 12 to 16 YEARS

Vitamins A and D, capsules containing 10,000 Units vitamin A and 400 Units vitamin D, natural, from fish liver oil—1 capsule.
Vitamin C—400 mg.
Vitamin E, mixed tocopherols, 30 I.U.
Brewer's yeast powder, with B_{12}—1 tbsp. or 6 tablets.
Bone meal, raw—2 tablets.
"Nature's Minerals"—6 tablets.

TEENS AGE 16 to 20 YEARS

Vitamins A and D (10,000 A and 400 D per capsule)—1 capsule.
Vitamin C—500 mg.
Vitamin E—100 I.U.
Brewer's yeast with B_{12}—2 tbsp. or 12 tablets.
B-complex, 100% natural, from yeast concentrate—1 tablet.
Bone meal—3 tablets.
"Nature's Minerals"—5 tablets.
Kelp—1 tablet.

ADULTS 20 to 40 YEARS

Vitamins A and D (10,000 units A and 400 units D per capsule)—2 capsules
Vitamin C, with bioflavonoids—500 to 1,000 mg.
Vitamin E, mixed tocopherols—400 - 600 I.U. If you have not taken vitamin E before, start with 100 I.U. and increase by 100 I.U. each week. If suffering from high blood pressure, or rheumatic heart diseases, consult your doctor on the proper dosage for your particular condition.
Vitamin B-complex, highest available potencies of 100 percent natural B-complex, from yeast concentrate—2 - 5 tablets. The usual strength of *natural* B complex, does not exceed 10 mg. for most major B's.

Brewer's yeast—1 - 3 tbsp. of powder or equivalent in tablets.

Bone meal or calcium lactate—½ tsp. of powder or 3 tablets.

"Nature's Minerals"—3 - 6 tablets.

Zinc—15 - 20 mg.

Kelp—1 tsp. granules or 2 - 3 tablets.

Lecithin—1 tsp. granules.

B_{15}, for those who live in areas with heavy air pollution—50 - 150 mg.

OVER 40 YEARS OF AGE

Vitamins A and D (10,000 units A and 400 units D per capsule)—2 to 3 capsules.

Vitamin C, with bioflavonoids—1,000 to 3,000 mg.

Vitamin E, mixed tocopherols from vegetable oils—600 I.U. - 1200 I.U.

Vitamin B-complex with B_{12}, highest available potency of 100 percent natural B-complex from yeast concentrate—4 - 6 tablets (see note on natural B-complex potency in "20 YEARS to 40 YEARS").

Brewer's yeast or primary grown food yeast—1 - 3 tbsp. of powder, or equivalent in tablets.

Bone meal or calcium lactate—1 tsp. of powder or 3 tablets.

"Nature's Minerals"—3 - 6 tablets.

Kelp—1 tsp. granules or 2 - 3 tablets.

Zinc—20 mg. for women and 30 - 50 mg. for men.

B_{15}—50 - 150 mg. for those who must live continuously in areas of heavy air pollution.

Important tips on taking vitamins and supplements

1. Again, we must stress that the above suggestions are only a very general outline of the supplementary needs for the average individual. There is, however, no common or average person, biochemically speaking. As Dr. Roger J. Williams stressed so expertly, "Individual human beings have great diversity in human nutritional needs." There-

fore, please understand that the above suggested dosages are only given as a very general guidance, referring to *minimum* doses used by most nutritionists and doctors who specialize in preventive and therapeutic uses of vitamins.

The above dosages are for more or less healthy individuals. I say more or less, because no one seems to be completely healthy any more.

2. In conditions of ill health, your vitamin and mineral needs are different; usually they are increased considerably. Also, specific isolated B vitamins are used therapeutically for many conditions of ill health. For specific therapeutic dosages of vitamins, minerals, herbs, etc., see my book, *How To Get Well*, where the complete therapeutic dietary and supplementary program is outlined in detail for most of our common diseases.

3. Vitamins and supplements to be taken during pregnancy and lactation are listed in Chapter 3.

4. The amount of vitamin C for children, even small ones, can be increased considerably during colds and infections. Children 1 - 6 years old can take up to 500 mg. a day, and after 6 years, as much as 1,000 mg. a day. Those over 12 can take 2 or 3 times that much.

5. If you or your child suffers from a serious disease, it is not wise to doctor or medicate yourself, even with vitamins. Let your doctor, upon a careful examination and nutritional and metabolic evaluation of your condition, determine the exact dosage and the duration of the vitamin therapy specifically prescribed to fill your individual needs.

6. All supplementary vitamins and minerals should be as natural as possible. Vitamin C should be preferably made from fruit or vegetable sources, although this is not possible with higher potencies. Vitamins A and D must come from fish liver oil, or possibly vitamin A from lemon grass for those strict vegetarians who object to using any animal products. Vitamin E must come from vegetable oils, and vitamin B-complex from concentrated yeast, rice polishings, etc. Minerals and trace elements, likewise,

should be from natural sources such as bone meal, dolomite, kelp, egg shell, milk, etc. "Nature's Minerals", which are recommended for all ages in this chapter, are made from 100 percent natural sources, such as: ocean oyster shell, egg shell, dolomite, yeast concentrate, kelp, black strap molasses, garlic, watercress, alfalfa, carrots, Irish moss, horsetail plant, bran, dulse, prune powder, etc. "Nature's Minerals" contain no bone meal, no milk or wheat products, no synthetic minerals, and no artificial colorings, flavorings, or preservatives. They are sold in health food stores.

7. As a general rule, all vitamins and food supplements should be taken with meals, or immediately after meals. They are better utilized with foods. For little infants, cod liver oil and vitamin E should be given right after breast feeding or bottle feeding, but orange juice and/or vitamin C can be given with water about midway between feedings.

8. All the dosages for all ages as recommended in this chapter are to be taken *daily*, unless specified otherwise. Divide the suggested daily amounts equally among three meals, or between two meals if this is more practical.

9. Take all vitamins and supplements suggested in this chapter *continuously*. If you use larger doses of vitamins for therapeutic purposes, such as those outlined in *How To Get Well*, and in several chapters in Parts Two and Three of this book, especially high doses of isolated synthetic B-complex vitamins, they should be taken only *for the duration of the therapeutic program*. This is usually 1 to 2 months. After a 4 - 6 week interval, the therapeutic program can be repeated, if needed. The reason for this recommendation is that some vitamins are cumulative (such as vitamins A and D) and some vitamins, like isolated vitamins from the B-complex, if taken in therapeutic megadoses and for prolonged period of time, can cause vitamin imbalances in the body. Also, the continuous ingestion of isolated synthetic B vitamins in large doses may cause deficiencies of other B vitamins, and/or interfere with the body's own synthesis of these

vitamins in the intestines. Brewer's yeast (B-complex) and plain fish liver oil (A and D) can be taken continuously, even in large doses. However, even therapeutic doses of all vitamins can be taken on a continuous basis if so prescribed by your doctor.

10. The adult doses of vitamins and other supplements, as suggested in this chapter, can be taken by the whole family, men as well as women. Those members of the family who are exposed to a greater degree of physical or mental stress, or larger level of environmental pollution and stresses, should take more of vitamins C, B, E, and B_{15}, and more brewer's yeast and "Nature's Minerals," to counteract the effects of stress.

11. The supplements and vitamins, as suggested in this chapter, are for individuals who adhere to the Airola Optimum Diet as described in Chapters 3 and 4. Those who eat nutritionally less adequate diets or live on a "regular" American diet, with plenty of sugar and white flour products and other overprocessed, denatured, demineralized, and devitaminized supermarket-type foods, will need much more supplementary vitamins and minerals in order to optimize their nutritional intake. For example, white sugar and white flour products rob the body of B vitamins. So, if you eat lots of sugar and white bread, take more brewer's yeast and B-complex vitamins to compensate for the deficiencies. Smoking destroys vitamins C and B in the body and also cuts down on vital oxygen supply to the brain and tissues. Therefore, smokers should take more vitamin C, vitamin B, and vitamin E. Of course, if you smoke, please turn to Chapter 28, "What Smoking Does To Women." Chances are that after reading the chapter you will join the growing number of ex-smokers.

10

The Development Of Character

Mental, emotional, social, and spiritual development of the child

"Train up a child in the way he should go, and when he is old, he will not depart from it."

The Bible.

Character is not something a child is born with; neither is it something that can be taught. What is it, then? It is a slow, gradual process of development and growth motivated and influenced by the attitudes, principles, standards, and values in the child's immediate and then gradually expanding environment and, most importantly, by the positive example of his parents and other members of his family. A child's character is rooted, fed, and cultivated by the character of the parents. As only good soil can produce good plants, so only good character in parents and proper emotional and moral nourishment of the family and environment can produce good character in their children. Thus, the influence and the example of parents are of paramount importance to the development of their children's character. The mother's role is especially significant since she spends the most time with the child during his early, most impressionable months and years. There is much truth to the old adage that "the hand that rocks the cradle rules the world."

Thus, raising children becomes a responsibility of supreme magnitude. Parents are not only molding and shaping the future character of a new human being, but also, collectively, the future of the nation and the destiny of humanity. Not only is this an immense responsibility, but a most difficult task. As Winston Churchill said, "It is easier to win two wars than to raise two children." And, he spoke from his own firsthand experience. Or as an old Chinese proverb says, "It is easier to rule a kingdom than a family."

Parents should make every effort to create a "good soil" in which their children can take root and grow—not only in respect to the immediate family environment, but the total environment. This is not always easy, but it can be done if values and priorities are clearly perceived.

During the early years of my marriage, while my children were small, I was extremely fortunate to have had insight regarding the vitally important influence of a child's environment on his entire life. We lived in Canada at the time. I had a successful professional career. We lived on a beautiful 100-acre farm in the country, with private lake and all, where we built a lovely home. We had five precious young children, four girls and one boy. Everything seemed to be the acme of success and perfection. But not *everything*.

We lived thirty miles away from the nearest church; twenty miles away from the high school. Our grade school was a so-called one-room country school with a total of eleven children in all eight grades—sensitive, shy, impressionable first graders all day in the company of tough seventh and eighth grade bullies. Most of our neighbors for miles around employed rather rowdy, foul-mouthed, heavy drinking and tobacco-smoking farm hands and transient laborers, with whom my children frequently came in contact. As much as we loved the beautiful Ontario countryside, I realized that we would be doing our children a great disservice if we allowed them to grow up in this type of an environment, which may have set the course for their entire lives. So, we sacrificed our lovely farm, I gave up my flourishing career, and we moved to sunny Arizona. I went to a real estate office and studied a map of the city. I found the place in the most livable citrus-growing area of the town where grade school, high school, and church were all in the same block. I circled the area around that block within a walking radius of half a mile, and said, "I want you to find me a house within this circle." They did.

I have never regretted that move. During the most impressionable years of our children's lives, we created an opportunity for them to grow and develop in an environment which was conducive to intellectual, moral, social, and spiritual development and growth. We are now reaping the rewards of parental pride and joy of having well-adjusted, well-balanced, healthy, and successful children with high moral and spiritual values. Any of the personal sacrifices that we made to accomplish this are richly compensated for by the abundant blessings which come with having happy, successful, and loving children.

So far in this book we have dealt primarily with the biological functions and the physical and nutritional aspects of motherhood and childhood. Most of the remaining chapters will deal with specific physical health problems of children and women. But a child is much more than a physical entity. He is a complex physical, mental, and spiritual being. The purpose of his coming to this planet is the development and perfection of all the various attributes of his total personality—not only the physical aspects of it, but the moral and spiritual fiber of his being.

The parents' efforts to help develop emotional, intellectual, and spiritual faculties in their children are even more important than feeding them good foods and giving them the right vitamins. Teaching children to become better human beings; to be more loving and compassionate, to be fair, honest, and trustworthy; helping them to develop moral courage, self-confidence, and self-respect; teaching them courtesy, politeness, and good manners, to be friendly and generous; encouraging their individuality and originality; helping them to be imaginative and creative, to be industrious and self-reliant, to be kind and loyal, to be obedient and willing to submit to authority, whether it is at home, school, or work; teaching them to be patient, openminded and tolerant; to be reliable and responsible; to be unselfish and willing to help others—developing these and many other positive personality traits in your child is of paramount importance for their total character growth. These personality traits do not come automatically, neither are they learned in special courses in schools. They are instilled and implanted in your child's character during his early childhood, mostly by the positive example and the influence within the family, but also through human contacts and relationships in school, church, and the child's immediate environment. It is a slow, gradual building process.

In assisting the child's character building, motherly intuition, inspiration, and spiritual insight are the best guides, of course. But, since so many of today's young mothers have come to depend on "expert" advice, I will try to give some tips as to what to look for as the child begins to grow and develop, not only physically, but also sexually, mentally, emotionally, and spiritually. Wise parents must and can help their child in this development.

Here are a few tips as to what parents can do, as well as what they should avoid, to maximize the process of the child's growth and development.

From birth to one year

At this early age, the baby will already show some signs of mental and emotional development. The most important contribution you can make to the development of his character at this time is to show him unlimited and unconditional love. Follow the advice of the great Tagore, who said, "I do not love him because he is good, but because he is my little child."

For the first few years of life, all the impressions the child soaks into his receptive mind are from his home. His home is his whole world. Make it a place of contentment, security, love, peace, and happiness. Smile at him, talk to him, sing to him. Cuddle him, love him, show him that you enjoy being with him. Spend time with him, play with him, respond to his needs and moods. Reassure him if he is frightened; calm him if he is disturbed. Be gentle, friendly, warm, loving. Remember: contrary to what some pediatricians or child-care experts may tell you, you cannot spoil a child with too much love! Surrounding your baby with an atmosphere of genuine warmth, affection, gentleness, kindness, peace, and love at this impressionable age will have a tremendous positive effect on his future mental, moral, and social development.

By the end of your baby's first year, you may begin to show, in a very kind and tolerant way, of course, that obedience to certain simple daily routines is expected of him. Most babies will begin to show very early some signs of selfishness, thinking of their own pleasure first, but, at the same time, they realize that they are almost completely subject to the will of others and are responsive to parental approval or disapproval.

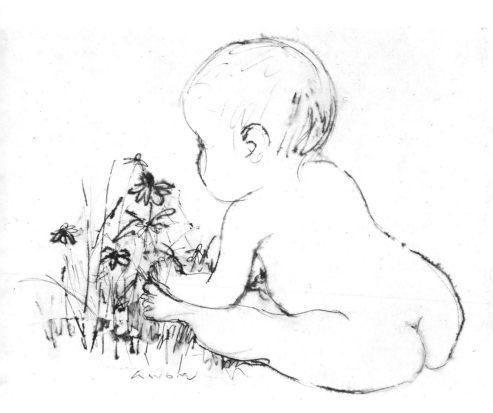

From one year to three years

These two years are the most important for a child's mental, emotional, and social development. He is now exposed to a multitude of impressions in the new wider world that he has entered. He will try to feed himself with a spoon and will hold a glass. He will try to walk. He will try to speak. Do not force or try to speed up these developments. Let him take his time. He will improve in time, when he is ready. If the baby is sucking his thumb, do not stop him with a constant "no-no!", but offer him more to eat and direct his attention to something else. Often, this is a sign that he feels the need for more security and affection.

If the child shows *definite* signs of being left-handed, refrain from doing anything about it. At first, however, children may pick up things with either hand, seemingly haphazardly, so there is nothing wrong with placing the spoon in his right hand, if he happens to put it first in his left, at least until he shows a definite preference. Many of the left-handed individuals are not that way because of the specific inherited characteristic following the Mendelian Laws, but because parents neglected showing and teaching them at a very early age.

Be careful how you speak to a child. The tone of your voice is most important as it conveys to the child your actual feelings. Also, watch what you say, not only to him, but to others in his presence, because he will pattern his speech after yours.

Encourage good comradely relationships between him and other children in the family or neighborhood. Teach him good manners, politeness, gentleness—mostly by your own example, of course.

The child's mental and intellectual curiosity knows no bounds as he nears the age of three. He drives you mad with questions. His curiosity and imagination are incredible. This is all very important for his total development. Answer his questions truthfully. He may ask questions about sex differences, or where babies come from. Tell him the truth in a simple and brief manner, like, "babies grow inside mother's tummy"; do not tell fairy tales or stork stories. And, be calm, unemotional, genuinely helpful, not disapproving. When the child is older, you will teach him more, and he will be able to understand it better.

A child of this age often shows signs of jealousy and sibling rivalry. He can be jealous of a new baby. He seems to want the exclusive love of someone as dear and important to him as his mother and father. Assure him that you love him as much as ever. After the age of three, he will lose some of his dependence on parents' affection and will feel more secure.

Teach your child obedience, but gain it not by force nor demands, but by friendly, but firm requests. Make sure your requests are reasonable. Be sure not to set standards too high for his age and ability. Respond with warm praise and affection to his efforts to please you. Establishing and enforcing standards for young children does not mean parents should be dictators. The parent-child relationship should be based on mutual love and respect. *Children must be taught early the meaning of responsibility and respect for parental authority. This will help them so much in establishing friction-free human relationships in the outside world when they grow up.*

Do not be confused by the advice given by some well-meaning but very unrealistic child-care experts who tell you that you should not dictate to or enforce any demands on a child, but let him learn by his own experiences and mistakes. This may be true to a very limited extent. But take, for instance, this example: A father may say to a three-year-old, "Daddy doesn't want you to play in the street because a car might hit you." The child may or may not be hit by a car, but you don't want him to learn this by finding out for himself. He should learn to obey simply because his father or mother said so. And for the child of this age, this is usually reason enough. He can understand the respect for parental wisdom and authority if he is secure enough in their love and affection for him. Three years old is still too immature to understand the abstract

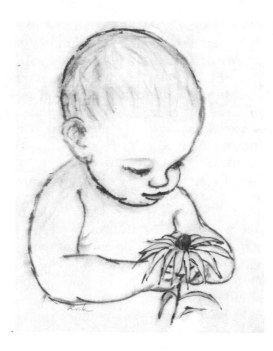

differences between right and wrong. But, he *is* fully aware of the difference between approval and disapproval from those he loves. He wants their approval and will do all he can to gain it. As far as his thinking is concerned, the standards of right and wrong are set by the parents, and he respects these standards and is loyal to them, because he knows that they are set by those who love him. As Francis Bacon said, "Happy are the families where the government of parents is the reign of affection."

Keep this in mind, however: moralizing, at this age, is a much less effective way to influence your child than the loving, warm, and kind atmosphere at home where he feels secure, warm, and loved. No amount of teaching in school or Sunday school in later years can be as important as these early impressions a child receives in his first world—his home. Make *your* home a place which your child will remember as Thomas Jefferson did his. He said, "The happiest moments of my life have been the few which I passed at home, in the bosom of my family."

From three years to eight years

This is a period of great curiosity and endless questions. Your child's vocabulary increases by about five hundred or more words a year. He loves to hear stories, but also likes to tell them. Sometimes, he confuses facts with fancy. His imagination can be amazing and amusing. Some children are little actors with tall tales to tell. Don't be disturbed by his innocent lies—he just enjoys the sensations he creates. Don't make him feel guilty, but encourage him to always tell the truth.

By American standards, at the age of five your child is supposed to go to school. Some parents even try to get their little ones to school before that. I feel that this is far too early an age for a child to enter into the rigid world of disciplined intellectual studies. His mind is not ready for that, and psychologically he is still not prepared for such a forced, scheduled life. He is still in a stage of playful discoveries on his own. The home is still the most important school in the world for him. This is the time for great mental and emotional receptivity for him, but not in the intellectual, organized manner. I believe that one of the main reasons why we have so much of the "Johnny can't read" problems is because we send our children to school too early. In many European countries and in Russia, children enter school one or two years later than in America, yet these children, in just a few short years, bypass American children in scholastic achievements—and by the time they finish grade school, they are on the level of our junior high school, as several actual tests and comparable studies have demonstrated. When a child is really ready for learning and his intellectual curiosity as well as learning capacity is enormous (at the age of seven or eight) he plunges into studies with great eagerness, and learns fast. On the other hand, if he is forced to enter school too early, he develops a "psychological allergy" towards studies, a turn-off rejection syndrome, and will be a poor learner throughout school. Johnny can't read not because he is too dumb to learn, but because he subconsciously doesn't want to learn.

Five or six years of age is not the time to shift the parents' responsibility for a child's education to the school even if a working mother may be in need of a babysitter. He needs to be with those whom he can trust and those whom he admires and loves. Teach him at home, read to him, converse with him. If you speak a second language, now is the time to teach it to him in conversation. Encourage him to draw pictures, paint, play musical instruments, play games that require thinking and decision-making. It the child's imagination and appreciation for music, color, and nature (plants, animals, flowers) are recognized and encouraged at an early age, an important foundation will have been established upon which the intellectual, moral, and spiritual growth of later years will flourish.

When your child is three, he can begin to participate in daily prayers; for example, just a simple little prayer at bedtime. Do it with him, show him an example. Faith and prayer are the greatest powers known to man, and fortunate is a person who was taught early in life to rely on them. By the time he is eight, or even before, he will begin to show a real curiosity in spiritual matters. He may ask questions about God: who is He, where is He, etc. By the age of eight, he is able to understand the story of the Creation, the beauty of the divine plan for our lives, and the wisdom of living the Golden Rule. Make a short devotional or prayer moment, in which children can participate, a daily occurrence in your family. Again, example is the best teacher, *the only teacher*. Remember, the home, not the church, is the foundation of the child's spiritual feelings and orientation. His experiences at home are imperative for the development of such qualities as compassion, generosity, kindness, helpfulness, honesty, obedience, tolerance, responsibility, and unselfishness. Keep in mind that all the above are traits of the character, not lessons that can be taught. To be of value, they must be genuinely felt, not practiced for ulterior motives. Only by parental example, by experience and lessons at home at an early age, will these traits become an established part of his character and total personality make-up.

From eight years to twelve years

This is the time for massive intellectual development. The years between eight and twelve are often referred to as the "memory period" because the average brain seems to retain information more readily at this period than at any other. At this time, your pre-adolescent child grows into a full-fledged and mentally-developed individual, with the ability to reason, reflect, discuss, and debate. He now has a highly developed ethical sense and is able to see the difference between right and wrong.

Girls are generally two years ahead of boys in their emotional and physical, as well as sexual, development. The average girl in America *begins* puberty at about the age of eleven, and completes it with the onset of menstruation at about thirteen.[1] The average boy reaches puberty about two years later. But, of course, there is no rule about it. Some boys and girls, all perfectly normal, mature earlier than others. Excessive meat and other animal protein in the diet promotes an earlier sexual maturity and faster physical growth—both of which are actually undesirable features as far as the total physical and emotional health is concerned (see more on body weight and premature sexuality in *Questions and Answers*).

This is also the time when your child's behavior can become troublesome. Don't be too critical. He will go through a period of self-doubt, sometimes even guilt, especially since he knows that better behavior is expected of him. By being too critical you reinforce guilt processes in the child. The child must learn to discipline himself, since self-discipline must be the basis for his future moral behavior. Encourage his efforts to improve himself and be very understanding, tolerant, and flexible in enforcement of your own standards. Now is the time when your child examines your standards critically and sets his own standards for himself. Don't worry, if you have done a good job so far, and have shown him plenty of love and good examples, his own standards will be as high or higher than yours.

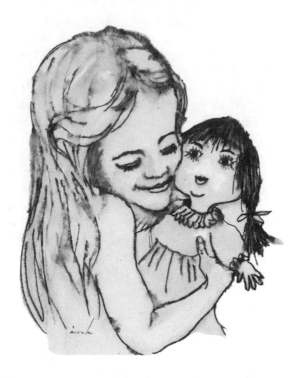

The power of example is, especially now, the most important tool that parents can use to influence their children for good. In one real-life story, a young man was being pressured by his friends to smoke a cigarette. After repeatedly declining, he was asked by his friends why he didn't give in. His reply was simple: "My dad has been offered cigarettes many times in my presence, but he has never accepted."[2] The same magazine gave another illustration of the power of positive example. A young boy was asked to give a public talk about the kind of family life he thought to be ideal. The talk he gave was beautiful and moving, and the audience marveled, wondering how he ever prepared such a magnificent talk. The boy answered, "I just described my own home life."

Don't miss the opportunity at this most important time in your child's life to influence him by example. Make his home and his environment such that the influence will be for good.

I am reminded of Dorothy Law Nolte's widely quoted classic expression of this principle:

CHILDREN LEARN WHAT THEY LIVE

If a child lives with criticism, he learns to condemn.
If a child lives with hostility, he learns to fight.
If a child lives with ridicule, he learns to be shy.
If a child lives with shame, he learns to feel guilty.
If a child lives with tolerance, he learns to be patient.
If a child lives with encouragement, he learns confidence.
If a child lives with praise, he learns to appreciate.
If a child lives with fairness, he learns justice.
If a child lives with security, he learns to have faith.
If a child lives with approval, he learns to like himself.
If a child lives with acceptance and friendship, he learns to find love in the world.

From puberty through adolescence

This is the time when girls and boys develop into women and men, the time between childhood and adulthood. It is also referred to as the "teens."

This is a difficult age, mainly because parents look at the boys and girls still as children, and the boys and girls look upon themselves as adults—both forgetting that actually they are neither one. They are too old to be children, and too young to be adults. So, their life is actually a normal and natural see-sawing back and forth between childhood and adulthood.

As I said earlier, girls mature physically and sexually about two years earlier than boys and reach puberty sooner. Breast development is usually the first sign of sexual maturity in girls, well before the appearance of hair in the pubic or underarm areas. Then comes menstruation, at about thirteen. But most boys do not begin with the first sign of sexual maturation, nocturnal emissions, until about fifteen, two years later than the average age for the onset of menstruation. The biological or spiritual significance of this age difference in maturity I could never understand, but it certainly creates some problems in boy-girl relationships during adolescence. Girls don't want to associate with still babyish boys of the same age, and seek companionship with older adolescents. Developing sex glands may cause immature sexual behavior such as excessive self-stimulation of genitals (see "Masturbation" in Chapter 21). Also, some girls may think that they are ready for sexual experiences with male partners and cannot understand why grown-ups do not condone such behavior.

While during pre-adolescence the mental development moves at an accelerated speed, during adolescence it is the physical development that seems to go faster. There are sudden and rapid increases in height and weight. Many girls reach their full adult height before sixteen, many, but not all, boys before eighteen. Some boys continue growing until the age of 25, especially those with late sexual development.

During this age period, preferably just at pre-puberty, the parents should discuss with their children the changes that are occurring in their young bodies. Do it in a natural, helpful, and frank way. The father may explain to the boy the reasons for his "sudden" sexual maturity and what it means. Sex education should begin at home with parents, whom growing adolescents can trust and relate to. The mother can explain to the girl the purpose of menstruation and impress upon her, preferably before menstruation begins, that it is a natural and normal process. Give her the necessary instructions for proper hygiene and care of her body. You can find reliable information on reproduction and sexual functions in any good encyclopedia. Emphasize at this point the importance of good nutrition for the optimal sexual and reproductive development.

Social and emotional maturity must be encouraged by parents during the formative years of adolescence. As the child is now entering the greater, contemporary world, social maturity will be important for his well-being and happiness. One of the important aspects of social and emotional maturity is the willingness to submit to authority—in school or at work, or to governmental and law enforcement agencies. This is not easy for an adolescent when he suddenly feels his own independence and self-assertion and wants to show it off. Remember, although his independence and self-reliance should be encouraged, he still needs and wants your parental advice and guidance—although he may not always want *you* to know that!

Most normal adolescents are rebellious at times. But they have a good concept of what is right and fair, and can discipline themselves if encouraged in their independence and not criticized too harshly. They are responsive to the fairness and logic in the Golden Rule of conduct—"Whatsoever you would that men should do unto you, do ye even so unto them."

Raising children is not easy. At times, it seems that even when you are doing everything right, you have nothing but problems. All the love, work, and effort you put in seems to be wasted. Your child is rebellious, ungrateful, doesn't want to talk or share his feelings with you, ignores you. "Where did I go wrong?" asks many a parent. Don't despair! Try not to let yourself become angry, hurt, or disappointed. An adolescent goes through a certain age when the assertion of his own self and independence is very important to him. If you persevere and show him genuine love, concern, and understanding, he will come back to you and will show appreciation for the forgiveness and understanding you showed during his troubled and trying times.

Some adolescents, entranced by their fast developing brain power, seem to go through a stage of overmagnification of their selfworth and overestimation of their intellectual capacity. Mark Twain illustrated this well with an anecdote from his own adolescent years. He wrote:

"When I was a boy of fourteen, my father was so ignorant I could hardly stand to have the old man around; but when I got to be twenty-one, I was astonished at how much he had learned in seven years."

An adolescent can be self-opinionated, rebellious, egotistical, ungrateful, disobedient, distant, and difficult to communicate with. But, remember, love conquers all, and if you show lots of unconditional love, forgiveness, warmth, kindness, and forebearance to your child, the final triumph of emerging as a successful parent will be assured.

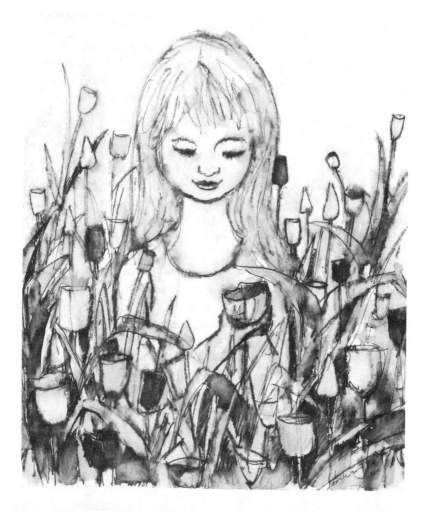

11

Love And Sexual Behavior:

Emerging Womanhood

Here is one of the letters I received from a very young girl, a reader of my Question and Answer column in one of the magazines. It illustrates what effect the "sexual revolution" and parental permissiveness has had on the minds of our children.

"Dear Dr. Airola: My mother receives your magazine every month, so, I have the chance to read it. I believe it is a very informative magazine and I enjoy reading it very much. As I understand, it is supposed to be about the natural things in life.

In the June issue, you published an article on birth control, titled "Birth Control: A Biological Perspective." In many ways, it was a great article. In most respects you are very right. However, I do disagree with you on one statement. You state that this is a "promiscuous age." As a reader, I feel I have the right to question that statement.

I have been told by an authority of the law that the age of consent in North Carolina is twelve years. If two consenting adults perform the act of sexual intercourse, is it really promiscuity? I am very sorry to say that the article containing your statement about promiscuity contradicts the whole purpose of your magazine.

In hopes of an honest reply, I ask you: What is more natural than sexual intercourse? Does it really make any difference if two people are married to one another or not?"

My answer read as follows:

"There is a severe lack of logic in several of your

conclusions and statements:

(1) Just because the age of consent in North Carolina is, as you say, twelve years, it does not mean that: a) twelve-year-olds are considered adults; or b) that they can freely indulge in sexual intercourse upon reaching that age.

(2) In using the term "sexual promiscuity," I did not refer to all sexual intercourse between consenting adults, but to the lack of *discrimination* in sexual liaisons— indiscriminate hopping into bed with partner after partner, without consideration of physical, psychological, or social consequences of such behavior.

(3) I agree with you that sexual intercourse is *natural*. But this does not mean that we can "do it" indiscriminately, without exercising self control, discipline, and consideration of those with whom we live and associate, or without having a thorough understanding, preparedness, and willingness to accept the possible long-term effects of such acts. Defecation is natural, too, yet we exercise great discrimination and control as to when and where we perform this perfectly natural act.

(4) Your naive question, shared by so many today, "does it really make any difference if two people are married to one another or not?", proves better than anything else that this *is*, indeed, an "age of promiscuity." It *does* make a difference. Human sexual intercourse is an expression of love. That's where we human beings, created in the Divine image, differ from animals. Sex is a beautiful and divinely sanctioned act, but only between two responsible adults bound not only by temporary infatuation or physical attraction, but by genuine love, total commitment, and fidelity in a monogamous, permanent relationship."

What is promiscuity? Dr. Allan Gerson, a California psychologist, defines it as "sexual intercourse at least once a week with a different partner at least every third time."[1] So, according to the "new morality" standards, sex every second week with a different partner at least once a month is not promiscuous. No wonder after two decades of "sexual revolution" and unprecedented permissiveness from authorities and parents, more than half of all unmarried teenagers in America engage in regular sex, with the disastrous result that not only does their loveless, uncommitted marathon sex cheapen and demean the sacred nature of masculinity and femininity, but sexually-transmitted diseases (STD) are now a "number one American health problem," an epidemic beyond control. The Communicable Disease Center reports that the VD rate in the twelve-to-twenty age group is triple that of the rest of the population, and that the typical high school student in Los Angeles, New York, or other big cities will have VD before his diploma. Ten to fifteen million Americans are stricken by venereal disease each year!

Venereal disease is particularly devastating to women. Over 275,000 young women in the United States, infected with gonorrhea each year, are threatened with sterility and major surgery because of pelvic inflammatory disease (PID).Over 300,000 new cases of the "new" VD, *herpes progenitalis*, appear each year. Herpes is linked to cervical cancer and severe brain damage and death in babies born to infected mothers. The matter is complicated by the fact that 85 percent of affected women have no symptoms of these diseases until the infection is advanced beyond the possibility of cure. Gonorrhea can blind a newborn, and active herpes infection at the time of delivery requires a Caesarean section to protect the infant from infection or even death.

What causes such an epidemic? Most investigators agree that immorality and promiscuity are the major causes for the STD epidemic. The wide availability of penicillin has given a false belief that VD is so easy to cure that it shouldn't be feared anymore. The Pill has extended sexual freedom, and the only birth control method that could be somewhat helpful in preventing VD infection, the condom, has fallen into disfavor. But unbridled promiscuity is, no doubt, the main cause, especially promiscuity among adolescents and children, *where over fifty percent of all new cases of VD can be found.*

But what causes promiscuity?

A series of studies conducted by Dr. Gerson showed that the causes of promiscuous behavior lie in the child-parent relationship. Promiscuous subjects viewed their fathers and mothers negatively. They characterized them as being dominant, forceful, hateful, threatening, firm, aggressive, and distant.[1]

This again shows the tremendous responsibility that is placed on the shoulders of parents. Chapter 10 began with the Biblical quote: "Train up a child in the way he should go, and when he is old he will not depart from it." Young children today are exposed to a massive amount of propaganda in movies, TV, books, and magazines, which pictures sexual liberation and promiscuity as an essential part of the modern "good" life. They are under pressure from their schoolmates. Children want to be popular, and those who do not wish to participate in what everybody else seems to be doing are called sissies and are left out. Temptations are enormous. They want to be part of the gang. Parental attempts to intervene and defend old-fashioned virtues are often dismissed with, "But, Mom, this is not the Victorian era, you know—it's the eighties!" So, how can you follow the Biblical admonishment to "train them"?

You may find yourself in the situation where your young daughter informs you that she is moving in with her boyfriend. "Live together without being married?!" "But, Mom, a marriage license is just a piece of paper! This is a New Age, and we have alternative lifestyles now!"

So, what can you do? Perhaps not much *now*, if you haven't prepared your daughter for successful and ful-filling womanhood earlier. Like I said, the preparation should have begun in the cradle; even before—in the womb. Actually—before conception!

Throughout this book I have stressed the importance of parental influence on the future emotional, mental, social, and spiritual character of the child. In the very first chapter, I explained that, contrary to what hereditists tell you, even the physical law of heredity can be superseded by the higher spiritual laws, and that with a conscious maternal influence, expressed in thoughts, wishes, feelings, and desires, before and during pregnancy, as well as during early infancy, the mother can reverse many of the heredity and natural tendencies and fashion the moral, intellectual, and spiritual fiber of her child. Then, throughout the child's infancy, his emotional, intellectual, physical, and moral attributes, trends, and capabilities are formed by the constant influence and example of the parents, and especially by the mother who nurtures the child at her bosom. Later, it is for parents to decide what TV shows their young, impressionable child sees, what book he reads, what company he keeps. Without supervision and control, we cannot expect our children to grow the way we want. Mental, intellectual, and moral nourishment for their minds should be as closely planned and supervised as the nutrition for their bodies. Optimal nutrition for the body will produce optimal health. Optimal nutrition for the mind will produce well-balanced, well-adjusted, and happy children, with a healthy dose of self-respect as well as self-discipline.

Oh yes, self-discipline! That's where it's all at! If children have the ability to exercise self-discipline, they can more easily confront and counteract the negative forces in their environment. They can control their own behavior and face temptations without succumbing to them.

And how can they *learn* such self-discipline? They can't! Self-discipline is the result of parental influence and example as well as the kind of parental discipline that was used in the home during the child's upbringing. If the child was raised in an atmosphere of love, trust, and respect for parental authority, he will have a high degree of self-esteem and self-discipline. Love-oriented and love-based discipline in the home, enforced with kindness and fairness, but, nevertheless, *enforced* through what is called natural consequences, will help the child to grow up with a sense of self-esteem and self-discipline.[2] Because of some misdirected child-care experts' advice of a couple of decades ago, we now have a whole generation grown up without strong parental influence and discipline. Permissiveness and lack of clear authority and discipline in the home are, to a great degree, responsible for the fact that today one child in nine can be expected to appear in juvenile court before the age of eighteen; suicide has become the second leading cause of death among young Americans between the ages of fifteen and twenty four; and every year, *one million* children run away from home.[3] Our schools have turned into jungles of crime, violence and vandalism. Last year, school children committed 100 murders, 12,000 armed robberies, 9,000 rapes, and 204,000 aggravated assaults against teachers and each other. Over $600 million worth of school property was vandalized. Nationwide, over 5 million youngsters use illegal drugs and 500,000 teenagers are alcoholics.[4] It seems the three R's of today's American education have become Rape, Robbery, and Riot.

The cause for such an alarming increase in juvenile delinquency, teenage crime and drug abuse, teenage runaways, and sexual promiscuity, can be found in the broken-down American family structure.[5] We must restore the family to the high standards of its divine institution, where children are reared in an atmosphere of love, affection, respect, trust, mutual dependence, and obedience. *Obedience* and *dependence* are becoming dirty words in the new-age vocabulary. Yet, these are the imperative characteristics of the strong and stable family life that will help to develop in sons and daughters the high degree of self-esteem, independence, self-reliance, and self-discipline, which are so much missing in our present promiscuous and permissive society.

Fortunately, the sexual liberation movement may be coming to an end. Very recent national polls show that there is a definite shift away from indiscriminate sex and sexual promiscuity, away from sexuality for sexuality's sake. An incredible seventy-two to eighty-seven percent of those polled disapproved of adultery, homosexuality, and casual sex among adolescents. As one dedicated female liberationist remarked recently, "People found that instant sex was about as satisfying as a sneeze." And Barbara

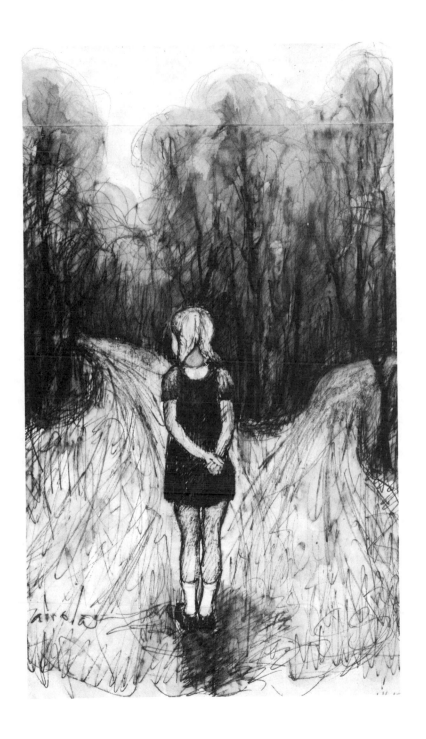

Seaman, author of *Free and Female*, says "The backlash is against carnal sex because a lot of people were hurt."

For a girl, promiscuity, sex without love, sex only for gratifying pleasure without interpersonal attachment and commitment, destroys self-respect and leads to loneliness. A wise and responsible mother must teach her young daughter, as she grows into womanhood, that her body is the temple of her spirit and should be kept clean and undefiled. She should save herself for her husband with whom she can then have a joyous sexual relationship as an expression of deep love in an atmosphere of mutual trust, respect, and total commitment.

What about the constant pressure from friends to "go all the way"? Tell your daughter that the loss of a few friends is much less serious than the loss of self-respect. She can win new and better friends standing firmly by her principles; but lost self-respect is not easily regained. A girl who gets pregnant against her wishes (and in the U.S. there are one million unwanted pregnancies a year!), or contracts a venereal disease, can suffer a severe psychological trauma and a feeling of inferiority that can last a lifetime, affecting negatively her future relationship with her husband and her children. Clearly, the price for momentary pleasure is too high to pay. And, if she is forced into marriage because of an unwanted pregnancy, such a loveless marriage may lead to countless problems that can be all traced back to that one evil—promiscuity.

Sex is a wonderful gift. It can and should be enjoyed to the maximum in the context of a loving, committed, permanent relationship. Chastity is a prerequisite for a perfect, satisfying relationship which can only be built on such virtues as purity, fidelity, and trust. Social customs vary and change, but our relationship to our Creator and his eternal moral and spiritual laws has not and will not be changed. The maintenance of high moral and spiritual standards is more important today than ever before in human history. It is the only hope we have for the cure of human ills that plague the world today.

Part Two
Children's Health

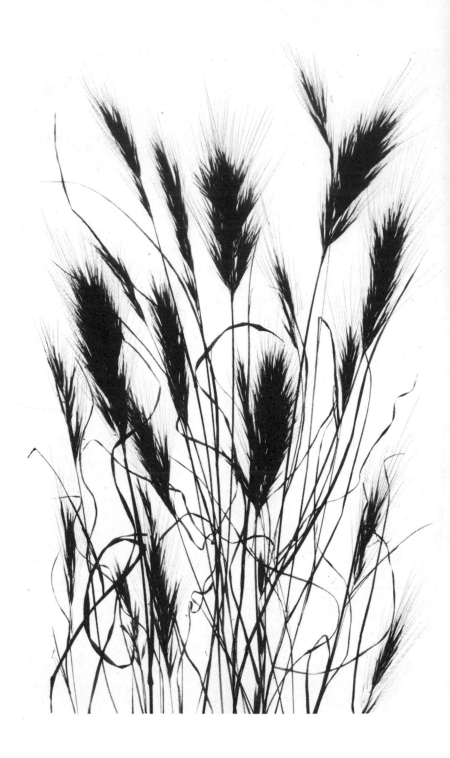

12

Allergies

Most allergies in infants are caused by early feeding of foods, solid or liquid, other than mother's milk. A baby's digestive system lacks the necessary digestive enzymes and is unable to effectively digest any foods other than breast milk. Thus, if fed foods it cannot digest efficiently, the infant's body reacts to them as if they were toxic matter, and develops an immunological rejection response. Usually this takes the form of gastrointestinal disorders such as colic or diarrhea, but skin rashes and eczema are other common symptoms. The foods that most commonly lead to severe allergic reactions are cow's milk and milk products, eggs, chicken, citrus fruits, tomatoes, soya products, wheat, and corn; although virtually any solid food fed to an infant before the age of six to eight months may contribute to the development of allergies—immediately or later in life. Total reliance on breast feeding for at least six months, with the gradual addition of solid foods thereafter will prevent most allergies in children, as well as later as they grow into adulthood.

The above conclusions are substantiated by a great deal of research and clinical observation.

Dr. E.R. Kimball conducted an extensive study of 1378 children and found that the longer the duration of the babies' breast feeding, the lesser the incidence of allergy. In babies breast-fed for a minimum of six months, the incidence of allergies was reduced to zero percent (if the mother didn't suffer from allergies).[1] It was also found that in the rare cases where babies developed allergies when fed breast milk alone, the allergy subsided and disappeared as soon as the foods to which the baby was sensitive were eliminated from the nursing mother's diet.[2]

The most common allergen—the food that most infants cannot tolerate and develop allergy to—is cow's milk. This fact notwithstanding, cow's milk is the most common ingredient in baby formulas. In one study of 172 infants under two years of age, 109 were found to be sensitive to cow's milk.[3] The symptoms varied from an array of gastrointestinal problems to skin disorders. Dr. S.S. Freedman, another researcher, reported 49 cases of violent allergic reactions in the form of atopic eczema in children who were fed cow's milk at an early age.[4] As early as 1936, the *Journal of Pediatrics* reported that "The general incidence of infantile eczema is lowest in the breast-fed infant. In the partially breast-fed it is twice as frequent as in the breast-fed, and in the artificially-fed infants, seven times as great."[5]

Not only is cow's milk the most common allergy-causing food, but feeding cow's milk in early infancy contributes to gluten intolerance later in life. Swedish study of infants who were fed cow's milk early in life showed that although after a time some of them developed a certain level of tolerance to cow's milk, they also developed allergy to gluten when wheat was introduced into their diet. This study illustrates the hypothesis that early intolerance to certain foods may "set the stage" for later development of a sensitivity to other foods.[6]

How allergy develops

Dr. S. Freier says that the infant's body is not genetically nor biologically programmed to utilize large quantities of foreign protein. The proteins supplied by formula feeding, and especially by cow's milk and meat at an early age, are foreign to the digestive system of the infant and lead to an allergic reaction. "Quite apart from the increased danger of infection, a considerable proportion of infants suffer from hypersensitivity brought about by the impact of a large quantity of foreign protein at a time of life when the intestine is designed to receive mother's milk only. It should not be forgotten that the large-scale use of cow's milk in infant-feeding is less than a hundred years old. Solids and semi-solids were introduced into infant-feeding no more than 50 years ago, while the ill-conceived advice to rush in with meat on the tenth day of life has become fashionable only recently...These very fundamental changes in infant-feeding habits may be responsible for an increase in infantile gastrointestinal allergy."[7]

Cow's milk contains four major proteins: casein, serum albumin, beta-lactoglobulin, and alpha-lactalbumin. Most infants are allergic to one or more of these forms of protein, most commonly beta-lactoglobulin and alpha-lactalbumin.

The quantity as well as quality of foreign protein is crucial. As I said in Chapter 7, cow's milk contains almost three times more protein than mother's milk. Also, the protein in cow's milk is 85 percent casein and 15 percent whey protein (lactoglobulin and lactalbumin), while mother's milk casein content is only 40 percent, 60 percent being the whey protein fraction. Being water soluble, whey proteins are much easier to digest, while casein is the curd-forming protein which is more difficult to digest. We must remember that it is the inability to properly, effectively, and speedily digest certain foods that predisposes an infant to the development of allergies. Cow's milk was designed for calves who have four stomachs containing digestive bacteria or the casein-curdling enzyme, rennin, neither of which is found in the human stomach.[8] Therefore, when cow's milk is consumed by the human infant, it is coagulated in the stomach by digestive acids to form rather hard, rubbery curds which are not as readily digested as the soft, flocculent curds which are produced from human milk.[9]

In addition to the excess quantity and undesirable quality of foreign proteins in artificial feeding, there are other factors that may also contribute to the development of allergies in infants.

Cow's milk, even when it is diluted to minimize its high protein content, still contains excessive amounts of calcium, which weaken the infant's ability to digest milk proteins due to the calcium's buffering effect on the stomach acids. Thus, undigested proteins cause undue stress on the baby's kidneys and can lead to toxemia.

Not only do protein-rich foods such as cow's milk, meat, eggs, cheese, chicken, etc., contribute to allergic sensitivity if fed to the infant before the age of 6 - 8 months, but any solid foods, such as grains, fruits, and vegetables, may be causatively involved.

The symptoms of allergy

How do you know when your baby is showing allergic reactions to certain foods?

The most common symptoms are:
- frequent vomiting
- large, often water stools
- chronic rhinitis (runny nose, mucus)
- abdominal pains, colic
- atopic dermatitis, eczema
- asthma

Also, when your baby shows lethargy, weakness, irritability, excessive crying, restlessness, or prolonged pallor, a possible allergy to foods may be suspected—although none of the above symptoms alone are necessarily indicative of allergy, but may be connected with other health disorders.

What to do

Dietary prophylaxis, or prevention, is the best way to protect your baby from becoming crippled for life by allergies. Here are some important general guidelines:

1. Begin allergy-preventive program during pregnancy. Avoid all foods that you know you are allergic or sensitive to. Sensitivity to foods can be transferred from mother to child.

2. Your infant should not be given any other solid or liquid foods except breast milk until at least the age of 6 months. The early feeding of any other food will increase the baby's chances of becoming allergic to some of them.[10]

3. When supplementary foods are added to your infant's diet—from the age of 6 months and later—avoid, if possible, feeding such common allergens as cow's milk, wheat, soya, eggs, and chicken. These foods—potential

allergens—should be withheld for at least the first 9 months of the infant's life, preferably for one year.[2,11]

4. When solid foods are eventually added to the diet, watch for possible allergic reactions (symptoms mentioned earlier). As I said before, the main cause of food allergies is the baby's inability to properly digest certain nutrients. Undigested food becomes, in effect, "a foreign" matter in the body, causing toxic reaction. The simple, logical, common-sense cure for allergy is to eliminate the offensive food from the diet. How do you determine which food is the culprit? Experimenting with *one food at a time* is the best way to determine which food is the offender. This can be done by two different processes. One, leave a suspected food out of the diet for a week and see if allergy symptoms disappear. If they do, you have found the offending food. Two, make a meal of one single suspected food and watch the reaction. Usually, a violent reaction follows if a large quantity of an allergen is eaten alone.

5. If the allergen is identified, it is wise to leave it out of the diet for as long as possible, but not necessarily forever! It is quite common for a child to "outgrow" his allergies and later tolerate foods to which he was allergic earlier.

6. Allergy in adults should be traced in the same manner, except that adults can improve their body's tolerance to allergens (improve the digestion of foods) by taking digestive enzymes such as hydrochloric acid, pepsin, pancreatin, ox-bile, etc., in tablet form. Also, specific supplementary vitamins and minerals, especially vitamins A, C, D, E, pantothenic acid, manganese, and calcium, can help increase the body's tolerance to allergens as well as assist in food digestion by activating the digestive enzymes. Infants and young children, however, should not be given any supplementary digestive enzymes or vitamins (except those mentioned in Chapter 9).

7. The orthodox medical approach to allergy is oriented towards removing symptoms rather than eliminating the underlying causes. Conventional doctors use

antibiotics, antihistamines, vaccines, hormones, desensitization, and even psychotherapy to treat allergy. I do not approve of such an approach. Avoidance of allergens—abstinence from foods one is allergic to, or, in mild cases, cutting down on their use—is the only sensible and logical way to deal with allergies.

The most absurd and tragi-comical situation in American medicine today is that there are over 20 million people in this country who are under some kind of medical treatment for allergies. Many millions more are treated for "diseases" (such as digestive disorders and indigestion) which are, in truth, nothing but food allergies— misdiagnosed. And yet, much of the expense, misery, and suffering could be avoided if mothers would follow the advice in this chapter and abide by a few simple, common-sense rules, especially by returning to exclusive breast feeding, which would virtually eliminate this condition from the American scene in just one generation. If children are breast-fed and properly nourished from infancy through adolescence, they will be strong and resistant to allergens and will be able to digest practically any natural foods.

8. So far, the discussion in this chapter has dealt with infant *food* allergies, the common causes and treatments of same. However, infants and children may have other than food allergies: allergies to pollens, dusts, animal hairs, environmental chemicals, food additives, etc. The proper approach to such allergies is: first, the allergen must be correctly identified, either by you, the parent, or by the doctor, perhaps with the help of allergy tests; second, all efforts must be made to eliminate the identified allergen from the infant's food or environment; and third, strengthen and increase the infant's tolerance to the allergens by increasing his general resistance and raising his total level of health by following the dietary and other health improving programs suggested in this book. Also, taking large doses of vitamin C (see Chapter 9 for correct dosage for different ages) can help tremendously, since vitamin C is an excellent detoxifying and anti-allergenic agent.

13

Infant Anemia

I have a special chapter on anemia among mothers, and women in general, in Part Three of this book, but here we'll explore the issue of anemia in babies.

It is well known that breast-fed babies are not susceptible to anemia, while bottle-fed babies often are.[1] Since it is also known that human milk contains only a little iron, why then are breast-fed babies immune to anemia?

There are many answers to this question:

1. Although the iron content of human milk is low, there is, nevertheless, almost twice as much iron in mother's milk as in raw cow's milk. Thus, infants fed formula based on cow's milk without iron fortification get only half as much iron as do breast-fed babies. But even when artificially-fed babies receive more iron than breast-fed babies, because of their formula being fortified with supplementary iron, they are still more likely to become anemic.[2] This is, in part, because the absorption of supplementary iron is very uncertain. Supplementary iron also destroys vitamin E in the formula as well as in the infant's body, thus contributing further to anemia since vitamin E deficiency is one of the known causes of anemia. When an infant's blood is deficient in vitamin E, the red blood cells are destroyed by exposure to oxygen.[3]

2. Iron is not the only trace element involved in preventing anemia. Proper levels of copper, manganese, and zinc are also important for the normal blood-building process. Mother's milk has higher levels of a utilizable form of these trace elements than does cow's milk. There is about three times as much copper in human milk as in cow's milk.[4]

3. Most commercial formulas are made from skimmed cow's milk, with vegetable oils added as the source of fat.

Vegetable oils have a high level of polyunsaturated fatty acids that further lowers the serum tocopherol (vitamin E) level, since the metabolism of polyunsaturated fat requires larger amounts of vitamin E than the metabolism of fat from mother's milk. And, since vitamin E is essential for iron absorption, as well as for protection of red blood cells from destruction by oxidation, this is one of the obvious causes of hemolytic anemia among bottle-fed babies.[5] Human milk from healthy mothers has ten to twenty times more vitamin E than does cow's milk.[6, 12]

4. Breast milk also contains large amounts of two specific substances, *lactoferrin* and *transferrin*, which are not found in cow's milk, but which are important for the prevention of anemia. Lactoferrin is an iron-binding protein which not only improves the iron metabolism, but also inhibits the growth of harmful E. coli bacteria in the intestines, preventing infections and malabsorption of nutrients.[7] Transferrin acts as a transportation vehicle of iron from mother to infant.[1, 13]

5. Adequate amounts of ascorbic acid (vitamin C) are needed for the absorption of iron and prevention of anemia.[8] There is about twice as much vitamin C in mother's milk as compared to cow's milk.[9]

6. Finally, many infants who are fed formulas based on cow's milk become allergic to milk. This allergic sensitivity to cow's milk not only causes poor absorption of minerals, including iron, but also can cause gastrointestinal irritation and bleeding, which, in turn, contributes to anemia.[10]

As you can see from the above, there are many reasons why a breast-fed baby is better protected against anemia than the artificially-fed baby.

Mother-infant anemia relationship

Although the superiority of breast feeding over artificial feeding for prevention of nutritional anemia is well established, even breast milk cannot always be relied upon to provide all nutrients needed by the baby, including iron. If the expectant mother adheres to the Optimum Diet as described in Chapters 3 and 4 of this book, a full-term infant will store enough iron to last six months, especially if the mother's diet is also optimal during the lactation period. The Optimum Diet during lactation will also ensure an adequate supply of other minerals and vitamins necessary for efficient blood building and the prevention of anemia, such as copper, manganese, zinc, vitamins C, E, B_6, A, B_{12}, etc. But, if the mother-to-be eats an inadequate diet during pregnancy, and is anemic herself as a result of nutritional deficiencies, her baby will probably be anemic also.[8] This means that the most important factor in preventing infant anemia is an optimal diet for the mother-to-be during pregnancy.

Again, the adequacy of the mother's diet for the purposes of anemia prevention must not be measured by its iron content alone. Many other nutritional factors are vitally involved in preventing anemia. If the diet is deficient in B vitamins the stomach cannot secrete sufficient hydrochloric acid to absorb iron, even if it is present in the diet in adequate quantities. Lack of protein, zinc, and vitamins C, E, and folic acid can also lead to anemia in babies.[8]

Another significant factor in the prevention of infant anemia is the hemoglobin iron concentration in the placenta at the very moment of birth and if it is allowed to be transferred to the baby. If at the time of delivery the umbilical cord is allowed to drain much of its valuable iron-rich blood before being clamped (see Chapter 6), the baby will have a greater store of iron than he otherwise would. It would have a considerable influence on iron requirements during the early months of infancy.[11] This is why premature babies usually have no stores of iron in the body. However, even premature babies, if they are breast-fed, rarely develop anemia, although breast milk furnishes only about 1.5 mg. of iron per quart.[12]

How long is a breast-fed baby protected?

How long can the mother be sure that her breast-fed baby is protected against anemia? Can a baby rely on the iron in mother's milk for longer than the usually-recommended five or six months? And, even for this period, what evidence is there that the baby will stay healthy on an exclusive diet of mother's milk?

First, all babies, as well as all mothers, are different. The nutritional value of mother's milk varies considerably. With the exception of definite cases of inferior quality of mother's milk, the baby is perfectly safe nutrition-wise on an exclusive breast milk diet for six months, or even as long as eight months. Supplementary foods should not be, as a rule, introduced before that age. Even if you would give your baby iron-rich foods at an early age, his digestive system is not able to properly utilize it.[13] As I stated in Chapter 7, infants do not have the special digestive enzymes to properly digest any other foods than mother's milk for at least six to eight months. Therefore, unless your baby shows clear signs of anemia, you can safely breast-feed him at least to the age of six to eight months.

How can you tell if your baby is anemic?

The most obvious symptoms of iron-deficiency anemia (the most common form of nutritional anemia) in infants or adults are general pallor, or the colorlessness or paleness of the skin, and a feeling of tiredness and being "out of sorts." The baby may also have digestive problems such as diarrhea or colic. He may cry a lot, be fussy, and difficult. The anemic baby is less resistant to colds and infections as well.

Of course, if these definite signs of anemia are present (not just concerns and remarks of a worried, meat-eating grandmother when she hears that your baby is not getting meat), it would be wise to consult a doctor and request a test to determine if the baby's hemoglobin level is within the normal range for his age. Again, most doctors will probably suggest that unless you start giving your baby solid foods, and preferably meat, at the age of two or three months, he will become anemic. Don't be alarmed. Many doctors are too busy to keep up with the newest research. You can show him this book, or refer him to the extensive research on the unadvisability of early feeding of solid foods compiled by the La Leche League International.[1] Or, you may choose to overlook his ignorance and gently request the hemoglobin test. He may be surprised to find that most breast-fed babies (almost 100% of them) are not anemic at all, even though they are on an exclusive mother's milk diet and even if the lactating mother does not eat meat. According to many of the world's foremost experts on infant nutrition, notably Drs. E.R. Kimball and G.J. White, breast-fed babies, in general, do not become anemic. In fact, the above doctors stated that they have never seen a case of anemia in a child who was completely breast-fed for the first six months and then started on the gradual supplementation of solid foods of high nutritional quality.[1,14]

What are normal and abnormal hemoglobin levels? Ordinarily, the baby's hemoglobin level at birth ranges from 18 to 20 gm., and then gradually decreases over the next eight to ten months. Usually, by the end of the fourth week of life, the hemoglobin level has dropped to about 15.4 - 16 gm., sometimes even lower than that. By the end of the fourth month, the normal range could be about 10 - 15 gm. But, anywhere from 9.8 to 12.6 gm., between the ages of two and twelve months, could be considered in the normal range.[15,16] Most pediatricians would consider a hemoglobin level below 10 gm. at the age of six months or earlier as abnormal.

If baby is anemic...

The most likely causes of anemia in babies are:
(1) Insufficient storage supply of iron received at birth due to deficient diet of mother during pregnancy.
(2) Cutting of umbilical cord too early, before most of the blood in the placenta is transferred to the infant (see Chapter 6).
(3) Lactating mother's severely deficient diet during breast feeding.
(4) Artificial formula feeding.

(5) Baby's poor assimilation of iron and other blood-building nutrients.

(6) Other health disorders that interfere with normal blood-building process.

If the lastly mentioned two causes are suspected, the baby's doctor must diagnose and treat the conditions involved. If anemia is related to nutritional deficiencies caused by an inadequate diet of the nursing mother, baby's formula, or baby's diet, steps should be taken to improve the diet and optimize the levels of iron and other blood-building factors in mother's and/or baby's diet. Here are a few of the things you can use:

Green juice (see Recipes and Directions) is a vegetable juice made from green leafy vegetables such as parsley, alfalfa, comfrey, turnip greens, beets, and carrots. It is one good way to get easily assimilable iron, as well as other trace elements. Babies tolerate it well, too. This juice can be given even before the age of six months, if needed, beginning with ½ teaspoon and gradually increasing to ½ cup a day by the age of six to eight months. Do not use spinach or other vegetables rich in oxalic acid.

Blackstrap molasses is another good source of biologically-active and easily-usable iron. As soon as the baby can eat grains (see Chapter 8), oatmeal, millet, and hulled sesame seeds will be excellent sources of organic iron.

Brewer's yeast is a superior source of iron and all other important blood-building elements. The baby can be given small amounts of brewer's yeast at a very early age, even after the first four weeks, if needed, and the amount of brewer's yeast can be increased gradually to 1 or 2 tbsp. a day, by the age of twelve months. Especially if the baby is bottle fed, brewer's yeast should be added daily to the formula. Brewer's yeast is such an excellent source of easily-assimilable iron that anemia can not only be completely prevented, but also corrected if a few teaspoons of brewer's yeast powder is added daily to a baby's formula or used as a supplement to the mother's milk. Even at a later age, during childhood and adolescence, a daily intake of brewer's yeast, plus eating the Optimum Diet as recommended in this book, is the best preventative against anemia.

Bananas are an excellent anti-anemia food. Serve them raw and mashed to your baby, even at an early age, if anemia is suspected of diagnosed. Bananas are particularly beneficial, as they contain, in addition to easily-assimilable iron, folic acid, and even traces of vitamin B_{12}, both extremely important in prevention and treatment of anemia.

Raw egg yolks are another good source of organic iron, as is liver, for those who are not vegetarians.

Inorganic iron salts, often prescribed by pediatricians for anemia, are to be avoided. Not only are they very poorly assimilated, if at all, but they can destroy important vitamin E, thus actually *causing* anemia, or going to the other extreme, they can cause hemosiderosis, a fatal disease resulting from storage of excessive iron.[8] Inorganic iron supplements can be toxic to young babies. In fact, dozens of young children die annually from eating iron supplement tablets prescribed by obstetricians for their mother, mistaking them for candy.

Even taking iron salts, and such inorganic iron supplements as iron sulfate, during pregnancy, is not only potentially dangerous to the mother, but also can bring about miscarriages or premature births, and may cause malformations and mental defects in babies as well as contribute to infant anemia.[8]

Iron-rich fruits and vegetables, as well as their juices, are, by far, the best nutritional approach to anemia in older children and adults. Fruits especially rich in iron are: apricots, unsulfered raisins, peaches, bananas, prunes, apples, and blackberries. Iron-rich vegetables are: turnip greens, spinach, beet tops, beets, and dulse. Most whole grains and beans are also very good sources of dietary iron.

14

The Hyperactive Child

Millions of American children are afflicted with a disorder that was virtually unknown a hundred years ago in the pre-chemical era—hyperactivity, or what is medically termed as *hyperkinesis*. Official medical sources estimate that there are five to seven million children suffering from hyperactivity and learning disorders. In the biological medical vocabulary, we often refer to certain ailments as "civilization diseases," especially in regard to cancer and heart disease. But perhaps hyperkinesis is the most obvious civilization disorder. Although the epidemic growth of the number of children with hyperactivity and learning disorders has baffled medical science until recently, the pioneering work of Dr. Ben F. Feingold, Chief Emeritus of the Allergy Department of San Francisco's Kaiser Foundation and the Permanente Medical Group, has shed much light on the origin and the solution of this problem.[1] And, as every mother of the hyperactive child knows, hyperactivity *is* a very serious and enervating problem.

Symptoms

The most observable symptoms of the hyperkinetic child are:

- *Hyperactivity.* Unnatural, constant, high-gear activity, or as one mother describes her child, "he is *never* still, constantly on the move; can't sit still even ten seconds."
- *Aggressiveness.* Attacking, fighting, hitting everyone in his path, adults or children, especially little brothers and sisters.

- *Destructiveness.* Breaking toys, tearing books, smearing paint on clothes and walls, throwing foods, clothing—anything!
- *Bad temper and bad moods.* The hyperkinetic child doesn't have many friends in school.
- *Extremely short attention span.* No sooner does he start to do something, than he almost immediately loses interest and switches his attention to something else.
- *Nervousness.* Biting nails is one of the typical nervous symptoms of a hyperkinetic child.
- *Rebelliousness, disobedience and disrespect.* He cannot take orders, advice, or suggestions from anyone: parents, teachers, or friends.
- *Learning disorders.* Because of many of the above symptoms, especially short attention span, hyperactivity, and disobedience, the hyperkinetic child is usually below average in school work; often he is a poor reader. In severe cases, he may be several grades behind scholastically, although by all indications he possesses a high I.Q.

Causes

In recent years, there has been much work done by medical researchers, especially in the United States and Australia, as to the causes of hyperactivity, mostly regarding Dr. Ben Feingold's theories.

Dr. Feingold found that the "trigger factors" of many behavior problems are strictly nutritional. Highly-processed, man-made foods with artificial colors and flavors and other additives and preservatives are the most common cause of hyperactivity. He also indicated natural salicylates in some unprocessed fruits and vegetables. Foods containing natural salicylates include: almonds, apples, apricots, cherries, cranberries, cucumbers, grapes, nectarines, oranges, peaches, peppers, pickles, plums, prunes, raisins, tangerines, and tomatoes.

Dr. Feingold, as well as several other doctors, such as Dr. Arnold Brenner and Dr. Richard Sledden, who tried Dr.

Feingold's dietary plan, found that 60 to 70 percent of hyperkinetic children show a significant improvement when dietary "trigger factors" are eliminated.

In my own observations and studies, I have found that although the "trigger factors" discovered by Dr. Feingold are without doubt some of the major causes of hyperactivity, there are several other vital factors involved, which may be responsible for those 30 to 40 percent of cases that do not respond to Dr. Feingold's treatment.

In respect to hyperactivity, as in respect to any other human illness or disorder, we must shun simplistic answers and solutions. Health problems, both in terms of causes as well as therapy, are usually very complex. Often many contributing causes are involved and intertwined. Therefore, the holistic healing approach, which takes into consideration all of the possible contributing causes and healing alternatives, is always the most effective.

On the basis of my extensive research of presently-available scientific studies and clinical observations, here are the basic contributing factors of hyperactivity and learning disorders in children, in order of their importance:

1. Processed foods, drinks, or condiments that contain artificial colorings and flavorings, even so-called U.S. certified colors.[1, 7]
2. Other man-made chemicals, additives and preservatives[6]—especially monosodium glutamate (MSG, also known as "Accent"), sodium benzoate, butylated hydroxyanisole (BHA), and butylated hydroxytoluene (BHT); likewise, toxic chemicals present in polluted air, water, and food, especially lead,[2] mercury, cadmium and carbon monoxide.
3. Refined white sugar and refined white flour and everything made with them.[3] Excessive sugar in the child's diet contributes to the development of hypoglycemia (low blood sugar), which is one of the common contributing causes of hyperkinesis.
4. Caffeine-containing beverages, such as colas, tea, and coffee. Chocolate also contains caffeine.

5. Allergies. The most common allergens are: cow's milk and cheese, wheat (even whole wheat), eggs, chocolate, and citrus fruits and juices.
6. Hypoglycemia. Whether it is related to allergies, excessive sugar in the diet, or other causes, hypoglycemia is one of the common contributing causes of hyperkinesis.
7. Nutritional deficiencies. Many hyperkinetic children suffer from severe nutritional deficiencies, although they have plenty to eat. The average American supermarket-bought diet of overprocessed, canned, and frozen foods is so lacking in vital nutritive elements, especially vitamins, minerals, and trace elements, that it may lead to chronic nutritional deficiencies. Result: overfed but undernourished children.
8. Such environmental factors as loud noises or noise inaudible to the human ear (infrasounds),[4] and artificial light, such as fluorescent room lighting. Studies show that changing the lighting to a type of light spectrum more like that of the sun improved the hyperactive behavior immediately.[5]
9. Drugs. Many commonly used prescription and nonprescription drugs can trigger hyperkinesis in children.[8]
10. Lack of authoritative discipline and clear, defined rules of family life and expected behavior. Children, even at a very early age, must know exactly what is expected of them and what they can and can't do. Some system of reward for good behavior and punishment for misbehavior is a must. Undisciplined and left on their own, children feel neglected, disoriented, confused, and tend to react with irrational behavior.
11. Deprivation of love and affection. Sometimes, hyperkinetic symptoms, especially destructiveness, rebelliousness, and bad temper, are expressions of deep-seated feelings of insecurity and of being unloved or unwanted.

Holistic treatment

As you can see from the above, hyperactivity in a child can be a complex health disorder caused by many contributing factors, singularly or in combination. Therefore, the most effective treatment should be a total holistic approach, taking into consideration all possible contributing causes and eliminating as many of them as possible.

I shall suggest a mode of action, listing my recommendations with numbers corresponding to the above-mentioned eleven contributing causes of hyperkinesis.

1. Eliminate from the child's diet everything that contains artificial colors and flavors. *You must become an avid label reader.* Do not give your child any processed, bottled, or canned foods or drinks before you read the small print of contents on the label and are assured that they do not contain artificial flavorings or colorings.

2. The above rule of thumb also applies to *all* man-made chemicals, preservatives, and additives. Since most processed, prepared, pre-packaged, or canned foods sold in supermarkets or restaurants today are loaded with many chemical additives, the only way to make sure that your child's diet is free of all chemical additives is to buy only fresh, natural, unprocessed foods and prepare all food yourself. For example, it is almost impossible to find a restaurant today that is not using MSG in food preparation. Also, all the oils used in restaurant cooking and frying contain BHA and BHT. If lead poisoning is suspected and/or diagnosed, large doses of supplementary zinc and vitamin C should be added to the list of suggested supplements that follows under Number 6.

3. Eliminate all refined white sugar and white flour from child's diet. That means: all commercial ice cream, cookies, cakes, donuts, candies, soft drinks, bread, etc. Sounds almost impossible? It is, admittedly, not easy. But, in the long run, it will be well worth the effort.

4. All caffeine-containing beverages and foods must be strictly avoided. You wouldn't think of giving your two or four year old a cup of coffee, yet many mothers allow small children to drink cola beverages without realizing that they contain huge amounts of caffeine. Here is a list of beverages and drugs that contain caffeine:

Brewed coffee, 1 cup	100-150 mg. caffeine
Tea, 1 cup	60-75 mg. caffeine
Cola drinks, 1 glass	40-60 mg. caffeine
Aspirin or Bromo-Seltzer, 1 tablet	32 mg. caffeine
Excedrin, 1 tablet	60 mg. caffeine

Caffeine, just like an excess of sugar, causes severe disorders in a child's sugar metabolism and contributes to the development of hypoglycemia—a condition in which the brain does not receive a sufficient amount of oxygen, causing many of the hyperkinetic symptoms and learning and behavior disorders.

5. Hyperactivity, especially aggressiveness, bad temper, and bad moods, are often caused by unrecognized allergies. A hyperkinetic child should be checked for possible food allergies, and if it is found that he is allergic to certain foods, they should be eliminated from his diet. Cow's milk should be the first suspect, especially if the child was formula-fed as a baby.

6. If your child is hyperactive because of low blood sugar (hypoglycemia), you must follow the dietary restrictions as described in my book, *Hypoglycemia: A Better Approach*, which is available from health food stores or from the publishers of this book.

7. Feed your child the Optimum Diet of nutritious foods as described in Chapters 3, 4, and 8 of this book. Make sure he receives plenty of fresh vegetables and whole grain products. Whole-grain cereal should be eaten at least once a day. Millet,

buckwheat, whole rice, or oatmeal cereals are best. Also, beans, peas, or lentil soups and homemade bread, raw nuts and seeds—these are all important preventive and health-building foods. Avoid large amounts of fruit juices, even homemade, but let your child eat fresh, whole fruit. Most fruit juices contain too much concentrated sugar, as well as natural salicylates, which can put too much stress on the child's digestive system, as well as distort his sugar metabolism. Don't force him to drink the traditional orange juice every morning! He will be better off without it. Add to his diet protective vitamins and supplements according to his age, as suggested in Chapter 9. Here are specific vitamins and supplements that can help your hyperactive child:

Brewer's yeast—1 tsp. to 1 tbsp.

B-complex vitamins, with B_{12} (100% natural formula, made from yeast)

B_6—25 to 100 mg.

B_3—25 to 100 mg.

C—200 to 1,200 mg.

Pantothenic acid—25 to 100 mg.

E—50 to 400 I.U.

A—5,000 to 10,000 units

"Nature's Minerals"—2 to 5 tablets

B_{15}—50 mg.

These are daily dosages, which should be adjusted to the age of the child—the older the child, the larger the dosage.

8. Make sure that your child has not picked up the habit of listening to unbearably loud music. Quiet, soft, mellow music is conducive to quietness and gentleness in disposition, while loud music can make a child irritable, nervous, and ill-tempered. See that your child does not have fluorescent lighting in his room or spend too much time in rooms that are artificially lighted. The amount of natural daylight your child receives has a definite effect on

his behavior. Dr. John Ott's studies show that sunlight improves behavior in hyperactive children.[5]

9. Since many prescription and non-prescription drugs can contribute to hyperkinesis, do not allow your hyperactive child to take any drugs except in cases of medical emergency, and then only if prescribed by a physician who is aware of your child's condition.

10. You will find them in every city, in every town: hundreds of young men and women who move aimlessly from place to place, can't hold a job, can't stay in school long enough to complete their studies, can't develop a responsible relationship; who have no desire to stay in contact with their parents; who are undisciplined, disoriented, confused, and insecure. They come from homes where "enlightened" parents raised them without discipline, according to the dictates of modern pediatricians and psychologists. They have never learned respect for elders, for authorities, for the law, not even for their parents. Hence, not being disciplined at home, they haven't learned to discipline themselves. Psychologists have finally changed their minds and now realize the need for strict parental guidance and discipline, but a generation of misled parents—and their unfortunate children—must pay the high price for this scientific experiment.

To raise a self-respecting, self-reliant, disciplined, confident, and well-balanced young man or woman, you must train him or her throughout childhood to respect parental authority and abide by the clear-cut rules and responsibilities of communal living as a family unit. Children must know exactly what their duties as well as their rights are, what is expected or not expected of them, what they can and what they cannot do. They must be punished for disobedience and misbehavior, and rewarded for exceptional behavior and actions. By punishment, I don't mean beating them! Suspension of special privileges or allowances is an effective and educational form of punishment. All-the-while, make sure your child understands that discipline and rules are designed *for his own good*, that they are motivated by his father's and mother's deep love and concern for his future welfare and happiness.

11. Finally, make sure that your child does not harbor feelings and fears—justified or imagined—that he is unloved, unappreciated, or unwanted. Shower him with all the love and affection he is entitled to! A hyperkinetic child needs even more love than a normal, healthy child. He is starved for love—he craves it! A child without love is worse off than a child without food. Love is the best nourishment, the best medicine, the best comforter. Plenty of parental love is imperative for the optimum health and happiness of the child.

I know that if you follow the 11-point program outlined above, you can expect dramatic changes in your hyperkinetic child's behavior. During the last several years, I have had an opportunity to suggest this holistic program to several parents of hyperkinetic children, and *all* of them were amazed at the results. Hyperactive children became calm, their school work improved, and they became well-adjusted, harmonious, and obedient children, popular with their classmates and with teachers.

I will admit that this 11-point program isn't easy to follow, but every parent of an improved hyperkinetic child will concur, it is well worth the effort.

Re: The Feingold Diet for Hyperactive Children

Those who are interested in learning more about the pioneering work on diet for hyperactivity by Ben F. Feingold, M.D., mentioned earlier in this chapter, should obtain and read carefully his excellent book, *Why Your Child is Hyperactive*, published by Random House, New

York, N.Y., 1975. It is available from most book stores, or directly from:

> Feingold Association of the United States,
> 2941 Wilson Ave.,
> Redding, Calif. 96001

The Association will also be happy to supply you with the newest research material on hyperactivity, as well as answer your questions regarding the Feingold Diet.

Keep in mind, however, that the dietary approach, important as it is, may not always be sufficient to help each case of this condition. The *total*, holistic approach, as advocated in this chapter, is best to achieve fast and lasting results in the treatment of hyperactivity.

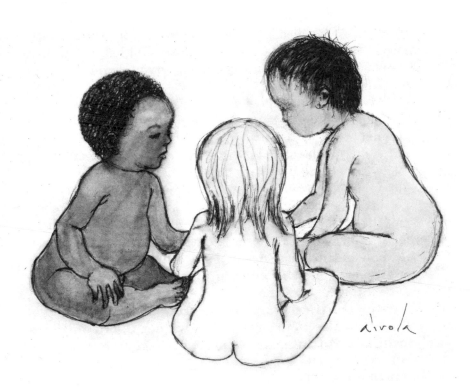

15

Infant Obesity

The following question appeared in one of my magazine columns:

"Dear Doctor: My pediatrician says that my 8-month-old baby is 4 pounds overweight. He weighs 28 pounds. We—my husband, my parents, and myself—and most of our friends think he is a cute looking baby, perhaps a little plump and pale, but nice and cuddly. He has a good appetite. I've nursed him for four months, but now he is on formula and also gets a lot of other foods such as cereals, fruit juices, mashed potatoes, and some commercial baby foods. How can I help him to lose weight? Or, rather, should I? He seems to always be hungry and cries if I don't feed him."

My answer to her was as follows:

Pudgy babies, like their overweight adult counterparts, are not healthy. Overweight is often the result of malnutrition. Bottle-fed babies and babies on commercial baby foods are especially likely to be undernourished. Overfed, but undernourished! Let me explain.

Ideally, a baby should be breast-fed for at least eight months to a year. Breast milk supplies optimum nutrition for infants without excess calories. Consequently, breast-fed babies are almost never obese. With artifical feeding, it is different. First, commercial formulas contain, as a rule, more calories than mother's milk: more fat, more sugar, more protein. Encouragement to drink the entire content of the bottle also contributes to the higher caloric intake of artificially-fed infants.[1] Second, although the artificially-fed baby is getting more calories, he is getting less of the important vitamins and minerals, especially iron, and other trace elements that are present in mother's milk. Consequently, trying desperately to get the missing nutrients, the baby will eat more and more. But, since you are filling him up with nutritionally-deficient, but calorie-rich foods, he is getting fat. Thus, as you can see, a baby can actually be overfed but undernourished.

It is significant that you, as well as the baby's grandparents, think that your overweight baby is "cute." In our prosperous culture, we often equate fatness with cuteness, especially in children. Ours is a so-called "clean-plate society," where a mother cajoles her children into finishing every last bite or spoonful. As the mother stuffs her children with mashed potatoes and gravy, she always reminds them to think of "all the starving children around the world." So, we have fatter and fatter babies and children, and, consequently, fatter adults. In fact, over half of our population is overweight and 30 percent of the adults and 20 percent of the teenagers are actually obese!

To prevent this national problem of obesity, we must start with infants. Several studies indicate that a too high caloric intake in infancy and childhood can lead to the growth of excessive numbers of fat cells in the body, which may be permanently fixed in number throughout life.[2, 3] Studies showed that the number of fat cells developed during infancy persisted throughout life, regardless of diet. That is, when an infant is overfed, he develops a much larger number of fat cells in his body than a normal infant. That excessive number of cells will remain with him for life and cannot be reduced by dieting in later years.[4] "Those fat cells will be waiting to be filled throughout life," says Dr. Sarah Short, associate professor of nutrition of Syracuse University in New York. Thus, the so-called "healthy, plump baby" is likely to become the obese adult. A study of overweight children revealed that most of them had been overweight since infancy.[5]

Although the fat-cell theory is still debated among the scientists, there is a united consensus among pediatric experts that fat babies are not healthy babies, and that a tendency towards overweight during infancy may set a pattern of life-long overeating and a chronic problem of excess weight. It is also well known that fat babies have more health problems than slim or normal weight babies. They have more respiratory ailments, and are more susceptible to colds, diabetes, and communicable children's diseases, and even heart disease.

Mothers of fat babies often complain, "He is always hungry! What can I do?" Yes, if once you have allowed him, by overfeeding and improper nutrition, to become fat, he will always be hungry. How *can* you get your overweight baby to lose weight?

First, what you *cannot* do. You cannot use any kind of fasting or reducing diet for your infant or child! Forcing young infants and children to go on a reducing diet can have irreparable physical and, especially, psychological consequences. Dieting is harmless only if it is accompanied by a complete understanding and conscious will and desire to discipline one's own eating habits. Without such an understanding and deliberate desire, dieting becomes starvation. You cannot very well cut down on the amount of foods the fat, but undernourished, child obviously craves.

The solution? *You must improve the nutritional quality of the infant's diet*. Follow the advice on infant feeding in Chapters 7 and 8. Give him vitamin supplements as suggested in chapter 9. If you feed your child according to the dietary principles of *Optimum Nutrition* as outlined in this book, his improved diet will supply the optimal amounts of all the minerals, vitamins, and other nutrients he needs, and *he will stop overeating*. His excessive craving for food will disappear because the optimal diet of nutritious foods will supply him with adequate amounts of all the nutrients he needs.

Prevention of chronic obesity must begin right after birth. Exclusive breast feeding for as long as possible is the best way to prevent infant obesity. When the infant is weaned, he must adhere to the Optimum Diet, as recommended in Chapters 3 and 4 of this book. It is the parents' responsibility to keep the cupboards and refrigerator free of all sugar and sugar-containing products, and processed, canned, calorie-rich, but nutritionless junk foods that contribute to obesity. Parents must also encourage children at an early age to be physically active, play games, participate in sports, work, etc. Vigorous physical activity is an essential adjunct to proper nutrition in a meaningful preventive program against overweight.

16

Colic

Almost every mother—and father, and the rest of the family, too—has been through the following, all-too-familiar and frustrating (I am tempted to say "classic") experience:

Soon after the feeding, sometimes even before it is finished, the baby begins to stir uncomfortably. He stiffens his legs and pulls them up, drawing his thighs up on his abdomen as if in intense pain, screams piercingly, and continues shrieking and wailing for two, three, or four hours, with hardly a respite. His abdomen becomes distended with gas and he may pass gas from the rectum or by burping. But neither gas relief seems to stop his discomfort and frantic screaming. The desperate mother tries a pacifier, or rocking, or a drink of water, or more burping, turning him over, changing him—but nothing seems to help! Finally, when the mother's and father's nerves are raw and screaming too, mostly from a combination of fear, rage, exhaustion, and frustration at being unable to command the situation or help the poor baby, the frantic screaming stops and the baby falls into a limp sleep.

According to reliable studies, most small babies (one doctor estimated as many as 80 percent) go through this routine, which is called *COLIC*. It usually starts between the second and sixth week of life and usually lasts about three months. This three-month pattern is so regular that the condition is commonly-referred to as the "three-month colic."

The babies seem to be regular in terms of the exact time of day that they perform this routine. Lucky are those parents whose babies have their colic in the daytime and sleep peacefully in the evening and night. My sympathy goes to parents whose baby sleeps happily all day and cries half the night! Most babies seem to become uncomfortable after the evening feeding.

The following common observations about colic can be made, for what they are worth, since they do not solve the mystery of colic:

- Colic seems to be perfectly harmless to the baby. It doesn't matter how uncomfortable and how much in pain he looks when he screams, after he finally tires himself out and takes a long nap, he awakes happy, and is himself again. And he is growing and developing well, being perfectly healthy by all the normal signs.
- Colic most often begins after a feeding, sometimes right after, sometimes half an hour or so later.
- Both breast-fed babies and formula-fed babies are subject to colic, although formula-fed babies are more susceptible.

What causes colic?

Every pediatric text I read says that the cause is unknown. Many speculations have been offered by various writers, but none seem to fit all colic sufferers, or even many of them.

The most logical guess would be that colic is a disorder of the digestive system, but the regular disappearance of colic at three months throws researchers off and suggests that it could be a developmental condition. Dr. T. Barry Brazelton, of the Childrens' Hospital Medical Center, Boston, suggests that at an early stage of his development, the baby has no other means to relax tensions and let off emotional steam but by crying. Gradually, he replaces these crying periods with sociable interaction with his parents and with other attractions of his environment.[1]

However, as I plowed through a massive amount of research material in preparation for this chapter, and as I remembered my own experiences as a father of five children, and the many sleepless nights due to their colic, I became more and more convinced that the psychological or tension theory is wrong, that colic is a true physical problem. There is no question that during an "attack," the baby suffers physical pain, gas, and cramps. Is he faking or creating these symptoms deliberately to draw your attention, or relieve tension, or let off emotional steam? Not likely.

There is much evidence and clinical research which shows that breast-fed babies do not suffer from colic as frequently as do artificially-fed babies.[2] (See Chapter 7.)

There is also much evidence that in a breast-fed baby, colic may be caused by the baby's allergy to certain foods the nursing *mother* eats. The quality of the mother's milk is affected by her diet. Some babies are extremely sensitive to the changes in their mother's menu. Certain foods bring immediate reactions in the babies in the form of gas and digestive distress. According to Lendon H. Smith, M.D., a famous pediatrician, the most commonly-offensive foods in this regard are garlic, onions, cabbage, beans, chocolate, fish (especially tuna), eggs, corn, and wheat.[3] Some mothers reported to me that broccoli, cauliflower, and citrus fruits can also give babies colic-indigestion. This sensitivity of the baby to certain foods in the nursing mother's diet explains why at a certain time of the day he is perfectly happy with breast milk, at other times he is not. When the baby is nursed after the mother ate the meal which included the offensive foods, the milk will contain the substances that are disagreeable to the baby's digestive system. One nursing mother told me that when she took B-complex vitamins, her baby cried with colic every day for two weeks. She discontinued taking the vitamin, and the baby's crying stopped immediately. She tried B-vitamins again, and the colic returned within six hours.

Bottle-fed babies are often allergic to some ingredient in the formula, usually to cow's milk. Changing formulas and using either goat's milk or soy milk may be helpful in solving the problem. The infant may be sensitive to vitamin drops, or even to a specific sugar in the formula. Lactose, or milk sugar, is usually the best tolerated sweetener. The reason breast-fed babies suffer less often from digestive disorders and colitis is that mother's milk contains several protective factors that help prevent gastrointestinal disorders in infants. Recent studies show that both colostrum and breast milk contain secretory IgA, as well as other substances which may protect infants from enterocolitis and other intestinal disorders.[4] None of these protective factors are found in formulas, of course. Lysozyme, an antimicrobial enzyme, is present in appreciable quantities in human milk and may produce a bactericidal effect.[5] The bifidus factor in breast milk, a group of nitrogen-containing polysaccharides, promotes the growth of the beneficial bacterial flora in infants' intestines, particularly *Lactobacillus bifidus*, which lowers the pH of the intestinal tract and, thus, inhibits the growth of *E. coli*, yeast, and *Shigella*.[6, 7] Lactoferrin, which is also present in human milk, inhibits the growth of *Staphylococci* and *E. coli*.

The combined effects of all the above-mentioned protective factors in mother's milk are responsible for the fact that breast-fed babies are not as likely as bottle-fed babies to be colicky.

What can you do?

1. First, don't be alarmed or scared if this is your "first time around." Recognize the fact that *most* babies get colicky. Some are worse off than others, but the condition is fairly common and it doesn't seem to do the baby any permanent harm. On the contrary, it seems to most often occur in babies that are rather active and lively and who are developing and growing well. And, remember, the condition will probably be gone by the time the baby is three months old, if not before. Also important: don't feel guilty or blame yourself for the baby's obvious suffering.

2. Second, try to make it as comfortable as possible for the baby during a crying period. A pacifier can be helpful in some cases, although some parents disapprove of them. The colicky baby is usually more comfortable on his stomach. Sometimes, a hot water bottle can be helpful. Don't have it too hot, though, just warm enough to be held

against your arm without discomfort. Wrap the bottle in a diaper or towel before laying the baby on it, or against it. Of course, show him all the love and attention he deserves during his time of distress. Rock him, pat him, cuddle him, massage his back gently, hold him tightly against you, walk, talk, or sing to him. Don't be afraid to spoil him by showing him extra attention.

3. There are some herbal teas that are mild enough and can be helpful to baby during colic. Camomile is soothing for the stomach and intestines. Peppermint helps digestion. Catnip can help the baby to sleep. Make teas very mild (see Recipes & Directions) and give the baby a teaspoonful or two before the feeding that is normally followed by colic distress. If made mild enough, herbal teas cannot harm the baby even at a very young age.

4. The Biochemic tissue salt, *Mag. Phos.,* which can be obtained in most health food stores, can be of great benefit for colic. Give two little tablets in a teaspoon of warm water.

5. Take a look at your own diet and see if you are eating some of the most commonly-offensive foods, drinks, or vitamins mentioned earlier. Eliminating them one at a time can help to determine which one is causing trouble.

6. If your baby is on formula, try to substitute it for a day or two with a yogurt or acidophilus milk formula. You can make your own yogurt from whole raw milk (it must be whole, not skimmed) using yogurt culture bought in a health food store. Or you can make your own acidophilus milk by using acidophilus tablets or culture, also sold in health food stores. When milk is curdled, place it in a blender and run until curds are all liquified and milk is smooth. Mix 50-50 with boiled, then cooled, water, and feed by bottle. Such a milk is virtually predigested milk and often not only cures the colic problem, but prevents its recurrence by cultivating the beneficial *Lactobacillus acidophilus* and *Lactobacillus bifidus* bacteria in the intestines.

If you breast-feed your baby, you may try to give him a few drops of liquid acidophilus culture (sold in health food stores) with a spoonful of boiled, then cooled, water before or after nursing. Many mothers have found this to be very effective.

Yogurt and acidophilus formulas are well tolerated by all babies, healthy or ill, but are especially useful for infants suffering from enteritis, diarrhea, constipation, gas, allergy to milk, colitis, and other disorders of the digestive tract.

Note: homemade yogurt or acidophilus milk, made from raw goat's or cow's milk is best (See Recipes & Directions). If commercial yogurt or acidophilus milk is used, add ½ cup of thin cream to each quart as they are usually made from skimmed milk. If acidophilus or yogurt formula is given for more than a few days, add 2 tbsp. of lactose (milk sugar) to each quart. Lactose is sold in health food stores and drug stores.

Not all crying is colic

Of course, you must understand that not all crying is symptomatic of colic or a digestive problem. Crying is about the only way the baby can communicate with his environment at this age. He can cry for a number of reasons. He may be hungry, or cold, or too hot, or wet, or uncomfortable, or a safety pin is sticking him, or the flies are biting him, or noises are irritating him, or the light is too bright—or he is just missing you and wants a little love and attention! Give it to him! The more love and attention you show to your baby now, the better adjusted he will be, and the problems of raising him later on will be minimized.

17

Acne

Adolescent acne, or *Acne vulgaris*, is not only the most common form of chronic skin disease, but also a most torturous and agonizing condition, which manifests itself during the age when growing and sexually-maturing adolescents are painfully conscious of their appearance.

Acne is a disorder which usually sets in at puberty. According to the National Center for Health Statistics (NCHS), it affects as many as 86.4 percent of all pre-teens and teenagers! It may be mild and brief, or severe and chronic, but in one form or another, most adolescents suffer from it. The most frequently affected areas are the face, chest, shoulders, and back.

In mild cases, acne manifests itself as a few pimples and/or blackheads, or whiteheads. In severe cases, when sebum (lubricating oil from sebaceous glands) is trapped and clogs the pores, it forms infected cysts. Acne can affect extensive areas with large infected cysts which can seriously damage the skin and leave permanent scars.

What causes acne?

Although orthodox medicine considers the *Bacillus acnes* to be a cause of acne (still being Pasteur-oriented as they are, and always on the look-out for a bacteria or virus as the cause of all ills), the holistic medical view of this seemingly limited skin disorder is more comprehensive and more than "skin deep." Although germs known as *Bacilli acnes*, more specifically *Staphylococcus aureus, Staphylococcus acnitis*, and *Corynebacterium acnes*, can be found, along with several other varieties of germs, in the *comedones* (irritated and inflamed blackheads and pimples), they are, according to a newer biological medical concept, a *result* of acne, rather than the cause. The germs only flourish in the greasy, clogged sebaceous glands, where excessive oils, trapped by the overgrowth of the horny layer of the skin, stagnate and change chemically to become a desirable medium for bacterial growth. But the *primary* causes of acne are the underlying metabolic, biochemical, glandular, and hormonal conditions which contribute to the pathological developments in the skin and excessive oil, or *sebum*, production.

The following are the known underlying contributing causes of Acne vulgaris:

(1) Excessive and accelerated sex hormone production during puberty, resulting in excessive sebum production.

(2) Malnutrition and/or nutritional deficiencies.

(3) Allergy to certain foods, beverages, and drugs.

(4) Menstrual irregularities.

(5) Constipation.

(6) Anemia.

(7) Lack of exercise.

(8) Physical and mental stresses and lack of rest and relaxation.

Let's take a look at these contributing causes, one at a time.

Excessive sebum production

Since acne is a puberty-related condition, it has long been known that excessive secretion of oil by the sebaceuos glands is effected by the sex hormones which begin to pour into the system at the beginning of sexual awakening. Sebaceous glands produce more lubricating oil after the onset of puberty and continue to do so for as long as ten or more years, or until physical and sexual maturation is complete.

But, since the increased hormonal output during puberty is perfectly *normal and natural*, and acne is clearly an *unnatural and an abnormal* pathological condition (clear, healthy skin is the "birthright" of every healthy individual—even during puberty), the question can be asked: why would such a natural function as sex hormone output lead to such an unnatural, pathological condition as acne?

There is a logical answer to this logical question: the *normal* activity of sex glands, even during puberty, does not cause acne—the *abnormal* activity does! Normally, sexual maturity is a slow and gradual process. Sexual glands in both male and female begin to mature early, but do not begin to secrete hormones until the child reaches the age of 14 to 16. In our culture, however, sexual maturity is accelerated and the age of puberty is lowered by several years. It is now common that menstruation begins at the ages of 10 to 12, whereas only a few generations ago, it was 3 to 4 years later. The reasons for this premature sexual development are many: early mental and physical sexual stimulation in our sex-oriented and permissive culture; overeating—especially the excessive consumption of meat and milk products; massive use by pre-adolescents of such items as sugar, salt, strong spices, drugs, caffeine-containing foods and beverages, alcohol, and tobacoo—all nerve and endocrine gland stimulating and irritating substances.

All the above-mentioned factors contribute to earlier sexual maturity by stimulating the pituitary gland as well as sex glands to earlier sex hormone production. When sexual development is normal and not accelerated by dietary factors, overeating and conducive environment, as it is now in most "primitive," underdeveloped countries, such as India, China, Central and South America, etc., acne is a very rare occurrence. When sexual maturity is natural, slow and apportioned to the body's general growth and development, the sex hormones do not cause excessive sebum production. But when sexual growth is premature or accelerated, and the balance of the various sex hormones not yet stabilized, it leads to abnormal biochemical reactions by the underdeveloped body. Acne is one of these abnormalities.

That hormonal imbalances contribute to acne was

demonstrated by a study conducted at the University of Oklahoma Health Sciences Center. The majority of women who took oral contraceptives in which *progesterone*, rather than *estrogen*, was the dominant hormone, were affected by severe acne. They showed marked improvement when they switched to an estrogen-dominant preparation.[1] Many women experience acne flare-ups following discontinuation of birth control pills.

Malnutrition and nutritional deficiencies

I have had an ample opportunity in my capacity as a naturopathic physician as well as nutrition consultant to observe that vegetarian and other health-food oriented teenagers only seldom suffer from acne. There is massive clinical and empirical evidence that overeating, improper diet, as well as nutritional deficiencies caused by eating nutritionless, processed, and denatured foods, are definite contributing causes to acne.

Overeating and consequent adolescent obesity are definitely contributing factors to acne and other skin disorders. Eating such "junk" foods as sugar in every form, white bread, cookies, ice cream, candies, chocolate, deep-fried, greasy foods, and drinking sugar- and caffeine-containing cola-type beverages are other dietary factors definitely linked to acne. Vitamin and mineral deficiencies caused by such diets, especially deficiencies of iron, zinc, and vitamin A, are directly tied to the development of acne.

Excessive salt in the American diet is another acne-related factor, Dr. Edward Caul of Evansville, Indiana, says that the tendency towards the formation of comedones (whiteheads and blackheads) is increased by excessive *sodium*, and formation of pustules and cysts is increased by excessive *chlorine* in the diet.[2] Common salt, sodium chloride, contains both sodium and chlorine. As is well known, our teenagers are notorious for their consumption of highly salted nuts, crackers, potato chips, peanut butter, popcorn, pretzels, relishes, etc.

Chocolate and cocoa, so favored by the adolescents in

America, are other common culprits. Chocolate and cocoa are derived from the seeds of the South American cocoa tree and contain the acne-stimulating ingredient, *Theobromine Dimethylxanthine*, which is chemically similar to caffeine, the nerve stimulant present in coffee, tea, and cola drinks. That means that you should never use chocolate bars, chocolate-coated candies, chocolate ice cream, chocolate milk or milk shakes, chocolate cakes, chocolate icing, chocolate cookies, chocolate donuts, chocolate custards. You must also avoid cola drinks which normally contain *cocoa* and *cola*, among other harmful ingredients.

Allergy to foods and drugs

It has been shown that allergy to certain foods and drugs is often a major contributing cause of acne. One recent report in the *Medical Tribune* linked the development of common acne with allergy to certain animal and vegetable proteins.[3]

By a strict elimination diet, instituted after careful testing for food allergies, some doctors have achieved over 70 percent "good to very good" results if the diet was strictly followed.

The most common allergens (foods that acne sufferers are most likely to be allergic to) are: wheat products, milk and cheese products, tomatoes, mustard, pepper, and paprika. But *any* food can be an allergen to some people. Therefore, if you have "tried everything" and failed to effect a betterment in your acne condition, a visit to an allergist to determine the sensitivity or possible allergies to acne-causing foods, may be in order. By the elimination of the offensive foods or drugs, a dramatic improvement in acne is often evidenced. By taking large amounts of vitamin C, B_6, and A, you can also increase your body's resistance and its ability to counteract the toxic and acne-causing effects of allergens.

Menstrual irregularities

It has been the observation of many a dermatologist as well as many women who have never visited a dermatologist, that acne is often time-related to the menstrual cycle. Some teenagers, as well as more mature women, have an acne breakout a week or two before menstruation; their skin seems to completely clear up after the menstrual period. Those who suffer from more severe acne may experience a noticeable flareup of their acne condition before menstrual periods. This is related to the hormonal output which changes during the monthly cycle. Prior to menstruation, more progesterone than estrogen is produced to prepare the lining of the womb for the fertilized ovum. If pregnancy does not occur, the hormone-prepared womb lining is then shed away in what is known as menstruation. After the menstrual period, hormonal output is changed again—less progesterone, more estrogen—until the time of ovulation!

These menstruation-related causes of acne have been helped dramatically by oral administration (sometimes intravenous) of vitamin B_6 (pyridoxine) and by the external use of vitamin B_6 cream.[4] Every individual seems to need different doses of B_6 for effective control of acne; some take as much as 400 mg. or more a day; some require much less. B_6 can also help to eliminate another common problem associated with menstruation in some women—water retention. Although B_6 is considered to be harmless you should clear it with your doctor if you need to take larger than normal doses.

Constipation, anemia, lack of exercise

Chronic constipation is one of the main causes of excessive systemic toxicity. When our "usual" detoxifying organs, such as kidneys, are overloaded, the body uses the skin—our biggest eliminative organ—to throw off many systemic toxins. The result: skin eruptions, rashes, eczemas, and acne.

Lack of exercise contributes to internal sluggishness and poor elimination, which in turn contributes to the skin eruptions.

Anemia, especially associated with excessive blood loss during profuse menstruation, as well as dietary-caused iron-deficiency anemia, have been linked to the appearance of acne in some teenage girls.

Physical and mental stresses

Testosterone is a male sex hormone which has been known to stimulate acne development when it is secreted in excessive amounts during puberty. But testosterone production is not limited to the sex glands, neither is it limited to males. The adrenal glands of both boys and girls produce a small quantity of testosterone under the influence of excessive physical, and especially emotional and anxiety-type *stress*. Many teenagers are stressed by fatigue due to lack of sleep or rest, or due to worries and anxieties.

Therefore, sufficient sleep, relaxation, and peace of mind are good preventatives, as well as treatments for acne. Many have noticed that acne improves during the relaxation of a summer vacation spent at the beach with moderate exposure to the sun and sea-water swimming.

Zinc—the nutritional anti-acne miracle

While most orthodox dermatologists still insist that diet has nothing to do with acne, subject their patients to strong antibiotics, especially tetracycline, and recommend skin peeling, irradiation, or treatment with cortisone-based medication, some avant-garde physicians around the world have begun to suspect and clinically prove that dietary abnormalities—excesses or deficiencies—play a significant role in causing acne. They have also found that a nutritional approach in the treatment of acne offers the best results so far.

Of all the specific nutrients associated causatively as well as therapeutically with acne, *zinc* seems to be the most important.

Studies at the prestigious Swedish University Hospital at Uppsala demonstrated that a zinc deficiency may be the primary factor in causing acne. A group of 64 acne patients participated in the study. After only 4 weeks of 45 mg. daily zinc supplementation, 65 percent of the pimples disappeared, and after 12 weeks, 87 percent of the acne was cleared up![5]

In the United States, zinc deficiency is quite common, mostly due to the soil depletion and the fact that whole grains (the best food source of zinc) are not widely used in the American diet. Some daily diets in hospitals as well as in average American households have been found to contain only 4 to 7 mg. of zinc—well below the recommended 15 to 20 mg.[5] By the way, both copper-type I.U.D.'s and hormones in birth control pills can reduce the amount of zinc in the blood.

I have many letters in my files from readers of my book, *How To Get Well*, in which I recommended zinc for acne, who report that their acne was "miraculously" cured in a few weeks by taking 20-30-40 mg. of zinc a day—after years of unsuccessfully trying everything else!

Other nutritional factors related to acne

Two vitamins have been used successfully to treat acne: niacin and vitamin A. Taken in doses of 100 to 200 mg. a day, niacin produces facial flush, and has been found to be more effective in acne treatment than niacinamide, which does not produce the flush. Vitamin A, which is a well-known "skin vitamin," is also useful in the treatment of acne, when taken in doses of 100,000 to 150,000 units per day. Let your doctor determine the proper dosage for you. The length of treatment with either of these vitamins in large dosages should not exceed one month. Treatment can be repeated after a one-month interval. Some doctors advocate the use of a water-soluble form of vitamin A, since natural, fish-liver-oil based vitamin A, is often poorly utilized, contains too much oil and iodine, and is less effective in acne treatment.[2]

B-complex vitamins and B-complex-rich brewer's yeast have also been used successfully in the treatment of acne.[6]

Garlic, garlic oil, and garlic preparation (capsules and tablets) have likewise been used effectively in the treatment of skin disorders such as eczema and acne.[7]

Although the following is not exactly a natural, nutritional factor, it is, nevertheless, a vitamin treatment, and should be mentioned here. It is vitamin A acid,

retinoic acid, marketed under the names of Retin-A and
Tretinoin (as Retin-A cream, 0.1% concentration, or Retin-
A gel, 0.025%), available only by prescription.[2]

Holistic approach to acne

It must be evident from the material presented in this
chapter that there are many underlying causes of acne;
hormonal,nutritional, allergic, environmental, pathological, etc. The holistic treatment for acne must, therefore, begin with the *elimination of the underlying
causes*. If, beginning at birth, the child is raised in ac-
cordance with the nutritional and other lifestyle principles
advocated in this book, the likelihood of his developing
acne will be minimal. Exclusive breast feeding during
infancy and adherence to the Optimum Diet with a
minimum of meat and animal proteins during childhood
will prevent premature puberty and prevent the excessive
hormonal insult on a body too young and undeveloped to
handle such an excess. Breast feeding and the Optimum
Diet are also likely to prevent the development of allergies,
constipation, nutritional deficiencies, and anemia—other
common underlying causes of acne.

However, there are those who do suffer now and are
tormented by this "embarrassing" disease. What can they
do to alleviate or correct the condition? Here are some
helpful hints from the bag of a holistic practitioner:

1. *Diet.* Avoid all refined and processed foods; avoid
(or eat sparingly) meat, fish, fowl, cow's milk and cheese.
Avoid also wheat and wheat products, salt, coffee, tea, cola
drinks, sugar in every form, chocolate and cocoa, and
orange juice. Eliminate from the diet all foods that you are
possibly sensitive or allergic to. Do not eat fried or greasy
foods and avoid an excess of fat in the diet, even an excess
of vegetable oils. The emphasis in the diet should be on
raw foods, especially fresh fruits and vegetables and
sprouted seeds, such as alfalfa, soybean, and mungbean
sprouts, and whole-grain cereals, such as millet and brown
rice.

2. *Hygiene.* Twice-daily washing of oily skin is recommended. Use natural soaps sold in health food stores. Do not use commercial cleansers for face or affected parts. If skin is too oily, use a drying soap or lotion, or aloe vera gel, which are sold in health food stores and drug stores. Expose the face to the sun and fresh air as often as possible.

3. *Cosmetics.* Cosmetics can give you acne! *Acne cosmetica* is a well-known term among dermatologists. It is acne caused by any of the various cosmetics, lotions, and creams used by most women today. Many cosmetics contain harsh synthetic materials that irritate the skin and cause acne-like rashes and lesions, as researchers found at the well-known acne clinic at the Hospital of the University of Pennsylvania in Philadelphia.[8]

4. *Constipation.* If constipated, follow the anti-constipation program described in Chapter 31. Many skin problems, including acne, disappear when elimination is improved.

5. *Cleansing fast.* A one- or two-week cleansing juice fast is extremely helpful in ridding the system of the accumulated toxins and restoring health, including the health of the skin. Follow the detailed instructions for fasting as outlined in my book, *How To Keep Slim, Healhty, and Young, with Juice Fasting.*[9]

6. *Eliminate stresses.* Since acne can be caused and is always aggravated by emotional stresses, imbalances, and anxieties, plenty of rest, relaxation, and peace of mind are essential in the holistic program for acne treatment. Get plenty of sleep at night. Avoid all undue stresses and worries.

7. *Avoid smoking and alcohol.* Smoking is a great skin-destroyer and excessive use of alcohol definitely aggravates acne.

8. *Vitamins and supplements.* The following supplements should be taken daily in addition to the diet suggested earlier. The doses listed are for adults; children up to the age of 18 should take ½ dose:

> Vitamin A—50,000 to 75,000 units daily for one month. Can be repeated after a one-month interval.
> Zinc—20 - 50 mg.
> Vitamin E—200 - 400 I.U.
> Vitamin C—1,000 to 3,000 mg.
> Vitamin B₆—50 - 100 mg. (especially for acne caused by menstrual irregularities.)[10]
> Niacin—200 - 400 mg.
> Pantothenic acid—300 - 400 mg.
> B-complex, high potency
> Dolomite or bone meal—2 - 3 tablets
> "Nature's Minerals"—5 tablets
> Acidophilus culture, liquid—1 tbsp., or equivalent in capsule.
> Brewer's yeast—1 - 2 tbsp. powder.

The above-mentioned supplements are sold in health food stores.

9. *Herbs.* The following herbs have been used effectively in treatment of acne: dandelion, burdock, red clover, golden seal, chaparral. Use these herbs, separately or mixed, in the form of tea: steep 1 tsp. of dried herb or the content of 2 - 3 capsules in a cup of boiling water for 15 minutes. Strain and sweeten with honey.

10. *Healing masks.* The following healing packs or masks, used externally, have been reported to be effective:

- grated cucumbers
- oatmeal cooked in milk
- a mixture of sulfur and black molasses
- aloe vera
- yogurt
- cooked creamed carrots
- vitamin E, mixed with raw egg white
- lemon juice

Masks are left on for one-half hour, then washed off with cold water. (See Chapter 32 for detailed instructions on how to make and apply masks.)

18

Worms

Worm infestations are not limited to the primitive or "developing" countries, they are common among children even in the United States. There are many different kinds of parasitic worms that live and multiply in human bodies. They most often infect the intestines, but some types are found in other organs, in the blood, in the lymphatic system, in the skin, and in the muscle tissue.

Most worm infections are passed from person to person through food, water, or soil contaminated with human feces that contain worm eggs and/or through direct body to body contact.

The most common intestinal worms affecting children are pinworms, roundworms, hookworms, and tapeworms.

Pinworms

Pinworms (sometimes called threadworms or seat-worms) are small parasitic worms, about a quarter of an inch long. They look like thin white threads. They are the commonest variety in small children, although they may affect adults as well.

Pinworms live in the lower intestine, but come out into the anal region at night to lay their eggs. They cause intense itching between the buttocks, which is the principle symptom of their presence. Their crawling can also be felt, and in small children, sometimes mild abdominal pain, diarrhea, and nausea can accompany the condition. The child's sleep is badly disturbed. Since he tends to scratch the area, the eggs are sometimes lodged under the finger-nails and cling to the hands. Unless the hands and nails are scrubbed constantly, the child may infect other children and members of the family or set up a cycle of re-infecting himself.

After the pinworms are discovered and treatment initiated, it is important that the towels, bedclothes, pajamas, and underwear of the infected child be boiled for twenty minutes or so at least twice a week. The toilet seat also should be scrubbed with soap after each time he comes in contact with it.

Roundworms

The giant intestinal roundworm is a fairly common parasite, especially in children. It looks very much like an earthworm. The diagnosis is usually made when a worm, or many worms, are discovered in the child's feces. Roundworms usually do not cause any symptoms unless the child has a great number of them.

Roundworm infection is spread through contaminated foods. The feces of infected persons contain many worm eggs. The worm itself is pearly white in color, and may be, in the adult state, up to 8 - 12 inches long.

Hookworms

Hookworms are about one half inch long and derive their name from the hooked teeth by which the adult worms fasten themselves to the lining of the small intestine where they suck the victim's blood. Hookworms are common in some parts of the Southern United States, in Asia, and in Africa.

Hookworm disease is contracted by going barefoot in soil that is infested by larvae which develop from eggs that are produced by a female worm in the human intestines and passed out in the feces. Larvae are able to burrow into the skin of the feet and enter the bloodstream. Several weeks later, the larvae reach the intestines as adult worms.

Diagnosis of hookworms is made by examining a feces specimen in which the eggs can easily be seen.

When present in large numbers, hookworms cause anemia, weakness, underweight, and malnutrition, and may retard normal physical and mental development of the child.

Treatment

Medical doctors use various drugs in treatment of worms. Most of the medical treatments are effective, and should be considered, unless parents have a strong objection to toxic drugs.

The following harmless, or relatively harmless, biological and herbal treatments, both ancient and modern, have been reported to be effective in removing intestinal worms:

1. *GARLIC.* Garlic has been used since early history by the Chinese, Greeks, Romans, Hindus, and Babylonians for the purpose of deworming. It has also been used by biological medical practitioners in modern times, especially in Russia and Japan. Garlic has been used in the United States in the past by practitioners of folk medicine and is recommended for that purpose by most herbal text books. Both fresh garlic and garlic preparations can be used for treatment. Children should be given as much raw crushed garlic as possible by mouth, mixed in some liquid or juice to improve palatability. If children refuse to take raw garlic, try garlic preparations, garlic oil pearls, capsules, or tablets. Or why not try an ancient method of garlic medication: place a couple of cloves of fresh garlic in each shoe—yes, shoe! As the child walks, the cloves are crushed and the worm-killing garlic oil is absorbed by the skin and carried by the blood into the intestines. Garlic possesses a powerful penetrative force. Within 10 - 15 minutes of its being rubbed on unbroken skin it can be detected in the breath. The worm-expelling effect of garlic was demonstrated in many clinical studies in Russia.

2. *SODIUM CHLORIDE.* Sodium chloride, or common table salt, is a simple, time-proven remedy for pinworms. Children who develop worms are often deficient in sodium chloride. A heavily salted diet for a week or two has been known to be effective against pinworms.

3. *ALMOND BRAN AND FIG JUICE.* This is Dr. Royal Lee's formula in tablet form, available through health food stores or through chiropractic or naturopathic

physicians. Dosage: 4 - 6 tablets orally. Children, half dose.

4. *ARECA NUT (BETELNUT)*. This herb has been used by prominent herbalists for tapeworms. Dose: 2 - 4 drachms.

5. *PINKROOT, WORMSEED, AND WORM-WOOD.* These herbs are commonly recommended by herbalists for expelling all types of intestinal worms.

6. *MALE FERN (ASPIDIUM)*. This herb is used mainly for expulsion of tapeworms. One tsp. of dry fern roots is steeped in 1 cup of boiling water for 30 minutes. Cool, and drink 1 or 2 cups during the day, a good mouthful at a time.

7. *PUMPKIN SEEDS.* This completely harmless and beneficial food has been used in folk medicine for expelling worms. Grind them in a seed grinder and give to your child by spoon, sprinkle on foods, or mix in juices or drinks.

Whether using natural, herbal, or medical treatments for expelling worms, make sure you follow the instructions regarding sanitary procedures and washing of clothing, bedclothes, towels, underwear, etc., given earlier in this chapter.

19

The Circumcision Decision

I received the following letter from one of the readers of my column on holistic health:

"Dear Dr. Airola:

I am expecting a child in four months. If it is a boy, should he or should he not be circumcised? My best friend just became the mother of a little boy and she said that the labor room nurse brought a consent form to sign, and when she was uncertain of what to do, the nurse told her that if she refused to sign, her son would be 'laughed at in gym class when he grows up.' So, she signed. Somehow, I don't feel that circumcision is right. If there is no valid functional purpose for the foreskin, then why is it there? The reasoning that the protective foreskin of such a delicate and sensitive organ is unnecessary and expendable doesn't seem logical to me. Can you enlighten me on this puzzling question?"

Circumcision (Latin work meaning "a round cut") is the removal of the protective foreskin, the prepuce, which covers the head of the penis. Until very recently, it was practiced only as a religious or tribal ritual, usually among Jews, but also among Mohammedans, Ethiopians, Indian Moslems, and some tribes of Africa. Since circumcision was introduced to the United States at the turn of the century by the Jews who immigrated here in large numbers from Eastern Europe, it has been commonly practiced, even among Gentiles. In Europe, circumcision is practiced only very seldom except by the Jews. In Russia, the Orient, Scandinavia, and Central and South American countries the practice is virtually nonexistent. In Australia, where circumcision did catch on to some extent, it was soon viewed with disfavor by the medical community. The Australian Pediatric Association passed the following resolution at a meeting in 1971: "The Australian Pediatric Association recommends that newborn male infants should not, as a routine, be circumcised."

Usually, circumcision is done shortly after birth, but sometimes it is performed during adolescence or even on adults. In the United States, circumcision is usually performed while the newborn is still in the hospital, generally on his last day before going home, by the physician attending the delivery.

The Jews justify their practice of circumcision by the interpretation of the passage in the Bible (Genesis 17:9-27) where Abraham, at the age of 99, and his son, Ishmáel, at the age of 13, were commanded by God to be circumcised. Since then, circumcision has been performed on all Jewish male infants on the eighth day after birth, as a sign of the everlasting covenant between God and the seed of Abraham. It is a symbolic religious act to insure protection against "the wrath of God" (Exodus 4:24-25). It also served as a mark of belonging to the people of Israel. No uncircumcised male was allowed to marry a daughter of Israel—thus, the purity of the race was preserved.

The practice of circumcision was abandoned by Jews who were converted to Christendom. In the New Testament, circumcision is clearly renounced by St. Paul. "Watch out for those wicked men, dangerous dogs I call them, who say you must be circumcised to be saved. For it isn't the cutting of our bodies that makes us children of God, it is worshipping him with our spirits. That is the only true circumcision." (Philippians, 3:2-3, *The Living Bible*)

The apparent reason that circumcision became widely practiced in the United States is that some studies showed that Jewish women had a considerably lesser incidence of cervical cancer than the non-Jewish women in America. This was attributed to the fact that Jewish males are circumcised, are more hygienic, and do not contribute to the vaginal infections and irritations through smegma, which uncircumcised men supposedly do. Smegma is a white, creamy substance which is secreted by the sebaceous glands of the foreskin. This material is thought by some to irritate the cervix of the uterus and possibly initiate tumor formation. Although a growing number of doctors dispute this theory, the present American vogue of circumcision—often rather forcefully and persuasively brought to the attention of expectant or new parents by hospital nurses and doctors—is based on this largely unsubstantiated medical hypothesis. Apparently, it has never occurred to those who originated this theory that although it is true that Jewis women have less cervical cancer than non-Jewish women in America, the incidence of cervical cancer is even less in many countries where the whole male population is uncircumcised—such as Japan, Germany, Switzerland, Finland, Sweden, Russia, China, or Central and South American countries. Obviously, there must be some other reasons why American non-Jewish women have a higher rate of cervical cancer. Americans have more of any kind of cancer as compared with most other countries; in fact, we lead the world in cancer statistics. In Chapter 25 on breast cancer, I explained some of the causes for this. Recent scientific studies show that cervical cancer is more prevalent among women who began an active sex life at a very early age and who have had a multiplicity of partners. Also, most Jewish people (including Jewish women), even though living in America for generations, retain many of their own dietary customs, which are, on the whole, much less cancer-producing than the diets of non-Jewish Americans.

A study made in England showed no difference in the circumcision status of the husbands of 54 cervical cancer patients and 54 control subjects.[1] A convincing study made in India showed that the Parcee women and the Indian Christian women, whose men are uncircumcised, suffer less frequently from cancer of the cervix than the women of the circumcised Indian Moslems.[2] Investigation in Kenya, Africa, revealed no significant differences in the number of cases of cervical cancer in women of tribes whose men were or were not circumcised.[3] Curiously enough, in Ethiopia, where 90 percent of the males are ritually circumcised at birth, the incidence of cervical cancer is higher than in countries of Europe where the male population is largely uncircumcised.[4]

The other common reason for advocating infant circumcision is that it supposedly prevents the development of infection of the foreskin. However, infections are mostly due not to the presence of the foreskin, but to the practice, advised by doctors, of pulling back the foreskin of young boys for daily washing. This practice is definitely harmful, and unnecessary. Many doctors now agree that the practice of pulling back the foreskin at an early age to wash out the smegma does more harm than good. At the Vancouver Birth Center, doctors now counsel mothers to leave this foreskin alone, and, as a result, they now have a 100 percent reduction in infections.

In countries where circumcision is not routinely practiced, mothers never disturb the foreskin of the baby boys and the infection problems is virtually nonexistent. In England, doctors have been telling mothers for years not to pull the foreskin back, since this practice is believed to be the primary cause of infections.[5] When the baby is born, there is a membrane that adheres to the head of the penis and keeps the foreskin tight. This membrane is for protection against bacteria and should not be destroyed, but left intact. As the penis grows, the membrane thins out and gradually tears away from the head and disappears. This developmental process usually is completed by the age of four, when the foreskin can be retracted completely. Washing is necessary only on the part of the penis that can be comfortably uncovered by gently pulling the foreskin back.[6] The mother can do it herself, or she can teach the boy to wash himself under the foreskin when he takes a bath. According to Drs. Howard S. King, M.D. and Richard I. Feinbloom, M.D., "With proper hygiene, there is not need to be concerned about uncleanliness and proneness to infection.[6]

An occasional foreskin infection can occur. If it does, here is a simple and perfectly natural remedy, used and recommended by Joyce Prensky, mother of two boys, and printed in *Mothering* magazine:[5]

Dilute 1 tablespoon cornstarch in ¼ cup warm water. Soak cloth or cotton in this solution, then hold next to the foreskin for about 3 minutes. Repeat 3 times a day. Cornstarch is sold in any supermarket.

Those who have used this simple treatment report that the swelling usually goes down the first day, and the infection disappears in a day or two.

Interestingly, a current survey showed that over 90 percent of American male infants are now circumcised, while more than 50 percent of surveyed New York obstetricians feel that the operation is unnecessary.[7] A North Carolina study also showed that about half of surveyed pediatricians and urologists were against circumcision.[8]

If, after reading all the information on circumcision presented herein, you decide to have your baby boy circumcised anyway, you should wait until he is at least eight days old. Vitamin K, which is a natural blood coagulant and helps in healing, does not enter the bloodstream of the infant until the eighth day of life. Circumcision before the eighth day could lead to excessive bleeding and/or post-operative infection.

Before you make your decision, please investigate carefully the evidence in support of circumcision presented by its advocates. My studies of the subject didn't turn up any valid scientific or statistical proofs that would justify this ancient tribal and religious custom, which is such a traumatic and painful experience for a newborn baby. About the only reason most circumcision advocates give for continuing this practice is that you may wish your child to be one of the crowd. Even this may not be anything to consider since the circumcision fad is dying out rapidly and more and more young, new-age mothers reject it as unnatural. They want their child to be left with his foreskin intact as nature and God created him. Perhaps after one more generation, being *un*circumcised will mean *being* one of the crowd, even in America. On a world-wide scale, being uncircumcised is being "one of the crowd" *now*, since less than 10 percent of all males are presently circumcised.

20

Immunization: A New Look

I receive a large number of letters regarding vaccinations from worried young parents, especially those who are "into" a natural way of living. As the federal government's and the medical establishment's drumbeating in favor of mass vaccinations grows louder, parents are having second thoughts about immunization. They are worried about possible adverse reactions. Reports about serious disease and even deaths caused by vaccinations— long ignored or soft-pedaled by establishment press—are finally reaching the public. Concern is not limited to the United States. Headlines from Europe, England, and Australia show the same reaction: more and more parents refuse to vaccinate their children. And this worries doctors as well as—or especially—drug companies.

To combat this reluctance, the American Academy of Pediatrics has just released a film, *A Gift, An Obligation*, which stresses in glowing terms the importance of childhood immunizations. It is significant that the film was produced with financial assistance from a drug company which is commerically involved with vaccines. School boards across the country are launching a mass campaign to force vaccinations on all children by refusing to admit unvaccinated children to school. Health departments and fast-food restaurants have joined hands in various parts of the country to cajole young children into receiving immunizations before starting school. The prize: A free order of french fries for the first 1,000 who receive their shots! In Saginaw County, Michigan, the children receive a "Good Patient Certificate" as well as the coupon for the fries.

As the pressure on parents is mounting, their doubts regarding the safety and wisdom of childhood immunization are increasing proportionately.

Most letters I receive are from concerned parents who simply don't know much about the pros and cons of vaccinations, but who feel that innoculations with toxic drugs and live viruses and bacteria is a rather unusual way of preventing disease. Some letter writers have had personal negative experiences with immunizations and have seen children suffer the agony of vaccination complications. Here is an excerpt from one such letter:

"When my first daughter was only six months old, we decided to travel to South America. We were advised that to obtain a visa we must all be vaccinated for smallpox. This trip never materialized—my daughter was so sick from the vaccination that she almost died. She was violently ill for six months, and has been a sickly child ever since. In spite of such a sad experience, I let my pediatrician convince me to have my second daughter immunized. The day she got her first DPT shot (diphtheria, tetanus, whopping cough), she was very sick with pain and high fever, and cried all night. Her reaction to the second DPT shot was even worse. Her entire thigh became red and swollen, she had diarrhea, refused to nurse, and was sick for several days. I am now reluctant to take her for the third shot."

Some more militant objectors to "herd immunizations" look upon vaccination mania as modern witchcraft and a political, rather than a medical, issue. They refer to the recent grand fiasco with a nationwide swine flu immunization program, which had clear political overtones, at the cost of dozens of innocent lives and millions of taxpayers' dollars.

However, when faced with pressure from schools and pediatricians, these parents, although in principle against compulsory immunizations, are still in doubt as to the right course in this confusing and controversial issue, and are looking for some authoritative approval of their stand, not willing to accept full responsibility for their decision.

Let me say right at the beginning that I cannot advise in any individual case regarding electing or rejecting vaccinations. No one but the recepient, or the child's parents, can make the decision to permit or refuse immunization. I will try, however, to present some objective information regarding the pros and cons of vaccinations so that the educated reader will be better equipped to make an intelligent choice. The ultimate responsibility for examining both sides of the story and deciding whether to place the child in the long lines forming for immunizations still lies with each mother and father.

Immunization: natural versus artificial

When an infant is born, he is protected against the threat of viral or bacterial infections by an inherited supply of antibodies and also by the immunological factors that he continues to receive from his mother's breast milk. Gradually, as the child is subjected to various toxins and viral and bacterial insults from his new environment, food, water, and air, his body will be building up its own defensive system, and developing its own immunological mechanisms. Thus, natural immunization results when the body is challenged directly by the health-threatening factors. If the child's general health level is excellent and his natural resistance high, he will be able to resist even the common infectious childhood diseases. They cannot take hold in a body which enjoys the optimum level of health, but are met and defeated by the body's strong immune system. However, if the viral and bacterial insult is stronger than the defensive mechanism, infection will occur—again, the severity depending on the level of the general health and resistance. When an infection occurs, the body's natural response is to quickly manufacture antibodies that attack the invading intruder. When the battle is over, and the invader is defeated, the antibodies remain in the child's body ready to attack and defeat the same virus or bacterium if it challenges the body again, perhaps many years, or even decades, later. This is called natural immunization.

During their childhood, most children are subjected to a variety of mild bacterial and viral infections. This only helps to build up and strengthen their immune systems and develop the body's own defensive and healing mechanisms. Thus, trying to keep the child so isolated and protected that he would have a minimal opportunity to be subjected to, or come in contact with, "disease-causing" viruses or bacteria, would really be doing him a disservice. It is well known that children who "grow up on the street," in what some look upon as unsanitary conditions, playing with a large number of other children, many of whom have colds and other infections, develop stronger immune systems and have more resistance to infections later in life than children who are deliberately kept isolated and protected from others.

Artificial immunization, as advocated and practiced by medical orthodoxy today, is based on the premise that the body's immune system can be stimulated to produce active antibodies by injecting into it attenuated (weakened) live or dead viruses of disease-causing bacteria. The proponents of the artificial form of immunization claim that it is as solidly effective as natural immunization. Although the viruses or bacteria in vaccines are killed or weakened enough so they can't produce disease, the body's response in producing antibodies still takes place. Thus, antibodies produced as a result of vaccination remain in the body and can protect it by attacking the live viruses or bacteria if and when the body is subjected to it.

Shaky foundation

The practice of artificial immunization is based on the Pasteurian germ philosophy of disease, the postulation being that every disease is caused by different germs or bacteria, and in order to cure the disease, we must (1) find and identify the disease-causing germ, and (2) direct the treatment at the destruction and elimination of it. This hypothesis has been the basis for world-wide immunization programs since, according to this germ theory, infectious diseases are caused by transmission of pathogenic organisms from one host to another.

This grossly oversimplified theory is now seriously questioned by a growing number of doctors and researchers. Professor Gordon T. Stewart, a leading epidemiologist from Glasgow University, Department of Community Medicine, writes that "The germ theory has become a dogma because it neglects the many other factors which have a part to play in deciding whether the host/germ/environment complex is to lead to infection."[1] Questioning the effectiveness of whooping cough vaccine, Dr. Stewart writes in the *British Medical Journal* that "of 8,092 reported cases of whooping cough, 2,940 (36%) were fully immunized, while only 2,424 (30%) were definitely not immunized."[2]

Dr. Rene Dubos, renowned microbiologist at the Rockefeller Institute for Medical Research, appealed for a "need to re-examine the entire germ theory of disease." He stated, "Most human beings carry throughout life a variety of microbial agents, potentially pathogenic for them; only when something happens which upsets the equilibrium between host and parasite does infection develop into disease. In other words, infection is the normal state, it is only disease which is abnormal."[3] Dr. Dubos writes about a group of Danish physicians and other internees who were imprisoned in German concentration camps during World War II. He says, "It was remarkable indeed that most of the prisoners of war overcame their microbial maladies shortly after their return to a normal environment and often without the help of specific therapy. Even in cases of TB, a rapid recovery was the rule, though no anti-microbial agent was then available for its treatment."[3]

Dr. Dubos expresses the new view, held by an increasing number of doctors that so-called pathogenic bacteria are not always, or even ever, the cause of disease. Or, in the words of Dr. Dubos, "Viruses and bacteria are not the cause of disease, there is something else."[4] Bacteria, although almost always present in the environment, and even in the organism itself, remain completely harmless until "the equilibrium between host and parasite is upset." In other words, the resistance of the host organism must be lowered and the body's normal defensive mechanism broken down by such environmental factors as physical and emotional stresses, malnutrition, and nutritional deficiencies, etc., before the ever-present bacteria can become pathogenic.

The Pasteurian germ theory of disease seemed logical and simple at the time it was so quickly accepted by the medical orthodoxy. But, as time goes by, its validity is questioned more and more. It is evident, as two of the world's most prominent investigators of the immunization hazard, Drs. Archie Kalokerinos and Glen Dettman, of Australia, recently wrote: "Sometimes the disease is present without the germ, and more often than not, so-called pathogenic germs are present when there is no indication of disease."[5] As the fiasco of the Pasteurian germ concept of disease becomes more and more evident the investigators would be wise to resurrect the nearly-forgotten remarkable scientific works by the contemporary of Pasteur, the true medical genius, Professor A. Bechamp. Bechamp's research showed that the basic element of all organic matter was the microzyma. Through the enzymatic evolutionary processes and fermentation, the microzyma is the precursor of other factors including RNA and DNA, as well as viruses and bacteria. Thus, according to Bechamp, what we call pathogenic bacteria, are actually endogenously (or sometimes exogenously) developed dormant bacterial precursors of what he calls microzymian evolution. This development depends not on the presence of dormant bacteria per se, but on the nutritional status of the cell, or what we now refer to as the biochemical microenvironment. The much-adulated Pasteur not only plagiarized the work of Bechamp, but distorted the great scientific discovery of Bechamp to suit the scientific mood of the 19th Century medical establishment, which was on the lookout for a plausible philosophy of disease.[6] Thus, for one hundred years, medical science was based on the witch hunt for disease-causing germs, and the responsibility for one's health was moved from the individual himself (the "innocent victim of vicious germs") to the modern doctor equipped with powerful drugs and injection needles with which to fight the disease-causing intruders. Had the Bechamp discoveries been understood and incorporated into the medical teachings one hundred years ago, millions of people would have been spared the suffering or the agonizing deaths caused by mass immunizations and we would have a much healthier mankind who would have been educated in the Bechamp concept of disease—i.e., the individual himself is responsible for his ills by a wrong way of eating and living, which upsets the equilibrium in his body's biochemical microenvironment, weakens the resistance, and prepares the biological milieu suitable for bacterial growth, and development of disease.

The effectiveness of artificial immunization

The proponents of mass vaccinations claim that artificial immunization programs around the world can be credited with the sharp decline in the prevalence of our most killing infectious diseases, which used to plague the world in the pre-immunization era. This may surprise the reader, but the actual statistics and records from around the world show that this is a totally unsubstantiated claim. Actually, most of the major infectious diseases had declined approximately 90 percent *before* the introduction of compulsory immunizations and antibiotics.[7] According to most investigators, the reason for the decline was improved hygiene, sanitary engineering, and better nutrition.[8] It is well known that smallpox has practically disappeared in all areas of the world, both in countries with compulsory vaccination as well as in countries where smallpox vaccinations were never instituted.

William Howard Hay, M.D., in his testimony to the Medical Freedom Society on the bill to abolish compulsory vaccinations, said that he had an ample opportunity to observe firsthand that vaccinations did not offer any protection in epidemic situations. He supervised an epidemic

of 33 cases of smallpox of which 29 victims had vaccination histories "and a good scar to prove it," some of
them vaccinated within the previous year. He also reported
on a study of Cook County, Illinois Hospital, where one
half of the nursing staff was vaccinated against diphtheria, and the other half was not. Diphtheria broke out
soon afterwards, infecting both immunized and unimmunized, with the total of cases much higher among the
vaccinated.[11]

The *Journal of the American Medical Association*
reported that of the 18 cases of paralytic polio and 2 deaths
from polio reported in the United States in 1977, 3 of the
victims had received polio vaccine and 10 had been in close
contact with recently-immunized people.[9] This revelation
shows that immunizations not only do not guarantee protection from disease, but might actually cause them.

As far as the effectiveness of the whooping cough
vaccine is concerned (whooping cough vaccine is a component of the triple DPT baby shots), Dr. Edward B. Shaw,
a distinguished University of California physician, has
stated, "I doubt that the decrease in pertussis (whooping
cough) is due to the vaccine, which is a very poor antigen
and an extremely dangerous one, with many very serious
complications...The decline in pertussis began long before
the widespread use of vaccine."[10] Dr. Shaw also seriously
questions the conventional view that the decrease in polio
is a result of the polio vaccine.

The effectiveness of rubella (German measles) vaccination is of special concern to women because for some
reason women appear to be especially susceptible to the
rubella virus. When the disease is contracted by a woman
during the first three months of her pregnancy, it is
known, in a large percentage of cases, to produce birth
defects in the child, especially mental retardation, congenital heart defects, blindness, and deafness.

Dr. John M. Leedom, associate professor of medicine at
the University of California, has been involved in studies
of the effectiveness of rubella vaccination for some time.
He says that there are certain doubts as to whether im-

munization really protects the unborn child from birth defects. "Ideally," Dr. Leedom notes, "the recipient of the vaccine doesn't become sick or even infected with the strong virus challenges. But, this doesn't seem to be the case with the rubella vaccine."[12] U.S.Army experiments, as well as similar carefully-controlled studies done by Dr. Leedom at Pacific State Hospital, indicate that vaccinated persons are not fully protected from German measles infection. They are still capable of becoming infected with the wild virus, should they become exposed to it, even though they may not always show the clear signs of sickness. An article in *Lancet*, the prestigious British Medical Journal, stated, "Immunity to infection by rubella virus, whether the result of natural infection or from attenuated vaccine, is by no means absolute. Subclinical infections may ensue and this is more likely in those whose immunity is vaccine-induced than in those who acquired it from natural infection."[13]

On my recent nationwide research and lecture tour of Australia, I became acquainted with the work of Dr. Beverly Allan, a medical virologist at the Australian Laboratory of Microbiology and Pathology in Brisbane. Dr. Allan conducted studies on the effectiveness of rubella vaccinations which gave overwhelming evidence that immunization did not offer any protection at all. Army recruits were vaccinated with the attenuated rubella virus, to which they produced rubella antibodies. They were then sent to a camp which usually has an annual epidemic of rubella; 80 percent of these so-called immune recruits became infected with rubella. The same results were shown in a consecutive study which took place at an institution for mentally retarded people.[14]

The health hazards of immunizations

While the *effectiveness* of artificial immunizations is still in doubt, there is not doubt whatsoever about their potential and real health *hazards*. Vaccinations can be extremely dangerous and cause many health disorders, including the very disease they are purported to prevent.

British statistics show that smallpox attained its maximum mortality after vaccination was introduced. Many doctors question the wisdom of compulsory vaccinations, since all vaccines are toxic and can pose a serious health hazard to susceptible individuals, especially the very young and very old. Some of the adverse reactions to vaccines are just as bad, or even worse, than the disease itself. As Dr. Robert Mendelsohn, Medical Director of the International American Hospital in Zion, Illinois, said, "With some immunizations, the risk of taking the shots may outweigh their benefits."[15]

Diphtheria

Diphtheria is one of the diseases where the risk of the immunization seems to outweigh its benefits. During the four years from 1941 through 1944, the Department of Health in Scotland admitted that there were 23,000 cases of diphtheria among immunized children, more than 180 of which proved fatal. On the other hand, in Sweden, diphtheria virtually disappeared without any immunizations, and in Germany, where compulsory mass immunization of children was introduced in 1940, the number of cases increased from 40,000 per year to 250,000 by 1945, virtually all among immunized children. Many other countries in Europe showed a striking increase in cases of diphtheria after compulsory immunization. For instance, the increase in France was as much as 30 percent, in Hungary, 55 percent, and in Geneva, Switzerland, the number of cases tripled after compulsory immunization was enforced in 1933.[32]

Flu vaccine

The swine flu mass vaccination in 1977 was one of the examples where zealous medical bureaucrats overreacted to a supposed danger which, in fact, never really existed. Although there had never been any proof of swine flu among human beings, or that it could be transmitted from human to human, the government, with the blessing of the medical establishment, ordered innoculations on a national scale. No consideration was given as to the possible danger to the lives of small children or elderly. The outcome was that at least 30 people died as a direct result of the vaccinations, and thousands of persons suffered severe health damage.[16] One of the most serious reactions was Guillain-Barre Syndrome, a serious paralyzing condition. On the basis of the governmental surveilance, 565 persons suffered severe paralysis from swine flu shots.[15] Encephalitis is another severe neurological reaction to the flue vacination, which is an even more serious disease than the flu itself.

Measles

Measles is one of the most common childhood diseases, and may serve a very useful role in building up an immunity against more serious diseases in adulthood. Although the seriousness of measles should not be overlooked, it does not have the dread implications of smallpox, tetanus, or diphtheria. Contrary to popular belief, measles doesn't cause blindness; it can cause photophobia, a temporary sensitivity to light, which is treated simply by pulling down the window shades and keeping the lights low.

The primary reason for wanting to prevent measles cited by proponents of measles vaccinations is that it causes encephalitis. This risk, however, is minimal, especially if the patient is given good care with lots of rest. On the other hand, the measles vaccine itself can cause not only encephalitis, but also many other serious complications, such as SSPE (subacute sclerosing panencephalitis), loss of muscle coordination, impaired speech function, personality changes, mental retardation, learning disability, hyper-activity, rage outbursts, aseptic meningitis, hemiparesis, and epileptic seizures that can lead to coma and death.[15,16] Dr. Robert Mendelsohn speculates that "the current epidemic of hyperactivity in children may have its origin, at least in part, in the measles vaccine."[15] Atypical measles, with measles-like rash, high fever, and even pneumonia are other serious side effects of measles vaccinations.[17] Recently, the *Journal of the*

American Medical Association published warnings by two doctors from Buttersworth Hospital in Grand Rapids, Michigan, who treated a 17-year-old girl with atypical measles, who had received "killed virus" measles vaccine 14 years ago. Doctors said that about 600,000 children received this type of vaccine in the early 1960's and that as many as two thirds of them, or 400,000 are in danger of developing the severe atypical measles. They said that there was no certain time limit between immunization and the onset of atypical measles. Australian scientists have also implicated measles vaccination with the risk of developing multiple sclerosis. They found that MS sufferers have a higher than normal proportion of the measles antigen in their blood.[13]

While the dangers of measles vaccinations are so great, how effective a protection against disease does it offer? The World Health Organization did a study and found that while in an unimmunized, measles-susceptible group of children the normal rate of contraction of disease was 2.4 percent, in the control group, that *had been immunized*, the rate of contraction rose to 33.5 percent.[18] Unable to explain the surprising findings, the physician who conducted the study said, "Maybe there were bad batches of vaccine."

It is more difficult to explain the outbreak of measles in January, 1977, in a Massachusetts high school. Investigation by the Center for Disease Control revealed that of 47 cases of measles infection that occurred in students aged 13 to 18, 25 victims (53%) had a history of immunization with live attenuated measles vaccine and immune globulin prior to 1966. The editorial note in the same report adds, "this outbreak illustrates that measles can occur in communities in which a high proportion of students are reportedly vaccinated.[19]

German measles

The German measles (rubella) vaccinations remain very controversial throughout the world. While their effectiveness is more vociferously questioned by a growing number of doctors and medical journals, including *Lancet*, and the *Australian and New Zealand Journal of Obstetrics and Gynecology*,[20] it is becoming apparent that serious health risks are connected with the vaccine.

Dr. P.F.H. Giles writes that 1 - 2 percent of vaccine recipients develop arthritis and arthralgia, which are often mistakenly diagnosed by doctors, who are unaware of vaccination history, as rheumatic fever and rheumatoid arthritis.[21] Up to 50 percent of women vaccinated with rubella vaccine reported side effects, mostly mild, but arthritis occured in 10 - 15 percent. The *Australian Medical Journal* reports an additional risk from rubella vaccination—myositis, inflammation of the muscle tissue.[22]

Polio

Polio vaccine has now been implicated as the major cause of polio (paralytic poliomyelitis) in the United States by no lesser an expert than Dr. Jonas Salk, the man who introduced the original polio vaccine in the 1950's. He writes in *Science Abstracts:* "Live virus vaccines against influenza and paralytic poliomyelitis, for example, may in each instance cause the disease it is intended to prevent; the live virus vaccines against measles and mumps may produce such side effects as encephalitis...The live virus polio vaccine is now the principle cause of polio in the United States and in other countries...Contrary to previously held beliefs, about poliovirus vaccines, evidence now exists that the live virus vaccine cannot be administered without risk of inducing paralysis...The live poliovirus vaccine carries a small inherent risk of inducing paralytic poliomyelitis in vaccinated individuals or their contacts."[23]

Kaiser Hospital in Walnut Creek, California, reported in January, 1979, that the father of a young boy who received the polio immunization, was stricken with polio himself. The doctors from the Communicable Disease Center felt that he contracted the disease from his child's diapers.

DPT—Tripple antigen shots

One of the most common forms of child immunization in the U.S. today is DPT, or triple antigen vaccine, combining diphtheria, pertussis (whooping cough), and tetanus vaccines. Doctors advocate giving DPT shots to infants as soon as possible after the age of 2 months; then giving several booster shots as the child grows up.

The *British Medical Journal* published the following letter from Rosemary Fox, Secretary, Association of Parents of Vaccine-Damaged Children:

"Two years ago, we started to collect details from parents of serious reactions suffered by their children to immunizations of all kinds. In 65 percent of the cases referred to us, reactions followed "triple" vaccinations. The children in this group total 182 to date; all are severely brain-damaged, some are also paralyzed, and 5 have died during the past 18 months. Approximately 60 percent of reactions (major convulsions, intense screaming, collapse, etc.) occurred within 3 days, and all within 12 days. During the period 1969-74, when 64 deaths resulted from whooping cough, 56 cases of severe brain damage followed whooping cough vaccination."[24]

Pharmaceutical companies, in their instructions to doctors, warn that "triple vaccine should not be given if there is any illness or ill health (including allergic disorders) in the child. Other contraindications are familial neurological disease, history of convulsions, or evidence of other abnormality of the central nervous system." How would any one know if a two-month-old baby has any of the mentioned contraindictions, other than a family history of neurological disease, until it is too late?

Dr. Glenn Dettman, of Australia, says that triple antigen injections are especially risky if the infant is deficient in viamin C. "We have shown that triple antigen injections given to scorbutic children (children deficient in vitamin C) can result in massive immunological insults which may cause death."[34]

Immunizations and multiple sclerosis

Multiple sclerosis is a rapidly-increasing disease in most civilized countries. It also has defied all attempts by scientists to decipher its origin. Now, however, medical scientists are beginning to lean towards a causative relationship between vaccinations given to children and MS. Research carried out at the University of Colorado showed that smallpox vaccinations given to small children could be contributory causes of multiple sclerosis later in life.[25] Actually, the University of Colorado scientists didn't discover anything new; many other researchers from various parts of the world have reported on a possible link between vaccinations and multiple sclerosis. In 1967, the *British Medical Journal* published studies by Stovicek (1959), Palffy and Merei (1961), McAlpine, et al. (1965), Zintchenko (1965), and various German authors on an apparent connection between not only smallpox vaccinations, but also typhoid, tuberculosis, tetanus, polio, diphtheria, measles, and even anti-rabies vaccinations and the development of multiple sclerosis several years, even decades, after the original vaccination.[26]

Reye's Syndrome

"Even though Reye's Syndrome is not a common disease, medically speaking, it is a very important one," writes Robert Mendelsohn, M.D., in his "Ask the Doctor" column in the *San Francisco Chronicle*.[27] "Reports linking immunizations to Reye's Syndrome continue to appear. In an epidemic affecting 22 children in Montreal, 5 had received vaccines (measles, German measles, DPT, and Sabin polio vaccine) within the three weeks prior to their hospitalization. While the Center for Disease Control has been quick to suggest a relationship between Reye's Syndrome and certain flu outbreaks, they have not, to my knowledge, given equal time to a consideration of an association between this disease and the flu vaccine itself."[27] Reye's Syndrome is a newly-discovered, often-fatal disease involving the brain and the liver.

Vaccinations and cancer

The cancer-producing effect of vaccinations has been demonstrated in animal studies.[28] Whether there is a similar danger potential for humans is unknown, but, as Dr. Carlton Fredericks, renowned American nutritionist, says, "For children, at least, this possible risk certainly outweighs any preventive benefit."[28]

One scientist who is concerned with long-term effects of artificial immunization on the general health, and specifically its relation to many of our common so-called diseases of civilization, is Dr. Robert W. Simpson, of Rogers University in New Jersey. At a recent seminar, sponsored by the American Cancer Society, in St. Petersburg, Florida, Dr. Simpson stated that "immunization programs against flu, measles, mumps, polio, etc., actually may be seeding humans with RNA to form pro-viruses which will then become latent cells throughout the body. Some of these latent pro-viruses could be molecules in search of diseases, which under proper conditions become activated and cause a variety of diseases, including rheumatoid arthritis, multiple sclerosis, lupus erythematosus, Parkinson's's disease, and perhaps cancer."[29]

Alan H. Nittler, M.D., one of the pioneers of preventive medicine, expressed fears similar to Dr. Simpson's, when he wrote, "Unfortunately, we do not know if by using vaccinations we have just suppressed the outward manifestation of the disease and forced it inwards, only to have it come out some other time, in more virulent form, when it is not allowed to escape from the body via a cleansing program."[30]

Re-evaluation long overdue

It is not easy for a doctor who has been indoctrinated in the Pasteurian germ concept of disease from the very first day of his medical schooling, to allow any doubts regarding the very foundation of established medicine. Yet, as can be seen from extensive factual and reputable data presented in this chapter, an open-minded doctor should feel no guilt for asking himself a question: Could Pasteur possibly be wrong, and Bechamp right?

One of the leading bacteriologists of our time, renowned physician, Professor of Bacteriology at the London School of Hygiene and Tropical Medicine, and formerly Director of the Public Health Laboratory Service, Sir Graham S. Wilson, M.D., L.L.D., F.R.C.P., D.P.H., had to re-evaluate his view on vaccinations after being presented with irrefutable facts. He wrote in his book, *The Hazards of Immunization:*

"The risk attendant on the use of vaccines and sera are not as well recognized as they should be...The late Dr. J.R. Hutchinson, of the Ministry of Health, collected records of fatal immunological accidents during the war years, and was kind enough to show them to me. I was frankly surprised when I saw them, to learn of the large number of persons in the civil and military population that had died apparently as the result of attempted immunization against some disease or other. Yet, only a very few of these were referred to in the medical journals...And further, when one considers that such accidents have probably been going on for the last 60 or 70 years, one realizes what a very small proportion would have ever been described in the medical literature of the world."[31]

One of the great immunologists of all time, Sir MacFarlane Burnet, has also cast serious doubt regarding the flimsy platform upon which the germ-disease theory is based. He wrote, "When I was younger and had time to read an occasional long and scholarly book, I read Creighton's *History of Epidemics in Britain*...a true scholarly study of epidemics by a man who did not believe in the Pasteurian germ theory of disease. Until I read Creighton, I didn't realize how naive were the early bacteriologists: diphtheria bacillus is found in diphtheria, therefore, diphtheria bacillus causes diphtheria; but when one finds a diphtheria bacillus in a healthy throat, it must be something else, a diphtheroid bacillus. To an intelligent and sophisticated historian such a statement was logically beneath contempt."[33]

Clearly, re-evaluation of the very basis upon which immunization practice stands is long overdue. The

Pasteurian theory that bacteria cause disease cannot pass the rigid test of modern investigation. Repeating what one of our leading scientists, Dr. Rene Dubos, said, "Viruses and bacteria are not the causes of disease, there is something else."[4] Dr. Rene Dubos continued, "Most human beings carry throughout life, a variety of microbial agents, potentially pathogenic for them; only when something happens which upsets the equilibrium between host and parasite does infection develop into disease." Which means, that not the bacteria, but the "upset equilibrium"— the broken down health and lowered resistance on the part of the host carrier of the parasite—is the real cause of disease.

Natural disease prevention

Consequently, the logical common sense approach to prevention of diseases would be not to try to identify and destroy the bacteria, but to increase the health and resistance level of the host organism to the point where bacteria would have no chance of survival or doing any harm. Dr. Bernard Rimland, of San Diego, expressed this concept brilliantly in a recent communication to *Science News*: "Looking for the germ or virus involved [in disease] is merely a search for one of many potentially precipitating events. It is more constructive to consider diseases as a set-back for the body's usually formidable defenses than as a victory for the attacking microbes. Medicine has generally taken the opposite view, and it has proven to be a faulty strategy. It is far better to fireproof a structure than to spend a great deal of time and effort trying to decide whether the fire was started by a match or a cigarette."[34]

In various other chapters of this book, as well as in my other writings, the factors that can improve the general level of health and raise the body's resistance to all diseases, including those which established medicine is now trying to immunize against, are described in detail. The basic philosophy of biological medicine is that "the healthy body never becomes sick—only the already sick body (that is, the body whose resistance has been weakened) gets sick." With proper nutrition, pure natural food and water, vitamins, exercise, fresh air, rest, relaxation, and a positive, health-oriented outlook on life, we can build an optimum level of health and such a strong resistance to disease that we can enjoy superb health and resist diseases and infections. As I stated repeatedly before, an Optimum Diet during pregnancy and lactation, and breast feeding the infant for a year or more, are very basic requirements for a healthy and disease resistant child.

One of the nutritional factors which is specifically involved in protecting (immunizing, as it were) from infectious diseases mentioned in this chapter, is vitamin C. Dr. A. Kalokerinos and Dr. Glen Dettman have worked with the Aboriginal children in Australia who suffered such poor health that the infant mortality rates exceeded 172 per 1,000 in some areas. They found that almost all of the children suffered from severe vitamin C deficiencies. By "correcting scorbutic status" of these children (giving them large doses of vitamin C), they succeeded in reducing death rates drastically. These Australian doctors also observed that many of the infant deaths were directly related to the immunizations they received.[35] Their further studies showed that administering large doses of ascorbic acid prevented these deaths. Dr. Kalokerinos writes, "Some Aboriginal infants displayed a second adverse reaction to immunizations: the immunizing agent acting as an immunological insult and predisposing to serious and sometimes fatal infections."[35] Large doses of vitamin C—500 mg. or more—are needed, sometimes by injection.

The reason vitamin C is so effective in preventing infections of all kinds is that it neutralizes the toxins produced by bacteria. Dr. Irwin Stone, in his book, *The Healing Factor: Vitamin C*, cites ten studies showing the remarkable effectiveness of vitamin C in inactivating bacterial toxins.[36]

One of the other very important factors in increasing the body's resistance against all infections is keeping the intestinal canal in such a healthy condition that the beneficial lactic acid producing bacteria, which normally live there, thrive and multiply. Avoiding putrefactive foods, such as meat and other animal proteins, and using plenty of lactic acid fermented foods, such as soured milks (yogurt, acidophilus milk, kefir, etc.) pickled vegetables, and sourdough breads, will help these bacteria. Dr. W. Sandine, professor of microbiology, Oregon State University, says that with good nutrition, and, in particular, an ample supply of lactic acid-producing organisms, our body produces its own antibiotics.[37]

Garlic is another natural antibiotic and immunizing agent. It has been shown in many studies to not only increase the body's resistance to most infectious diseases, even the common childhood diseases, such as whooping cough, diphtheria, flu, etc., but also to possess a miraculous therapeutic property in treatment of practically all human ills.[38] If children object to the taste and smell of garlic, odorless garlic capsules and tablets, such as Kyolic, are now available in health food stores.

Difficult decision

The information in this chapter is offered not with the intention of your indiscriminate following, but in hope that you will consider both sides of the controversial question of immunization and make a wise decision. Admittedly, making such a decision, which may affect not only the health, but the very life of your children, is not easy. On the one hand, by refusing vaccination, you may be (just may be, although many doctors now doubt it) increasing the risk of your child's contracting some of the communicable diseases, which can be serious. On the other hand, vaccination poses a real and definite risk to the health of your child, as the ample evidence presented in this chapter shows. Doctors have seen many cases where perfectly healthy and strong children who had never seen a sick day until they were vaccinated, responded to the toxic insult of vaccine by losing their general resistance and have been sickly children ever since. As Dr. Hay said,

"I couldn't put my finger on the disease they had. They just weren't strong. Their resistance was gone. They were perfectly well before they were vaccinated. They have never been well since."[11] And, as the many doctors' reports quoted in this chapter show, mental retardation, arthritis, multiple sclerosis, cancer, and even death may be caused directly by vaccinations. The fact that the California State Legislature has recently passed a law, the first of its kind, which provides up to $25,000 for medical expenses of children who suffer catastrophic reactions (how bad is catastrophic?) from required immunizations, shows that such reactions can't be all that rare! Perhaps the financial ruin of the California State Government caused by this legislation will force the authorities to take another look at the pros and cons of immunization.

It is true, as I said before, that the best immunization and protection against infections is the body's natural high level of resistance. In an ideal environment, where lifestyle is conducive to optimal health, where air and water are pure, where foods are natural, unprocessed, without toxic additives or pollutants, where stress factors are minimal, and where plentiful physical exertion is balanced by sufficient rest and relaxation—where, in other words, mental, physical, and biochemical environments are conducive to well-being and an optimal level of resistance to disease—artificial immunizations would be unnecessary. However, these ideal conditions hardly exist today. We are living in an increasingly polluted and stress-filled environment, and our level of natural resistance to disease has been steadily declining. Under *these existing* conditions: Should we, or should we not, vaccinate our children?

Difficult question to answer, indeed. Only *you* can answer it. You must weigh the pros and cons of immunization, natural and artificial, the risks, and the benefits of both, then take the inherent parental responsibility of electing or rejecting vaccinations. Since no two individuals are alike, and every child's health and resistance status is different, you should consult with your pediatrician or your family doctor, who is better equipped to evaluate the risks versus the benefits of the procedure in your child's specific situation. Try to find a doctor whose mind is not closed by dogmatic prejudice.

If you and your doctor's final thinking on immunization is that the potential harm of *some* immunizations is lesser than the possible benefits derived, it may help you to know that most doctors think that the dangers involved with tetanus immunization are apparently minor, compared with the severity of the disease; thus, tetanus vaccinations may be justified as the lesser of the two potential evils. Immunization against German measles (rubella) is considered quite ineffective, while smallpox, polio, measles, whooping cough, and diphtheria innoculations are considered to be most dangerous.

In any case, I do not endorse *compulsory* immunizations. I believe that every parent should have the right to make his own choice. In case you didn't know, there are federal laws which exempt those who do not wish to be immunized because of conscientious objections based on personal beliefs as well as when innoculations are medically contra-indicated. Thus the present nation-wide drive by school boards to bar the admittance of unvaccinated children is illegal. Doctors who routinely vaccinate each child are playing Russian roulette since it is well established that there is always a certain percentage of children with so low a resistance that the outcome of the vaccination will be fatal. As an article in the *International Medical Digest* stated, "There is no sound basis for the assumption that every child or infant must be innoculated with every available vaccine; on the contrary, there may be a valid reason for omitting any or all available antigens. Each patient is an individual, and deserves evaluation on this basis, rather than as an epidemiologic statistic…The incidence of vaccine-induced morbidity has increased alarmingly. The profession must re-evalute the principles, purposes, and hazards of immunization and reassess current procedures."[39]

If you choose to vaccinate

If, taking into consideration all the available evidence regarding the health hazards versus the benefits connected with immunization, you choose to vaccinate your child, there are some proven prophylactic measures you can take which will minimize the harmful effects of vaccines, help to neutralize their toxic effects, and increase the body's chances to withstand the health-damaging insult of the antigens.

Here are some of the measures advocated by the holistic and biological medical practitioners:

1. Vitamin C is the most important protector. Adults can take up to 10,000 mg. of ascorbic acid or sodium ascorbate daily, even more in acute or severe conditions; children, up to 5,000 mg.; and infants, 100 mg. to 1,000 mg., depending on age. These protective doses of vitamin C should be taken daily, one or two weeks before vaccinations, as well as several weeks after the innoculations. Medical literature is filled with reports on studies which show that vitamin C can neutralize and destroy toxins in the body and increase the body's resistance to virtually any bacterial toxins as well as drug insults.[5,34,35,36,40,41] It would be advisable, on the day of vaccination, to administer vitamin C intravenously, in addition to oral doses, to maximize its protective effect.

2. Other protective vitamins and supplements are:

   Vitamin A—50,000 to 75,000 units
   Vitamin B-complex, high potency
   Zinc—30 - 50 mg.

These are the daily adult doses for a two to four week period; children's doses are half of this, and infants' one quarter or less, depending on age (see Chapter 9).

3. In addition to the above-mentioned protective supplements, some mothers have been giving for a few days after innoculation, 1 mg. of folic acid, 100 mg. of magnesium, 200 mg. of calcium, and 50 mg. of vitamin B_6, to help their babies' bodies combat the effects of vaccination if they seem a little rundown after the shots.[42] Again, the younger the infant, the smaller the dose.

4. Raw garlic, or garlic tablets or capsules, should be taken before and after the vaccinations. Garlic is a powerful neutralizer of poisons, and, along with vitamin C, is the best possible protector against bacterial and environmental toxins.[38]

5. The following herbal aid to counteract the possible undesirable side effects of immunizations is recommended by Joyce Prensky, author of the book, *Healing Yourself:* Bring 10 cups of water to a boil, add 3 tablespoons of echinacea root (Echinacea augustifolia) and simmer for 20 minutes. Remove from heat and add 3 tablespoons of peppermint leaves. Cover the pot, let stand for 5 minutes, and strain. Give your vaccinated child, beginning the day of vaccination, 1 cup a day, sweetened with honey, if desired.[43] Note that milk sugar (lactose) is the only sweetener that should be used for nursing-age infants.

6. Homeopathic doctors offer highly attenuated and totally harmless homeopathically prepared immunizing agents for most of the transmittable diseases, such as Hypericum for tetanus, Lathyrus Sativa for polio, and homeopathic form of attenuated diphtherotoxin for diphtheria. The same homeopathic medicines are used to counteract the undesirable side effects of conventional immunization antigens. Needless to say, you should discuss all medications, even homeopathic, with an understanding doctor. Homeopathic Information Service, P.O. Box 44, Chestnut Hill, Massachusetts, 02167, can supply you with more information regarding their methods and can refer you to doctors who practice homeopathic medicine.

21

Other Common Health Problems In Childhood

Here are, in a nutshell, natural, nutritional, and biological approaches to diseases, disorders, and health problems common during early infancy and childhood.

Please keep in mind that diets, vitamins, juices, herbs, and other natural alternative approaches mentioned in this chapter (as well as in other chapters of this book that deal with diseases and health disorders of any kind) are not offered as *cures* for disease, but only as supportive means of helping the body's own inherent healing forces and assisting its own healing activity. The principle of biological medicine and natural, holistic healing is that no food, no vitamin, no herb, no specific therapy or treatment—and, for that matter, no drug!—can ever cure disease. Disease can be cured only by the body's own healing and health-restoring power. Your body and your child's are equipped with the most extensive, elaborate, and effective healing mechanism known to science. The human body is designed as a self-healing mechanism and it always strives to maintain a high level of health and correct any of the disorders or ills that it is occasionally subjected to. The programs suggested here are aimed at helping the body's healing mechanism by eliminating the causes of disease and creating the most favorable condition for the body's own healing forces to bring about the actual cure. The treatments presented herein are not intended to *replace* conventional therapeutic approaches, but are to be used as an adjunct to other forms and methods of healing, including medical.

It is also important to realize that every individual's response to vitamins, specific foods, and other herbal or nutritional therapies is greatly different, depending on his specific condition, individual requirements and needs, age, health stature, his ability to assimilate nutrients, his emotional health, etc., etc. Therefore, we strongly advise that if you use any of the information in this book for therapeutic purposes, you do so in cooperation with a nutritionally-oriented doctor, abiding by his decision as to the advisability of using the suggested therapies for you or your child. Self doctoring, especially when dealing with health disorders of infants and young children, can be dangerous. In case of any serious illness it is wise to consult your doctor immediately.

Fever

Fever is one of the body's own defensive and healing forces, created and sustained for the deliberate purpose of aiding in the restoration of health. The high temperature speeds up the metabolism, inhibits the growth of the invading virus or bacteria, and literally burns the enemy with heat. Fever is an effective protective and healing measure not only against common colds and minor infections, but even against such serious diseases as polio and cancer.

Although the healing process of fever is well substantiated by medical research and has been looked upon as such not only by Hippocrates, the Father of Medicine, Galen, and other giants of old medicine, but also by many geniuses of contemporary medical science, such as Nobel Prize winner, D.R. Lwoff, and Dr. Werner Zabel, do not expect that your own family doctor or pediatrician will concur with the idea. He most likely was raised and educated in the Pasteurian era of medicine where fever is considered to be "bad," a disease condition, which must be controlled and "cured." Instead of letting the fever, the proper rest, lots of liquids, and temporary abstinence from food accomplish the health-restoring goal for which the body had initiated fever, conventional doctors suppress it with drugs. This only counteracts the body's own healing efforts and may help change the minor acute disorder into a serious chronic condition.

But talking about and accepting the philosophical principle is one thing, while dealing with fever of your own little baby is quite another! When your child suddenly develops a fever of over 100, which keeps climbing, what should you do?

First, it is quite common that small children run high temperatures with relatively minor infections. Childhood is the time when the body encounters all kinds of new bacteria or viruses, and the very first mode of response by the body to the intruder is a raised temperature. So do not be alarmed every time you find that your child has a temperature of 100°, 101°, or 102°. It *may* mean, of course, that your child is seriously sick, and if the temperature remains high for longer than 24 hours you should consult with your doctor. But, in nine cases out of ten, the fever is just a symptom, the *healing symptom*, of a cold or minor infection, and undisturbed, will accomplish its purpose and disappear on its own—leaving your child in better shape than before!

The normal temperature of a child, taken by mouth, is 98.6°F. Rectally-taken temperature (advocated for infants and small children) is normally about ½ to 1 degree higher, or about 99.1° to 99.6°F. Don't worry if your child's temperature is below normal. Some children just normally have low temperatures, like 97° or 97.6°F. If he acts and looks healthy, don't worry about his temperature being low.

What should you do if your child has a fever?

If the fever is only slight—101° to 102°—keep him in bed, well covered with blankets. He will probably feel chilly, and should be kept warm. Give him something warm to drink, such as orange juice diluted with warm water, or freshly-squeezed lemon juice in warm water, sweetened with honey. Herb teas are also good. Camomile, rosehip, or peppermint tea is good. They help to induce perspiration, which usually brings the temperature down. Slippery elm tea is excellent if the child is coughing.

Vitamin C can help the body in its healing activity and should always be given in case of fever. Give 100 to 300 mg. to small children, and up to 5,000 mg. to older children, spread through the day in smaller doses. Vitamin C can be mixed with fruit juices or water.

Biochemic tissue salt, **Ferrum. Phos.**, can be given for fever. Place 2 - 3 tablets under the tongue.

If your child develops a fever as high as 103 - 104°F, it should not be left at this level for too long. If it does not go down right away with large doses of vitamin C, you should call the doctor immediately. Until the doctor advises you, you must try to prevent the temperature from going even higher with a wet rub. Wet your hands in cold water (not ice water) and gently rub the child's exposed arms for a couple of minutes. Then cover his arms and rub his legs, then chest, then back, keeping all but the part being rubbed covered, to avoid chilling. If the fever does not go down, or even climbs, and the doctor is nowhere in sight, you may consider giving 1 tablet of "baby" aspirin (1¼ grains). This is just as an emergency measure. It is rare that a high temperature will not respond to fruit juice or herb teas and large doses of vitamin C in conjunction with a wet rub.

Colds

Colds and children seem to have an affinity for each other. Although breast-fed children and those raised on wholesome diets of natural foods are much less susceptible to colds, even they can come down occasionally with fevers, runny nose, cough, flu, tonsillitis, sinusitis, and minor-type respiratory infections. It is safe to say that every child will get a cold at one time or another—most likely many times.

No one seems to know for sure the real cause of colds. Conventional medicine believes that colds are caused primarily by a virus. Since no one has ever seen the cold virus, doctors explain that it is a so-called "filtrable virus," so small that it cannot be seen even through a microscope. The cold virus lowers the resistance in the mucus membranes of the nose and throat and then the other germs, the so-called secondary invaders, enter the picture and make the cold a more serious condition, which may develop into bronchitis, sinusitis, tonsillitis, and pneumonia.

The biological medical theory is that colds in early childhood are nature's own way to immunize the child and build up and strengthen his immune and resistance mechanism. That's why children at very young ages, between 2 and 6, have 4 - 5 times as many colds as do older children.

Colds by themselves are usually "harmless," i.e., they usually come and go without affecting the child unfavorably other than causing a certain amount of discomfort. There are the complications of colds, colds that are not nurtured properly, or suppressed by toxic drugs and antibiotics, that cause problems.

Of course, it is wise, when your child comes down with a cold, to make sure that it is not a symptom of a more serious condition. Many infectious childhood diseases have early symptoms that are similar to a common cold.

If, by all indications, you suspect that your child has a common cold, here are a few helpful suggestions that can help his body to correct the condition and restore health:

1. If the temperature is above normal, keep the child in bed. Follow the advice and directions suggested earlier under the subtitle *Fever*.

2. Do not force him to eat if he doesn't want to. Give him lots of liquids: fruit juices, herb teas, lemon water.

3. Give him lots of vitamin C. Vitamin C in large doses has an antibiotic action.[1] In acute conditions, children between 12 and 18 can take massive doses of up to 5,000 mg. a day, 500 mg. every second hour. Children under 12, 200 - 400 mg. every two hours, and 2 - 6 year-olds, about 100 mg. several times a day. Vitamin C can also be given intravenously by a doctor or nurse. The therapeutic value of vitamin C in treatment of colds is scientifically proven.[2]

4. Garlic is another effective natural antibiotic.[3] It can be taken internally—crushed or as a freshly-squeezed juice mixed with fresh vegetable juice, such as carrot juice. For

mouth and throat infections, keep a clove of garlic or a vitamin C tablet in the mouth—it is a very effective way to kill the invading germs in the throat, mouth, and nose areas. Garlic oil combined with onion juice, diluted with water, and drunk several times a day, has been found in several studies to be extremely effective for patients suffering from grippe, sore throat, and rhinitis.

5. If the child is constipated, and especially if he has been constipated prior to "catching" cold, a small enema of water, heated to body temperature, and mixed with freshly brewed camomile tea, can be helpful. A small infant should have no more than 2 ounces, a one-year old about 4 ounces, and a 5-year old or over, about 8 ounces. Older children can take an enema in the regular manner (see instructions in Recipes & Directions). For a small infant, it is easier and safer to use a rubber syringe with a soft tip of the same material. Fill the bulb carefully so that you won't be injecting air. Grease the tip with a little vaseline. Place the child on a waterproof sheet on a bed with an absorbant soft towel over it. Lay the child on his side with his legs pulled up against his stomach. Squeeze the bulb very slowly. If the child is big enough to sit on the potty, have it close at hand.

6. After the fever and cold has subsided and the acute condition is over, continue with juices and vitamins, and give your child plenty of raw fresh fruits to eat.

Finally, you can do a lot to help prevent colds in the first place. Feed your child a diet of optimum nutrition as recommended in this book. Give recommended vitamins and supplements regularly, especially vitamin C, cod liver oil, and brewer's yeast. See that he gets plenty of undisturbed sleep and rest. Avoid undue chilling; see that he always wears a head covering, or hat, especially in winter. (The current fad of exposing the head to the cold in winter and the hot sun in summer is responsible for more health problems than you can imagine.) And see that your child does not lower his resistance to colds with junk foods: sugared cereals, processed and canned foods, cookies, candies, soft drinks, etc.

Ear infections

Middle-ear infection (otitis media) is the most common ear problem in children. It is often associated with severe colds. Germs can spread from the throat up the eustachian tube to the middle ear and cause inflammations with severe earache. Also, ear infection is a common complication of tonsillitis, measles, or influenza. The symptoms, in addition to pain, may be fever, deafness, ringing in the ears, and, if the ear drum has perforated, a discharge from the ear.

Ear infections can be serious and doctors usually use antibiotics to combat infection.

Among the more natural approaches are:

1. Large doses of vitamin C, orally or intravenously.

2. Castor oil pack over the affected ear. Saturate a small cotton ball with castor oil (sold in drugstores) and push it gently into the ear. Cover the ear first with a small sheet of plastic, then a dry washcloth. Place a warm hotwater bottle or electric heating pad over the washcloth. Leave for 20 - 30 minutes. Then remove the heating pad, but leave the cotton ball inside. Keep the head warm at all times.

3. If the baby is on a cow's milk based formula, give him nothing but fresh mashed fruits, such as bananas or apples, plus fruit juices and 100 mg. of vitamin C twice a day, for one or 2 days. Also, give ½ tsp. of cod liver oil each day. Sometimes, ear infections can be associated with allergy to cow's milk. Older children should take a multi-vitamin-mineral tablet, children's strength, for a few weeks during all kinds of infections, in addition to the vitamin C and avoidance of possible allergens.

4. If your child is given antibiotic medicine for his ear infection, or for any other reason, give him lactobacillus acidophilus tablets or liquid during the duration of the treatment and at least two weeks after to counteract the effect of the antibiotics on the intestinal bacteria and help to re-establish a new intestinal flora.

5. Needless to say, optimum nutrition and avoidance of all refined, processed, prepared, and sugared foods and drinks, is imperative.

Tonsils and tonsillitis

Medicine has made many blunders throughout its illustrious history. Some of them have cost many innocent lives. Thalidomide and swine flu mass vaccinations are some of the most recent senseless acts of folly. Fluoridation of public water supplies will one day be looked upon not only as quasi-scientific nonsense, but a flagrant crime against humanity. Removal of tonsils on a mass scale is another of the irrational blunders in the recent past. A couple of decades ago, doctors removed tonsils by the millions at the first sign of infection or even minor swelling. Ludicrous as it may seem now, perfectly healthy tonsils were removed "to prevent tonsillitis." I remember vividly the front page story in my hometown newspaper in the late fifties about a large family with eight children, photographed as they were leaving the hospital, after all of them, including the parents, had undergone tonsillectomies—an act of family solidarity because one of the kids had swollen tonsils. The doctor in the report praised the "heroic" family, and urged other families to follow their example to prevent their childrens' tonsil problems later in life, once and for all.

Tonsils are a pair of flat, oval masses of tissue on each side of the entrance to the throat. They are a part of the very important lymphatic system which is the body's defensive mechanism in its fight against bacteria or toxic insult. Tonsils trap and destroy disease-causing bacteria and other impurities, help to overcome infections, and build up the body's resistance against disease. Unbelieveable as it may seem, doctors didn't know this then. They thought that tonsils were useless (just as some still think the appendix is) and without any beneficial physiological function—except of being a persistent source of bothersome infections. So, they cut these organs out, and threw them away.

Tonsils become swollen when there is an infection nearby. The swelling is an indication that the tonsils are laboring hard to destroy germs and protect the body. This is certainly a poor reason for removing them! Enlarged tonsils are *not diseased* tonsils, even if they are enlarged most of the time. They are only *overworked* tonsils. If you see that your child's tonsils are always swollen, take a good look at his general health condition and try to remove *the underlying* causes for the overworked tonsils—do not remove the tonsils!

Usually, even in perfectly healthy children, the tonsils gradually become larger until about the age of 9 or 10, then gradually decrease in size. Sometimes, tonsils are rather large throughout the teens, especially during colds, flu, or any kind of illness or infections. Do not rush to the doctor to ask him to remove your child's swollen tonsils. Be happy that they are swollen—they are working hard to protect your child and build up immunity and resistance for a long life.

However, there are times where medical intervention can be justified. Severe forms of tonsillitis, or throat infection, should be treated and not overlooked. As with any other organ, the tonsils may be so overloaded and infected for so long a time that they may break down and become a source of extensive toxicity for the body. In extreme cases, drug treatment or removal of tonsils is advisable. In most cases of tonsillitis, proper naturopathic treatments, such as juice fasting with cleansing enemas, followed by a cleansing, alkaline, raw vegetable and fruit diet, rest in bed, and lots of vitamin C and other vitamins, can be very helpful. Vitamin C—½ teaspoon of ascorbic acid powder dissolved in a glass of water—can also be used as a gargle. DAG as a gargle (made from Irish moss) is also beneficial. Keeping a clove of garlic or a vitamin C tablet in the mouth is a great help. Hot epsom salt baths, especially hot foot baths, are very effective (see *How To Get Well* for instructions on fasting, foot baths, etc.;[1] also, Chapter 2, in this book on fasting).

Skin disorders

From the time your child is born until his late teens, he will get one or another of the many skin disorders of childhood, from diaper rash to acne. Here are some of the most common skin disorders and what you can do about them, naturally speaking.

Diaper rash. Babies have sensitive skin, particularly in the diaper region. The most common form of diaper rash is small red pimples or patches of irritated red skin. Diaper rash can have many causes. Exogenous causes include infrequent diaper changes, overheated room or bed, allergic reaction to synthetic or plastic materials in disposable diapers or bedding, and diapers washed in strong detergents. Ammonia, which is formed by bacteria that thrives in the wet diapers, is a strong irritating chemical and prime contributor to diaper rash. Waterproof pants are very undesirable, although I know they are practical. The endogenous causes include a too-acid or too-alkaline urine or feces due to badly formulated formula or specific foods the nursing mother eats; diarrhea; or vitamin and mineral deficiencies and imbalances, especially in bottle-fed babies.

The corrective approach must be directed by the known or suspected underlying causes, which must be corrected or eliminated. Make sure the baby doesn't stay in wet diapers for too long. Avoid synthetic materials, especially plastics. The best diapers are pure cotton, nondisposable diapers, which should be washed in mild, natural soap and dried outside in the sun, if possible. In bad cases of diaper rash, it would be wise to boil the diapers in order to discourage the bacteria which make ammonia.

The best treatment for diaper rash is to expose the whole affected area to the air for as long as possible, several times a day, keeping the baby in a warm room. In the summertime, let the baby play (lay) outside in the nude. Just fold a diaper underneath him to catch some of the urine.

Baking soda and vinegar solutions have been used by some mothers. One such mother wrote to me recently:

"Dear Dr. Airola: I read recently in your column that you recommend using baking soda or vinegar as natural deodorants. I decided to try it for diaper rash. It works well. After washing the area with soap and water, I apply the baking soda solution (½ tsp. of soda dissolved in a glass of water) wth a piece of cotton, and the redness is soon cleared up. Also, fresh air and a dab of sun are helpful."

When diaper rash is caused by ammonia and a too-acid urine or feces, the alkaline baking soda (bicarbonate of soda) will be very beneficial. Using cornstarch powder on affected areas is also helpful.

Prickly heat. Small pink pimples around the neck and shoulder area, especially during hot summer weather, are usually referred to as prickly heat. In bad cases it can spread to the chest and back and even to the face.

Dusting with cornstarch powder or dabbing with cotton soaked in a baking soda mixture (½ to 1 tsp. of soda to 1 cup of water) are simple treatments for prickly heat. Of course, keeping the baby cool is also advisable. In warm weather, take most of the baby's clothes off and keep him in a well ventilated, but not drafty, area.

Vitamin C seems to be a very effective natural treatment for prickly heat. Dr. T.C. Hindson, a British dermatologist, conducted a double-blind test with 30 children who had suffered from severe cases of prickly heat for at least eight weeks. While only 2 children of the 15 that were given placebo medication improved, all but 1 of the 15 children on vitamin C were completely cured within two weeks.[4] Several other studies, some reported in the *Journal of the American Medical Association*,[5] showed that vitamin C is very effective in the treatment of prickly heat. The dose for children over the age of 8 is 250 - 500 mg. a day, under the age of 8, a half of that. Babies can be given 25 mg. of vitamin C dissolved in pure water, 2 - 3 times a day.

Insect bites

Insect bites that are itching (mosquito bites for instance) can be treated by the following simple, natural means, which help to minimize or eliminate the itching:

1. Apply a paste made of salt and water to the exact spot, or

2. Put a drop of lemon or lime juice on the spot, or
3. Apply a paste made from baking soda and a few drops of water, or
4. Apply aloe vera gel.

For a bee sting, first remove the stinger, if visible, with tweezers, and apply a paste made of baking soda as above. For wasp or hornet stings, rub a drop of vinegar on the spot after removing the stinger.

Eczema

It is a well-known fact, well substantiated by clinical studies, that breast-fed babies only seldom have problems with skin rashes, particularly eczema, while it is quite prevalent among artificially-fed babies. It is generally considered that a baby's allergy to certain constituents of infant formulas, especially to cow's milk, coconut butter, and sweetening agents, is a major cause of infant eczema. This type of eczema clears up rapidly when baby's formula is changed.

Sometimes, it is the lack of sufficient fat or oil in baby formulas that causes eczema. Formulas are frequently made from de-fatted soy milk or skim milk. These lead to a deficiency of linoleic acid and consequently cause the development of eczema.[6]

Deficiencies of B-vitamins, especially B_6 and B_2, often cause the development of scaly, dry and itchy eczema.[7] Babies can be given ½ to 1 tsp. of B-vitamin-rich brewer's yeast in their formula or as supplement to breast milk. Older children can take B-vitamins, both B_2 and B_6, as well as other vitamins of the B-complex, in tablet form. It is advisable to take high potency B-complex, plus 2 - 3 tbsp. of brewer's yeast daily. Salve containing vitamin B_6 has also been helpful in some cases.[7]

Eczema can also be caused by allergy to some material in clothing, especially that made from synthetic materials, as well as in the air and environment. Exposure to extremely dry air for a prolonged time, as in the winter when the home is heated by a dry air system or electric heat, is also one of the most common causes of extremely dry skin and eczema.

Other common causes of eczema, especially in older children and adults, are chronic constipation, faulty, sluggish metabolism, and poor elimination of toxic wastes from the body. Excessive salt in the diet, as well as strong spices such as pepper and mustard, may cause eczema in some individuals.

The natural approach to the treatment of eczema must begin with diagnosing the possible underlying causes and then eliminating them.

A 100% raw diet of optimal nutrition with emphasis on sprouts, and raw fruits (except citrus) and vegetables is a good cleansing diet that can be given to children at any age beyond infancy. Raw potatoes are especially beneficial. This diet can be complimented with brewer's yeast, 1 tbsp. of cold-pressed olive or sesame seed oil, honey, and raw goat's milk, preferably in the form of homemade yogurt or kefir (see Recipes & Directions).

All salt, sugar, chocolate, and caffeine-containing beverages should be avoided. No refined, processed, or cooked foods.

Avoid washing affected areas with regular soaps or shampoos. Bathe affected parts often with plain water. After a bath, you can rub the affected parts with a slice of cucumber. An acid-type soap, sold in health food stores, can be used, if you feel soap is necessary.

For external application, do not ever use mineral oils, especially those labeled as "fine baby oils." Such oil can pass through the skin, enter the blood, and absorb fat-soluble vitamins A, D, E, and K, before being excreted in the feces, thus robbing the body of these vitamins.

You may use some of the following for external application:

- Lanolin cream with vitamin A & E
- Homemade Formula F Plus (see Chapter 32)
- Aloe vera, fresh jel or cream (sold in health food stores)
- Whey powder (dust affected parts)

Older children can take the following vitamins and supplements daily (young children half dose):

C—1,000 - 3,000 mg.

A—50,000 units for one month, then reduce to 10,000

Cod liver oil—1 - 2 tsp.

B-complex, high potency, with B_{12}

B_6—50 mg.

B_2—50 mg.

PABA—50 mg.

Calcium lactate—3 - 4 tablets

Brewer's yeast—1 - 2 tbsp. of powder or equivalent in tablets

"Nature's Minerals"—3 - 5 tablets

Whey powder—1 tbsp. (can be mixed in drinks or food)

Kelp—1 - 2 tablets or use granules in food

Lecithin—1 - 2 tsp. of granules

Herb teas have been used effectively in some cases. The best herbs are: comfrey, burdock, juniper berry, solidago, wild pansies, elecampane, celandine.

French herbal healer, Maurice Messegue, developed a very successful natural treatment for eczema, which he used on thousands of patients with a reported 98 percent rate of cure.[8]

Here is the Mességué treatment:

Make an herbal extract in the following manner: boil a quart of water, using a glass or enamel pot, then let it cool until lukewarm. Drop in a handful of each of the following herbs: artichoke leaves, elecampane (flowers and leaves), celandine (leaves—fresh if possible), chicory (roots and tips), broom (flowers), lavender (flowers), and nettle (leaves—fresh, if possible). Let the mixture soak for 4 to 5 hours. Strain and pour into a clean bottle for storage until use. The extract will retain its effectiveness for eight days.

The extract is used for an 8-minute foot bath each morning before breakfast, and an 8-minute hand bath in the evening before dinner. The bath is made in the following manner: boil 2 quarts of water and let stand for 5 minutes. Add ½ pint of the herbal extract to 2 quarts of boiled water. Take foot or hand bath as hot as you can tolerate. The bath preparation can be kept and warmed for the next bath, without boiling or adding more water.

(Maurice Messegue, *Of Men and Plant*, Macmillan Company, 1973).

Dry skin is improved by using olive oil. You can gently rub even very young infants with olive oil. Use only fresh cold-pressed olive oil sold in health food stores. You can use it on the head too; it is a good stimulant for healthy lustrous hair growth. Cod liver oil is also good for flaky and dry skin, taken internally and rubbed on externally.

Sunburns. If your baby happens to be accidentally sunburned (you should always take care not to leave your baby in the sun unprotected for more than 5 - 10 mintues), use vitamin E. Just squeeze the vitamin directly from the capsule and spread over the burned area as soon as possible. PABA ointment is good to use as protection against sunburn. So is aloe vera gel.

Diarrhea

A healthy, normal baby may have as many as 6 - 10 bowel movements a day; but as long as the stools are well formed (even though small) he is not having diarrhea. It is common that a breast-fed baby has a movement after every nursing. It is also not unusual that breast-fed babies skip a whole day, or even two or three days—sometimes a whole week! Yet, regardless of how frequent or infrequent the evacuation, if the feces are well formed, not too hard and not too watery, you shouldn't be concerned. Some babies assimilate mother's milk so well that there is not much residue left. Formula-fed babies, as a rule, have more frequent bowel movements. As the baby grows, the number of movements decreases.

Diarrhea exists only if the stools are liquid, watery, "explosive," and completely unformed. If of short duration, diarrhea in a breast-fed baby could be caused by something the mother ate which the baby does not tolerate. Or it could be a mild intestinal infection. The normally yellow color of the feces turn greenish when there is diarrhea. The odor is usually also different. Mild diarrhea of short duration is common in young infants and should not be a cause for concern. In bottle-fed babies, diarrhea is often

.aused by excess sugar in the formula. When sugar is eliminated, the condition is often corrected immediately. Also, lack of sufficient unsaturated fats in artificial formulas often can cause diarrhea.

A recent study, conducted by Drs. S.A. Larsen, Jr., and D.R. Homer at the Kaiser Foundation Hospital in Hayward, California, confirmed statistically what many doctors had observed clinically for a long time: that nursing can prevent serious intestinal infections and other gastro-intestinal disorders in babies. Of 107 babies treated at the hospital for diarrhea, weight loss, and other gastro-intestinal disorders, only 1 was breast-fed at the time of admission. All others had been on the bottle for at least a month, and more than 70 percent had never been breast-fed.

The lack of B-vitamins, especially niacin, in a nursing mother's diet can give chronic diarrhea to a breast-fed baby. If the mother takes B-complex vitamins with extra niacinamide , and if the baby is given some brewer's yeast powder in addition to milk, the diarrhea often disappears.[7]

Diarrhea in infants *can* be a serious condition if one of the following symptoms accompany it: pus or blood in the stools; vomiting; distended abdomen; fever of 101° or more; baby appears to be sick and is losing weight. A doctor should be consulted in such cases.

Here are some measures you can take if diarrhea is persistent but baby is seemingly doing well without having any of the above-mentioned symptoms which can signify a more serious condition.

1. If the baby is breast-fed, continue breast feeding. Give him some water between feedings to prevent dehydration. If the baby is bottle-fed, dilute each bottle to half strength. When his movements become normal, go back to full-strength formula. Add brewer's yeast powder to the formula: ¼ tsp. at first, gradually increasing to ½ tsp. for each bottle.

2. A nursing mother should eliminate any foods from her diet that she just started eating at the time of the onset of diarrhea in her baby. Also, she should take 1 - 2 tbsp. of

brewer's yeast a day, plus high-potency B-complex vitamins for a couple of weeks.

3. If the baby is on a mixed diet—breast milk plus solid foods, or formula plus solid foods—omit all solid foods until the diarrhea is over. In reinstating solids, go slowly, one food at a time, trying to determine which of the foods is a possible cause of the diarrhea. Cooked rice and homemade applesauce are well-tolerated by children who have diarrhea. They're also healing foods.

4. The following natural aids can be used in mild forms of diarrhea:

- *Carob flour or powder.* Add 1 tsp. of carob to every bottle, or, if the infant is breast-fed, give ½ tsp. mixed with water or skim milk, twice a day, between feedings.
- *Tea made from dried blueberries.* It would be smart to sun dry some blueberries when they are in season to keep for such an emergency (some herb houses may sell them). Soak 1 tbsp. of dried blueberries in 1 cup of hot water overnight and give baby 1 - 2 tsp. of strained liquid every 2 - 3 hours.
- *Cinnamon tea* is another effective herbal for diarrhea.
- *Peppermint tea.* Usually the essence of peppermint is used, 15 drops in 1 cup of hot water. Give 1 - 2 tbsp. at a time.
- *Garlic* is an excellent treatment if diarrhea is caused by intestinal infection. Crush a garlic clove and give a few drops mixed with water. Older children can take a clove with every meal, finely chopped and mixed with some food or drink. Also, garlic capsules or tablets sold in health foods stores, such as Kyolic , are effective.
- *Lactobacillus acidophilus.* If your child has been receiving antibiotic therapy, his diarrhea may be caused by the drug, which disrupts the whole digestive system by killing the beneficial bacteria in the intestines. Give the child lactobacillus acidophilus tablets or culture to help restore the intestinal flora. Older children can use yogurt, kefir,

or other cultured milks in the daily diet.

- Cornstarch mixed with fresh apple juice (contains pectin) is an old remedy from folk medicine, as is barley or rice water.

Constipation

As I said before, *frequency* of evacuation in very young infants is not an indication of diarrhea or con-stipation. It's the *consistency* of stools that is important to watch. Only if stools are hard, dry, and difficult to pass can the condition be classified as constipation. Breast-fed babies sometimes evacuate every second, third, or fourth day. No problem. Even after several days, *if the stool is not hard*, they are not constipated.

Breast-fed babies almost never are constipated. But in bottle-fed babies, constipation is quite common. Cow's milk and sugar in formulas are the most likely factors. Re-placing regular sugar with lactose, or milk sugar, can help; also cutting down on the amount of milk in the formula. You may try to add stewed, pureed prunes to the formula. If the child is older, you can add flax seed puree to his diet. Soak 1 tbsp. of raw whole flax seeds in a cup of water overnight, then liquify in the blender. Even small babies can be given ½ to 1 tsp. of this puree occasionally, as needed. A mixture of 1 tbsp. of homemade yogurt, ¼ tbsp. of yeast, ½ tbsp. of lactose, ¼ tsp. of magnesium oxide powder, and 1 tbsp. water, can be given to older infants and children.

One nursing mother wrote about the close relationship between her diet and the baby's bowel movements. She normally ate yogurt every day for breakfast. However, at one time, she stopped using yogurt. The baby became constipated a few days later, and didn't get better until the mother started to eat yogurt again. The connection was noted on two different occasions.

Bedwetting

The exact cause or causes of bedwetting (medical term: nocturnal enuresis) are still unknown. There are many theories. The Canadian neurobiologist, Roger Broughton, found that REM (Rapid Eye Movement—the deep sleep stage) period was delayed when bedwetting occurred in children under his study.[10] He also found that nervous or hyperactive children are most likely to be bedwetters. These children had a faster heart beat, and higher respiration rate during the entire sleep cycle than did the control subjects.

Dr. Lendon H. Smith, in his book, *Improving the Child's Behavior Chemistry*, speculates that bedwetting may be related to excessive sugar consumption. Since sugar consumption in the evening causes a sudden drop in the blood sugar level during sleep, the nervous system doesn't have enough energy to give the cerebral cortex, "area of social concern," the message that the bladder is full.[11] Dr. Smith also feels that excessive excitement, worries, or fears during the day can cause a child's blood sugar levels to fall during sleep and contribute to bedwetting. Thus, hyperactive children are more likely to also be bedwetters.

It appears that there are a few cases of bedwetting caused by physical abnormality in the urinary system. These cases can be corrected by appropriate surgery. However, most doctors feel that perhaps less than 3 percent of bedwetters have surgically-correctable abnormalities of the urinary system. They feel that the problem is largely psychological and that psychotherapy, or simply showing more loving attention to the bedwetter, is the most effective approach.

Here are a few other approaches that may be helpful in solving your young child's bedwetting problems. All of the following treatments for bedwetting have been used by doctors, patients, or parents, found to be successful in some cases, and reported in medical literature.

1. Self-hypnosis, or hypnotic treatment by a clinical hypno-therapist. A study by Karen Olness, M.D., assistant professor of medicine and of child health and development at George Washington University, Washington, D.C. (reported in *Clinical Pediatrics*, March 1975), showed that

self-hypnosis can be a very effective way to correct bed-wetting. Of 40 children, age 4½ to 16 years, half boys and half girls, 31 were cured completely of bedwetting, 23 in the first month of treatment.[12] Call your local medical society for the name of a doctor who specializes in such therapies.

2. Special exercises to strengthen the muscles of the urinary tract that control urination. The exercise is simple: urinate and stop—urinate and stop—over and over, until finished.

3. Vitamin-mineral supplements: magnesium, B-complex, plus multiple vitamin and mineral supplement, childrens's strength.

4. Herb tea made from cinnamon sticks or powder, sweetened with honey and drunk in the morning and early afternoon. Some children like chewing on cinnamon bark or sticks.

5. Eliminate allergens. Bedwetting has often been connected with allergies. By eliminating all foods that your child is suspected or known to be allergic to, and giving magnesium and vitamins A, D, C, and E, you may discover that his bedwetting will be cured.

6. Eliminate all sugar and foods with artificial colorings and flavorings. Especially avoid giving sweets or sugared foods or drinks to your child in the evening before going to bed.

7. Make sure the child empties his bladder before going to bed.

Warning to mothers and fathers: Avoid scolding, threatening, or humiliating a bedwetter! This will only aggravate the problem and may contribute to the development of a fixation complex that becomes incorrectable. Above all, do not be alarmed **too soon.** All children are bedwetters at some time. If the child is less than 4 years old, you should not even consider it a problem. Even if he is 5 or 6, it would, perhaps, be wise not to make a big issue of it. Show lots of attention and love to your child, and the problem will probably clear up by itself in a short time.

Professor Thomas Anders of Stanford University School of Medicine wrote in **Medical Times** that 5 to 17 percent of children between the ages of 3 and 15 have this disorder, which *disappears with maturity*. It is only if a child is constantly humiliated, threatened, and scolded that this common and relatively minor disorder is likely to continue into adulthood.

Child masturbation

It is important that parents have a thorough understanding of a child's sexual development. Such an understanding can help prevent the development of sexual fixations, inhibitions, and dysfunctions in children as they grow up, so that they can grow sexually healthy and can have satisfying sex lives as adults.

It has been generally thought that sexual interest and sexual feelings in children begin at puberty, when he or she develops the capacity to reproduce. Recent studies show, however, that children actually have sexual feelings as early as at birth. Thus, erections in baby boys are quite normal and frequent during diapering or bathing. They continue throughout the whole childhood. Correspondingly, a baby girl's vagina begins to lubricate within a few days after birth, too. This indicates that both boys' and girls' sexual systems are functioning normally. Now, do not confuse these *sexual* systems with the *reproductive* systems, which will not begin functioning until puberty.

As the child grows, he will discover that there is pleasure in touching and fondling his sexual organs. If anxious parents respond in an overly-negative manner at this time by pulling the child's hand away, or spanking his fingers, or telling him "not to do this," etc., he will develop a feeling of shame or guilt about his sexual organs which may have a paralyzing effect on his future sexual attitudes and functions. If, however, parents permit the child's curiosity to take its normal course, and let this sexual growth process develop in a natural way (provided that his interest is not all-consuming), this may help him or her to develop a positive attitude about sex and a successful sexual responsiveness in adult life, without complexes, fears, and fixations.

It is good to keep in mind, however, the following scientific facts as well as long-established teachings of the world's oldest religions:

1. Although occasional masturbation is considered to be totally harmless by most doctors today, excessive masturbation does drain unnecessarily some of the vital physical, emotional, and creative energies. The loss of zinc, by excessive masturbation, may lead to zinc deficiency. The Bible clearly condemns those "who cast their seed upon the ground." Dr. R.S. Clymer,[13,14] Dr. B.P. Randolph,[15] and Dr. G.E. Poesnecker[16] have, in their extensive research and writings on the subject, expressed a rather convincing working hypothesis which postulates that during normal sexual intercourse between a man and a woman, provided it is conducted with love and affection, there is an exchange of electro-magnetic energies; this exchange, which depends on intermixture of the male and female sexual fluids exuded during intercourse and the electric vibrations received during such a sublime experience, is vital for man's, and especially woman's health, well-being, and emotional, intellectual, and spiritual development. Thus, while the utilization of the sexual creative energy will aid in the building and perfecting of the physical, mental, and spiritual structures of the human being, the neglect to properly utilize such a constructive energizing process through sexual intercourse could lead to the opposite.

2. Hindus and Yogis refer to semen as a "vital force" and teach   that conservation of the substance by moderation leads to better health, more energy, and is conducive to spiritual development. Balance and moderation are keys to optimum health in every aspect of life—the discharge of seminal fluids is no expection.

3. The modern sexologists claim that the danger of "too much" masturbation is minimal because "the body will automatically stop responding when it has "had enough." This may be true. However, tampering (playing) with such important endocrine glands as the sex glands, and interfering with their normal activity (the normal

activity being affected by the loving interaction with the opposite sex) can have undesirable effects, both physiologically and psychologically. Dr. Paul Ricchio expressed this thought succinctly. He said, "Masturbation has been treated too lightly in the past...No one in his right mind would knowingly play with his thyroid, adrenals, and pituitary gland just for the sensation that it would bring; the sex glands certainly deserve the same consideration."[17]

In summary, I think that the truth about masturbation is somewhere between the exaggerated views upheld on one extreme by some strict religious dogmas which look on it as a major sin and some misinformed individuals who believe it to be a cause of insanity, blindness, and total physical and mental deterioration , and, on the other extreme, the contemporary sexologists who teach that it is a totally harmless and actually desirable "alternative" form of sexual expression. Indeed, there are serious, respected doctors today who tell mothers that "adolescent girls should be actively encouraged to explore their own bodies" and they actually should be taught how to masturbate in order to develop a satisfactory sexual response in adult life.

It is not my desire to impose my opinions or judge the opinions or beliefs of others, but after making a rather thorough study of the subject, my conclusion is that parents, when noticing their young children's interest in touching and fondling their sex organs or older children's masturbation, could respond in the following manner:

1. Do not dramatize or exaggerate the importance of the event by overreacting, displaying a horrified expression on your face, and telling the child that "his fingers will fall off," etc., etc. Such actions can only result in feelings of shame, guilt, and fear in the child and may have a damaging effect on his future sexual attitudes and development.

2. Try to communicate your disapproval in a gentle, loving way. For example, you could say that sexual feelings are beautiful and natural, but that sexual parts are private and sacred parts of the body which God created for special uses when he grows up.

3. It is also very important to impress upon the child that although people do occasionally experience self-pleasuring, eventually, as they grow up and get married, they will prefer other kinds of sexual pleasures with a person of the opposite sex.

4. Finally, parental example and a stable family structure are the best guarantees that a child will have a healthy and normal sexual development. Observing his mother's and father's affection and loving relationship on a daily basis will help a child to grow and develop into a gentle, loving, considerate person, with healthy and normal sexual desires and responses.

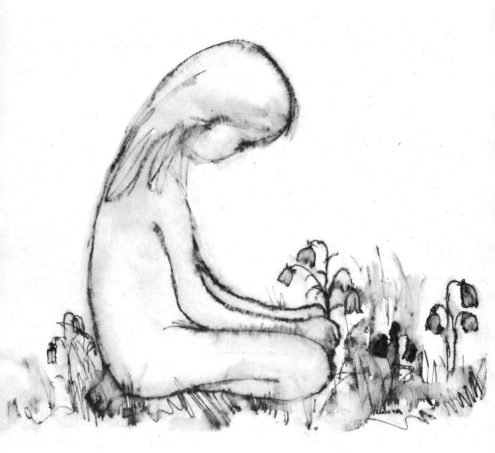

Part Three

Specific Female Health Problems

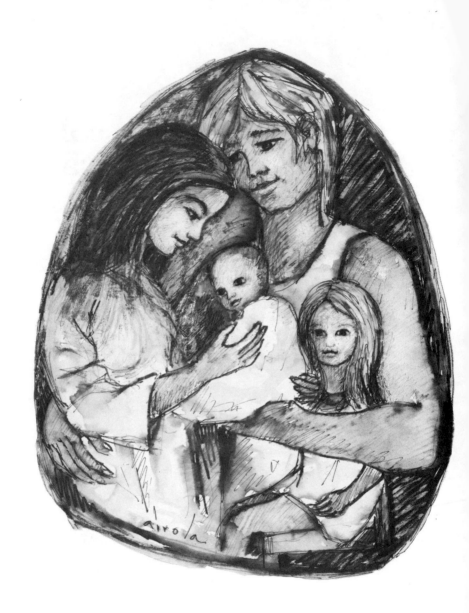

22

Birth Control: Natural and Unnatural

Birth control, the deliberate effort to prevent pregnancies, has been practiced for as long as mankind has existed on this planet. Whether or not we approve of it, it is a fact of life we must accept as inevitable and deal with intelligently. The issue of birth control will not disappear by sweeping it under the carpet, as has often been done, especially in certain religious circles. Only by open, scientific, objective discussion of the pros and cons of birth control and various forms of contraceptives can we avoid the possible grave damage to health, even to life itself, that some of the currently-popular birth control methods present.

Discussion of the controversial birth control issue, with its moral, religious, sociological, and political implications, is a precarious endeavor. There are those who think that the sole function of sex is procreation. Others think that the world population growth, if not controlled, will soon overwhelm the planet's capacity to sustain life. Others feel that the primary function of sex is enjoyment and pleasure and, therefore, birth control is as natural as sex itself. Without moralizing, taking sides, or passing judgement on the views and opinions of others, I will try to present an objective overview of existing birth control methods, their effectiveness, and safety, so that those who desire to practice birth control can choose a contraceptive technique that is most suitable for their individual needs and is not in conflict with their religious or other beliefs.

Motives

The motives and reasons for birth control are legion. Some wish to prevent conception because of potential health problems for the mother or child. Indeed, today even young women often suffer from a long line of serious degenerative conditions which make pregnancy a risky undertaking with potential health damage to themselves or their offspring. In fact, any woman who lives in a heavily chemicalized and polluted environment or who is smoking, drinking and/or using drugs on a rather regular basis, is hardly fit to be a prospective mother.

Some may not be in financial or social position to allow for the birth and proper care of children. Many women of child-bearing age are either studying or working outside the home. Many "can't afford" a child. Just the thought of coming up with several thousand dollars in doctors and hospital fees that having a baby costs today makes many a couple think twice before considering the "luxury" of having children.

Then there are couples who feel they have all the children they want or can afford to properly raise and educate, and, therefore, wish to limit the size of their family. Others feel that the earth is overpopulated already and do not want to contribute to the real or imagined overpopulation crisis.

The so-called Sexual Revolution of the 60's and 70's, of which I spoke earlier in the book, and the easy availability of birth control pills has contributed to sexual promiscuity among adolescents and teenagers. According to surveys, there are eleven million sexually-active teenagers in America today. Incredibly, 17 percent of fourteen-year-old children were found to be sexually active! There are also 600,000 babies born a year to teenagers! Unless the sexual counter-revolution, which is currently on the way, will halt this unbridled promiscuity (which is often disguised behind deceptive euphemisms of "new morality" or "alternative lifestyle"), the easy availability of contraceptive devices may be a blessing.

Whatever the reasons or motives, imagined or real, birth control is obviously an existing reality to be considered seriously. And, judging by the fact that it has been practiced rather widely since the beginning of the human race by virtually all civilized as well as primitive peoples, birth control is a fact of life, whether we approve of it or not. A survey by the National Center for Health Statistics showed that in 1973, 70 percent of American women of childbearing age, or their sexual partners, were using some method of contraception.

In this chapter, I will examine the various possible methods of contraception from the medical and natural-health point of view. Those who choose for one reason or another to use contraception *should know* the pros and cons of each method regarding their effectiveness and safety.

As the chapter title suggests, I consider some birth control methods to be natural, and some unnatural. Since nature intends all species to multiply, it is obvious that all methods of birth control must involve some thwarting, or at least circumvention, of nature. However, as it is not easy to "fool Mother Nature," procreation is difficult to avoid. Also, most of the artificial, unnatural methods to prevent conception are very harmful and dangerous to the health. It is clear that with something as serious as changing basic biological processes, one should exercise great caution.

The Pill

Millions of women around the world are taking the "Pill" every day. It is estimated that up to 20 million women use it in the United States alone, although recently the number of Pill users has gone down as the Pill-cancer connection becomes more and more publicized.

The oral contraceptive was developed some 25 years ago, and most women had been taking the Pill without fear, convinced that it was harmless. One Pill manufacturer used to distribute a brochure in which he stated,

"When taken as directed, the Pill does not interfere with your state of well-being." This brochure is not distributed any more. Instead, the Pill manufacturers are faced with hundreds of lawsuits from women who were misled into believing that the Pill was completely safe. The evidence that oral contraceptives are extremely dangerous drugs which can play havoc with a woman's sexual and reproductive life and cause serious health disorders, including cancer, is mounting. Obviously, anything powerful enough to drastically alter normal biological processes is powerful enough to do other things to the body as well.

Here is a list of some of the *less* serious, although bothersome, side effects of oral contraceptives:[1,2,3,4]

- Increased susceptibility to vaginal and bladder infections
- Lowered resistance to all infections
- Cramps
- Dry, blotchy skin
- Mouth ulcers
- Dry, falling hair, and baldness
- Premature wrinkling
- Acne
- Sleep disturbances
- Inability to concentrate
- Migraine headaches
- Depression, moodiness, irritability
- Darkening of the skin of upper lip and lower eyelids
- Sore breasts
- Nausea
- Weight gain and body distortion due to disproportional distribution of fat
- Chronic fatigue
- Increase in dental cavities
- Swollen and bleeding gums
- Greatly increased or decreased sex drive
- Visual disturbances
- Amenorrhea (failure to menstruate)
- Blood sugar level disturbances which complicate diabetes or hypoglycemia.

More serious complications caused by oral contraceptives are:

- Eczema[1]
- Gallbladder problems[2]
- Hyperlipemia (excess fat in the blood)[5]
- Intolerance to carbohydrates leading to "steroid diabetes," which can lead to clinical diabetes[6,11]
- Strokes[6]
- Seven to ten times greater risk of death due to blood clots[6]
- Jaundice, liver damage, and liver tumors[6,15]
- Epilepsy[5]
- High blood pressure[7]
- Kidney failure[7]
- Edema[8]
- Permanent infertility[9,13]
- Varicose veins[12]
- Thrombophlebitis and pulmonary embolism[12]
- Heart attacks[12]
- Cancer of the breast, uterus, liver, and pituitary gland[6,9,10]

Oral contraceptives contain the synthetic sex hormones, estrogen and progesterone, also chemically-referred to as progestin, mestranol and ethinyl estradiol. The mestranol-containing Pill is considered most likely to be causatively related to liver tumors. Uterine and breast cancer is thought to be produced or aggravated by synthetic estrogens in oral contraceptives.

The most recent findings show the adverse effect of oral contraceptives on the cardiovascular system, especially in women over thirty. High blood pressure, blood clots, strokes, and heart disease are definite side effects—sometimes leading to death. Studies conducted at Oxford University by Dr. Joel Mann, showed that women between the ages of 40 and 44, who take the birth control Pill, increased by five times their chances of dying from a heart attack.[12]

Recent studies have indicated that women exposed to

the Pill during or *before* pregnancy have a significantly higher incidence of malformed babies. A study conducted by the Birth Defects Institute, New York State Department of Health, showed that while only 4 percent of the mothers of normal children had been exposed to hormone treatment (the Pill), 14 percent of the mothers with malformed children had a history of exposure.[16]

Clearly, oral contraceptives *ARE* dangerous drugs and should never be used by anyone concerned with their health or the health of their children! Most of the above-mentioned side effects may never be experienced by the majority of Pill users, but some certainly will be. And who knows, the side effect you suffer may be a stroke, blood clots, heart attack, or cancer. So, why take the chance? *There are* perfectly natural and safe methods of birth control, as I will show later in this chapter.

However, women who, for one reason or another, in spite of my warnings and the conclusive medical evidence, decide to use birth control pills should have an extensive clinical examination and give a responsible doctor a thorough personal and family history to determine the likelihood of the more serious complications. For those who have a family history of any of the above-mentioned serious side effects, especially cancer, heart disease or thrombophlebitis, taking oral contraceptives is like playing Russian roulette!

Nutritional protection

If you have taken the Pill in the past and are worried about possible side effects turning up in the future, or are taking it now, in spite of all the warnings and your better judgement, what can you do to counteract somewhat its health-damaging effects?

Improved nutrition and taking special vitamins and supplements can help to ward off the worst. Many of the side effects of the Pill are directly linked to nutritional deficiencies which it induces.

Here are the most important anti-Pill-damage supplements:

Vitamin B_6

Nausea, mental and emotional changes, and edema are due to vitamin B_6 deficiency induced by taking the Pill. A daily dose of 50 - 100 mg. of B_6 should correct this.[1,17]

Vitamins A and C

Pill-caused lowering of vitamins A and C levels in the body leads to decreased resistance to infections.[1,10] Taking 1,000 - 2,000 mg. of vitamin C and 10,000 - 25,000 units of vitamin A daily may be needed to improve resistance to infections.

Biotin

Biotin deficiency caused by the Pill contributes to eczema, depression, fatigue, dry hair, and hair loss.[1] Two or three tablespoons of brewer's yeast powder or 150 - 300 mcg. of biotin in tablet form can be taken daily.

Vitamins B_1, B_2, and B_{12}

These B vitamins are depleted by continuous use of the Pill and should be added to the diet. Brewer's yeast is the best natural source of all B vitamins.[1,14]

Folic Acid

This is another of the B-complex vitamins that is lowered in the body by the Pill.[15,18] 1 to 2 mg. a day is sufficient.

B-Complex

The Pill interferes with tryptophan (essential amino acid) metabolism. This can be corrected by taking one high-potency B-complex tablet and/or 2 - 3 tbsp. brewer's yeast every day.[7]

Iron and zinc

These are two of the most important minerals to help counteract the damaging effects of the Pill.[19,20] Approximately 15 mg. of zinc and 20 mg. of iron can be taken daily by all Pill users.

Selenium and Iodine

These are two specific protective trace elements that can help to minimize the carcinogenic effect of the Pill (see Chapter 25). The usual dosage is 50 mcg. of selenium and 2 - 3 tablets of iodine-containing kelp daily. Kelp and dulse are the best natural sources of iodine, and brewer's yeast is the best natural source of selenium.

All the above-mentioned vitamins and minerals are sold at health food stores.

Pill and the pre-adolescent

An alarming fact connected with the Pill is that girls at younger and younger ages are using it. Often, with the blessings (and even insistance) of worried mothers, girls are put on the Pill at the time of their first menstrual period. If the Pill can cause all the before-mentioned severe biochemical, hormonal, and pathological disorders in adult women, just imagine how devastatingly injurious it can be to the young, tender, undeveloped body of a twelve or thirteen-year-old child!

The sad part of the situation is that too many mothers are unaware of the long-term health-damaging effects of the Pill, and think that by permitting their adolescent daughters to use the Pill, they are doing them a favor—as well as protecting themselves against the possible risk of social embarrassment. They may be unknowingly, in ignorance, crippling their dear children for life! The following anecdote illustrates humorously the unfortunate manner in which some mothers (and grandmothers) view the subject:

A 68-year old grandmother, while in her doctor's office for a checkup, requested a prescription for the contraceptive pill. The doctor said:

"The Pill, at your age?"

"My age is none of your business," snapped grandmother. "Just give me the Pill."

Reluctantly, the doctor wrote the prescription.

When the grandmother visited his office a few months

later, the doctor, remembering the Pill prescription, asked with a derisive grin:

"How are you doing with the Pill, Mrs. Jones?"

"Oh, just great!" said grandmother. "I sleep like a baby."

"Sleep like a baby?! Those aren't sleeping pills, you know," said the alarmed doctor.

"I know, silly," she said slyly. "But, I have a 13-year-old granddaughter and every morning, before she goes to school, I crush one Pill and mix it with her orange juice. And now I sleep like a baby!"

Weight gain and the Pill

During various natural hormonal changes that occur in a woman's life, she has a tendency to gain weight. Such weight gain periods are adolescence, pregnancy, and menopause.

Artificially induced drastic hormonal changes have the same effect on the body—weight gain. In fact, weight gain is one of the most common reasons for dissatisfaction with birth control pills. It seems some women are more concerned about their figures than the potential carcinogenic and other dangerous effects of the Pill.

Here's how the Pill causes weight gain:[21]

1. It increases the appetite by the anabolic and androgenic actions of *progestin* in the Pill.

2. *Estrogen* in the Pill causes fluid retention.

3. *Estrogen* also causes localized fat deposits in some women. This is related to the Pill's so-called feminizing action. Some women experience an increase in fat tissue over the thighs, hips, and breasts.

Although weight gain caused by fluid retention (edema) is easily corrected if the Pill is discontinued, the fat deposits caused by the Pill are not lost as readily as the excess water.

Smoking and the Pill

After keeping their heads, ostrich-like, deep in the sand as far as the serious health dangers connected with birth control pills are concerned, the Federal Food and Drug Administration (FDA) finally, in 1978, after almost 25 years of universal and massive pill use and probably millions of deaths due to such complications as heart attacks, liver rupture, blood clots, and cancer, issued a warning and established a new "patient information" statement to be given to women by doctors who prescribe oral contraceptives. It includes information regarding increased risk of heart attacks and other circulatory problems, such as strokes, for women who smoke while taking birth control pills.[22] This warning was based on two recent studies that alarmed even the hard-headed FDA. The warning states that "Women who should not take the Pill, *in addition to those who smoke*, are those who have had blood clotting disorders, cancer of the breast or sex organs, unexplained vaginal bleeding, a stroke, heart attack, or angina pectoris, or who suspect they may be pregnant...those with scanty or irregular periods." The FDA also warns that "more serious side effects, while less frequent, can be fatal."

Cancer and the Pill

As early as 1966, studies linked birth control pills to cancer[23] especially of the uterus. Other studies showed that the risk of developing cancer of the breast, liver and pituitary is increased in women who take the Pill, especially if they are between the ages of thirty and forty.[9,10]

Dr. Otto Sartorius, director of the Cancer Control Clinic of Santa Barbara General Hospital in California, reported that "After a two-year study of two hundred young Santa Barbara women, there are indications that a *majority* of those women who use the Pill for birth control, are sustaining irreversible and permanent breast damage, and are exposing themselves to an approximate three-fold increase in the risk of developing breast cancer. The breast, under stimulation from the Pill, becomes nodular, firm, enlarged, and sometimes tender. Cysts, microcysts, papillomas, and inflammatory reactions may be seen—the direct result of overstimulation of the breast by estrogen and progesterone."

"If I were a girl," Dr. Sartorius says, "I would not be on the Pill. The Pill is producing abnormal changes in the breast and I know I wouldn't want them in my breast. What will happen to millions of women with these breast changes? I worry about this"..."Estrogen is the fodder on which carcinoma grows," states Dr. Sartorius.

Cellular studies also show ductal and glandular hypertrophy and hyperplasia of the supporting tissues.[22]

Dr. Roy Hertz, of the National Institute of Health, after noting that breast cancers have been induced in five different species of animals treated by the powerful synthetic hormones used in oral contraceptives, stated that "by 1971, breast cancer may start to occur increasingly among women who take oral contraceptives."[22] He was right! Breast cancer is now the leading cause of cancer deaths among women!

I shudder when I think that there are millions of young, unsuspecting, adolescent girls in this country who are popping birth control pills like candy, totally unaware of the grave risk of cancer that they pose.

Intra-uterine devices

Next to the oral contraceptives, intra-uterine devices (IUD's), are presently the most popular birth control method. They are made in many shapes (shields, loops, and coils) and from diverse, more or less toxic materials such as plastics and copper. IUD's have been used since ancient times—yet the exact mechanism by which they work is unknown. The intra-uterine device, as the name suggests, is inserted into the uterus. Its continual presence there prevents, either by mechanical interference, or by its toxic action, the attachment of the egg to the uterine wall, and thus, prevents conception.

IUD's are almost as harmful as oral contraceptives. Not only is their failure rate higher than that of the Pill (4.1% vs. 3%) but the side effects may include: cramping and pain, especially increasing during the menstrual period; tubal pregnancy; spontaneous abortion; uterine bleeding; blood poisoning; bowel obstruction; cervical infection; anemia; and perforation of the uterus. The devise can even become imbedded in the uterus. The latter problem frequently leads to hospitalization and even death.

On the positive side, although users of IUD's are five times as likely to be hospitalized as the Pill takers, mortality related to oral contraceptives is four times greater.[5]

It has been shown that complications caused by IUD's result less from the device itself than the technique of placement, and only a highly-skilled specialist should perform the task. Furthermore, it is difficult to train women to check themselves for the proper position of the IUD.

Recently, the FDA approved a new intra-uterine device that releases progesterone for one year. Called Progestasert, it is a T-shaped device with a curved polyethylene inserter, which supposedly greatly diminishes the risk of perforating the cervix of uterus.[24] The new device assures a lower pregnancy rate—about 2.5%, as compared to 4.1% for other IUD's. Since this new IUD has been available a very short time, its side effects are not known, but I predict they will be even worse than for the earlier types of IUD's. Being progesterone (powerful synthetic hormone) medicated, they no doubt will have, in addition to the usual side effects caused by IUD's, the serious complications associated with oral contraceptives that contain the same hormones.

Diaphragm, jelly, cream, foam, etc.

Spermicidal jellies, creams, suppositories, tablets, or foams are sometimes used alone, but since their effectiveness is not considered very high, they are generally used in conjunction with a diaphragm. Together they form a fairly reliable, although somewhat inconvenient and messy, contraceptive. The major drawback is the difficulty of insuring that the diaphragm will remain in the proper position. It must be fitted by a doctor and refitted every year, or after a pregnancy, or gain or loss of ten pounds. Some women have pelvic conditions that rule out the use of the diaphragm. It also may become dislodged during intercourse if the woman is on top. The diaphragm, when used with jelly, cream, or foam, must be left in place for at least six hours after intercourse to be effective.

Although to my knowledge no research has been done to determine the degree and frequency of toxic and irritating effects of spermicidal chemicals on the genital tissues, this can pose a very serious health hazard. Some women are extremely sensitive to these irritating chemicals. Also, these toxic chemicals may be absorbed through the mucuous membranes of the vaginal tract and poison the entire body. Internal or external use of strong chemicals should always be approached with caution.

Condoms

Personally, I feel that birth control should be primarily the man's responsibility. When used properly, high-quality condoms are almost 96 percent effective. What is more important, they are 100 percent safe! They are, of course, more bothersome than some of the more dangerous methods, but they have absolutely no health-damaging side effects to either the man or the woman. They decrease penile friction somewhat, some brands more than others, but this is considered by many to be a benefit since it tends to prolong intercourse.

Condoms are also the only contraceptive that offers a reasonably good protection against veneral disease, although contraceptive creams offer some protection, according to clinical studies reported in *Advances in Planned Parenthood*. This is not a minor advantage, considering that the exploding venereal disease epidemic is the number one infectious disease problem in the United States—10 to 15 million new cases are reported each year! This means that one in every twenty sexually-active adults (and children) contracts venereal disease!

Condoms have been used for centuries and come about as close to being a natural birth control method as is commonly available, outside of the fertility awareness method described later in this chapter. In the past, condoms were made from the skins of sheep intestines, but now the rubber variety is most common. Condoms which are sold in the United States (in every drugstore) are usually of very high quality and are well-tested. Although the pre-lubricated kinds are more comfortable, they may involve questionable chemicals, so the ideal is to use the non-lubricated brands.

The condom is the only contraceptive used by the *man*. However, in this age of the Pill, I have found American men to be so "spoiled," that they won't be bothered with the condom. In my seminars, when this question comes up and women complain that their men refuse to use it, my usual response is: "If a man objects to the small inconvenience of putting on a condom, and is willing to subject his woman to the serious and proven risk of dying from cancer, heart disease, or stroke by insisting that she use oral contraceptives, he is not a man—he is an inconsiderate, selfish beast who does not deserve a woman!"

The failure rates for all the above-mentioned contraceptives, according to current figures obtained from the Planned Parenthood Federation of America, are: 3% for the Pill, 4.1% for the IUD, 4.3% for the condom, 5% for the diaphragm, and 14.8% for jelly and foam barriers.

Some new, but dubious, medical innovations

According to a report in the West German Medical magazine, *Praxis-Kurier*, aspirin may act as a birth control pill for men. After only a week of taking aspirin doses normally given for headaches, the male test subjects were virtually sterile. This may partly explain the dramatically-increased incidence of sterility among men in the United States in recent years. More aspirin is consumed in the United States than anywhere in the world! Aside from the possible side effects, such as stomach ulcers and hemorrhage, aspirin can hardly be recommended, since the aspirin's biochemical action causing sterility is still unknown.

A new tablet contraceptive, *Encare Oval*, was developed in West Germany and recently made available in the U.S. The effervescent tablet is inserted into the vagina, where it covers the cervix and kills the sperm. In studies involving 11,000 women in Europe since 1969, the tablet has been found to be 99 percent effective, according to Dr. H.Brehm, professor of medicine at the Gynecologic Clinic in Cologne City Hospital in West Germany. Although claimed to be "safe physically and chemically" and without "strong side effects or dangers," anything strong enough to kill sperm is strong enough to irritate the delicate tissues of the vagina and cervix. Therefore, the vaginal pill may, on a long-term basis, turn out to be just as harmful as the rest of the unnatural birth control methods.

An improved diaphragm may be available soon. The new device is a small sponge with microscopic pores which, when inserted into the vagina, would trap any sperm that try to swim through it. Since use of the sponge requires no cream, jelly, or drugs, it might be a good alternative to the conventional diaphragm, which is messy, inconvenient, and has a comparatively high percentage of failure. A new sponge is inserted once a month, and removed occasionally for washing with plain water. At present, this new device is being tested at the University of Arizona, in Tucson, and also on two thousand volunteers worldwide.

A radically new birth control chemical has been developed by Dr. Harry Kent of Rutgers University in New Jersey. It contains no hormones of which the ill-famed Pill is made, and needs to be taken only eight days each month. It is called **Kentsin**, and, according to its discoverers, the new contraceptive interferes with the ovulation cycle and has no harmful side effects. It is both safer and cheaper than today's Pill, but is not expected to be on the market until 1980 or later, as tests, sponsored by the National Institute of Health, still continue.

Perhaps the most dubious of all recent medical innovations in the field of birth control, is the anti-pregnancy vaccine which was developed at the All India Institute of Medical Sciences in New Delhi. The principle on which the vaccine supposedly will work is that it produces antibodies to a hormone essential to the maintenance of pregnancy. The vaccine is still in the early stages of testing at research centers in a number of countries.

Some new, more natural techniques

In Russian studies with 800 women, vitamin C was found to be a 96 percent effective contraceptive.[25] The vitamin C tablet, 250 - 500 mg., is not taken orally, but is inserted into the vagina ten minutes before intercourse, its contraceptive effect supposedly lasting half an hour. Further research by the Aquarian Research Foundation of Philadelphia seemed to confirm this, but they recommend it only in conjunction with cyclic methods to be discussed later. Further studies are warranted before this method could be confidently recommended, although the biochemical principle—the ascorbic acid neutralizing the sperm, or creating a biochemical milieu where sperm can't survive—seems sound.

A similar contraceptive device was developed by the California Rabbi, Dr. Bronner. It is a bullet-shaped suppository which contains citric acid, glycerine, and malic acid. Its contraceptive action is based on the assumption that it will lower the pH in the vagina to less than 4.0— and "conception is impossible below pH of 4.0," claims Dr. Bronner. The suppository is encased in cocoa butter which melts from body heat when the suppository is inserted, thus releasing the citric acid. It takes a few minutes to heat the cocoa butter. According to Dr. Bronner, his contraceptive is "natural, edible, non-irritating, and harmless." Of course, the effectiveness of this device has never been tested or proven by scientifically accepted methods.

Another frontier of harmless contraceptive research involves the use of light. Scientists at the Roch Reproduction Clinic in Boston, Massachusetts, have found that if a woman sleeps with the lights on during the night at certain points in her menstrual cycle, her hormones are regulated in such a manner as to make conception impossible.[26] This approach, which is still in the experimental stage, is interesting, although it is doubtful that it can ever become useful and practical, nor anything more than a fascinating scientific curiosity.

Still another experimental technique, which is in the same class as the light approach, is the use of temperature regulation of the testicles. One on-going experiment has shown that keeping the testicles especially warm (in comparison to the rest of the body) could cause male sterility in just a few weeks. Conversely, keeping the testicles cold can enhance fertility. Dry heat, microwaves, infrared rays, ultrasound, wired pouches, hot baths, saunas, and even athletic supporters have been successfully used to achieve this sterility effect.[27] Obviously, some of these warming methods, such as microwaves, would not be advisable. Again, I don't see any practical application of this discovery, except as a possible means of increasing male fertility by cold showers and especially by cold sitz-baths, which are described in my book, *How To Get Well*, page 238.

Other alternatives

Coitus interruptus, or withdrawal, is an ancient, but ineffective, and rather frustrating form of birth control. If this method is used, ejaculation should definitely follow (away from the vaginal area, of course, to avoid possible conception), in order to prevent prostate trouble that can result if sexual fluids are not released. The unreliability of the withdrawal method relegates its use to emergencies.

The FDA recently approved the controversial "morning after" pill of diethylstilbestrol—with the warning that it should be only used in serious emergencies, such as rape, or medically inadvisable conception, since DES is known to cause vaginal cancer.

Abortion, as a method of birth control, is being practiced more and more widely, especially in some oriental countries, but also in the U.S., ever since it was legalized in many states.

From a biological and holistic health point of view, abortion is unnatural. Only sick women, unable to produce healthy offspring, abort (miscarry) spontaneously. Once experiencing abortion, the body will be less likely to carry a pregnancy to full term. Thus, miscarriages are frequent in those who have undergone previous surgical abortions. Abortion is, as any surgery, a severe shock to the body, and the anesthetics used can cause further problems. Only in cases of rape or where the poor health of the woman does not allow for the possibility of a healthy delivery, or if a continued pregnancy would mean a serious threat to the health of the mother, can abortion be justified.

Sterilization—vasectomy for men and tubal ligation for women—is becoming more and more popular as a method of birth control. An unbelievable 1.3 million Americans are sterilized each year! This does not include a growing number of hysterectomies performed for other than birth control purposes. Although in 1970, 80 percent of all sterilization was done on men, the proportions have changed as tubal ligations are becoming simpler. Now, 51 percent of sterilizations are performed on women.

Sterilization methods are not considered reversible (some attempts have been made, but with limited success), so a decision for such a drastic and irreversible method of contraception must be made with great care. The chances of successful reversal of female or male sterilization have improved with new micro-surgery techniques developed recently. Even so, only a small percentage of sterilized females can count on their fertility being restored. For males, the possibility of restoration of fertility is even more uncertain. A man's body, after a time, develops antibodies which destory sperm. This process often continues even after surgical reversal of the vasectomy, leaving him sterile.

Although surgical sterilization is too new to be scientifically assessed as to its possible long-term side effects, it is known already that male hormone levels are lowered, the libido eventually decreases, and there is often an accumulation of fat in various parts of the body.[1] Anything that so drastically interferes with the glandular system's normal function is bound to have undesirable side effects, both physically and, especially, psychologically. Clearly, this is one of the most unnatural methods of contraception and we must view it with great caution.

Herbs and birth control

Various herbs have been ascribed contraceptive properties by folk medicine. Although many travelers to "primitive" cultures have reported oral herbal contraceptives being used by women in various tribes, surprisingly little scientific research has been done to determine the contraceptive value of these different herbs. I know of only one such research at present. It is in regard to a plant called *Lithospermum rederate* (root) and *Semen Lithospermi* (seeds). The research is being done at Indiana University under the direction of Breneman and Carmack.[28] *Lithosperma* (root or seeds) has been used by Nevada Indian tribes in the form of a tea to prevent conception. The tea must be drunk over a period of several months. In studies with mice fed alcoholic extract of this plant, the animals exhibited decreased weight of the sex organs and of the thymus and pituitary glands, as well as cessation of the normal estrus cycle.[29] Also other researchers used this plant on rabbits and rats and concluded that *lithosperma* appears to inhibit the action of gonadotropin in the ovary.[30] Indiana University studies showed that one of the body's hormones inhibited by *lithosperma* is oxytocin, which is involved in controlling uterine contractions.

Cherokee women used the spotted cowbane root, *Cicuta maculata*, also called beaver's poison. It was well known, however, that if a woman ate of this root for four days, she became permanently sterile. It is so toxic that it can be deadly if eaten in excessive amounts.

Beowawe Indian women drink false hellebore tea daily, made from the fresh root, to prevent conception. A tea of the cured root supposedly ensures sterility for life.

And another Indian tribe from Nevada uses an herb called stoneseed for the same purpose. Infusion from the root of the plant is drunk daily for six months to effect permanent   sterility.

Other plants credited with contraceptive properties are milkweed (the whole plant), Indian turnip, ragleaf bahia, cramp bark, dogbane (roots).

The following herbal "morning after" birth control is practiced by rural residents of India's Rajasthan state: carrot seeds are chewed by the woman for several days after intercourse. The New Delhi scientists claim that it really works. The seeds supposedly act just like estrogenic agents in inhibiting implantation of a fertilized egg in the uterus.[30]

In my recent travels in Australia, I found confirmation of the reports that Australian aborigines use wild yams for contraception. The analysis of the plant shows it to be high in estrogen-like hormones.

In Morocco, women eat raw castor beans, which are extremely poisonous. They eat one bean for each year they wish to remain infertile.[31] Castor beans are also used in some other African countries and in India for the same purpose.

As I studied the available literature on contraceptive herbs, the following thoughts kept recurring:

1. All of the herbs, roots, seeds, etc., used for contraception seem to work by stopping menstruation and producing sterility. Since all contraceptive herbs that I've studied are more or less toxic, the sterility seems to be accomplished by poisoning the whole body, and, thus, making it unfit for reproduction. You see, nature is extremely wise. If a woman is sick, poisoned, weak, or otherwise unhealthy and not likely to give life to a healthy offspring, ovulation ceases in order to prevent conception and giving birth to a defective baby. It is nature's way of preserving the quality and life of the species.

2. Consequently, toxic herbs, which alter and interfere with the body's basic biochemical and hormonal processes are, then, a no better means of contraception than the Pill or other chemical contraceptives, *even though they are natural*. In our New Age counter-culture, everything synthetic and "establishment" is automatically rejected and

everything natural is favored. Nature does grow many *toxic* plants, some of which can be used as medicines in minute amounts. But, using poisonous plants for such a non-medical reason as birth control—toxic plants that may affect the health of the future mother for life by altering the vital functioning of her reproductive system—does not seem rational to my common-sense mind. Therefore, until contraceptive herbs are found which are not only 100 percent effective, *but also 100 percent safe and non-toxic*, I hesitate to recommend them for birth control—especially in view of the fact that we *do* have 100 percent natural and 100 percent safe birth control methods already available. Keep reading!

The total fertility awareness method of natural birth control

Now, finally, we are coming to a birth control system that can be recommended. Known separately as cycle, ovulation, rhythm, mucus, and temperature birth control methods, they are all essentially the same and are based on the sound concept—actually a proven fact—that there are only certain days of the month (menstrual cycle) when impregnation is possible. Conception can occur only during ovulation, the time when the female ovaries release the ovum, which travels to the fallopian tubes and uterus and can there be fertilized by the male's spermatozoa. A few days before actual ovulation and two or three days after ovulation are *unsafe days*, the only days of the month when conception can occur. The difficulty is in determining the exact time when ovulation occurs. Each of the various cyclic methods claims to do that the most effectively. Actually, by far the best and safest natural birth control is to use a *combination* of all these basic cyclic methods—calendar or rhythm method, the basal body temperature method (BBT), and cervical mucus or ovulation method—*simultaneously*! Or, what I call a

TOTAL FERTILITY AWARENESS METHOD.

Billings ovulation method

This ovulation method was discovered by an Australian husband and wife team of doctors, Drs. John and Evelyn Billings.[32,34] It is appropriately called the Billings Ovulation Method. The ovulation method is approved by most churches, including the Roman Catholic Church, and is actively endorsed and supported by many official health groups, such as the Natural Family Planning Research Center in California, which is engaged in a long-term study of the ovulation method on grants from the National Institute of Health and the Department of Health, Education and Welfare.

The Billings Ovulation Method is based on the observation of the quantity and quality of vaginal mucus discharged through each menstrual cycle. The mucus originates from cervical gland-like crypts. In the beginning of each cycle (in the first few days after menstruation) when the hormone estrogen level is low, the vagina feels dry and the mucus is scant, sticky, and opaque, due to the presence of a large quantity of cellular matter. This can be confirmed by the woman's examining finger. In the middle of the cycle (8 - 10 days after menstruation) the estrogen levels begin to increase as the body prepares for ovulation, and the quantity of the mucus increases. It becomes thinner and clearer in appearance. As estrogen increases in the system, the mucus becomes clearer and more slippery. The estrogen level peaks right before ovulation (about one day before) when the mucus will be most profuse (up to ten times what it was earlier) and also very clear and slick, and so stretchy and slippery that you may be able to stretch an unbroken shimmering thread of it between your thumb and forefinger. It resembles raw egg white in quality and it produces a definite lubricating sensation. Ovulation occurs at the peak of that sensation.

The purpose of the lubricating mucus just before and during ovulation is dual: a) to facilitate intercourse, which is biologically designed to preferably occur at this time to assure conception and procreation: and b) to prolong the life of the sperm cells. Abundant fertile mucus nourishes the sperm, guides them upwards towards the ovum in the uterus, protects them from the acid pH of the vagina (mucus is alkaline) and keeps them from being destroyed by phagocytes (blood cells that can eat or destroy foreign matter or bacteria).

These changes in the quality and quantity of cervical mucus during the cycle can be easily recognized by every woman, simply by feeling with her fingers at the exterior of the vagina. By learning to recognize the differences in the mucus and by keeping careful records or charts of the change in the mucus during her cycle, a woman can predict effectively those exact days when she may be fertile. The couple can then use this knowledge to prevent conception by abstaining from intercourse during that time, which is normally about seven to eight days—four days before and three days after the ovulation.

The calendar or rhythm method

This method is based on the mathematical calculations of your individual menstrual cycle and an approximate estimation of the ovulation date. First, keeping careful records of your menstrual periods for six to twelve months, you determine the length of your personal cycle. The cycle length varies in different women, but is usually between 21 to 35 days. The rhythm method is rather uncertain if your cycle is irregular. Therefore, I would not advise reliance on this method exclusively. But, if you are very regular (the same length menstrual period each time) you can predict your fertile days pretty well. Ovulation occurs approximately fourteen days before menstruation begins. Here is an approximate chart of the length of the cycle and the first fertile day, counted from the first day of menstruation:

If cycle is:	First fertile day is:
22 days	4th day
24 days	6th day
26 days	8th day
28 days	10th day

30 days	12th day
32 days	14th day

Beginning from the first fertile day, you must abstain from intercourse for 7 to 8 days to prevent conception.

Basal body temperature method

This method is based on the biological fact that the temperature of most women, measured right after awakening in the morning, undergoes changes throughout the cycle. Before ovulation, the temperature is average or low, but immediately after ovulation it rises several tenths of one degree over what it was before ovulation. By a careful charting of the temperature every morning, the exact day of ovulation can be determined with relative accuracy. Although the temperature may vary slightly each day, it will rise noticeably during and after ovulation, often as much as one degree.[33]

The basal body temperature (the temperature of your body at complete rest) must be taken each morning, using a special basal thermometer (sold at drug stores), and recorded on a graph. Usually before ovulation, the temperature is around 98 degrees or just below. Right after the ovulation, it rises as much as 0.6 degrees. Generally, it is a sudden rise in one day, but occasionally it is a gradual rise over a period of several days. Three or four days after your temperature reaches the high point, you become infertile and may resume intercourse.

The drawback to the BBT method is that it doesn't tell you when ovulation is coming. It only tells you when it has occurred. Thus, the unsafe time *before* ovulation is more difficult to determine. Therefore, the BBT method should preferably be combined with other cyclic methods, such as the calendar rhythm method and/or the ovulation method.

Sympto-thermal method

This method was developed for exactly the reason mentioned above. In addition to the basal temperature changes, it combines other symptoms that are characteristic during the cycle, such as irritability, pain, breast tenderness, edema, etc. They are all combined into one integrated method of achieving fertility awareness.

Consequently, as I said before, the most effective and accurate natural birth control method is a *Total Fertility Awareness Method* (TFAM), where all the above-mentioned methods based on the physiological, hormonal, and biochemical changes during the female cycle are *combined* and used *simultaneously*. There is a good book which describes all the above-mentioned cyclic methods in detail, in simple, easy-to-understand language and in practical terms. Every woman who chooses to practice cyclic natural birth control should acquire *The Cooperative Method of Natural Birth Control*, by Margaret Notzinger. It is available from The Book Publishing Co., Summertown, Tenn., 38483. They also sell basal thermometers as well as graph charts that can be used to record the basal body temperature.

Summary

As our planet becomes more and more overpopulated, there will be an increasing demand for effective birth control methods. The need for birth control is accentuated by our new social, moral, and marital concepts, as well as by the fact that more and more women in this era of physical degeneration are unable to carry and deliver healthy offspring.

There are many reasons why couples might wish to practice birth control. I am neither recommending and endorsing, nor discouraging and condeming, the practice. I have simply reviewed the alternatives from the viewpoint of a natural, holistic health approach. I believe that every woman and every man should know the facts about the available contraceptive methods.

I think the message in this chapter is loud and clear: stay away from all harmful, toxic, health-damaging contraceptive techniques! The most popular birth control methods, although relatively effective, are anything but safe. At this writing, *all* oral contraceptives and IUD's are extremely dangerous. A growing number of deaths are attributed to the use of both, in addition to such serious side effects as breast and uterine cancer, heart attacks, strokes, etc.

Foams, jellies, vaginal tablets, and medicated suppositories that are strong enough to kill sperm, are strong enough to cause irritation and damage to the delicate mucus membranes of the sex organs.

Tubal ligation and vasectomy, although 100 percent effective, are too new to be properly assessed as to their long-term side effects. But we do know already that in the male, hormone levels are decreased, the libido is lessened, and body fat is added as a result of such drastic surgical insult on the body.[1] We must view with great caution anything as unnatural as surgical methods of contraception.

Which leaves us with only two methods which I can personally condone. Both are well tested, safe, totally harmless and natural: the condom, and/or the Total Fertility Awareness Method, as described in this chapter. The fertility awareness method has the added attraction of being the only non-sexist form of birth control. It requires the love and understanding of both partners, where neither one is required to bear a health burden or assume the exclusive responsibility. And since sexual intercourse is not the only way to make love, even those few unsafe days during the month can be, with love and imagination, as fulfilling as the rest.

Obviously, each individual must assume responsibility for whatever method is chosen. For those who for one reason or another wish to practice birth control, the information presented in this chapter should help to choose a contraceptive technique or method that is best suited to their individual needs, taking into consideration physical, psychological, religious, and moral implications. For them, it must be comforting to know that with the right method and a proper mental attitude, contraception need not pose a serious threat to health.

23
Holistic Approach To Menstrual Problems

In our culture, the female menstrual period has been synonymous with pain, discomfort, and stress for both mind and body. The menstrual syndrome range from cramps, sore breasts, backache, and edema, to depression, tension, irritability, and faintness. But these menstrual symptoms are not really natural nor necessary. In some other, more "primitive" cultures, those of Central American Indians, Chinese, and Hunzakuts, women do not experience these side-effects of menstruation.[1, 2] It has also been noted that improved environment and nutrition have a beneficial effect on all menstrual disorders. In this chapter, we will examine the causes, prevention, and biological and nutritional therapies for menstrual difficulties.

The total approach to menstrual problems

It has been scientifically and empirically shown that most menstrual difficulties are due to deficiency, excesses, or improper metabolism of female hormones. Vitamins E, B_6, C, PABA, and folic acid affect estrogen levels and metabolism. Zinc, copper, and calcium metabolism play a role in some menstrual afflictions. Because of the bleeding, there is also a loss of iron. Thus, it is obvious that nutrition should play a vital role in the prevention and treatment of most menstrual disorders. Strangely, with the exception of iron, this simple fact of biochemistry is seemingly ignored by the medical establishment.

All parts of the body are interrelated, and the general

state of health of an individual determines the ability of the body to withstand stress of any kind. A specific weakness or disorder is only a manifestation of a general breakdown with special vulnerability in that area. This also applies to menstrual difficulties of all kinds, whether they are cramps, anemia, edema, or depression. Therefore, a general health-building lifestyle and diet must be pursued. The person who relies on a pill or single therapy to "correct" the condition, without a radical change in diet or lifestyle, can expect inevitable relapse. In Biological Medicine, we do not treat symptoms, making them temporarily disappear—we try to determine the underlying causes, and, by removing them, we assist the body's own healing mechanism to correct the condition. Of course, specific biological and nutritional therapies aid this process, but we merely wish to emphasize the *total approach* to health in trying to correct any disorder.

Physical and spiritual perfection?

In the past, some of my activity was in capacity of a nutrition adviser for several ashrams of young people, members of some of the most popular spiritual movements in California. I had an exceptional opportunity to observe firsthand how severe menstrual problems and irregularities may result from extreme nutritional fads and the resultant nutritional and hormonal deficiencies. I have been consulted by many young women who, for example, had very irregular menstruation, and many who had no menstruation for as long as three or more years. One twenty-six-year-old girl said she hadn't menstruated since the age of sixteen.

In most cases such as these I have found that the women have been involved with heavy drug use, plus a variety of extreme dietary fads. Many of those who didn't menstruate at all had lived on a pure fruitarian diet or other deficient diet for several years. When, after some time of eating nothing but fruits, their menstruation stopped—and males on the same diet became impotent—they were told by their leaders (gurus or masters, whatever the case may be) that menstruation is a sign that the toxic body was trying to throw off poison from the system with the menstrual flow, and that now that their bodies were cleansed and purified, there was no more need for menstruation—they had achieved the ultimate in physical and spiritual perfection. You have to know how much blind faith in, and reliance on, their "perfect masters" these young devotees have, to be able to understand how they can fall for such obviously ridiculous and unscientific reasoning. The truth of the matter is that, according to both the scientific and Divine order of nature, when the human body is weakened and its health potential severely lowered by some environmental factors—inadequate nutrition, disease, or severe emotional or physical stress— such a body will be deprived of its ability to reproduce. This natural law is aimed at preventing the individuals with inferior health from impregnating or conceiving and producing defective or imperfect offspring. This protects the species from physical degeneration. Ovulation ceases and menstruation is disrupted or stopped in females; in males, the spermatozoa and sex hormone production is impaired and they become impotent. I am sure everyone has observed either in their own lives or among those they know intimately, that when a person is severely ill and weak, normal sexual activity will be the first body function to be deranged. To me, this is one of the easiest natural laws to understand: only healthy and vigorous individuals are given the privilege and ability to procreate. Yet, there are some writers who insist that *all* menstruation is abnormal, the result of a toxic body. I cannot see any explanation for this illogical conclusion other than an attempt to explain and justify the lack of menstruation among women who chose to follow the severely deficient, bizarre diets advocated by these misinformed and misguided "experts."

Dietary indiscretions

In most cases, when these sexually and physically devitalized young people stopped their dietary indiscretions and adhered to an Optimum Diet of vitalizing foods—with emphasis on grains, seeds, and nuts, milk and milk products, vegetable oils, brewer's yeast, lecithin, kelp, and other supplements—their reproductive disorders were quickly corrected. Girls began menstruating again and young men became virile. A pure fruitarian diet, with the exclusion of all grains, seeds, and nuts, is perhaps the most perverted and unnatural diet that has ever been invented. I emphasize this because there are so many young, sincere, beautiful, and idealistically-oriented people who are attracted to such a diet, perhaps picturing it to be an aesthetically pure "Garden-of-Eden" sort of diet. Nothing could be further from the truth. Grains, nuts, and seeds are the true Staff of Life—the Divinely designed basis of man's diet—as given in Genesis 1:29: "Behold, I have given you every herb bearing seed [(grains)], which is upon the face of all the earth, and every tree, in which is the fruit of tree yielding seed [(nuts and seeds)]; to you it shall be for meat." Grains, seeds, and nuts contain the germ of life, the potent reproductive power which affects the reproductive capacity and power of human beings—in addition to being the most nutritious of all health-building foods, storehouses of high-quality proteins, fats, minerals, vitamins, and natural energy- and vitality-giving carbohydrates. The healthiest and most virile peoples of the world—Hunzas, Abhkasians, Bulgarians, Vilcambambans, Yucatan Indians—all use grains and seeds as the basis of their diet. In my travels around the world, nowhere have I seen people who eat only fruit. Even in the most Garden-of-Eden-like places, where a variety of wild-growing fruit is available for picking, the natives cultivate stony hills with sweat and toil, to grow some form of seeds, such as corn, beans, millet, or rice, for their dietary staple. Their instinct tells them that without seeds, optimum health and long life cannot be obtained.

Such an Optimum Diet, with an emphasis on grains, seeds, and nuts, and a variety of vegetables and fruits, is also recommended by the most respected of all independent nutrition research forums: The International Society for

Research on Civilization Diseases and Environment. Of course, this Optimum Diet also excludes all devitalizing and refined foods such as white flour and sugar in all forms, canned and processed supermarket-quality foods, tobacco, alcohol, soft drinks, etc. Only natural, whole, and preferably organically-grown foods should be eaten to build up the body as quickly as possible. All grains, seeds, and nuts, are useful but the best are: millet, buckwheat, rice, corn, almonds, sunflower seeds, and sesame seeds. The next most important food group is vegetables, eaten mostly raw. Fruits should be eaten primarily in the morning to assist the body's own cleansing process. Milk, particularly fresh, raw goat's milk, or lactic acid fermented milks such as yogurt and kefir, are also health-building foods in the Optimum Diet, which is described in detail in my books, *How To Get Well* [2] and *Are You Confused?*,[3] and in Chapters 3 and 4 of this book.

Special supplements for menstrual problems

Brewer's yeast is a miraculous food containing high-power nutrition, including 40 - 50% high-quality proteins, a large amount of natural B-complex vitamins, zinc, selenium, and other trace minerals, and nucleic acids—all important in eliminating menstrual difficulties.

Cold-pressed vegetable oils are also essential for the health of the reproductive organs. Olive and sesame oils are most likely to be pure and cold-pressed. Oils should never be used for cooking, baking, or frying—heated oils are carcinogenic. The best way to eat oils is in salad dressing. One tablespoon a day is sufficient.

Kelp is another dietary supplement of general value, but specifically for menstrual difficulties, since it is an excellent source of iodine and minerals. Iodine-rich kelp is especially recommended in excessive menstruation.

Lecithin is important, but since both lecithin and brewer's yeast are high in phosphorus, adequate calcium should also be taken, whether in food form or in concentrated food supplements, such as calcium lactate, dolomite, or bone meal tablets. This is especially important because of the previously-mentioned need for calcium during menstruation, which we will discuss in detail later.

Iron-rich foods should be emphasized to balance the loss through menstrual bleeding. Apricots, eggs, liver, whole grains, seeds, legumes, nuts, grapes, raisins, beets, spinach, prunes, and bananas are rich in iron.

An adequate amount of high-quality protein also should be obtained. For many reasons discussed in Chapter 3, meat is not a recommended protein source, despite the promotion of that image by the meat industry. Buckwheat, millet, sunflower seeds, pumpkin seeds, sesame seeds, soybeans, peanuts, and almonds are good sources of high-quality proteins. Milk, natural cheeses, eggs, and fish are also excellent sources. Fertile eggs are particularly beneficial for healthy reproductive functions. Vegetables—especially green leafy vegetables, avocados, and potatoes—are also good sources of high-quality protein. Fresh wheat germ is an excellent protein food—but make sure it is really fresh. And, of course, the previously-mentioned brewer's yeast is a superior source of high-quality proteins.

If juices are used, they should be those which will aid the body in correcting menstrual problems, particularly anemia. Green juice (from a variety of green vegetables—see Recipes & Directions) red beet juice, and dark fruit juices such as grape, prune, cherry, and black currant, are recommended. Dilute all sweet fruit juices with water, half and half.

The Optimum Diet can and should be supplemented with the specific nutrients, plus vitamins and minerals, mentioned in this chapter for menstrual difficulties.

Hypoglycemia and menstruation

Many of the common symptoms of menstruation are simply due to low blood sugar or hypoglycemia, which is aggravated during the menstrual period. If an individual suspects she has hypoglycemia, the diet should be modified to fit that for hypoglycemia as outlined in my book, *Hypoglycemia: A Better Approach*.[4]

Anemia and menstruation

One of the effects of profuse menstruation is anemia due to loss of blood. The diet must be supplemented with vitamin B_{12}—up to 50 mcg. or even as high as 200 mcg. daily, under a doctor's supervision. The main consideration is, however, iron. Iron-rich foods, listed earlier, are best, as iron supplements are not always well absorbed. Chelated forms may be best; they are sold in health food stores. Vitamin C helps to absorb iron from food sources, but dietary vitamin C is often destroyed by smoking. Smoking, by the way, also aggravates menstrual problems. For over 5,000 years, the Chinese have successfully used the herb Dong Quai (related to ginseng, and available at health food stores) to counteract menstrual anemia.[5]

Irregular and abnormal flow

Suppressed, obstructed, delayed, slow, irregular, and excessive bleeding are some of the common menstrual problems. Irregular or profuse bleeding can be caused by thyroid deficiency and corrected by a natural source of iodine such as kelp.[6] Bioflavonoids also help correct menstrual irregularity.[7] Vitamins B_{12} (25 - 100 mcg. per day) and vitamin E (600 I.U. per day) are also helpful in restoring the normal cycle. A menstrual flow which continues to be heavy after 3 or 4 days has often been corrected by taking 600 units of vitamin E daily.[6] Because prolonged excessive menstruation can be a symptom of uterine cancer, a physician should be consulted immediately if excessive menstruation does not respond to the vitamin and/or mineral therapy suggested here.

Herbal remedies for menstrual problems

Here are the herbs used most often by experienced herbalists for various menstrual problems:[2,8,9,16,17]

Amenorrhea (failure to menstruate, or obstructed and delayed menstruation): pennyroyal, catnip, desert tea (Ephedra Viridis), blue cohosh, motherworth, black cohosh, false unicorn, licorice, holly thistle. These herbs are also effective for facilitation of menstruation at menarche, post partum and menopause.

Dysmenorrhea (painful or difficult menstruation—cramps, nausea, etc.): cramp bark, wormwood, pennyroyal, peppermint, catnip, red raspberry leaves, black cohosh, mugworth, life root, ginger, parsley, balm. Castor oil packs and ginger packs are also helpful.

Menorrhagia (profuse, excessive bleeding during menstruation): lady's mantle, witch hazel, amaranty, red raspberry leaves, solomon seal, cramp bark, white oak bark. Tea from white oak bark can be also used as a douche for excessive bleeding. Take douche on a slant board and try to retain for 15 - 20 minutes.[18]

Herbs are best taken in the form of an infusion, or tea. Place 1 tsp. of diced herbs, or the content of 1 or 2 capsules of powdered herbs, in a cup. Pour boiling water over, and let it steep for 10 - 15 minutes. In an acute condition, at the start of distress, take 1 cup every hour. Normally, 2 - 3 cups a day is sufficient, preferably taken several days prior to onset of menstruation, if time is known.

Homeopathic herbal remedy, Hamamelis Virginica (Witch Hazel), 6X, 8 tablets 2 - 4 times a day, is effective for any hemorrhage, including the excessive menstrual bleeding.

Chinese herb, Dong Quai, is used by many herbalists to normalize disorders.

Premenstrual edema

Premenstrual edema, swelling, and soreness are experienced by many women. These symptoms are usually relieved by the administration of vitamin B_6—50 to 150 mg. a day—especially during the ten days preceding menstruation.[10] Also, taking 2 - 3 bone meal tablets or calcium lactate or calcium orotate tablets daily during the 10-day period before menstruation begins can prevent menstrual cramps and edema.[6] Excessive salt intake may aggravate the condition. Garlic, watermelon, watermelon seed tea, kidney bean pod tea, parsley tea, cucumber juice, and bromelain (pineapple enzyme), as well as exercise, are all helpful in relieving edema, which is usually the cause of swelling and soreness.

Mental state and menstrual difficulties

The irritability, moodiness, melancholia, and depression, which often accompany menstruation, are problems perhaps more serious than we realize or admit. Deficiency or improper metabolism of hormones is part of the cause of the mental changes. Mental and emotional stresses contribute to this common menstrual syndrome. Also, hypoglycemia can be a major contributing factor, as stated earlier.

Vitamin E is well-known to be important both to the adequate production and to proper metabolism of the sex hormones. Due to refining of foods, vitamin E is usually not adequate in the average American diet.[11] The trace mineral selenium (found in foods such as brewer's yeast, wheat germ, sesame seeds, kelp, milk, most cereals, and vegetables), has a "sparing" effect on vitamin E.[12] However, synthetic estrogen, (such as in oral contraceptives), inorganic iron, and chlorine, interfere with vitamin E activity and absorption. Drinking chlorinated water and/or swimming in chlorinated pools (and all public pools are heavily chlorinated) may contribute not only to vitamin E deficiency and hormonal disorders, but also to the development of cancer.

Herbs which aid hormone production and metabolism include sarsaparilla, black cohosh, elder, unicorn, and licorice. Licorice also combats low blood sugar,[13] which can cause all the psychological effects associated with menstruation and, as mentioned previously, is common during the menstrual period.

Caution: herbs listed in this chapter for menstrual disorders should *not* be used during pregnancy, or if pregnancy is suspected.

Abnormal mineral metabolism is often associated with the menstrual period. Copper is often high and zinc low during menstruation.[14] Estrogen medication (or the birth control pill) raises the copper level and lowers zinc level in the blood. Zinc deficiency can lead to depression and psychosis, and elevated copper contributes to the "blues" of the period. Zinc supplementation would, thus, be important during the menstrual period. The usual dosage is 10 to 30 mg. daily. Nutrition in general, has a very powerful effect on our mental state, and at a stressful time like menstruation, this is particularly true.[15]

Menstrual irregularities and the birth control pill

Upon going to the doctor, women, especially young girls, who experience menstrual irregularities—a very short or very long time between periods, or "skipping" of periods for one or several months—are often put on birth control pills to "normalize" the menstrual cycle. The Pill usually accomplishes this almost miraculously. But this approach is a typical orthodox medical approach of treating and eliminating the symptoms without considering the underlying causes of the disorder. Obviously, when there are consistent menstrual irregularities, something is radically wrong with the functions of the reproductive or sex organs, and even with the general health of the patient. The Pill will not correct the basic underlying cause of the problem. In addition, the patient is subjected to the danger of severe side effects from the treatment. The contraceptive pill is known to cause many serious disorders such as phlebitis, varicose veins, heart disease, stroke, high blood pressure, and even cancer (see Chapters 22 and 25).

Menstrual pain and cramps

Aches, cramps, and pains associated with menstruation (aside from edemic soreness) are often due to calcium deficiency.[6] Since dietary calcium in the American diet is much higher than in the diets of other peoples, it would seem difficult to account for this. However, we also eat large quantities of meat which has 22 times more phosphorus than calcium—and, as every nutrition student knows, these minerals should be in approximate balance.

Thus, excessive meat consumption leads to calcium deficiency, which accounts for such calcium-deficiency disorders as periodontal disease, dental caries, and osteoporosis, which are so prevalent in this country. Perhaps this explains why lacto-vegetarians or vegetarians very seldom complain of menstrual pains and cramps.

Calcium absorption is also dependent on sufficient hydrochloric acid and proper levels of vitamin D and magnesium (approximately half the amount of magnesium as calcium is needed). Cod liver oil is the best source of vitamin D.

The homeopathic cell salt Mag. Phos. (available in health food stores or homeopathic pharmacies), is one of the most effective cell salts for menstrual cramps and pain.

Bioflavonoids were found to be helpful in relieving menstrual pain in some women, according to a French clinical team.[7]

Finally, hot "sitz baths" or shallow hip baths, are an old biological remedy for many disorders in the pelvic and hip region. The water should be as hot as can be comfortably borne and the duration of the bath should be 10 to 15 minutes, taken daily. This is not a regular bath, just a submersion of the hip and pelvic region. Juniper needles or chamomile flowers added to the water would be beneficial.[2]

24

Vaginitis:
A Natural Approach

Vaginal infections and problems of various kinds have become a major female disorder in recent years. Vaginal complaints have been around a long time but only within recent years have the so-called infectious kinds sky-rocketed. Now virtually every woman experiences multiple occurrences of the yeast, fungus, or virus-type infections that cause one or all of these symptoms: intense itching, swollen and red vulva, a burning sensation during urination, thick, white, offensive, curdy discharges, patches in the vaginal area, and pain during intercourse. Intermittently called *Moniliasis, Trichomonas vaginalis,* or *Thrush,* vaginitis is also known as *Candidiasis,* from the Candida organisms associated with it.

There are many dozens of kinds of these "infections" and doctors have difficulty diagnosing specific varieties, generally just referring to the collection of symptoms as "vaginitis." Doctors are also mystified about the cause of the problem. A number of leads give one an idea of how to avoid most of these vaginal afflictions, however. The nutritional approach, even in this specific area, has been tried very successfully.[1] We will discuss the nutritional approach to vaginitis a little later in this chapter.

A growing problem

Until recently, only diabetic and pregnant women were subjected to repeated vaginitis attacks.[2] The acid-alkaline balance of the vaginal fluid, the glycogen (sugar) content of the vagina, and changes in the lining cells of the vagina during the menstrual cycle or pregnancy are known to affect the susceptibility to vaginitis. Candida organisms normally exist all over the body—including the mouth, intestines, and vagina—and, generally, present no problem. Generally, washing the genitals with soap and water will keep Candida organisms under control, but the wearing of tight pants and underwear made from synthetic fabrics will provide good chances for Candida to proliferate. Several researchers have advanced some probable causes of the excessive flourishing of Candida and symptoms of vaginitis that accompany it.

The noticeable increase in vaginal infections came at the same time that antibiotics were introduced. Antibiotics not only kill the so-called harmful bacteria, but also the beneficial ones, which play a decisive role in keeping the Candida population down.[2] Pantyhose, tight pants, and underwear made of synthetic fabrics and worn in several layers, provide a warm, moist environment in which Candida multiply.[3] Actually, all tight underwear is biologically unsound. The panty is a relatively new innovation. Just a few generations ago, and throughout history, women never wore underwear, which was a good practice since it allowed good ventilation and kept this vital area of the body dry, preventing infections.

Tampons have also been indicted as a source of irritation and contamination as they do not allow a free drainage of the vaginal fluids.[2] They are also treated with chemicals which can irritate the delicate linings of the vagina. Detergents, if not rinsed out of underwear thoroughly, can irritate the skin, and in fact, almost any kind of irritation can break down the resistance of the body in that area.

A hotly debated point among doctors is whether or not the birth control pill causes vaginal infections—both by the deficiency of vitamin B_6 it induces and the chemical imbalances of the vagina, similar to those occurring during pregnancy, it can create. I, for one, feel that the causative relationship between the Pill and vaginal infections is well established (see Chapter 22).

Vitamin remedies

One of the most effective remedies for vaginitis is the intake of a large amount of all the B vitamins—about 100 mg. of B_1, B_2, and B_6, and 200 mg. of B_3, as well as pantothenic acid and the rest of the complex, supplemented with vitamin B-rich foods such as brewer's yeast.[4] Administration of the large doses of B-complex should not be for more than two months duration, but it can be repeated after a two-month interval. Relief from the itching sensations has been reported with the application of a B_6 salve directly to the affected area.[5] Vitamin B_6 and pantothenic acid seem particularly effective, since they stimulate the production of antibodies and white blood cells.

There are other vitamins which seem important in the control of vaginitis. Vitamin C is well known for its ability to render bacteria harmless and inhibit further growth, as well as strengthen the body's immune system and prevent further infections, when taken in large doses.[6]

Vitamin E (as little as 200 I.U. daily) has a good healing effect in vaginal infections, especially the inflammation and itching, according to some studies.[7, 8]

Garlic is another natural substance that should be used for any kind of infections, including vaginitis and urethral infections, both in male and female. Raw garlic is best, but even garlic pills and tablets can be used. A peeled, raw garlic clove can be inserted directly into the vagina. It has a definite antifungal and antibacterial effect and, according to many reports, can clear up some forms of vaginal infections in a couple of days.[9] Some women have reported to me that by inserting one or two garlic pearls in the vagina they obtained relief from itching within minutes.

Vitamin A has been especially effective in many cases, being vital to the health of the mucus membranes (including those of the vagina). One study reported good results with 50,000 units per day.[10]

Of course, a complete nutritional program, as described in Chapters 3 and 4 of this book, will strengthen the entire body against local weakness, and is just as important as any specific aids.

Douches

There are other sources of relief besides nutrition and vitamins. Douches are, of course, the oldest and most tested approach. Most often recommended is a douche of 2 tablespoons of apple cider vinegar to 1 quart warm water, twice per day.[11] Other variations include 1 teaspoon of salt plus 1 teaspoon of 3% hydrogen peroxide in 1 quart of water.[12] When taking a douche, the tip of the appliance should be inserted and the vaginal opening well-sealed with the hand so the water fills, stretches, and cleans all parts of the vagina. A teaspoon of lactic acid or acidophilus in a quart of water;[13] chlorophyll (especially wheatgrass juice)—a few tablespoons to a waterbag; [14, 15] and douches of herbs—golden seal (½ to 1 teaspoon)[16] as well as squaw vine, bayberry, blackwillow, bethroot, bilberries, and slippery elm[17]—are usually recommended as effective douches. All of these herbs possess antiseptic properties and relieve the inflammation. Squaw vine is very soothing on the vaginal tract and was used for centuries by North American Indian women. To prepare the herbs, take 1 oz. of cut or powdered herbs to 1 pint of boiling water, steep for 15 - 20 minutes, strain, and when infusion is lukewarm, place it in a douche bag.

Danger of excessive douching

We are brainwashed by the media commercials to think that sweet-smelling bubble baths, feminine deodorant sprays, deodorant tampons, and disinfectant and deodorant douches are indispensible for happiness and success in love and marriage. Now, both women and doctors are beginning to realize that feminine hygiene is a dangerous myth, that rather than *prevent* discomfort and infections, deodorant and disinfectant sprays and douches actually *cause* irritations and infections. A recent study of 348 women showed that those who used deodorant sprays and douches had a higher incidence of vulvovaginitis (inflammation of the vulva and vagina) than non-users. Dr. Gideon G. Panter, a prominent New York City gynecologist and a faculty member at the New York Hospital, Cornell Medical Center, says that "Douching only washes away the natural mucus and upsets the vaginal ecology ... Doctors are seeing more irritations of the vaginal area now than they have ever seen before, due to the increased use of commercial hygiene products."[22]

It seems clear that in order to prevent vaginal irritations and vaginal infections, excessive douching should be avoided. In cases of medically diagnosed vaginitis, a short-term use of a herbal or acidophilus culture douche (or other therapeutic douche prescribed by the doctor) can be useful, but as soon as the condition is corrected, all douching should be avoided. Plain soap and water is all you need for keeping the vaginal area clean. The vagina cleanses itself naturally. Glands located in the cervix secrete a mucus substance that bathes the vaginal walls and washes away trapped debris and germs. Merely wiping the lips of the vagina or washing between the legs with a mild, preferably unscented, soap and water is sufficient to keep the sexual organs clean.

Saline bath: a simple preventive and therapeutic aid

Dr. Gideon Panter recommends a simple, do-it-yourself treatment for those who have a tendency for mild, recurring vaginal infections and itching: a saline bath. Take a half cup of table salt and dissolve in a bathtub of water. Soak in this salty bath, and specifically wash your vaginal area, by inserting your finger into the vagina and letting the salty water enter into the vaginal canal. "The saline bath will reduce the population of any invading or

excessive organisms and enable your own body's defense
mechanism to do a better job in fighting the infection.
Nine out of ten times a few of these baths at bedtime will
clear up the infection and save a trip to the doctor's office,"
says Dr. Panter.

Suppositories

Various suppositories have been used with success in
the treatment of vaginitis. One recommendation is the
insertion of a gentian-violet suppository (a tampon is
suggested in conjunction, to prevent staining of clothing
by the dye). Most effective herbal suppositories use golden
seal in a base of cocoa butter[14] (formed into a two-inch
oblong on waxed paper and allowed to cool in the refrigerator), but other herbs which also seem to help are squaw
vine, slippery elm, yellow dock, chickweed, black cohosh,
and mullein (usually a mixture).[17] The insertion of the
suppositories should be done for several consecutive
nights, with douches during the day for greater, quicker
effects. Dr. Stuart Kabnick, of Philadelphia, developed a
biologically-effective vaginal suppository called "cabasil"
(available in some health food stores as well as through
some doctors). Cabasil also comes in oral tablets and oral
and douche powder forms as well. Many have found
remarkable relief with its use.[18]

Made famous by "new age" women's groups, yogurt,
put into the vagina (as well as taken orally), has relieved
many.[19] Its bacteria are similar to those naturally present
in the vagina that keep Candida from multiplying.
Acidophilus culture works on the same principle.

Some doctors have found one other thing effective in
controlling vaginitis: Staphage Phage Lysate, which they
consider semi-natural, and about the best they can offer in
extreme cases. It is also used for infected males. It is
administered in a dosage of 0.1 cc intradermally for at
least 12 weeks, and as long as 24 weeks. It works by
increasing resistance to staphylococcus, which usually are
mixed with the Candida, and gives the body strong resistance to further infections. A reaction to the shots, ranging

from a fever to itching at the site of the injection, can be expected by some.[12]

Herpes

One other very common form of vaginal infection is **Herpes Simplex, virus Type 2,** which appears as small gray-white ulcerations or blisters at the vaginal opening. Temporary relief might be found in direct application of aloe vera gel, vitamin E, or B_6 salve, but the program is generally the same as for yeast infections. Oral administration of B-complex (especially B_6), calcium, acidophilus, and large doses of vitamin C around the clock produce some results. The following herbs have also been used in treatment of herpes: golden seal, black willow and ground ivy. [17, 20] A good bathing of the area with plain water a couple of times a day is extremely important and very effective in helping the body's healing activity. One physician also reported zinc oxide and witch hazel effective.[21] Dr. Milos Chvapil, of the University of Arizona, has developed a zinc medication inserted into vagina in a contraceptive sponge which is in the testing stage at present, but shows a definite promise as an effective treatment to suppress herpes infections. And at the University of California at San Francisco, researchers are testing Pacific red algae as a possible effective natural agent against **Herpes Simplex.** Dolomite powder, alone or mixed with zinc powder, sprinkled directly on sores, speeds healing, as reported by some users. Douching with water, to which vitamin C has been added (1 tsp. of ascorbic acid powder to one pint of water), has been tried by some with reported effectiveness.

Perhaps one of the most effective natural treatments of herpes is **Lactobacillus acidophilus** capsules. They are sold in most health food stores. Note: they must be **capsules**—not tablets, pills, or liquid acidophilus culture (all of which are too weak), but acidophilus capsules! At the first indication that herpes is going to erupt, take five capsules four times a day; or, if herpes sores are already erupted and you are frantic with pain, take two capsules every hour the first day, then reduce to four or five capsules four times a day. Lactobacillus acidophilus capsules are harmless, even in large doses. Some women take as many as ten capsules an hour the first day. Capsules may give you an additional health-promoting benefit by improving your digestion and assimilation of food. *Important:* Lactobacillus acidophilus capsules must be fresh. Therefore, when you purchase them, ask when the shipment was received. After one month, capsules are less effective for this purpose; and after two months of storage they are practically useless. Consequently, do not buy capsules in advance, but right when you need them. If you have any capsules left over, store them in your freezer. They may be useful for a month or so.

If the Lactobacillus acidophilus treatment is instituted early enough it often suppresses the outbreak completely and the blisters will not appear at all. Sometimes, after you have successfully aborted an attack, another will arrive very suddenly within a week or two. If so, just take the lactobacillus capsules again.

Avoiding excessive exposure to the sun, and eating a mineral-rich diet with emphasis on calcium-rich foods is also beneficial and can help prevent herpes infections.

It should be kept in mind that there are no drugs, not even antibiotic drugs, which can cure **Herpes Simplex** virus infections, since antibiotics are ineffective against viruses. Therefore, the above-mentioned natural and biological remedies are the only effective means of attacking this problem.

In conclusion ...

I wish to stress the importance of building and maintaining the body's resistance at the highest level, both for the prevention and correction of any illness. This applies also to such conditions as vaginal infections. Often, various fruitarian, some vegetarian, and other popular diets, which are too alkaline because they leave out all grains, create a pH condition in the bladder and vaginal fluids which is too alkaline. It is important, therefore, that your diet contain plenty of acid-forming grains, beans, etc., as suggested in Chapter 3 of this book. Bacteria and viruses do not thrive in an acid medium. When the bladder content is too alkaline, fresh cranberries or cranberry juice are extremely effective in changing the alkaline condition into an acid one.

In trying some of the remedies, mentioned in this Chapter, please keep in mind that no remedy is perfect for all—while one herb, vitamin, or douche is effective for one, the other herbs or vitamins may be effective for another. By trying and experimenting, you may find the effective therapies for you, suitable for your personal needs. Needless to say, your best bet would be to find a good biologically-oriented doctor and undertake the discussed therapies and nutritional and biological approaches with his cooperation and supervision.

For the list of such doctors, who are trained in natural approaches to healing, you may write to the publishers of this book, enclosing a long, self-addressed, stamped envelope with your request. The list will be sent free of charge.

Finally, it must not be forgotten that prevention is better than a cure. Although some kinds of vaginitis may develop without being transmitted from another person (mostly due to chemical imbalances or changes in vaginal fluids caused by improper diet, dietary deficiencies, oral and vaginal contraceptives, hormonal imbalances, mental and physical stresses, (etc.), many forms of vaginitis are transmitted only through sexual contact. One of the most dangerous forms of vaginal infection, *Herpes Progenitalis,* is caused by *Herpes Simplex virus, Type 2,* which is almost exclusively transmitted through sexual contact. There is no doubt that the so-called "new sexual morality" and indiscriminate sexual promiscuity have contributed greatly to the epidemic growth of the incidence of venereal and non-venereal vaginal infections. Clearly, renouncing sexual "freedoms" and unrestrained promiscuity is imperative if the unbridled vaginitis epidemic in this country is to be halted.

25

Breast Cancer Can Be Prevented

Breast cancer is the deadliest and most prevalent of female cancers. It is a leading cause of cancer deaths among women in the U.S. And, it is increasing at an alarming rate. Breast cancer is expected to strike 1 of every 14 American women. Almost 100,000 new cases are reported, and almost 40,000 women die of breast cancer each year.[1] Numbers are growing with every new year. The situation is considered to be "out of control," reaching epidemic proportions. Millions of women live in constant fear that they will be next to be stricken with this dreadful condition.

The medical establishment has nothing more to offer than mastectomy, or surgical removal of the breasts. Fortunately, breasts are readily accessible for surgical intervention, and consequently, the statistics for successful surgery and recovery are quite favorable—if the disease is caught in time, before it spreads to the inoperable parts of the body. The woman who recovers, however, is maimed for life by losing one or both breasts and a great deal of the surrounding muscle tissue.

Fortunately, I have very hopeful news for all those who still have their breasts intact, and, especially for all young girls and young women. There are many simple, inexpensive, scientifically-proven ways to improve the chances of avoiding or preventing breast cancer. A few specific nutritional measures can enormously increase the ability of any woman to protect her breasts from the growing threat of cancer. But, first, let's take a look at the many probable and proven causes of this dreadful disease.

Causes

1. *Failure to breast-feed baby.* One of the statistically-proven causes of breast cancer, of which I spoke before in the chapter on breast feeding, is the current fad of formula and bottle feeding instead of natural breast feeding. It has been shown that mothers who nurse their babies have a much lesser risk of developing breast cancer than mothers who chose to bottle-feed their babies.[2]

An interesting observation was made in South China, among Tanka women. Traditionally, they nurse their babies from the right breast only. How this rather peculiar and unnatural custom originated is not known. But what has been found by Dr. Roy Ing, a U.S. Public Health Service epidemiologist, and Dr. Nicholas Petrakis, professor of preventive medicine at the University of California, who studied the Tanka phenomenon, supports the contention that breast feeding prevents cancer of the breast.[20] In Tanka women, when there is diagnosable cancer of the breast, even after menopause, it almost always affects the left breast—the one that was not used for nursing.

2. *DES, or Diethylstilbestrol.* It has been shown by extensive research that diethylstilbestrol is a definite causative factor in cancer of the breast, uterus, and other reproductive organs.[3, 4] Most American women who eat meat on a regular basis get plenty of DES in their bodies to cause cancer. Diethylstilbestrol is a synthetic estrogen (female hormone), and it has been polluting most of our beef and poultry for the last twenty years. Stilbestrol is a cheap and powerful cattle fattener. USDA officials say that just sixteen cents worth of this synthetic hormone produces a weight gain worth about twelve dollars at the slaughterhouse. No wonder cattle and poultry growers use it so generously!

Although the cancer-causing potential of DES has been known for a long time, the FDA has allowed its use on cattle and poultry because of pressure from the industries. So, even now, with the DES-cancer connection well-established, the FDA allows its use on cattle, although now in the form of a pellet implanted in the animals' ears, rather than as a feed additive. The FDA believes that the pellets will leave no residue, but there is no proof they will not.

But, whether today's meat does or does not contain residues of DES, American women have been eating DES-containing meat for the last twenty years. And, it is well-known that DES, like most carcinogens, acts very slowly, possibly taking five to twenty years after exposure before the cancer is finally diagnosed.

For example, about twenty-five years ago, it was the medical fashion to give DES to pregnant women who were threatened with miscarriage, on the suspicion that the body's own deficiency of estrogen might be causing the problem. In 1972, reports began to appear that a large percentage of the daughters of DES-treated women began to develop vaginal cancers.[5]

So, if you have been getting traces of DES in your steak, or pot roast, or hamburger, or liver, three or four times a week, over a period of many years, it could have accumulated to a sizeable surplus of synthetic estrogen—which could induce a breast cancer in susceptible women.

3. *Estrogen replacement therapy.* Women who receive estrogen medication such as Premarin, either because of menopause, hysterectomy, or other reasons, have a twelve times greater chance of developing endometrial cancer and also a greater risk of breast cancer.[18] Yet, American doctors prescribe 48 million dollars worth of estrogen a year!

4. *Universal pollution.* The average layman, doctor, and even conventional cancer researcher in this country, is still convinced that the cause(s) of cancer is unknown. Billions of dollars are spent on so-called cancer research, aimed mainly at trying to find a virus that causes cancer. But actual causes of cancer have been known for a long time. The problem is, the causes are linked to our own eating and living habits—and we don't want to hear about such causes. We all hope that scientists will find a cancer-

causing "bug," which will eliminate our own responsibility and make our consciences clear.

The primary and ultimate cause of cancer is lowered or broken-down resistance of the body's own immunological, defensive, and repairing mechanisms, effected by physical, chemical, emotional, and/or environmental stresses, singularly or combined. The unprecedented chemical insult from the toxic environment, polluted air, water, and food, dietary abuses and consequent nutritional deficiencies, overindulgence, particularly in animal proteins and rancid fats, severe emotional stresses, faulty and health-destroying living habits—these prolonged stresses, singularly or combined—lower or break down the body's resistance to disease and pave the way for the development of cancer.[6]

The above-mentioned DES is only one of the hundreds of cancer-causing chemicals found in our food and environment. Artifical sweeteners, tobacco, nitrates and nitrites, coal-tar dyes in foods and cosmetics, radioactive strontium 90 and iodine 131 from fallout, excessive X-rays, cadmium, lead, and mercury in the air, food, and water, chlorine and sodium fluoride in your fluoridated and chlorinated tap water, hundreds of commonly-used drugs, household chemicals and cleaners, lead-containing paints, dry cleaning fluids, propellant in hair sprays, even common salt, coffee, and alcohol in excess—all these can cause cancer, individually, and especially in combination.

Therefore, it can be said that our massive chemical pollution and health-destroying eating and living habits are the basic causes of our steadily deteriorating health and the growing threat of cancer—not only breast cancer, but also lung cancer, cancer of the colon, cancer of the uterus, heart disease, emphysema, and hundreds of other degenerative and environmental diseases ranging from asthma and varicose veins to strokes and arthritis.

5. *Free radicals.* There is a direct causative connection between some dietary patterns and breast cancer. Dr. Nicholas Petrakis, of the University of California at San Francisco, made a revolutionary discovery in his study of

the cancer-prone breasts of the Caucasian-Americans and of cancer-resistant breasts of Japanese-American women. He pumped out the breast fluids of 1,500 women and found that the fluids from the breasts of the women who were cancer-prone contained a much greater amount of free radicals than did the fluids of the cancer-resistant breasts of Oriental women.[7]

Free radicals are the chemical by-products of deteriorated and rancid fats. They come from eating stale and rancid fat-containing foods, such as rancid oils, butters, seeds, and bread, aged meat, foods prepared in rancid oils, such as deep-fat-fried foods, etc. Most grains, nuts, and seeds contain natural oils, which are well-protected from oxidation by the skins or shells. But, as soon as the seed is broken and oxygen comes in direct contact with the oil, the deterioration (oxidation) begins, and harmful, toxic products of oxidation begin to form: peroxides, aldehydes, malonaldehydes, and free radicals. Therefore, in ground seeds, nuts, or grains (such as in bread), if more than one week to ten days old, sufficient peroxidation has already occurred to cause health damage and possibly contribute to the development of cancer.[8]

This is also true of meat. According to Dr. Raymond Shamberger—one of the most knowledgeable nutrition scientists in the world—of the famous Cleveland Clinic Foundation, as soon as an animal is slaughtered and the fat in the meat (beef contains up to 40 percent fat) is exposed to the air, the peroxidation process begins and carcinogenic malonaldehyde begins to form. Dr. Shamberger believes that malonaldehyde from aged beef is one of the contributing causes of cancer of the colon.[9] According to Dr. Petrakis, malonaldehydes and free radicals (fat molecules deformed by the action of oxidation) are contributing causes of the growing number of breast cancers.

6. *The Pill.* As I have already covered in detail in Chapter 22 on birth control, the oral contraceptives have been definitely linked to the increased risk of developing breast cancer. Studies by Dr. Otto Sartorius, Director of the

Cancer Control Clinic of Santa Barbara General Hospital in California, show that "women who use the Pill are sustaining irreversible and permanent breast changes. The cancer risk factor in women taking the Pill is 2.8 times greater the world around, than in women who do not use the Pill." If you have any doubts at all as to the cancer-producing effect of the Pill, as well as its other serious side effects, please read Chapter 22 in this book.

7. *Iodine deficiency.* Pioneering studies on the relationship between iodine deficiency in the food supply and breast cancer were first made by Dr. Bernard A. Eskin, Director of Endocrinology in the Department of Obstetrics and Gynecology at the Medical College of Pennsylvania. His extensive studies showed that breast cancer reaches its highest rate of occurrence in the areas where food supply of iodine is low. The connection between iodine deficiency and cancer is a roundabout one. Here is how it works.

Estrogen, perhaps the most important female hormone, influences almost all vital functions within a woman's body, as well as affects her mind. It is extremely important, however, that estrogen is present in exactly the right amounts. There is strong epidemiological evidence connecting breast cancer with an excess of estrogen— whether this excess is accumulated from synthetic sources, such as DES from foods, or from the body's own natural overproduction. The body wisely controls and maintains the right levels of estrogen in the system with the help of the thyroid hormone, *thyroxine.* Thyroxine is an antagonist to estrogen, keeps it under control, and prevents it from becoming excessive. The deficiency of iodine interferes with the healthy function of the thyroid gland and leads to a deficiency in the production of thyroxine, which, in turn permits the buildup of excessive amounts of estrogen in the body.

Japan and Iceland, for example, have a very low incidence of goiter (disease of the thyroid gland) and an equally low incidence of breast cancer. In Japan, iodine-rich seaweeds comprise a large part of the diet. Their death rate from breast cancer is five times lower than that of the United States.[5] Mexico and Thailand, on the other hand, have a high incidence both of goiter and breast cancer, in spite of the fact that most women in these countries still breast-feed their babies. It seems that even breast feeding cannot sufficiently protect the breast against cancer if the diet is grossly deficient in iodine. Statistical studies show that in the United States, the highest death rate from breast cancer is found in what is known as the "goiter belt" in the Great Lakes region, where soils are lacking iodine and foods grown on such soils are deficient in this important breast cancer protector. A study of Poland, Switzerland, the Soviet Union, and Australia, shows the same pattern: breast cancer death rates are highest in areas where goiter is endemic.

Dr. Eskin made extensive animal studies to confirm the above observation. He injected a powerful cancer-causing agent, DMBA, into two hundred rats. While all rats developed cancer eventually, the development was 25 percent sooner in the group of animals on the iodine-deficient diet than in the group that received sufficient iodine in the diet.

Dr. Wilfred Shute, the pioneering researcher on vitamin E, confirmed that both thyroxine and vitamin E play important roles in eliminating surplus estrogen, whether natural or synthetic, from a woman's body. Vitamin E seems to exert a normalizing effect on hormonal levels: increasing the hormone output in women who are deficient in estrogen, and lowering it in those who are prone to an excess.

8. *Selenium deficiency.* The selenium relationship to cancer is very similar to the iodine-breast cancer connection. It has been shown that cancer deaths are higher in areas of the United States, Canada, and other nations where soil is deficient or low in selenium, as compared to areas which are rich in selenium.

Dr. Gerhard N. Schrauzer, professor of chemistry at Revelle College, University of California, conducted a seven-year study of animals which showed that selenium is a definite protector against the development of breast cancer. Minute amounts of selenium added to the diet of mice which normally showed a 100 percent incidence of cancer, prevented cancer in an overwhelming majority of the laboratory animals—it reduced the incidence of cancer 90 percent!

It was shown by earlier human studies, conducted by Dr. Raymond Shamberger, that the blood of cancer victims always shows selenium levels below normal.[32] The researchers believe that selenium stimulates the immunological system in its work against the development of cancer.

In America, where the incidence of breast cancer is five times greater than in Japan, the average daily diet includes only 50-150 mcg. of selenium, while in Japan the average daily intake of selenium is 200-500 mcg.

Dr. Schrauzer said, "If the current average American selenium intake were increased by a factor of two, a significant lowering of breast cancer risk should result."[10] He recommended that Americans shift their emphasis from meat to more cereals and fish, which are high in selenium content. Brewer's yeast, kelp, garlic, and mushrooms are other excellent sources of selenium.

The exact mechanics of how selenium helps to prevent breast cancer and other forms of cancer is not known, but my theory is that being a powerful antioxidant and having a biological activity which is closely related to vitamin E, it can help prevent or slow down the formation of carcinogenic free radicals in the body, as well as help prevent the buildup of excessive estrogen in the system. Selenium is a great protector and detoxifier and helps to minimize the carcinogenic effect of all toxic chemicals. It also protects the liver and helps to regenerate it after damage, especially by cirrhosis. Many researchers believe that a selenium deficiency can, in addition to breast cancer, cause hypertension, strokes, and heart attacks. Studies show that where selenium in soils and foods is low, the rate for these diseases is high.[32]

How to prevent breast cancer

The causative relationship between nutritional deficiencies, faulty diet, specific environmental carcinogens, and breast cancer is well established and scientifically proven. By eliminating the causes, breast cancer can be prevented.

On the basis of the available information, here's what you must do in order to give your body the maximum protection against the threat of breast cancer:

1. Make sure your diet contains plenty of selenium.[10, 18, 32]   An excellent natural source of selenium is brewer's yeast, which is sold in all health food stores. Take 2-3 tablespoons of powder or 10-15 tablets a day. Make sure you're getting a genuine *brewer's* yeast, not a primary-grown yeast, such as torula, or other nutritional yeasts, which contain very little, if any, selenium. While taking brewer's yeast, take 1 or 2 tablets of calcium per day (500 - 1,000 mg.) to balance the excessive phosphorus in yeast. Other good sources of selenium are most grains and cereals, fish and shellfish, dairy products, eggs, mushrooms, garlic, and kelp. Garlic is, singularly, gram for gram, the richest food source of selenium. If its strong odor prevents you from using it regularly, you can use Kyolic, odor-free garlic tablets or capsules, available at health food stores. Garlic also contains another anti-cancer agent, germanium. Even with plenty of characteristically selenium-rich foods, however, it is difficult to obtain protective amounts of selenium if foods are grown in selenium-poor soils. Therefore, this vital mineral can be taken in supplementary tablet form, 25-50 mcg. a day. Health food stores carry selenium in the form of yeast concentrate; this is the best form of supplementary selenium. Note: Selenium is cumulative in the human body; therefore supplementary selenium should be taken with caution and in small dosages.

2. Make sure your diet contains enough iodine.[5] Iodine deficiency is actually not widespread today, since salt is iodized, but those who do not use a lot of salt (as no one

should) and especially those who cut down on salt for some medical reasons (such as reducing, for example) should supplement their diet with iodine. The best natural source of iodine is kelp or other seaweed. Kelp is sold in health food stores in granulated form or in tablet form. Take 2 - 3 tablets, or ½ teaspoon of kelp granules or powder a day. Kelp granules or powder can be used as a salt substitute in soups, salads, bread, etc.

3. The following specific vitamins and supplements, which have protective property against all cancers, but especially against breast cancer, should be taken daily:

- *Vitamin C*—1,000 - 3,000 mg. or more. Vitamin C is the most potent anti-toxin known. It can effectively neutralize or minimize the damaging effect of most chemical carcinogens in food and the environment, and thus be of great value in cancer-prevention programs.[11, 12] It will also help prevent the formation of free radicals which are causatively connected with breast cancer.

- *Vitamin A*—10,000 - 25,000 units. Vitamin A protects the body tissues from damage by carcinogens. The deficiency of vitamin A definitely contributes to the development of cancer.[11, 13, 14]

- *Vitamin E*—600 - 1,000 I.U. Vitamin E is a powerful antioxidant and will help prevent fat oxidation and formation of free radicals, which are known to be one of the causes of breast cancer. Vitamins C and E can help inhibit the activity of the enzyme, *hyaluronidase,* which is found in cancerous tissue. Vitamin E also increases oxygenation of cells, which is of crucial importance in the prevention of cancer.[5, 15, 16]

- *B-complex,* natural, made from yeast—3 - 5 tablets. Dr. Otto Warburg, Nobel Prize winner and director of the Max Planck Institute for Cell Physiology in Berlin, says that a powerful supply of B vitamins, especially pantothenic acid, niacin, and riboflavin, in the diet, is the best possible protection against cancer.[17]

- **Brewer's yeast**—2 - 3 tbsp. Brewer's yeast is the best natural source of B-complex vitamins, selenium, and chromium—all vital protective factors against breast cancer.[16, 18]
- **Lecithin**—1 - 2 tsp. of granules. Choline and inositol, the lipotropic factors in lecithin, are of special protective value against breast cancer because they can help in hepatic degradation of excess estrogen.[18]
- **Vitamin B₁₅ (pangamic acid)**—100 - 200 mg. The ultimate cause of all disease, including cancer, is oxygen deficiency in cells. Chronic oxygen deficiency contributes to the formation of cancer cells. B_{15} increases the body's resistance to oxygen deficiency.[6]

4. Limit the intake of folic acid to 100 - 400 mcg. and PABA to 30 mg. daily. Both of these vitamins can exacerbate cystic mastitis and, thus, contribute to the possible development of breast cancer.[18]

5. Eliminate all rancid and stale foods from your diet. As I mentioned earlier, all rancid foods contain carcinogenic substances and free radicals, which have been shown to be causatively connected with breast cancer. [7, 8] Eat only *fresh* foods, as recommended in Chapters 3 and 4.

6. Avoid excessive amounts of meat, especially beef, in your diet. Beef is one of the main sources of free radicals. Also, see Chapter 3 on harmful effects of excess of any kind of animal protein in the diet.

7. Eliminate all sugar from your diet. The excess of refined sugar in the American diet is, perhaps, singularly the most health-destroying dietary factor. It also contributes to the threat of breast cancer.[18]

8. Finally, two main factors causatively connected with the increased risk of breast cancer, mentioned at the beginning of this chapter, are the oral contraceptives and failure to breast-feed babies. Therefore, remember: if you have children, breast feeding will not only contribute to better health for them, but will also lessen your chances of

getting breast cancer.

As far as the oral contraceptives are concerned, they are definitely a major cause of breast cancer and, therefore, should never be used.

The above-mentioned prevention program, if followed, will not only improve your chances of avoiding the disease every woman fears the most—breast cancer—but will also improve your health generally.

Other ways to reduce cancer risk

The risk, not only of breast cancer, but of all forms of cancer, can be diminished if you follow these recommendations, which are supported by the National Cancer Institute, and the international concensus of cancer experts:

- Eat *less* beef, lamb, and pork, and *more* grains, and fresh vegetables and fruits—this is what the Senate Select Committee on Nutrition and Human Needs urged recently after several years of hearings and testimonies from nutrition and cancer experts.[19] An international diet survey showed that those who developed cancer of the colon (the most prevalent cancer in the United States except for lung cancer) and the rectum ate more meat than comparable persons free from these cancers. The fiber-rich Optimum Diet of natural foods, as advocated in this book, is the best cancer-prevention diet there is.
- Don't overeat—keep slim. Obese persons have a higher than normal risk of developing cancer of the breast, endometrium (lining of the uterus) and gall bladder, as compared to people of normal weight.[18, 21]
- Don't smoke. Two-pack-a-day cigarette smokers are at least 20 - 30 times more likely to develop lung cancer than non-smokers.[22]
- Avoid excessive X-rays. It has been scientifically proven that not only therapeutic X-rays, but even those used diagnostically by doctors, dentists, and chiropractors, can contribute to the development of

cancer and leukemia. Leukemia in children is often caused by pre-natal abdominal X-rays received by the mother during pregnancy.[23] Ironically, even X-rays used in mammography—X-rays used for detection of breast cancer—can, in themselves, contribute to the development of cancer. Dr. John Bailar, epidemiologist and editor of the Journal of the National Cancer Institute, said that radiation emitted during the exams might cause some cancer later. "This problem is particularly acute for women under 50, for most of whom this risk is actually greater than the expected benefit. Women under 50 should not be screened by mammography except in the most unusual circumstances," said Dr. Bailar.[31] At present, about 270,000 women over 35 are being examined annually by mammography at 27 breast cancer detection centers across the nation, sponsored by the National Cancer Institute and the American Cancer Society.

- Eat less salt. Yes, even common salt, sodium chloride, if used in excessive amounts, can contribute to the development of cancer of the stomach.[6, 24]
- Avoid excessive exposure to the sun, especially if you have a fair complexion. Risk of skin cancer can be increased by overexposure to the sun's ultraviolet light. Three hundred thousand new skin cancers are diagnosed each year and 5,300 people a year die from it.
- Avoid long or frequent exposure to household chemicals: solvents, cleaning fluids, detergents, paint thinners, pesticides, garden and lawn chemicals, paints, etc. They all contain potential carcinogenic chemicals.[22]
- Avoid all artificial sweeteners. One after the other, they have all been causatively connected with cancer.[33]
- Avoid smog, car fumes, factory exhausts and cigarette-smoke-filled places. Ozone, carbon monoxide, nitrogen dioxide, and other photochemi-

cal pollutants, plus lead, cadmium, mercury, etc. in polluted air have all been indicted as definite carcinogens.[25]

- Do not drink or use in food preparation regular tap water if it is chlorinated and fluoridated. Both chlorine and sodium fluoride have recently been found to be causatively linked to cancer, even in such small amounts as in treated water, if it is used for prolonged periods of time.[26, 27, 28]

- Finally, for the prevention of cancer, a peaceful, relaxed, positive mental outlook on life, a health-oriented, rather than a disease-oriented state of mind, and the avoidance of undue mental and emotional stresses, worries and fears, may be just as important as the avoidance of physical carcinogens. More and more valid scientific research indicates that certain types of people—people with a lowered ability to deal with severe emotional conflicts and stresses, people with uncontrolled anxieties and worries, those with traumatic emotional experiences or losses, those with feelings of loneliness, inadequacy, hopelessness, and desperation, people who could be classified generally as hopeless or unhappy—are more predisposed to succumb to cancer.[34] Researchers from New York University and the University of Rochester Medical Center, who made extensive studies of this subject, emphasized that although such a negative state of mind may not cause cancer in and of itself, it increases the biochemical vulnerability and sets the stage—creates the favorable milieu—for cancer growth.[35]

26

Varicose Veins: Prevention and Treatment

Varicose veins affect many women's lives, not only physically, but also emotionally. Although men are affected by varicose veins, this condition is far more common among women. Also, men are less concerned about the aesthetic aspect of varicose veins since it is easier for them to keep their unsightly veins covered.

The purpose of veins is to drain the capillary beds and body tissues of "used" blood and return it to the heart. Venous blood from the head and neck returns to the heart by the force of gravity. But from the legs, venous blood must be moved up against the force of gravity with the help of the rhythmic sucking action of breathing, muscular contractions of the extremities, and the valves located in both the deep femoral and superficial saphenous veins. The valves prevent the back flow and provide an indispensable "lift" to the upwards moving blood.

A varicose vein is one in which the valvular system has broken down, and when one valve breaks or weakens, the next valve is put under pressure and becomes subject to breakage or weakening, and so on. This is why varicose veins tend to increase in number as time goes on. When the valves no longer prevent back flow of the venous blood, the abnormal pressure dilates the superficial veins, causing stagnation and pooling of the blood. This results in permanently dilated veins, which are not only unsightly, but also painful.

It is estimated that one out of seven adults in North America has varicose veins. By contrast, the condition is rare—virtually unknown—in "primitive" countries where people eat more natural, fiber-rich diets and live more physically active lives.

Which brings us to the causes of varicose veins.

Constipation

One of the major causes of varicose veins is chronic constipation—another of our national epidemics. Constipation contributes to the development of varicose veins in two ways: (1) overloaded bowels press against the veins in the lower abdomen year after year, gradually breaking down the valves in the veins and allowing a reverse flow of blood,[1] and (2) constant straining at stools increases pressure in veins and breaks the resistance in the blood vessel walls.[2] Exercising extreme pressure in the bathroom is perhaps the main contributing factor. The return of the blood from the veins of the legs is blocked almost completely by heavy straining in the bathroom and tremendous pressure builds up in the veins of the legs. Over the course of many years this back-up of pressure contributes in a large part to the development of varicosities.

The major causes of constipation are: faulty diet of refined foods and lack of dietary fiber; the lack of sufficient exercise; excessive meat in the diet (meat is virtually fiber-free); lack of sufficient liquids; and vitamin and mineral deficiencies (see Chapter 31 regarding constipation).

Liver malfunction

Some authorities consider the breakdown in the proper function of the liver to be a contributing cause of varicose veins. A swollen, enlarged, or fatty liver slows down the return of blood to the heart. Dr. Alan Nittler has successfully treated varicose veins, even in pregnant women, by using a liver cleansing program in conjunction with a nutritional supportive program to improve the function of the liver.[3]

Vitamin E deficiency

A prolonged vitamin E deficiency has been linked to the development of varicose veins. Supplementing the diet with vitamin E has brought dramatic improvement in many cases. This vitamin helps prevent the formation of blood clots and, at the same time, helps to dilate blood vessels. Vitamin E also helps to dissolve or prevent the formation of fibrin, a material that makes the formation of blood clots possible. Thus, vitamin E can play a role in prevention of varicose veins. Varicose veins frequently appear during pregnancy, a time when the requirement for vitamin E is unusually high, and when there is a surplus of natural estrogen in the system. An excess of estrogen may contribute to the development of blood clots, and vitamin E can lower the excessive estrogen.[6]

Dr. Richard A. Passwater conducted an interesting study among the readers of *Prevention* magazine, who were asked to comment on their experience with vitamin E and the heart. Many readers (158 persons) sent unsolicited comments about their experiences with the beneficial effect of vitamin E on varicose veins. Not only had vitamin E eliminated the pain of varicose veins, but, in many cases, the varicosities completely disappeared, or at least greatly improved.[4]

Many American women are chronically vitamin E deficient, partly because the diet of refined foods supplies an inadequate amount of this important vitamin, and partly because many women take synthetic iron supplements on a regular basis and vitamin E is often destroyed in the body by iron supplements.

Lack of exercise

Physical inactivity in combination with too much standing or sitting is one of the major contributing causes of varicose veins, especially when combined with the causes mentioned earlier. Varicose veins are largely a circulation problem. Regular exercise will improve circulation and prevent too much venous blood collecting in the lower extremities and creating undue pressure. Drs. Eric P. Lofgren and Karl A. Lofgren, of the Mayo Clinic in Rochester, Minnesota, say that "exercise of the leg muscles, particularly the calf muscles, is essential for normal function of the musculovenous pumping against gravitational forces."[5] They add that regular walking can lower the venous pressure to about one-third that of the pressure during the standing position.

What can you do?

First, you must recognize that prevention of varicose veins is much easier than a cure. If an effective preventive program is instituted early, varicose veins will not develop. Nutritional deficiencies and the wrong diet of fiberless refined foods must be corrected. A regular program of exercise, even "simple" exercise such as walking, can help prevent varicosities. If you adhere to the Optimum Diet as recommended in Chapters 3 and 4 of this book, take all the supplements recommended, especially E and C with bioflavonoids, avoid too much sitting or standing, and exercise regularly, you can be reasonably sure that you will not be troubled by varicose veins.

What can you do to improve or correct the condition if it has already developed?

Here are several suggestions that will help:

1. Optimum nutrition, as recommended in this book and in my *How To Get Well* book, is essential. Emphasis should be on whole grains, seeds, nuts, vegetables, and fruits, up to 80 percent eaten raw. Especially beneficial grains for varicose veins are buckwheat (as in kasha—see Recipes & Directions) and millet. This is a diet rich in natural fiber and will help prevent or correct varicose veins.

2. Avoid constipation, one of the major causes of varicose veins. See Chapter 31 for a 7-point anti-constipation program.

3. Avoid too much sitting, and too much standing (such as at work where either sitting or standing for the whole day is required). Studies at Auckland Medical School showed that prolonged sitting in chairs is one of the main contributing causes of varicose veins. Sitting with crossed legs is especially dangerous.

4. Avoid tight clothing, especially clothing with tight

bands on the edges as on panties, stocking, girdles, etc. Anything that constricts the venous return high up can contribute to varicose veins.

5. A slant board is a very good help for varicose veins. Lie head down on a slant board and do some leg exercises two or three times a day.

6. The foot of your bed should be elevated slightly—3 - 4 inches.

7. Walking and swimming are the best exercises for varicose veins. One to two hours of walking daily should be your goal.

8. The following few simple exercises, which can be done even while sitting at the desk, can help prevent varicose veins: (1) flex the ankles up and down 10 to 15 times each; (2) extend the knee horizontally and bring it back into a right-angle position, also 10 to 15 times each. Repeat the exercises, one after the other, every 30 minutes, if possible. Dr. Charles A. Hufnagel, chairman of the surgery department at the Georgetown University School of Medicine, in Washington, D.C., says that such exercises "prevent the pooling of the blood in the veins, and accelerate the return of the blood out of the veins."[7]

9. Take the following vitamins and supplements daily:

E—600 to 1200 I.U. mixed tocopherols (increases elasticity of blood vessels and prevents clots).

C—up to 3,000 mg. (strengthens the integrity of blood vessels and improves their elasticity).

Rutin—500 mg. (European research indicates that rutin and other bioflavonoids can help reduce the symptoms of varicose veins as well as reduce blood pressure.)

B-complex, high potency (helps to revitalize the liver which is often sluggish and overworked in those who suffer from varicose veins).

Zinc—50 mg. (speeds the healing of affected blood vessels).

Brewer's yeast—2 - 3 tbsp. of powder, taken in pineapple juice (brewer's yeast is the best natural source of B-vitamins, high quality proteins, and important minerals, especially selenium and zinc, which are of specific benefit for those suffering from varicose veins).

Lecithin—2 tsp. of granules (prevents fat accumulation in the blood vessels and improves circulation).

Wheat germ (must be fresh)—2 - 3 tbsp. a day (a good source of B vitamins and vitamin E).

Multiple vitamin—mineral formula, natural.

10. Take 1 or 2 cloves of garlic every day, or, if you object to garlic odor, take odorless garlic preparations such as Kyolic (sold in health food stores). Garlic helps to dissolve fibrin in blood vessels and improves circulation.

11. Surgery is not a solution for varicose veins. When varicose veins are corrected surgically, without correcting the underlying causes for their development, they usually reappear in a relatively short time.

12. Using elastic supportive stockings may be advisable in severe cases. Elastic support garments do help to promote the brisk movement of blood through the veins and strengthen the muscle tone of the calf.[5] Especially in severe cases, at least initially, the wearing of supportive garments could be combined with walking.

13. The following herbs are beneficial and can help varicosities: white oak bark, marjoram, comfrey, marigold, coral root, witch hazel, yarrow, mistletoe. (See Recipes & Directions regarding the preparation of herb teas.)

14. Vitamin E salve can be used topically. Or squeeze a capsule of vitamin E and gently massage the oil over affected parts.

15. A poultice made from comfrey leaves and/or roots and applied topically has been reported by some sufferers to be very soothing and healing.

16. A vigorous daily dry brush massage, which is an easy and enjoyable self-treatment (see Recipes & Directions), can be very helpful, especially in mild cases of the condition. Dry brush massage is also an excellent preventive measure against varicose veins.

27

What Every Woman Should Know About Sexually Transmitted Diseases

Sexually transmitted diseases have reached epidemic proportions in the United States. According to the U.S. Public Health Service Center for Disease Control, they strike at least 10 to 15 million Americans a year—or one in twenty sexually active adults and children! *Gonorrhea* is the most prevalent—4 million new cases a year. *Nongonococcal urethritis* (NGU) affects 2.6 million persons. There are 300,000 new cases a year of *herpes progenitalis,* a vicious infection linked to cervical cancer and severe brain damage and death in babies of affected mothers. There are an estimated half million untreated cases of *syphilis,* the most dangerous of all venereal diseases, with at least 25,000 new cases added each year. Millions of others are afflicted with other, less dangerous, but often unbearably uncomfortable forms of VD, such as venereal warts, crab lice, scabies, trichomonas vaginalis, and fungal vaginal infections. Sexually transmitted diseases are far more widespread than any other communicable diseases—more than TB, measles, hepatitis, strep throat, mumps, and scarlet fever *combined!*

Worst of all, according to the U.S. Public Health Service, the prevalence of VD among teenagers in the 12-to-20 age group is *triple* that of the rest of the population! One of every two new cases of syphilis occurs in a teenager. Government Public Health Officials and infectious disease scientists at Johns Hopkins School of Public Health admit that the situation is "totally out of control."

What causes venereal diseases and why such a sudden, widespread epidemic? I will try to answer these questions at the end of this chapter, but first, let us look at the various forms of sexually transmitted diseases and familiarize ourselves with their symptoms, treatments, and complications.

Syphilis

This is the most dangerous of all venereal diseases. It can cause damage to the brain, spinal cord, heart, liver, blood vessels, or any other vital organ of the body, as well as to the bones, skin, nervous system, eyes, and teeth of fetus and newborn babies. It can cause insanity, paralysis, and death if not treated in time.

Syphilis is caused by a spirochete, a cork-screw-shaped germ called ***Treponema pallidum.*** It is transmitted by sexual contact or from a syphilitic mother to her baby during the birth process. Generally, the first signs of syphilis infection occur 20 to 30 days after exposure, but symptoms could appear as early as 10 days, or as late as 90 days after.

The progression of syphilis is divided into three stages. The ***primary stage*** is the initial sore (chancre) which lasts several weeks, and heals by itself, even if untreated. It can be a large, hard sore, up to ¼ inch in size, or only a very small painless pimple, usually on genitals, but sometimes on hips, breasts, or even fingers. The biggest problem with syphilis is that the small primary sore often goes unnoticed or unrecognized, especially by women, and since it soon heals by itself, the infected person is unaware of having the dangerous disease.

If not diagnosed and treated intensively at an early stage, syphilis will enter the ***secondary stage,*** often several weeks or months after the initial infection. This stage is characterized by a rash over the body, usually on the chest and arms, sores in the mouth, swollen lymphatic glands and joints, and a flu-like illness. But, if ignored, misdiagnosed, and untreated, even these symptoms will disappear by themselves and the syphilitic may think that he is well.

The *third stage* may become noticeable many years after the original infection—even as long as 20 or 30 years after. By then, the destructive damage to the vital organs, such as the heart and brain, is already apparent.

The person infected with syphilis can transmit the disease during the first and second stages, up to a year or more after the exposure. But a syphilitic woman can infect the fetus or her newborn baby with the disease at any stage.

The only reliable ways to diagnose syphilis are blood tests (VDRL, Wasserman, or FTA tests). Formerly treated by mercurial compounds, syphilis is now treated by antibiotics. However, even antibiotics are not always effective, especially if the disease is not caught at a very early stage.

Gonorrhea

With four million new cases a year, gonorrhea is the most prevalent of all sexually transmitted diseases. It is caused by gonococcus, a germ that enters the urethra in the penis in the male or the urethra and vagina in the female and causes inflammation of the mucus membranes. The usual early symptoms in men are pain on voiding and discharge of pus from the penis, but there usually are no early symptoms in women. The symptoms can appear any time between 2 to 30 days. Whether there are symptoms or not, gonorrhea is highly contagious in all stages. It is transmitted almost exclusively by sexual contact.

Almost 85 percent of infected women have no symptoms of gonorrhea until it is too advanced to be treated. There are no reliable blood or other tests to detect it early. If untreated, gonorrhea can cause severe pelvic inflammation disease (PID). Gonococci bacteria can enter the reproductive organs and cause permanent damage and sterility. Both womb and ovaries can be affected. Gonorrhea can also cause blindness, eye infections, and arthritis in the newborn.

The diagnosis of gonorrhea is usually made by Gram stain smear for men and culture in Thayer-Martin medium for women.

Penicillin or other antibiotics are the current standard treatment. However, gonorrhea is becoming increasingly resistant to drugs. When first discovered, penicillin was hailed as a drug which would eliminate gonorrhea altogether. In the 1950's, 150,000 units of penicillin would cure the disease. Today it takes 4.8 million units, or a 30-fold increase. And, Dr. Michael Spence, a Johns Hopkins University gynecologist and VD specialist, says that "we will soon be unable to treat gonorrhea without hospitalizing patients. The dose will be too big."[1]

To complicate the matter, more and more Americans are becoming allergic to penicillin, and each medication with the drug increases the risk of serious reaction, even fatalities. A young man recently died as a reaction to penicillin during treatment for his sixth case of gonorrhea.

Moreover, the female hormone changes caused by oral contraceptives as well as during menstruation or pregnancy, alter the chemical balance of the fluids in the reproductive tract and increase susceptibility to gonorrhea. Menstruation spreads it deep inside the pelvic organs.

Recently, a new, penicillin-resistant strain of gonorrhea affected Americans in fifteen states. The World Health Organization (WHO) called the new strain "beta-lactanase-producer," and its source was traced to the Phillipines, Thailand, and Hong Kong. Since penicillin is completely ineffective against this new strain of gonorrhea, a more powerful drug, *Trobicin,* has been used. However, doctors fear that the new drug may have even more serious side effects than penicillin.

NGU—Non-gonococcal urethritis

Non-gonococcal urethritis (NGU), also known as non-specific urethritis (NSU), or gleet, affects an estimated 2.6 million Americans and is described by some genito-urinary specialists as "the biggest problem in present day venereology."

NGU is caused by bacteria and is a highly contagious disease, infecting mostly young singles with an active sex life. It was largely ignored until recently, because many physicians believed that NGU was a mild and self-limiting condition. Now it is known, however, that non-gonococcal urethritis is a very severe disease. Untreated female carriers may give birth to babies with eye infections which may cause scarring and blindness. In men, the common symptoms are a gonorrhea-like irritation of the urethra, painful urination, and occasionally, a mucus discharge. However, many carriers have no symptoms at all.

Diagnosis of NGU is difficult. Lab tests with smears and cultures can be inconclusive. Antibiotic treatments are considered to be effective, but since there are so many symptom—free carriers, there is but little hope that the epidemic spreading of non-specific urethritis can ever be halted.

Herpes progenitalis

Herpes progenitalis, also called herpes, or *Herpes Simplex virus, Type 2,* (HSV-2) was identified only six years ago, and is caused by a virus. It spreads in near epidemic fashion, and possibly affects millions of Americans, with 300,000 new cases reported a year, chiefly among teenagers and young people.

The usual symptoms, one to six days after infection, are tender, painful sores or blisters on the genitals, often accompanied by swelling. Diagnosis can be based on the appearance of herpes sores as well as by pap smear and cultures. There are no effective treatments and, once infection is contracted, the condition is considered to be incurable. Doctors in Germany treat *Herpes Simplex, Type 2,* with a drug, "lupidon G," which reportedly destroys the virus, but the drug is not approved by the FDA for use in the United States, as yet.

Herpes progenitalis is especially dangerous to women. There is strong evidence that it may lead to cancer of the cervix. Research has indicated that a woman with herpes simplex of the genitals is eight times more likely to develop cancer of the cervix than a woman who has not been infected.[1] Herpes is also linked to severe damage in central nervous system, or even death, in infants infected during birth! Miscarriages are also often caused by venereal herpes.

It is important to realize that once you are infected with herpes, it may stay with you, in an inactive, latent condition, indefinitely, even though the active herpes sores may flare up and disappear with longer or shorter intervals. (See more on Herpes in Chapter 24.)

Trichomonas vaginalis

There are an estimated three million cases of this sexually transmitted disease, caused by a protozoa, a one-celled organism. Although not as dangerous as the above-mentioned venereal diseases, trichomoniasis (also called trich, vaginitis, or leukorrhea), can often cause unbearable suffering. Four to 28 days after the infection, the symptoms are copious discharge from the vagina, intense itching, burning and redness of genitals and thighs, and painful intercourse. In men, often there are no symptoms, although even symptom-free men can infect their sexual partners.

Diagnosis of trichomoniasis can be made by pap smear and microscopic examination. The medical treatments are not very effective and often dangerous. Commonly-used Flagyl tablets may cause cancer or birth defects, as shown in some animal studies.

Monilial vaginitis

This is another increasingly common form of vaginitis, which is also referred to as thrush, yeast, moniliasis, or candidiasis. It is caused by a fungus and the symptoms are similar to trichomoniasis: intolerable itching, skin irritation, and thick, cheesy, offensive discharge.

The commonly-used treatments, such as antifungal creams or suppositories and vaginal tablets, are not very effective and usually afford only temporary relief, while they may cause secondary infection by bacteria. Mothers who are infected can transmit the disease to their newborn babies. The usual symptoms in infants are mouth and throat infections.[1] (See Chapter 24 regarding natural treatments of various forms of vaginitis.)

Venereal warts

Venereal warts, also called genital warts or condyloma, are highly contagious warty growths usually appearing around the orifice of the rectum (anus), or the vulva. In severe cases, they can spread enough to block the vaginal opening. Venereal warts can be extremely painful. They also cause itching and local irritation. Recently they are becoming widely spread among homosexual men.

Venereal warts are cousins to the common plantar warts and are caused by a virus. There are no effective cures, but doctors usually treat venereal warts with such drugs as podophyllin tincture, 5-fluorouracil, bleomycin, or with electrodessication or surgical excision. However, none of these seem to offer a lasting cure and the reinfection (or recurrence) rate in those treated is up to 75 percent. Some doctors are now developing a vaccine against venereal warts, but it is too early to say if it will be a successful alternative to present conventional treatments.

Scabies

This is a very contagious skin condition caused by an insect (mite) which burrows under the superficial layers of the skin and causes intense itching. The diagnosis is usually made by noting extensive scratch marks, itching, and raised gray lines in the skin where the mite burrows. In addition to the genitals, scabies may infest the elbows, hands, breasts, and buttocks.

The conventional treatment is Kwell cream, lotion, or shampoo. Kwell is, however, quite toxic.

Pediculosis pubis

This is one of the most prevalent sexually transmitted conditions. It is an infestation of six-legged crab lice—the reason why pediculosis pubis is popularly called "crabs."

Usually, it is transmitted by sexual contact, but can also be gotten from infested bed linen or clothing. The symptoms are an intense itching, pinhead blood spots on underwear, and tiny eggs on pubic hair. The conventional treatment is the same as for scabies.

Other sexually transmitted diseases

There are many other bacterial, fungal, and viral infectious venereal diseases that can be transmitted by sexual contact and which are reported in increasing numbers by the Communicable Disease Centers:

- *Hemophilus vaginitis,* characterized by a chalk-white discharge and a strong odor.
- *Hepatitis virus B,* especially among homosexual men and *Group B beta hemolytic streptococcus infections* in women.
- *Gonorrheal pharyngitis,* a gonorrhea infection of the throat often associated with homosexuality and/or oral sex.
- *Amebic dysentery,* a "new" STD, transmitted by the oral-fecal route, especially, but not exclusively, by homosexuals.

The cause and the cure

What causes Sexually Transmitted Diseases and why such a sudden widespread epidemic?

"Public health officials are at their wit's end," says one VD expert from the University of Washington in Seattle, who investigated VD control programs around the nation. And what do our medical and governmental agencies do about the epidemic? For one thing, they are allocating more money for the "VD prevention" research. Then, they are trying to develop vaccines so venereal diseases can be "prevented" by mass vaccinations. One famous doctor, David Reuben, went so far as to propose a scheme to inject 4.8 million units of penicillin into every man, woman, and child capable of having sexual intercourse on a "National VD Day"! Doctors try to devise new and stronger bactericidal creams, jellies, and douches, stronger and stronger antibiotics and more effective drug treatments.

But, none seem to be willing to point the finger to the real causes (and how, by eliminating them, the VD problem can easily be solved): our heralded sexual freedoms and unbridled sexual promiscuity. We know what the problem is, but we "like the problem" as one of my playboy acquaintances says, and we don't want to change. We want to have our cake and eat it, too. Just like with cancer: we know all the causes of cancer—smoking, carcinogenic chemicals in food and cosmetics, excessive meat in the diet, artificial sweeteners, excessive X-rays, oral contraceptives and other synthetic hormones—but we don't want to change our cherished live-for-the-moment health-destroying lifestyle. We are hoping that science will discover a vaccine or pill that will prevent cancer and enable us to go on with the old health-destructive ways.

But, just as a cancer-preventive pill will never be discovered—*we'll have to change our lifestyle and eliminate cancer-causing factors in our environment to eliminate cancer*—so the Sexually Transmitted disease epidemic will never be stopped *unless we relinquish and renounce the new sexual morality and sexual promiscuity and go back to "old-fashioned" sexual and moral standards.* Yet, this kind of solution we do not seem to be looking for. Even the public health officials refuse to admit that sexual promiscuity is the cause of the STD epidemic. "Blaming STDs on the change of sexual standards is pointless," they say. "Sexually Transmitted Diseases are caused by germs, not sex, and the name of the game is germ control, not preaching."

Yet, "preaching" is what this country needs if it is ever to get out of this epidemic mess which, by official admission, is "totally out of control."

"New sexual morality," parental permissiveness and

lack of discipline, the breakdown of the family structure and single-parent families, working mothers and lack of parental supervision, false security given by the Pill, and the wide availability of penicillin—all these have contributed to sexual promiscuity unparalleled in human history. As one doctor said, "I am convinced that not only is everyone doing it, but doing it with an infected person." One Los Angeles VD specialist tells of a woman who infected 100 individual sexual partners in a short period of time! One traveling rock group member said he had sex with a different girl every night for two years. Group sex, wife swapping, orgies, especially among adolescents and even pre-adolescents, are the fashion of the day. Everyone infecting everyone else with one or more of the dozens of varieties of sexually transmitted diseases.

To halt and correct the dangerously spreading epidemic of VD, we must engage in a new "sexual counter-revolution." We must reject and abandon the liberalized standards of sexual behavior; we must repair the shattered network of communication, supervision, and discipline in the families, whose breakdown is responsible for so much of the adolescent sexual promiscuity; we must rediscover, dust off and glorify the "old-fashioned" standards of sexual conduct and premarital chastity and realize the great joy that comes from sex within responsible and committed exclusive relationships—then, *and only then,* we will be able to lick the growing problem of the uncontrolled epidemic of sexually transmitted diseases.

28

What Smoking Does To Women

I will come to smoking-related diseases, such as lung cancer, heart attacks, coronary heart disease, emphysema, and perinatal death (stillbirth) in a moment, but first, let me tell you of a very unique experiment I was engaged in about thirty years ago.

I conducted small educational workshops attended by about thirty or forty people, approximately 90 percent of whom were women. For several years, I astounded the audiences by almost invariably being able to tell which women in the groups were smokers. Mind you, that was long ago, and the percentage of women who smoked was relatively small. Standing in front of the group and looking at their faces for a few minutes, I was able to pinpoint several women in the audience who were heavy smokers.

How did I do it?

The following tell-tale signs gave me the clues: smoking women had a gray, dull, rough, masculine tone about their faces, which also showed an unusual amount of wrinkles for their age.

Needless to say, I stopped that practice eventually—the smokers didn't appreciate it.

The above came to my mind as, in the process of researching material for this chapter, I came across the early studies (1928) of Dr. Raymond Pearl of John Hopkins Hospital, which showed that oxygen deprivation caused by smoking results in acceleration of the aging process.

Smoking a pack or more of cigarettes a day over a prolonged period of time deprives all the tissues of the body, but especially the skin, from its needed oxygen by constricting the oxygen-carrying blood vessels. The skin, not receiving enough oxygen, will shrivel, wrinkle, and age at an accelerated tempo. It is very common that a woman who is a heavy smoker has a face that is as lined and wrinkled as that of a women who is twenty years older.

Beauty comes from within. Even if cigarette smoking were not dangerous to the health—which it is, and how!—it scarcely enhances feminine allure. Peaches-and-cream complexion and rosy, blooming cheeks are first to go. Enter the gray, dull, rough, masculine, wrinkled face and hands! Her breath and body reeking of stale smoke! Her nerves, sex life, sleep, digestion—all reveal damage resulting from the consistent oxygen debt. Slow but deadly poison—carbon monoxide—from inhaled smoke replaces the life-giving and beauty-building oxygen in her bloodstream and tissues. Oxygen is the basic and most important nutrient of all living cells. The energy-yielding process of cellular oxidation affects the health of every organ and gland, and every tissue cell in the body—including those of the face.

The *Annals of Internal Medicine* reported on an observation very similar to mine, made by Dr. Harry Daniell, an internist in Redding, California. He made a year-long study of visible damage of smoking. He made a clinical examination of faces for wrinkles of all persons between the ages of 30 and 70 who entered his office, and took photographs at random in 400 cases. The wrinkle score was compared with the questionnaire regarding smoking habits of each patient. The results were striking! The report said: "The association between cigarette smoking and wrinkling was striking in both sexes soon after the age of 30. It was related to the duration and intensity of smoking. Smokers in the 40-49 year age group were as likely to be as prominently wrinkled as a non-smoker 20 years older." That is, heavy smoking can make you look 20 years older!

And, if that alone will not stop you from smoking, let's now take a look at the *real* reasons why you should never smoke.

Cancer, coronary heart disease, and emphysema

The smoking rate among women has doubled in one generation. Not only are there more women smokers, but women are smoking more. The percentage of women between the ages of 18 and 35 who smoke more than a pack a day has jumped from 9 percent in 1965 to 25 percent in 1978.[1] Worst of all is that girls are beginning to smoke at a younger and younger age. A nationwide study conducted for the American Cancer Society showed that 27 percent of the girls between the ages of 13 and 17 smoke; of those 60 percent began smoking before the age of 13!! Dr. Benjamin F. Byrd, Jr., President of the American Cancer Society, blames it on "an all-pervasive smoking environment" and new social values which stress "greater individual freedom, earlier sex relations, drinking at an early age, and wide-spread use of marijuana."[1]

Along with the rise in smoking among women, more women are dying earlier, and from diseases that once were comparatively rare to them. Cancer of the lungs is one such disease. According to the recent survey by the National Cancer Institute, the number of women dying of lung cancer in the United States has nearly doubled in five years.[8] Heavy smokers (2-pack-a-day or more) are at least 20 to 30 times more likely to develop lung cancer than non-smokers.[2] Studies show that the death rate from coronary heart disease is 9 times greater among women who smoke than in their non-smoking counterpart. And, the death rate among women from emphysema (a deadly lung disease) is 5 times as high for those with a history of smoking as for non-smokers; if they smoke a pack or more a day, or at least 10 cigarettes a day since the age 25, the death rate is 7.4 times higher than among non-smokers![3]

Would switching to low-tar filter-tip cigarettes help? A statistical study from Oxford University in England shows that smokers who switched to filter-tip cigarettes have probably reduced their risk of getting lung cancer, but by trading tar for carbon monoxide, they have increased their risk of dying from coronary heart disease.

Smoking and premature menopause

Women who smoke are likely to undergo menopause at a younger age than non-smokers, according to the findings of two studies involving more than 3,500 middle-aged women in seven countries. Studies were made at the Boston Collaborative Drug Surveillance Program, as part of a continuing international research project, and reported in the prestigious British Medical Magazine, *Lancet*.[4] The researchers, Drs. Hershel Jick and Jane Porter, of Boston University School of Medicine, and Dr. Alan S. Morrison of the Harvard School of Public Health, said they noticed the relationship while exploring the link between smoking and heart disease.

The studies showed that the more a woman smokes, the earlier her menopause is likely to begin. This means that smoking causes premature aging, and the timing of the approach of menopause is linked to the biological and hormonal aging of the woman's body. Smoking may speed up the biological aging as much as ten years.

Nicotine in smoke affects the central nervous system, which is involved in regulation of the output of hormones involved in the menopause. Cigarette smoke also interferes with the enzymatic function connected with the action of various sex hormones. These are two possible mechanisms for the link between smoking and premature menopause.

Smoking and motherhood

A study at the Laval University of Quebec, Canada, found that smoking during pregnancy increased the risk of perinatal death (late miscarriage, stillbirth, and deaths of babies right after birth) by 24 percent. Also, the twelve studies cited by the U.S. Public Health Service showed a "significant relationship between cigarette smoking and an elevated mortality risk among the infants of smokers."

And in Sweden, the country with the lowest infant-mortality rate in the world, statistics showed that the risk of stillbirths and deaths occurring during the first year of life is 60 percent higher for babies of smoking mothers as compared with non-smoking mothers.

Recent research shows that several highly toxic substances from medication as well as from inhaled smoke are transmitted by the mother to the unborn baby through the placenta.[5]

For example, researchers believe that *nicotine,* a powerful drug in cigarette smoke, is transmitted directly to the fetus when a woman smokes. Nicotine reaches the bloodstream almost immediately as smoke is inhaled. As a reaction to the toxin, the adrenal glands release *epinephrine* (the "alarm reaction" hormone). This raises blood pressure, contracts the blood vessels, and decreases the flow of blood to the peripheral blood vessels and limbs. Today, an alarming number of infants and children have cardiac defects and high blood pressure, believed to be "transmitted" by mothers who smoked during pregnancy.

The British study where more than 2,000 pregnant women were monitored, showed that the overall rate of unsuccessful pregnancies (miscarriages, spontaneous abortions, etc.) among smoking women was almost twice that shown for non-smokers. The same study demonstrated that high blood pressure is a serious risk in pregnancy and that blood pressure increases if a woman smokes.[7]

Carbon monoxide, another deadly gas in cigarette smoke, robs the pregnant woman of precious oxygen. When inhaled—and cigarette smoke contains 640 times more carbon monoxide than is considered safe in industrial plants!—it prevents the body from using oxygen properly and leads to severe oxygen deficiency. It has been shown that there is also a 30 percent reduction in placental oxygen when a pregnant woman smokes.

So, here we have a disastrous, life-threatening combination: on one hand, nicotine stimulates the heart action and increases oxygen demand, while, on the other hand, carbon monoxide cuts down the available oxygen to the minimum! The result: birth defects, stillbirths, miscarriages, babies born with cardiac defects or developing cancer in infancy or early childhood.

In addition to nicotine and carbon monoxide, cigarette smoke also contains a number of strong carcinogens—polycyclic hydrocarbons—chemical substances that cause cancer. These chemical carcinogens can enter the fetal bloodstream when a woman smokes during pregnancy and cause cancer in the unborn baby—cancer which may not become diagnosable until early childhood. Dr. B.L. Van Duuren, Director of the Laboratory of Organic Chemistry and Carcinogenesis at the New York University Medical Center, says: "In view of the established evidence that polycyclic hydrocarbons do reach the placenta and cross to the fetus, the suggestion that a pathogenic relationship might exist between inhaled cigarette smoke during pregnancy and the incidence of child cancers cannot be denied."[3]

Smoking is risky not only for pregnant women, but also for nursing mothers. The current *Journal of the American Medical Association* reported a study which showed that nicotine is present in the breast milk of nursing mothers who smoke.[7] In addition, female smokers have a lower fertility rate than non-smokers.

The *Journal of the American Medical Association,* summarizing the results of forty years of research on habitual smoking among women of childbearing age, concluded that women who smoke during pregnancy risk the life of their unborn child since their rate of spontaneous abortion and premature or still-births is much higher than in non-smoking women. Also, babies born to smoking mothers, if they survive, have retarded growth and many suffer from birth defects and have an increased susceptibility to cancer, high blood pressure and heart disease.[7]

Smoking and teenage girls

As I mentioned before, the most distressing fact about the increased incidence of smoking among women is that more and more young girls smoke and at such a young age as eleven and twelve years. The American Cancer Society

Survey showed that 60 percent of teenage girls begin smoking before the age of thirteen! Just imagine: young children, subjecting their tender, vulnerable, sensitive, undeveloped bodies to the destructive and killing effects of deadly poisons and carcinogenic chemicals in cigarette smoke!

The reasons for this alarming increase in smoking among adolescent girls are many:

- An all-pervasive smoking environment, not the least part of which is parental example. If not for any other reason, this should be sufficient motive for parents to stop smoking.
- Irresponsible massive persuasive cigarette advertising! Girls are given the impression that smoking is sophisticated, smart, the "in" thing! Girls want to be popular and socially acceptable. They think that smoking will help make them popular. When will the parents of America unite and demand of their elected representatives in Washington that *all* cigarette advertising, by any media, be totally banned?!!
- The increased use of drugs, alcohol, and caffeine-containing soft drinks by adolescents. Children gulp cola drinks, which contain large amounts of the stimulating and addictive drug, caffeine, at an increased rate. Also, use of alcohol among children is on the increase. The use of these products leads to the use of other drugs, such as cigarettes. Drinking and smoking go hand in hand.
- The lack of parental guidance, supervision, and discipline. Parents must set the standards and codes of behavior—do's and don'ts—and see that children adhere to them. Parents have a right to prohibit their children from smoking, in or out of the home, up to the age of eighteen, and to enforce that standard.

The rewards of stricter parental discipline and supervision can be many. According to an American Cancer Institute study, teenage girls who smoke also tend to be more rebellious than their non-smoking peers. They are more likely to use marijuana regularly, drink alcohol (often excessively), hate school, and run away from home. The non-smoker, by contrast, tends to be quieter, more involved with school activities and athletics, and to do more reading.[1]

Conclusion

All cigarette packs carry a printed warning: "The Surgeon General has determined that cigarette smoking is dangerous to your health." But it says nothing about the hundreds of thousands of women dying of lung cancer, breast cancer, or heart attacks. It says nothing about babies born with cancer or congenital heart disease; it says nothing about black lungs and crippling emphysema; it says nothing about smoking teenage girls' addiction to drugs and alcohol; it says nothing about stillbirths and perinatal deaths!

Any way you look at it, smoking is not a very smart thing to do. And it is incompatible with the special responsibility which goes with a mother-wife role. As a giver and custodian of life, woman has a special responsibility to herself as well as to her children. A smoking woman's chances to give birth to a truly healthy baby are practically nil. If she is a heavy smoker, her own chances of dying of a heart attack are nine times higher, and of lung cancer twenty to thirty times higher than that of non-smokers. To fulfill her role as a responsible mother and companion of her husband, she must guard her own health as well as that of her family. Smoking is clearly incompatible with that goal. A woman must set an example to her children by renouncing smoking—an ugly, repulsive, destructive habit—which not only can wrinkle her prematurely and make her look and feel twenty years older, but also cause her to suffer from horrid diseases and may even lead to her death!

29

Depression: A New Epidemic

Although both men and children do suffer from depression, it is largely a female affliction. Twice as many women as men suffer from what one journal calls "the number one mental health problem in America today."[1] It is estimated that over 20 million men and women are afflicted with depression, and almost half of these are being treated for the disorder. Although most depressives struggle to live relatively normal lives, more than half a million of them are so incapacitated by severe depression, that they spend most of their time inside hospital walls. About 20,000 of these depressives commit suicide each year.

Dr. Nathan Kline, director of the Rockland Research Institute, New York State Department of Mental Hygiene, says that depression is "one of the most common of all serious medical conditions."[2] It is also "the most under-treated of all major diseases. Were pneumonia, diabetes, or any other important disease entity so often undiagnosed and so often untreated, the courts would justifiably be filled with patients suing for medical malpractice."[3]

Women are especially prone to serious and prolonged depression, according to Dr. Myrna M. Weissman, director of Yale University's Depression Research Unit. Such "sexual imbalance" in depression distribution can have an especially disruptive effect on the welfare of the children. "The depressed person lacks energy, is apathetic, and needs care—hardly a state for caring for children," Dr. Weissman states.[4]

The magnitude of the depression epidemic is evidenced by the fact that one out of every ten prescriptions written in the United States is for antidepressant drugs! And these antidepressants are not harmless. In fact, persons taking the most commonly-prescribed antidepressants such as imipramine and related antidepressant drugs (known as tricyclics) frequently complain of racing pulse, mouth dryness, low blood pressure, urinary retention, and occasionally heart blockage, jaundice, and even seizures resembling epilepsy.[5]

What is depression?

Doctors differentiate several categories of depression:
1. *Simple depression.* This is the mildest form, when the individual is blue and miserable most of the time, but his symptoms do not appreciably affect normal day-to-day functioning.
2. *Severe or endogenuous depression.* This is so severe a depression that the patient is totally incapacitated and normal functioning is impossible. Severe depressives need medical attention and, normally, hospitalization.

Doctors also differentiate between "normal" depression, and "clinical" depression. Everyone gets the blues occasionally. We all have ups and downs, good days and bad days, highs and lows. Shifts of mood are "normal," especially if they are motivated by current environmental causes and stresses, and as long as the depression or blues do not persist and do not interfere with normal daily activities, such an individual is not a "sick" person. It is only when the depression becomes so severe, and deep feelings of despondency hang on for such a long time, that performing normal activities is impossible without psychiatric or medical help, that it is classified as *clinical depression.*

Dr. Nathan Kline, one of the nation's pioneers in the treatment of depression, who was quoted earlier, defines depression as "the magnified and inappropriate expression of some otherwise quite common emotional responses."[2, 3]

There are also thousands of depressives who are classified as **manic-depressives**. "Manics" differ from other depressives in that they experience intermittent extreme highs and extreme lows—two extremes of mood, although the depressive phase usually occurs more frequently and lasts longer. Manics, when in the **mania phase,** feel elation, euphoria, and seem to have inexhaustible energy. Often they work or play until they collapse— and suddenly fall into deep depression and uncontrollable despondency.

The symptoms

The symptoms of severe clinical depression are many and varied, which often makes it difficult to make a correct diagnosis. There are both physical and mental symptoms. Although it is true that the basic problems are "in the head," it is also often true that real physical, biochemical, metabolic disorders are major contributing causes to the mental dysfunction.

Mental and emotional symptoms of clinical depression are:

- Deep despondency that hangs on for a long time, whether it is related to a known stressful situation, or comes out of the blue with seemingly no specific external trigger.
- Lethargy; a sudden or gradual loss of interest in job, family, or other former activities.
- Drastic change in mood and temperament; such as extroverted and socially lively individual suddenly becoming a reserved, quiet, introverted person.
- Unjustified and exaggerated fears of such inevitable factors as loss of youth, aging, infirmities, financial security, and world affairs.
- Hypochondria; fear of becoming sick, or imagining all kinds of non-existent diseases by maldiagnosing or exaggerating real or imagined symptoms.
- Phobias; exaggerated fears of anything and everything: flying, germs, people, driving, being poisoned by foods or drugs, being alone, etc., etc.

- Turning the slightest setback or misfortune into a catastrophic event with resultant intense mental anguish.
- Feelings of futility and worthlessness; the belief that one is not as good (or as rich, or as healthy, or as talented, or as beautiful) as anybody else; that she has been slighted by fate, and she has nothing of importance to contribute and largely lives a useless life.
- Feelings of loneliness and hopelessness.
- Constant feeling that something horrible is going to happen.
- Threats of committing suicide.

Physical symptoms of depression are:

- Headaches.
- Cramps and pains in the gut and chest.
- Intermittent diarrhea and/or constipation.
- Insomnia; sleep problems.
- Extraordinary quantity of dreams in which the depressed person casts herself as the loser: jilted at the altar, lost an important promotion or job, crashed in accidents, was cheated or robbed, etc.
- A loss of, or increased, appetite.
- Weight loss.
- Unexplainable chronic fatigue.

It is obvious that "normal," healthy people experience some of these symptoms of depression at one time or another. As I said earlier, everyone gets the blues or has good and bad days, *occasionally.* If any of the above-mentioned symptoms are triggered by an apparent exogenous or endogenous factor (such as a reaction to a known physical or emotional stressful situation) and if they are of short duration, disappearing in a short time and being replaced by normalcy, you have nothing to worry about. Only when you suffer from several of these symptoms and if they persist for such a long time that they interfere with the performance of your normal activities, do they become serious and symptomatic of clinical depression.

Keep in mind that almost any of the typical symptoms of depression could be actually related to some other ailment, such as hypoglycemia, high blood pressure, anemia, hypothyroidism, adrenal exhaustion, or diabetes. It would be wise, therefore, to have a thorough physical examination, including complete chemistry lab studies, metabolic and nutritional survey, and a 6-hour glucose tolerance test, before the correct diagnosis of depression is made and therapy of any kind is initiated.

The causes of depression

Just as there is a great variety of symptoms of depression, there also are numerous—ad infinitum—causes of this difficult-to-diagnose, but devastating and tragic disease.

There are, essentially, two schools of thought regarding the causes of depression. The psychoanalysts and behaviorists believe that depression is caused by some kind of a traumatic loss in early life which manifests itself later in feelings of guilt, inadequacy, self pity, and anger. This initial loss is normally reinforced over the years by too much sympathy from family and friends. Intensive psychotherapy (psychoanalysis) to unearth the underlying cause and then behavior modification are the prime therapies advocated by doctors who belong to this school of thought.

The second school, a newer, but fast-growing branch of medicine, is the biological school, or orthomolecular psychiatry. The biological school maintains that depression often has a biochemical basis. It maintains that a biochemical systemic disorder, the excess or deficiency of certain chemicals, minerals, and/or trace elements in the brain is the primary cause of severe or clinical depression.[6] As proof for this contention, they refer to the fact that various chemicals and drugs often bring dramatic improvement in depressives. They claim that a long list of minerals, vitamins, and trace elements are involved in the smooth running of the delicate and complex process of the central nervous system. Every minute there are millions of impulses to and from the brain, relayed with the help of these minerals and chemical elements (neurotransmitters), which must be present in the body in exact amounts and proportions. When there is an excess or deficiency of any one of many chemical elements, the nervous system cannot transmit proper impulses and electrical changes to the spinal cord or brain or from one nerve to the other. The result is mental dysfunction, confusion, and depression. This theory is gaining increasingly wide acceptance among biologically-oriented psychiatrists.

My own view is that behavioral and biological causes of depression are, in most cases, intertwined. It is also likely that behavioral causes are not necessarily related to some losses or traumatic experiences and guilts in *early* life. In our Western culture, especially in present-day liberated America, there are plenty of reasons—or what experts call "environmental factors"—*at any time in life* for so many women to feel depressed. Almost one of every two marriages ends in divorce. Many women have no children, or are forsaken by their grown children. Close ties with immediate and extended families (grandparents, aunts, uncles, and other relatives), which provided security and a loving environment in the past, are no longer part of our culture. In the pre-liberation era, a woman felt secure in her home surrounded by her loving family, with children, and later grandchildren. She was taken care of and protected. Now, divorced or unmarried, she is thrown into the competitive, dog-eat-dog, man's world, forced to work and support herself, lonely, insecure, unloved, unprotected, depending on no one but herself, childless, or forsaken by her grown children or other relatives. Sexual revolution and liberation may have brought some positive improvements in a woman's lot, but none of them can compensate for the negative factors produced by the revolution—such factors as insecurity and loneliness, which cause so much unhappiness, anguish, and suffering. Loneliness is a national epidemic. Loneliness and insecurity are not only major contributing causes of depression, but also of many other mental and physical disorders.

Environmental factors

There is no question that, in addition to biological and nutritional factors and the possible predisposing effect of traumatic emotional experiences in early childhood, the environmental stressful factors, or what Dr. F. Flack calls the "depressogenic environment" are definite contributing causes of depression.[7] Our rapidly changing lifestyles lead to uncertainty, confusion, and insecurity. Unhappy or broken marriages; disappointment in children (or parents); high-pressure jobs; open, loose, uncommitted relationships between young people today; personal tragedies such as serious illness or death of loved ones—all are important factors that can trigger a genetic defect, biochemical malfunction in the activity of the brain and central nervous system, or other biological cause of depression.

The National Institute of Mental Health conducted a poll of hundreds of patients with severe clinical depression and found that the following factors, listed in the order of importance, are the top ten precipitators or triggers of depression:[1]

1. Threat to sexual identity. Real or imagined threat to, or loss of, masculinity or femininity. For example, a woman's discovery that she cannot bear children, or the feeling that she has no sex appeal; or a man's discovery that he is impotent, or if he is rejected by women.
2. Breaks in close relationships. Example: divorce.
3. Instability, uncertainty, such as constant moving from one place to another, whether it is a local or long distance move.
4. Having a painful and repressed (secret) situation brought to the surface and being forced to face it.
5. Mild or serious physical illness.
6. Inability to do well at one's job.
7. Children's failure to meet their parents' expectations (affects *parents,* not the children).
8. Change in load of responsibility at home or at work.
9. Shift in social status, either upward or downward.
10. Death of an important or close person.

It is clear that excessive emotional or physical stress of any kind—even though it may not always be apparent—is involved in the triggering process of depression.

Biological medical approach

Much current research has been directed towards finding the exact cause of interference in the complex electric circuitry of the brain and central nervous system. It is known that nerve impulses are transmitted along the route of nerves, spinal cord, and brain, with the help of *neurotransmitters.* Neurons, or nerve cells, are separated from each other by a gap called the *synapse.* Until recently, it wasn't known how electrical nerve impulses jump the synapse. But now, biochemists and research psychiatrists have found that the presence of certain hormones and chemicals is imperative for effective neurotransmission. Epinephrine, or adrenalin, and norepinephrine (NE), or noradrenalin, are essential to neural transmission. Some scientists believe that a deficiency of NE in either the neuron itself or in the synapse, causes depression; and that an excess of NE causes mania—the euphoric high, the opposite of depression.

Doctors now use several drugs to affect the levels of NE, mostly to keep the levels up. One of the most current and very effective drugs is lithium carbonate (some European doctors use lithium orotate, which is reported to be even more effective). Actually, lithium is an essential trace element and normally present in man's environment, notably in mineral-rich, hard drinking waters. Exactly how lithium works is not known, but it has been shown in extensive clinical work that it is capable of correcting and preventing depression—in fact, often bringing striking results, especially in manic-depressives. Needless to say, since the exact mechanism and chemical action of lithium is still a puzzle, and we do not know its possible side effects on the other functions of the body, it should be used *with great discretion* and only upon prescription by a reputable physician. It is known that lithium medication can damage the kidneys. Personally, I do not advocate the use of drugs—either lithium carbonate or tricyclics and extremely dangerous MAOs (other commonly-used antidepressants)—in the treatment of mild, non-clinical, simple depressions, although I realize that drugs have their rightful place in the treatment of severe clinical depression. It is also important to realize that there are thousands of people who are not helped by these drugs, which suggests that in addition to an imbalance of NE, there may be other factors involved in maintaining the proper biochemical composition of nerve cells.

For example, it has been reported from such research centers as the National Institute of Mental Health of the Harvard Medical School that there is a difference in the levels of various hormones in the blood of "normal" and depressed people. Since we know that almost all physiological, neurological, and mental processes in women (more so than in men) are influenced by endocrine and sex hormones, it may give us a clue as to why so many more women than men suffer from depression.

There is a definite interaction between mind and body. It works both ways: a person's behavior, and especially mental and emotional stresses, can affect the quality and quantity of various hormonal secretions—and hormonal deficiencies (or excesses in some cases) can have a negative effect on nervous and mental functions. Which comes first: the chicken or the egg? In this case, the first could be either one. It is a vicious cycle.

Tryptophan and depression

The validity of the biological (biochemical) view of depression, both causatively and therapeutically speaking, has recently been demonstrated by the remarkable discovery that a common nutritive factor, the essential amino acid tryptophan, a component of such common foods as eggs and milk, can be a remarkably useful and safe therapy for some types of depression.

Medical reseachers first became interested in tryptophan because it is a precursor or a chemical forerunner of a substance in the brain called **serotonin.** Serotonin is one of the best known neurotransmitters and without adequate levels of it, impulses or messages along the brain and nerve pathways cannot be properly passed along. Doctors believe that a serious foul-up in the neuro-transmitting system could negatively affect behavior and personality.

Two British medical researchers, Bapuji Rao and A.D. Broadhurst, conducted a controlled clinical study to see if tryptophan would be effective in the treatment of clinical depression. They gave tryptophan in tablet form to nine depressed patients, and a popular antidepressant drug, imipramine, to seven others. All sixteen people in the study were suffering from depression severe enough to require hospitalization. To eliminate the possibility of a subjective evaluation of the results, the study was a so-called double-blind study—neither patients nor doctors knew who was receiving which medication.

The results of the study were more than encouraging. Both groups of patients showed major improvement over the four-week period. Moods improved and spirits lifted in all patients. The researchers concluded, as reported in the medical journal, that the natural tryptophan was just as effective as the prescription drug in relieving depression.[8]

Another study on tryptophan was a collaborative effort of nine Scandinavian doctors from Denmark, Finland, Norway, and Sweden. A total of 42 patients with serious, recurrent depression participated in a double-blind study. Again, the results were impressive. "Both the imipramine as well as the tryptophan group showed highly significant improvements ... with less frequent side effects in the tryptophan group."[9]

In another British study, tryptophan was used to compare its effect with electro-convulsive shock treatments—a standard conventional treatment for extremely depressed patients. Half of the patients received shock treatments twice a week, while the other half received a daily supplement of three grams of tryptophan and one gram of nicotinamide (vitamin B_3). Dr. David A.

MacSweeney, who directed the study, concluded, on the basis of the improvements of all major symptoms, that the tryptophan-vitamin B_3 treatment was superior to convulsive shock therapy in treating depression.[10]

As the above studies show, tryptophan, which can be found in most foods that contain complete protein, is, indeed, a God-sent natural substance that can be used to relieve and prevent one of our culture's most devastating and incapacitating illnesses—depression. Do not hasten, however, to draw what would seem to be a logical conclusion, that by including a generous amount of tryptophan-containing foods in your diet you can utilize the beneficial effects of tryptophan for depression (and also for insomnia, which yields wonderfully to the tryptophan treatment). Studies show that eating a tryptophan-rich, high-protein meal does not raise the level of tryptophan in the brain, even though blood levels of the nutrient do rise. On the basis of studies, scientists have found that in order to get tryptophan into the brain (where it is used to produce more serotonin) it has to be consumed by itself, without the other essential amino acids. This means that tryptophan must be taken in isolated form, as a supplement or medication. Most health food stores now sell tryptophan in a table form. To treat depression most doctors use doses of 3 to 9 grams per day. Lower doses are good for insomnia, but not for depression. *Caution:* About 25 percent of the patients with depression who take high amounts of tryptophan (over 4 grams per day) feel agitated and irritable. Therefore, the treatment with very high doses of tryptophan should only be done under supervision.

The total holistic approach

I have long maintained that the human body is a complex entity where physical, mental, emotional, and spiritual components are intertwined. The human body is also a *self-healing* mechanism, and always tries to correct any pathological dysfunctions and restore health. Our bodies are equipped with the most extensive and effective healing capacity and potential known to medical science. The best we can do is to *support* the body's own healing mechanism with all available means and create the most conducive environment for such healing to take place. Given such a holistic support from all directions—nutritionally, physically, emotionally, and spiritually—the body can heal itself and correct any disorders, including depression.

I have seen many examples of this. One of the most dramatic cases in my files is the recent case of a 27-year-old woman, Kathy M., from West Virginia.

Kathy said that she was perfectly healthy until the age of nineteen. My questioning revealed that at that time she was sick with a flu which was a nasty, lingering condition that lasted several months. However, not one of the dozens of doctors who treated Kathy during the eight years of her illness had ever questioned her about her past illnesses, and she had never connected this severe flu with her present "mental" disease.

After the flu, Kathy's menstrual period stopped. They resumed, irregularly, for a few months when she was twenty-two, but then stopped again, never to reappear. She also suffered from aches and pains "everywhere," persistent headaches, and extreme fatigue most of the time. All medical examinations and tests were negative. Gradually, doctors, her friends, and her parents started to insist that there was nothing wrong with her, that it was "all in her head." But Kathy knew better. She had constant cramps and pains in her stomach. She became a compulsive eater and soon added thirty pounds of extra weight. Her boyfriend of several years left her—he couldn't stand her constant complaints. She became more and more depressed, withdrawn, hostile. She knew that she was sick, that something was wrong with her. She had her headaches and severe stomach cramps to prove it, yet every doctor she consulted told her that she was healthy. She became more and more confused and despondent. She lost her secretarial job because she couldn't concentrate and made constant errors in her work. She felt that something terrible would happen to her—an accident, cancer, or even death. Her energy level was so low that she could hardly do anything; she mostly stayed in bed. Coffee gave her a little boost, but after awhile, even coffee didn't help. A year before she came to me, she made an unsuccessful attempt at suicide by taking a large dose of sleeping pills. Six months later, she finally volunteered to enter a local mental health clinic where she was given all kinds of tests and treated with rest and drugs. She felt better, and left the clinic after two weeks, but soon was worse than ever. She distrusted everyone, and refused to see any doctors.

When her mother called me for an appointment, Kathy refused to see me at first. I spent two hours on the telephone trying to convince her that her problems were real; that they were not mental, but physical; that judging from all the symptoms her mother had described, she most likely suffered from hypothyroidism and adrenal exhaustion; that her condition could be totally corrected if properly diagnosed and treated with natural hormones, supplements, and dietary changes. I finally convinced her to see me.

Although the glucose tolerance test (GTT) that I requested was marginally normal, it did show a rather flat curve, which indicates chronic adrenal exhaustion. Tests also showed a definite low thyroid function. I could clearly see the connection between her lack of menstruation, hypothyroidism, and adrenal exhaustion. This combination would explain most of her symptoms.

I outlined a comprehensive supportive program to normalize her body's biochemical and hormonal levels. In addition to the Optimum Diet and avoidance of all possible allergens (in her case: wheat and milk products in every form) she received a long list of vitamins and supplements to help her adrenal and thyroid function. She was given adrenocortical extract (ACE) injections twice a week, later reduced to once every two weeks. For the first two weeks, she received vitamins B_{12}, B_3, B_6, B_1, pantothenic acid, folic acid, kelp (iodine), zinc, and vitamin C intravenously, in addition to oral doses of high-potency B-complex. She also received lithium carbonate and tryptophan supplementation.

After only four months, Kathy's transformation is remarkable. She is no longer depressed, she smiles again, she has lots of energy, and she sleeps well. Last month she reported that she had a menstrual period, which gave a big boost to her morale. Kathy is now off ACE injections, has reduced her thyroid medication, but will continue to take heavy doses of vitamins and minerals. I have never seen a more grateful patient. Her "mental" illness miraculously disappeared when her body's biochemical balance was restored and nutritional deficiencies corrected.

Holistic supportive program

Here's what I suggest to those who suffer from simple or clinical depression (suffer from several of the most common symptoms mentioned earlier in this chapter):

1. First, have a thorough examination by a competent doctor, one who is nutritionally- and biologically-oriented. Depression could be a side effect of many organic disorders, or of medication taken for such disorders. The examination should include a glucose tolerance test and tests for all endocrine gland functions. If you cannot find a doctor who is nutritionally- and biologically-oriented, write to the publishers of this book and they will send you a nationwide Directory of doctors who practice nutritional and biological medicine. (Please enclose a long, self-addressed, stamped envelope with your request.)

2. After the condition is diagnosed, take injections or medications if prescribed by your doctor, and follow a comprehensive supportive program which will help your body and mind to heal and normalize all the vital physical, glandular, and nerve and brain functions. This supportive healing program should include:

    a. Optimal nutrition, as outlined in Chapters 3 and 4 of this book.

    b. Special vitamins and supplements in dosages set for your specific individual needs by your doctor. B vitamin deficiencies are typically involved in mental depression.[11] Here is the generalized list of daily vitamins and supplements I usually recommend for people with depression. (Your doctor can use this list as a skeleton from which to plan your individual program.)

C—3,000 - 5,000 mg.
A—25,000 units
D—1,000 units
E—400 - 800 I.U., mixed tocopherols
B-complex, 100% natural, from yeast concentrate—
    2 - 5 tablets
B_1—100 mg.
B_2—100 mg.
B_3—100 - 300 mg. (more if recommended by your doctor). Niacin is a "mood elevator".
B_6—100 - 300 mg.
B_{12}—50 mcg.
B_{15}—100 mg.
Folic acid—2 mg.
Pantothenic acid—100 mg.
Calcium—1,000 mg.
Magnesium—500 mg.
Zinc—30 mg.
Selenium—50 - 100 mcg.
Bone meal—5 tablets
"Nature's Minerals" (natural mineral complex)—5 tablets
Wheat germ, raw, fresh—1 - 2 tbsp.
Kyolic, Super Garlic Formula 101—6 tablets or capsules
Brewer's yeast—3 tbsp. of powder, or equivalent in tablets.
Kelp, for iodine—3 tablets
Lecithin—2 tsp. of granules

  c. Specific biological medicines, adrenal and thyroid hormones, lithium carbonate or orotate, neptone (mucopolysaccharides) and tryptophan, *if prescribed by your doctor.*

d. Extensive exercise program. Long walks, one to three hours a day, preferably in a pleasant, smog-free environment (woods, hills, park, by the lake, etc.) are especially beneficial and can change the mood from the blues and depression to peace and contentment. Bike riding, horseback riding, games and light sports are also very calming and soothing for the nervous system.

3. Rest and relaxation are imperative. Try to eliminate all triggering stress factors from your environment. A trip "away from it all" (like to an exotic beach resort), away from the usual sources of irritation and other predisposing factors, somewhere where you can rest, relax, and re-evaluate your life would do a lot of good.

4. Don't store up anger. Try to communicate your dissatisfactions or irritations to those involved *before* you explode with rage and then have the feelings of guilt and remorse that lead to depression.

5. Don't set unreasonably high goals for yourself then feel frustrated that you never reach them. Set very realistic, short-term goals, and stick to them.

6. Learn to enjoy the small pleasures and joys: chirping of a bird, the warmth of sunlight, the smile on a child's face, a soothing walk in the woods.

7. Finally, "get yourself together" by cultivating a positive state of mind. Do not indulge in disease-oriented thinking, but "think health." Think and talk about health, visualize yourself as enjoying perfect health and happiness.

Re-evaluate your life and put your priorities straight. Have faith! Even in the most despondent, dark moments of your life, when you feel lonely, insecure, unloved, and vulnerable, know that there is One who always loves you. He knows your needs and He will protect and help you, if you only ask Him to. Perhaps you *needed* this experience of depression and illness which might have a far-reaching effect on your future life. It may help you to put values and priorities in a proper perspective; it may bring enlightenment and understanding as to the true purpose of your life.

Thank God for this experience and ask for His guidance in the future. Thank Him for all the blessings you have and *they are many,* but they have been overshadowed by your tragic illness. You may have an understanding husband, loving children or parents, many friends who wish you well. You have a home, enough food to eat. You live in a free country where you have many opportunities; you are free to travel, pursue your interests. Think of all those around the world who are starving and homeless. Think of those who are in prisons, and those who are dying of dreadful and painful diseases. Perhaps then you will realize that *your* problems are minor indeed. Thank God for giving you new insight about your condition and a clearer understanding of what you can do about it after reading this Chapter. This insight was given to you because He loves you, and wants to help you. You are not alone. Have faith! Faith is the most powerful healing factor known to science. With understanding, faith, and hope, you cannot fail—you *will* be healed!

30

What Women Should Know About Anemia

Although anemia is not specifically a female condition, more women than men suffer from it, mainly because one common form of anemia, iron-deficiency anemia, is often associated with menstruation. Women whose menstrual flow is consistently heavy are especially vulnerable to iron-deficiency anemia.

What is anemia?

Anemia means deficiency of blood. Normally your blood is in a constant state of change. The bone marrow continuously produces red blood cells (erythrocytes) to replace those which are constantly being destroyed. The life span of a red blood cell is about 120 days. These blood cells derive their name and color from hemoglobin, the oxygen-carrying red coloring matter, or pigment, inside the blood cells. Hemoglobin gives your blood its red color. Red blood cells are microscopic—there are about 5 million of them per cubic millimeter of blood (the size of a large pinhead). The normal healthy blood count is anywhere between 10 and 15 grams (in 100 cc). Some doctors consider a count lower than 13 grams as indicating anemia.

Hemoglobin carries oxygen to every cell and organ of the body. Since a low hemoglobin level means less oxygen reaching the tissues of the body, the consequent symptoms of anemia are constant tiredness and being "out of sorts," lack of stamina, shortness of breath, headaches, dizziness, irritability, mental depression. Some anemic persons experience digestive disorders, discomforts in the abdomen, indigestion. Others complain of palpitations and pulsation in the neck. Menstruation is almost always affected. The disruption can go either way: the flow can be too heavy or very scanty. And, most anemic persons can be diagnosed by their pallor, or paleness, although general pallor is not necessarily always an indication of anemia.

What causes anemia?

Anemia can be roughly divided into two main groups: *primary anemia* and *secondary anemia.* In primary anemia, blood deficiency is caused by an excessive loss or destruction of blood resulting from injury, childbirth, bleeding hemorrhoids or peptic ulcers, or other trauma; or there could be an inborn or pathological weakness in the blood-building mechanism. Secondary anemia is caused by defective blood formation due to various dietary nutritional deficiencies or the body's inability to absorb and use the blood-building material which is present in the diet. This form of anemia is, by far, the most prevalent and the easiest to correct. Although iron-deficiency anemia is the one form of anemia with which most people are familiar, it is not necessarily the most common form. Deficiencies of *many* vital nutrients can cause anemia.

Folic-acid-deficiency anemia

This form of secondary anemia is common among pregnant women. Therefore, during pregnancy, it is important to supplement the diet with plenty of green vegetables, raw and/or cooked, which are excellent sources of folic acid.

Folic-and-deficiency anemia can be caused by a lack of vitamin C in the diet and an insufficiency of stomach acids. Even if the diet is rich in folic acid, it cannot be changed into a usable form unless there is sufficient vitamin C present.[1] But the most common cause of folic-acid-deficiency and the anemia associated with it is a diet of refined, devitalized food. Excessive alcohol consumption is another major contributing cause.[2]

The common symptoms of the anemia caused by folic acid deficiency are a sore mouth and tongue; sometimes there is an accompanying grayish-brown skin pigmentation. In women, a deficiency of folic acid may cause megaloblastic anemia of pregnancy, and spontaneous abortions, difficult labor, or high infant death rate.

In addition to avoiding refined foods and eating plenty of folic-acid-rich foods (deep green leafy vegetables, broccoli, asparagus, lima beans, potatoes, brewer's yeast, wheat germ, nuts), folic acid in tablet form may be advisable when a deficiency is diagnosed. Pregnant women should take folic acid supplement as a preventative: usually 0.4 to 0.8 mg. daily is sufficient. To correct a severe deficiency, 5.0 mg. or more is needed daily. In the United States, potencies higher than 0.8 mg. are available only by prescription. Folic acid should always be taken together with B-complex and B_{12} for its maximum effect.

Vitamin-E-deficiency anemia

Vitamin E deficiency is connected with anemia in the following causative ways:[2, 3]

- It prevents the absorption of iron.
- It inhibits the formation of hemoglobin.
- It causes oxidation and destruction of red blood cells by altering the essential fatty acid forming part of the blood cell structure.
- It reduces the life span of the blood cells.

Vitamin-E-deficiency anemia, just like folic-acid-deficiency anemia, is especially prevalent during pregnancy since there is an increased need for this vitamin during that time. Premature births are frequently the result of too little vitamin E during pregnancy.[4] Babies born to vitamin-E-deficient mothers can suffer from deficiency of this vitamin also, and are particularly susceptible to anemia.[3] Vitamin E deficiency can even cause blindness in babies. Mother's milk is the best protection against vitamin E deficiency and the anemia caused by it in infants, since breast milk of a healthy mother usually contains ten to twenty times more vitamin E than cow's milk. But even breast milk can be deficient in this vital vitamin if the mother eats a diet of refined foods which is inadequate in this nutrient.[2]

In addition to avoiding refined foods (such as sugar and white flour products), and taking fresh wheat germ and supplementary vitamin E, those who are suspected of having a vitamin E deficiency should also avoid excessive consumption of polyunsaturated oils (vegetable oils), especially for cooking or frying. Consumption of such oils increases the need for vitamin E.[15]

Vitamin-B$_6$-deficiency anemia

Both the number of red blood cells and the amount of hemoglobin can be adversely affected and decreased by diets deficient in vitamin B$_6$.

This form of anemia is especially common in women during pregnancy, but men and children can also be affected by it.

Vitamin-B$_6$-deficiency anemia is often misdiagnosed, mistaken for iron-deficiency-anemia, and treated with iron medication. This can have most tragic results since: first, this form of anemia cannot be corrected with iron; and, second, treatment with iron medication can so overload the system with iron that it damages the tissues and can cause dangerous iron storage diseases, siderosis or hemosiderosis, which can be fatal unless transfusions are performed or vitamin B$_6$ is quickly administered.[7]

Vitamin-C-deficiency anemia

Nutritional anemia (nutritional-deficiency anemia) can be caused by: (1) lack of blood-building nutritive factors in the diet, as discussed above, and/or (2) by the body's inability to absorb nutrients. For example, if the stomach lacks sufficient hydrochloric acid, the minerals, including blood-building iron, copper, magnesium, manganese, and zinc, cannot be properly assimilated, even if the diet is adequate.

Vitamin C is one vitamin that is vitally involved in absorption of minerals, especially iron. Several studies show that vitamin C promotes and enhances iron absorption—500 mg. of vitamin C a day nearly doubled the absorption of supplementary iron.[8] Vitamin C also increases the absorption of vitamin B_{12}, enhances and increases the rate of hemoglobin production, and is vital for the efficient use of folic acid by the body.[1, 2] Vitamin C also has a sparing effect on the body's use of vitamin E, and, thus, can assist in preventing anemia caused by vitamin E deficiency.[2]

Iron-deficiency anemia

Dietary deficiency of iron, contrary to popular belief, is not the chief cause of iron-deficiency anemia. Iron is so widely distributed in all natural foods that to produce anemia due to lack of iron in the diet one must live almost exclusively on refined and processed foods, which, unfortunately, many people do.

Iron-deficiency anemia can be caused, in addition to dietary lack of iron, by:

- The body's inability to utilize dietary iron (for many reasons mentioned earlier, including lack of hydrochloric acid). Because of their inability to utilize iron, bottle-fed babies often have iron-deficiency anemia, even though the formula contains plenty of iron.
- Dietary deficiencies of copper, manganese, vitamin B_1, B_2, niacin, choline, or pantothenic acid.[8, 9, 10] Copper is necessary for the synthesis of B_{12} by the liver.
- Dietary deficiency of vitamin C, which impairs the body's ability to absorb iron.[1, 8]
- Excessive blood (and, therefore, iron) losses during certain illnesses, such as bleeding ulcers or injuries, or during childbirth or excessive menstruation.

Iron is needed in the production of hemoglobin, in the manufacture of many enzymes involved in blood-cell production, and in the production of a substance known as myoglobin, which carries oxygen in muscle cells. Even a mild iron deficiency can cause lack of oxygen in the tissues with such immediate symptoms as chronic fatigue, headaches, and shortness of breath. Women of reproductive age and pregnant women are especially susceptible to iron-deficiency anemia; so are bottle-fed infants, young children, and adolescent girls.

If you avoid refined foods, adhere to an Optimum Diet, and take the special vitamin and mineral supplements as recommended in this chapter, you will be pretty well protected against iron-deficiency anemia.

Pernicious anemia

Pernicious anemia is largely a vitamin B_{12}-deficiency disease. However, it is only seldom caused by a dietary vitamin B_{12} deficiency, since B_{12} is present in many foods, such as liver, and even in purely lacto-vegetarian foods (brewer's yeast, sunflower seeds, soybeans, comfrey leaves, kelp, bananas, peanuts, concord grapes, raw wheat germ, pollen, milk, and eggs). Vitamin B_{12} is also synthesized in the liver and by beneficial bacteria in the intestines. The main cause of pernicious anemia is the body's inability to use vitamin B_{12} effectively. Normally, an intrinsic factor, an enzyme produced by the stomach, combines with vitamin B_{12} to produce an anti-anemic factor, which is then stored in the liver. In pernicious anemia, the stomach does not produce this intrinsic factor and, thus, vitamin B_{12} cannot be absorbed and utilized.

Since persons with pernicious anemia cannot easily assimilate dietary B_{12}, it must usually be administered by injection. In mild cases, if vitamin B_{12} is taken orally, supplemental hydrochloric acid, calcium, and vitamin C will promote its assimilation. Brewer's yeast (with B_{12}) plus other B_{12}-rich foods mentioned above are also essential, if accompanied by hydrochloric acid, calcium, and vitamin C.

Dietary considerations for nutritional-deficiency anemia

Aside from severe cases of pernicious anemia, which must be treated by injections, all other forms of nutritional-deficiency anemia respond rapidly to proper diet, digestive aids, and the special supplements outlined below.

Dietary emphasis should be on raw fruits and vegetables, especially those which are rich in iron and other blood-building minerals and vitamins: dark green leafy vegetables (spinach, alfalfa, comfrey, watercress, parsley, green onions, kale, broccoli, collards, chard, beet tops), okra, squash, carrots, radishes, beets, yams, tomatoes, potatoes (with jackets); and such fruits as bananas, apples, dark grapes, figs, apricots, plums, raisins, strawberries. Bananas are particularly beneficial as they contain, in addition to easily-assimilable iron, folic acid and traces of vitamin B_{12}—both factors extremely important in prevention and treatment of anemia.

Additional foods rich in iron and other blood-building elements are: sunflower seeds, pumpkin seeds, lentils, crude black strap molasses, rice polishings, wheat germ, pinto beans, black beans, almonds, sesame seeds (Tahini), peas, millet, egg yolks, and honey. Honey is also rich in copper, which helps in iron assimilation. Sunflower seeds contain almost as much iron as liver, and the iron content of pumpkin seeds even exceeds that of liver. Liver, usually prescribed by doctors in iron-deficiency anemia, would be an acceptable nutritional remedy *if healthy, non-toxic liver were available*; but, in this polluted age, it is not. Liver is a detoxifying organ, and livers of animals treated with hormones, antibiotics, and herbicide-filled feed, are storehouses of poisons and, thus, cannot be recommended.

The diet for anemia should also include a moderate amount of whole grains, especially millet, buckwheat, rice, rye, and a variety of beans.

By far the best dietary source of blood-building iron, as well as many other blood-building minerals and vitamins, is *brewer's yeast.* Regular intake of brewer's yeast is the best dietary protection against anemia as well as the best nutritional treatment of anemia.

Coffee and tea should be avoided, since caffeine in these beverages interferes with iron absorption in the body.

Vitamins and supplements for anemia

When nutritional-deficiency-anemia, as discussed in this Chapter, is present, the following corrective vitamins and supplements should be taken daily (adult dose):

Organic iron supplement, preferably in chelated form—10 - 20 mg.

B_{12}—25 - 50 mcg.

B_6—50 - 100 mg.

E—600 - 1,000 I.U.

C—1,000 - 3,000 mg.

Pantothenic acid—up to 100 mg.

Folic acid—0.8 - 1.0 mg.

B-complex, high potency.

Brewer's yeast—2 - 3 tbsp. powder (best taken 1 tbsp. at a time, mixed with grapefruit juice, and taken on an empty stomach, 1 or ½ hour before meal).

PABA—50 mg.

Crude black strap molasses—1 - 2 tbsp. (can be mixed with milk shake or in fruit juice).

Bone meal—3 tablets.

"Nature's Minerals"—5 tablets.

Kelp—1 - 2 tablets.

Sesame seeds (Tahini)—1 tbsp. (sesame seeds contain Vitamin T, which is beneficial in preventing and correcting anemia).

Betaine Hydrochloride—1 tablet after each large meal (promotes assimilation of iron and B_{12}).

Specific herbs and juices

The best juices for anemia are: green juice (see Recipes & Directions), fresh beet juice or beet juice made from beet powder (sold in health food stores), red grape juice, and juice from black currants, prunes, apricots, and blueberries.

Specific healing herbs are comfrey, dandelion, black currant leaves, raspberry leaves, yellow dock, fennugreek, and kelp. Herbs are best taken in the form of teas. Steep 1 tsp. dry herbs or 2 capsules in 1 cup of boiling water for 15 minutes; drink once or twice a day. Can be sweetened with honey.

31

How To Stay Younger Longer

We are living in the most exciting era of human history. Headlines announcing world-shattering events are an every-day occurrence. Age-long traditions are broken and discarded and totally new values are formed. The disorientation and confusion in virtually every area of life is bewildering. After shelving the stability of conventions and traditions such as family and religion, our youth are wandering aimlessly, looking for "alternatives." Gurus, masters, and other soul hunters are having a hey-day, offering expanded consciousness and higher awareness to morally destitute and spiritually impoverished seekers of truth. Meanwhile, overtaken by greedy commercial interests in virtually every field of human endeavor, our planet is becoming a more and more unlivable place, with air, water, food, and environment poisoned to the level where life in reasonable health is already impossible, and unless the mad race for self destruction is soon halted, all life will be extinct within a few generations.

Indeed, as I said, we live in the most exciting era in human history! Just imagine, witnessing all this first-hand! It is traumatic, it is tragic, it is disheartening—but you can't say it isn't exciting!

When the final history of humankind will be written, the end of the Twentieth Century will be known by many descriptive names. Off hand, I can think of the following fitting epithets:

- "The Slow-Extinction-Through Chemistry Era."
- "The Dark Age of the Unholy Alliance Between Medical Science and Food-Drug-Chemical Industries."
- "Inflation and Recession Era"—Ego Inflation and Moral Recession, that is.
- "The Era of the High-Protein Cult."

But, perhaps the most appropriate description of all for the second half of the Twentieth Century will be:

- "The Adulation-of-Youth Era."

For the first time in human history, old age and the wisdom gained from lifelong experience have become liabilities rather than assets. In our culture, we worship youth. We let them run the affairs of the nation, while old people are isolated in special old-peoples' homes and institutions where their experience and wisdom are wasted on playing checkers and shuffleboard.

As far as woman is concerned, living in our culture at this time is not easy. She is "over the hill" after forty, and chances of catching or keeping a man after that dwindle with depressing mathematical precision. The ideal woman, as popularized in all media, is a slim, teen-age-looking blonde starlet with lots of teeth and a big bosom. No wonder the plastic surgeons and a new kind of doctor, the so-called Youth Doctor, are making a fortune on the "adulation-of-youth" fad.

Gullible youth-seekers are being duped, exploited, and relieved of large sums of money in return for which they receive worthless treatments, shots, and injections which are supposed to restore their lost youth.

In this chapter, I will try to report to you only what is scientifically proven in the field of prevention of aging and preservation of youth. There is a legitimate special branch of medical science, gerontology, which has been researching the causes of aging and experimenting with the ways of extending life. There is also, what we call, accumulated empirical knowledge based on the studies of various peoples around the world known for their exceptional health and long disease-free lives. Most of my data and conclusions are derived from such studies. In my travels in many countries around the world, I have found that for thousands of years, natives have used certain herbs or natural foods and food substances to maintain their good health and attain a long life. Some of their special dietary factors have been proven by modern science to have age-preventive and life-extending properties. These rejuve-native secrets, secrets of how to stay younger longer, have nothing to do with drugs or injections. They are simple dietary and lifestyle factors that you can easily apply in your own home without going to expensive rejuvenation clinics or spas.

Vitamin C from roses

Medical scientists and nutritionists have long known that one of the main causes of aging, as well as many degenerative diseases and the visible aging processes in the skin, is the loss of strength, elasticity, and integrity of collagen, the connective tissue in the body.

Collagen, the substance which holds the cells together, is responsible for the stability and tensile strength of practically all the tissues of the body, including the skin, the muscles, and the tissues of all the organs. Wrinkles, flabbiness, discolorations, and other aging signs in the skin are all related to the deterioration of the condition of collagen. Scientific studies by Drs. J.W. McCormick, Johan Bjorksten, Roger Williams, and others, have shown that the deterioration in collagen is caused primarily by a deficiency of vitamin C in the tissues. Adequate amounts of vitamin C in the daily diet will help keep collagen strong and elastic, which, among other benefits, will produce tight skin and a smooth and lovely complexion.

I discovered the relationship between vitamin C and a lovely, healthy, and youthful complexion while traveling in Sweden in the late forties. Sweden has one of the best health records in the world, the lowest mortality rate, and healthy, beautiful people, with the most gorgeous complexions—in spite of the fact that they live in one of the most rugged and unfriendly climates in the world.

I found that Swedish women have their own secret of beautiful and youthful skin—wild rose hips! In the late fall, you can see thousands of women and children picking sacks full of rose hips (the cherry-like fruit of the rose) from acres of wildly-grown rose bushes. Then they take them home, dry them in a slightly heated oven, and use them as an essential part of the daily diet. They make soups, teas, jellies, and desserts from them. Rose hips are sold in every supermarket in Sweden (not just in health food stores) and you can order rose hip soup in virtually any restaurant in the country. In fact, rose hips are a Swedish staple food—in the humble cottage as well as in the King's castle.

How are rose hips related to your skin and beautiful complexion? They are an excellent source of important factors, specific vitamins, and minerals that are vital for keeping your skin and complexion healthy and beautiful.

- Rose hips are the richest known natural source of vitamin C, with the possible exception of acerola, containing 20 to 40 times more vitamin C than oranges!
- They have 25 times more vitamin A than oranges!
- They are extremely rich in bioflavonoids, co-factors in the vitamin C complex.
- They have 28% more calcium and 25% more iron than oranges![1]

Long before vitamin C was discovered, Swedes, guided by natural instinct, gorged on rose hips, saturating their bodies with vitamin C, *one of the most important health and rejuvenation vitamins.*

How vitamin C can keep you young

In addition to its all-important function of keeping collagen strong, elastic, and healthy, more and more research is turning up which shows that vitamin C is almost a miraculous substance for keeping you healthy and young.

The world-famous Nobel Prize winner, Dr. Linus Pauling, reported that vitamin C, if taken in large doses on a regular basis, can extend life 10 to 20 years. It can also prevent many of our common degenerative diseases, he believes.

Russian scientists have discovered that vitamin C has a profound stimulating effect on the adrenal glands. The adrenal glands secrete more than twenty steroid hormones, which are directly involved in keeping your vital bodily processes in a condition of high efficiency. It is generally agreed that a decrease in the output of these hormones—which normally begins in late middle life—is responsible for the symptoms of aging. Russian scientists have demonstrated that substantial daily doses of vitamin C have a rejuvenative, stimulating effect on all endocrine glandular activity, including the sex glands, and the hormones are once again produced at higher levels, similar to those found in younger people.[2]

Vitamin C is a marvelous detoxifier. It neutralizes most poisons, both those produced in the body and those picked up from food or the environment. It stimulates the production of antibodies and white blood cells and inhibits the growth of practically all pathogenic bacteria or viruses.

Vitamin C is also a first-class healer in practically every condition of ill health: atherosclerosis, cancer, arthritis, infections, high blood pressure, acute poisoning, pneumonia, influenza, and infectious hepatitis, to name just a few. In fact, those who have studied vitamin C claim that it is so universal in its preventive and therapeutic action, that it is often referred to as a medical panacea. It is virtually impossible to find a condition of ill health or diminished well-being that vitamin C would not affect favorably, very often with a miraculous healing effect.[3] Since old age is often accompanied by various conditions of diminished health, it stands to reason that vitamin C should be considered one of the most important rejuvenative tonics for anyone over forty years of age.

Vitamin C is non-toxic in reasonably large doses. We cannot get rose hips in this country to the extent Swedish people get them (although health food stores do sell rose hip powder and tablets) but we can take vitamin C tablets made from rose hips or other natural substances. Doses of

1,000 to 3,000 mg. can be taken on a regular daily basis; even more in cases of illness.

Colonic hygiene—secret of eternal youth

Of all the "secrets" of perpetual youth which scientists have discovered in their long search, none is more scientifically established than one which is based on the premise of colonic hygiene—or the perfectly and efficiently functioning digestive and eliminative systems. Poor elimination, chronic constipation, and intestinal sluggishness are the major causes of many, if not all, of man's ills, as well as of premature aging.

This was first discovered by a Nobel Prize winning scientist, Ilja Metchnikoff, the eminent Russian biologist, at the turn of the century. Dr. Metchnikoff's premise was as follows:

Your intestines house billions of beneficial bacteria which help your digestive system to break down the food you eat and, thus, aid in digestion and assimilation of nutrients. Also, these intestinal bacteria produce many important nutrients on their own, notably B-vitamins. Therefore, for optimum health, it is extremely important that there is always a plentiful supply of these beneficial bacteria. Metchnikoff discovered that soured milk products, lactic acid fermented milks, such as yogurt, kefir, or clabbered milk, not only contain bacteria similar to the intestinal bacteria—*Lactobacillus acidophilus* and *Lactobacillus bifidus*—but that they help feed the intestinal bacteria and help them to multiply. This inhibits the growth of the undesirable, putrefactive bacteria in the colon. Metchnikoff recommended eating soured milk products as the way to prevent constipation, improve the quality of intestinal flora, and assure good health and a long life.

Recently, the idea of constipation as being the cause of many diseases and premature aging, has not only been resurrected by Dr. D.P. Burkitt of England, but also universally accepted by the medical establishment. Dr. Burkitt stressed the word *fiber*, or rather the lack of fiber in the Western diet, as the major cause for disorders in the digestive tract, such as colitis and diverticulitis, varicose veins, and cancer of the colon. Dr. Burkitt based his conclusions on his study of many African tribes who live on a diet high in fiber, and who have no cancer of the colon, diverticulitis, or other disorders in the digestive and eliminative tract. The idea was picked up by other medical researchers worldwide and, suddenly, the need for *fiber in the diet* became the "in" thing. Even the American Medical Association, who scoffed for years at any suggestion that cancer of the colon could be related to the diet, acknowledged in an editorial in the ***Journal of the American Medical Association*** recently that a lack of fiber in the diet is, indeed, involved in development of bowel cancer.[4]

The bran fad is in full swing in America, and millions of people stuff themselves with this indigestible wheat fiber to prevent constipation and protect themselves from cancer. The problem is that, unwilling to change their dietary habits, Americans have ignored the most important aspects of Burkitt's findings. Burkitt emphasized that the disease-free people whom he studied, ate a diet of *natural* high-fiber foods, with plenty of unprocessed whole grains, vegetables, and fruits, and no, or very little, meat, sugar, or refined foods. Meat is one of the most constipating foods there is, because it is virtually fiber-free. But, since the idea of giving up meat does not appeal to the steak-loving Americans, they jumped at the idea of supplementing their diets with bran and, thus, preventing constipation while still continuing to eat meat.

However, in spite of the fact that the bran fad has been going on for years now, statistics show that the frequency of cancer of the colon is increasing. It is now the number two cancer in America, the first being lung cancer. The reason for this is that an excessive amount of meat in the diet not only contributes to cancer of the colon by causing constipation, but meat is carcinogenic in itself. In the process of meat digestion, carcinogenic ammonia is produced, which irritates the linings of the colon and contributes to the development of cancer, as discovered by Dr. Willard Visek of Cornell University.[5]

Excessive meat in the diet also contributes to the development of many other of our common degenerative diseases, such as atherosclerosis, heart disease,[6] arthritis,[7] and osteoporosis.[8] Excessive meat in the diet is also a direct cause of senility and premature aging. Amyloid, another chemical that develops during meat metabolism, interferes with cell regeneration and synthesis and, thus, causes the degenerative changes in the body that lead to premature aging, as discovered by Drs. Ph. Schwartz and R. Bircher, of Switzerland.[1] (See Chapter 3 for more information on the danger of excessive meat in the diet.)

How to prevent and/or correct constipation

Here are some helpful suggestions that will help you to prevent constipation, or if you are plagued by it already, help to correct it.

1. Eat a diet high in natural fiber. The Optimum Diet, as described in Chapters 3 and 4, is rich in natural roughage and will give you sufficient fiber without the need of taking extra bran. However, if your diet contains refined and processed foods and fiberless meat, then you should take 2 - 3 tbsp. of coarse wheat bran every day.

2. Drink plenty of liquids: water, juices, herb teas—6 - 8 glasses a day.

3. The following herbs, available in health food stores, are beneficial for preventing constipation: senna-pod or senna-leaf tea, alder, buckthorn bark, dandelion, slippery elm bark, cascara sagrada, mountain flax, and psyllium seed.

4. Avoid regular use of commercial laxatives. In an emergency, use herbal laxatives sold in health food stores.

5. If you suffer from a serious case of constipation, take 1 glass of Excelsior (see Recipes & Directions) each morning and evening.

6. Lack of sufficient exercise is one of the main causes of constipation. Exercise! Walk, jog, swim, ride a bike, dance—anything! Ordinary walking, two or more hours a

day, will remedy the problem in most cases.

7. Take the following vitamins and supplements each day:

> Brewer's yeast powder—2 - 3 tbsp. (take 1 hour before meal in grapefruit juice)
> Whey powder—2 tbsp.
> Flax seed—1 - 2 tbsp. (soak in water overnight and drink whole without chewing)
> B-complex—100% natural
> B_6—50 mg.
> B_1—50 mg.
> Lecithin—2 tsp. of granules
> A—25,000 units
> C—3,000 mg.
> Multiple vitamin-mineral supplement
> Olive oil—1 - 2 tbsp. daily
> Magnesium—500 mg.
> Dolomite—2 - 3 tablets
> "Nature's Minerals"—5 tablets

The rejuvenative miracle of brewer's yeast

The single most effective rejuvenative food is brewer's yeast. Here are some of its miraculous health-building, disease-preventing, and rejuvenative properties:

- Brewer's yeast is the richest natural source of B-vitamins. Most of the vitamins of the B-complex are directly or indirectly involved in keeping you young: B_1, B_2, B_6, B_{12}, PABA, folic acid, and pantothenic acid—they are all present in large quantities in brewer's yeast.
- Brewer's yeast is an excellent source of high-quality protein. Up to 40 - 50% of its weight is pure protein of high biological value.
- Brewer's yeast is one of the best natural sources of iron, zinc, chromium, and selenium. Zinc is involved in the healing processes and is important for the proper function of male sex organs and for prevention of prostate disorders. Chromium is vital for proper sugar metabolism. And selenium is one of

the true rejuvenators. Its function is similar to that of vitamin E and it enhances the vitamin E function in the system, helping to improve circulation and bring more oxygen to every cell of your body.

- Brewer's yeast is the best natural source of the nucleic acids, RNA and DNA. Up to 15% of its weight is nucleic acids. Nucleic acids are substances which are directly involved in keeping you young, contributing to effective cell rejuvenation and keeping the mental and physical processes at the peak of their youthful efficiency.

- Brewer's yeast is one of the few foods left in this polluted environment of ours which is relatively free from contaminants and toxic additives and residues.

As you can see, brewer's yeast is one of the most important foods you can eat if you wish to stay younger longer.

Make sure that the yeast you buy is true brewer's yeast. Not torula, not primary or nutritional yeast, or yeast number so and so, but real brewer's yeast. Although all nutritional yeasts are useful, only the real brewer's yeast contains sufficient quantities of the important trace elements, iron, zinc, chromium, and selenium.

You can take 2 - 3 tbsp. a day, or the equivalent in tablets. (See more notes on brewer's yeast and how to take it to avoid gas, in Chapter 3.)

Pollen, royal jelly, and honey

The discovery of pollen-rich honey as a life prolonger was made in the course of research in one of the longevity institutes in Russia. The famed Russian scientist, biologist, and experimental botanist, Dr. Nicolai Tsitsin, was engaged in research on longevity. The aim of his inquiry was to find ways of prolonging human life.

"We decided to send letters to 200 people claiming to be over 100 years old, with the request to answer the following three questions: what was their age; how had they earned their living most of their lives; and what had been their principle food."

Dr. Tsitsin received 150 replies to his 200 letters.

"We made a very interesting discovery. The answers showed that a large number of them were bee keepers. And *all of them,* without exception, said that their principle food had always been honey!"

But as sensational as this discovery was, this was not all!

"We found, continued Dr. Tsitsin, "That in each case, it wasn't really honey these people ate, but the waste matter in the bottom of the honey containers. Because most bee keepers were poor, they sold all of the pure honey on the market, keeping only the 'dirty residue' for themselves."

After a series of laboratory tests, Dr. Tsitsin discovered that the "dirty residue" of the honey was not dirt at all, but almost pure pollen, which falls off the bees' legs while they deposit their honey. Thus, Tsitsin discovered one of the most important rejuvenation secrets of Russian centenarians—pollen-rich, natural, unfiltered, and unprocessed honey!

Of course, the fact that honey and pollen are age-retarding and rejuvenating foods isn't really a Russian discovery; they have been considered such since time immemorial. Cave paintings from the Neolithic age show illustrations of honeycombs being gathered for food. Honey has been found in 3,000-year-old Egyptian pyramids. Pythagoras, the great Greek scientist, recommended honey for health and long life as early as 600 B.C. Many other Greek philosophers claimed that pollen held the secret of eternal youth. The original olympic athletes used unstrained pollen-rich honey for extra energy and vitality. Throughout the ages, honey and pollen have been regarded as *ambrosia*—divine foods with age-retarding and rejuvenating properties.

The miraculous rejuvenative property of pollen-rich honey is attributed to the fact that pollen is nature's own propagator of life. It is the male germ cell of the plant kingdom. Pollen, in addition to all known water-soluble vitamins—including B_{12}—and a rich supply of minerals, trace elements, and enzymes, contains *deoxiribosides* and *sterines,* plus *steroid* hormone substances. Pollen also contains a *gonadotropic hormone,* a plant hormone which is similar to the pituitary hormone, *gonadotropin,* which stimulates sex glands.

During the last three decades, much research has been done, mostly in Russia and Sweden, to uncover the medicinal and rejuvenative value of pollen and honey. Both have been found to be miraculous rejuvenators, largely by improving general health, preventing disease, increasing the power of the body's own immunological mechanism, and stimulating and rejuvenating glandular activity.

It has been demonstrated that natural, unprocessed honey:

- increases calcium retention (so important for staying younger longer);
- increases hemoglobin count and can help prevent or cure nutritional anemia (it is rich in iron and copper;
- has a beneficial effect on healing processes in such conditions as arthritis, colds, poor circulation, constipation, liver and kidney disorders, weak heart action, bad complexion, and insomnia;
- is rich in aspartic acid, an important amino acid which is involved in the rejuvenative processes, particularly in the rejuvenation of sex glands.

Now you can understand why pollen-rich honey is such an important health and longevity factor in the diet of all Russian centenarians.

In addition to honey and pollen, two other bee products have been associated with health and longevity: royal jelly and propolis.

Royal jelly is the food produced by the worker bees to feed the queen bee. It contains identified and unidentified substances that enable the queen bee to live twenty times longer than working bees, and produce 2000 or more eggs in a single day—which is greater than her own weight! Royal jelly is rich in all vital life factors, being an

especially exceptional source of pantothenic acid, known as a stress vitamin. Studies on royal jelly showed that:
- it speeds up the growth and increases the resistance to disease in test animals;
- it markedly increases the life span of fruit flies;
- it has anti-bacterial and anti-virus action, particularly against *streptococcus* and *staphylococcus*;
- it accelerates the formation of bone tissue;
- when applied topically, it helps heal wounds in half the time;
- it has a preventive effect against cancer;
- in human studies, it lowered cholesterol and accelerated healing in such conditions as hardening of the arteries, vascular disorders, and diseases of aging.

Propolis is the substance that is gathered by honey bees from the leaves and barks of trees, then secreted through their pharmageal glands. It is used as a binding material in building beehives. It was used by ancient civilizations over 2000 years ago as a natural antibiotic. Propolis has been recently re-discovered and is now available through the health food industry. It is used by many biologically oriented doctors as a natural anti-bacterial medicine. Ray Hill, in his book, *Propolis—the Natural Antibiotic,* says that propolis "offers the same immediate action as laboratory—produced antibiotics, but without toxic or other side effects."

Garlic and onions

At the end of the Second World War, when American troops finally confronted the Russian troops, American soldiers discovered that many Russian soldiers had their pockets filled with onions and garlic, and judging from the odor, they made good use of them. For several years, the Russian Army fought on a near-starvation diet because of a severe food shortage. But two things always seemed to be in good supply: garlic and onions. In addition to buckwheat porridge and black bread, garlic and onions comprised the Russian Army's staple ration.

While traveling in Russia, I enjoyed stopping at the villages and studying the life in the agricultural collectives, their methods of cultivation, preferred crops, etc. In addition to the collectively-owned fields, each family was allowed to have a large garden of their own, where they could grow anything they wished for their own use or for sale on the public market. I found that two vegetables completely dominated these gardens: cabbage (for sauerkraut) and onions!

Russian electrobiologist, Professor Gurwitch, discovered that garlic and onions emit a peculiar type of ultra-violet radiation called mitogenetic radiation. This radiation—the Gurwitch rays—has the property of stimulating cell growth and activity and has a rejuvenating effect on all body functions.

A great amount of scientific research has been done in various countries on the therapeutic properties of garlic and onions. Dr. A.I. Virtanen, Finnish Nobel Prize winner, discovered fourteen *new* beneficial substances in onions. Russian, German, French, Japanese, English, and American researchers have successfully used garlic to treat such varied conditions as high or low blood pressure, common colds, intestinal worms, cough, asthma, whooping cough, intestinal putrefaction, dysentery, gastrointestinal disorders, gas, tuberculosis, and diabetes.[9] American research has shown that garlic is a powerful agent against tumor formation in cancer.[9] Garlic contains germanium, a mineral that has both preventive and curative effect on cancer, as indicated by Japanese studies.

Russians discovered that garlic has antibiotic properties. They often refer to garlic as "Russian penicillin." Russian medical clinics and hospitals use garlic extensively—mostly in the form of volatile extracts that are vaporized and inhaled.

I found in my own practice that the most dramatic therapeutic use of garlic is, perhaps, in the treatment of high blood pressure. Almost without exception, blood pressure can be reduced in two weeks by 30 - 40 mm. by nothing but garlic therapy—including the generous use of raw garlic in the diet. High blood pressure is, of course, one of the causes of heart disease and strokes—two of our greatest killers. The fact that garlic has such a beneficial effect on reducing blood pressure makes it an important life prolongator. By counteracting intestinal putrefaction and improving assimilation of the essential nutrients from the intestines, garlic and onions improve health and prolong life. Not to mention the fact that garlic and onions also are most delicious foods!

During my recent trip to Japan, I met with the leading Japanese researcher, Dr. Satosi Kitahara, who discovered a new, exciting property of garlic—its ability to help remove toxic metals, such as lead, mercury, and cadmium, from the body. Considering the fact that environmental poisons are becoming a greater and greater threat to our health with every passing day, this discovery will have a far-reaching effect, and gives yet another reason why garlic should become an essential part of everyone's diet.

Worried about odor? Why not try an odorless garlic capsule or tablet, developed in Japan, called Kyolic. These capsules are sold in health food stores.

Buckwheat

During my recent meeting with one of the leading Russian scientists in the field of preventive medicine and longevity, the question came up regarding Russia's low incidence of cardiovascular disease and heart attacks. The Russian scientist said:

"We have a relatively low incidence of high blood pressure and cardiovascular diseases, and we attribute this in part to our regular eating or such foods as garlic and buckwheat. Buckwheat supplies *rutin,* a bioflavonoid, which we have found to have a blood-pressure reducing property, and a beneficial effect on the circulatory system."

Buckwheat, mostly in the form of a porridge, which they call *kasha,* is really the Russian national food. Wherever I've traveled in Russia, I have seen people eating kasha almost every day of their lives. Kasha is served to all personnel in the Russian Army several times a week, mostly with sunflower seed oil.

Buckwheat is an extremely nutritious cereal containing complete proteins, vitamins, and minerals—especially manganese and magnesium. It is low in sodium and very rich in potassium. The rutin in buckwheat makes it a very important rejuvenative and age-retarding food, as circulation problems and cardiovascular disorders are at the base of many aging processes. The protein in buckwheat is of very high quality, comparable in biological value to protein in meat and milk, as shown recently by a study of the U.S. Department of Agriculture. See Recipes & Directions on how to prepare this delicious and rejuvenative food, and also how to make delicious buckwheat pancakes.

Importance of effective assimilation

You have heard it said that "you are what you eat." This is only half of the truth. Surely we all realize the importance of eating wholesome and nutritious foods and taking all the special food supplements and vitamins mentioned so far in this chapter. But unless these good foods and supplements are properly and efficiently digested and assimilated into your system, they will not do you much good. So, actually, you are not what you eat, but *what you assimilate!*

I have found that natives in various countries known for their good health and long life use all kinds of natural aids to digestion and assimilation. Also, how you eat, when you eat, and how much you eat is important.

Here are a few tips that will help you to digest your food better and assimilate all the nutrients from it more effectively.

1. Eat slowly and chew well.

2. Do not overeat. Overeating will overload your digestive apparatus and result in ineffective digestion and assimilation. The less you eat, the better digested your food will be and the more nutrients your body will derive from it.

3. Do not eat unless you are hungry. Food eaten when

you are not hungry will have a poison-like effect on your body.

4. Do not drink excessively before or during meals, unless you are extremely thirsty. Liquids dilute the digestive juices and inhibit the digestion.

5. Use the following natural digestion enhancers in your diet regularly:

- Lime or lemon
- Chili and/or paprika
- Onion and garlic
- Papaya or pineapple
- Natural culinary herbs and spices.

Although we generally eat too much salt, *older* people should not go on a totally salt-free diet. A small amount of sea salt can be helpful in improving digestion, since it provides chloride needed for the production of the digestive aid, hydrochloric acid, in the stomach.

(See Chapter 3 for more information on proper eating habits.)

Vitamin E—rejuvenation vitamin number one

Of all the vitamins, vitamin E is the rejuvenation vitamin number one. This vitamin has been credited with being a miracle youth, virility, and vitality vitamin—a vitamin which can reverse the aging processes and keep you younger longer.

One of the leading American experts on aging—its causes and prevention—is Dr. Aloys L. Tappel, a biochemist at the University of California, and professor of food science and technology at Davis College. Dr. Tappel says that "Aging is due to the process of oxidation." He writes:

"Aging of our bodies appears to be influenced by an intracellular tug of war going on between two factors acting upon a third: intensity and duration of radiation-like effects, polyunsaturated lipids upon which they act, and the vitamin E available to protect them from excessive destruction."

Dr. Tappel says that as we grow older, the oxygenation of our cells is diminished and because of increased oxidation of fats, certain substances, called *free radicals,* are formed within our cells. These free radicals have a destructive effect on normal cell metabolism, causing damage and contributing to the aging processes. "Perhaps the reason some people look older than their years is that they have been more vulnerable to this damage than those who don't show their age," says Dr. Tappel.

Dr. Tappel's prescription for preventing premature aging is vitamin E. Vitamin E is the most powerful natural antioxidant. Dr. Tappel says: "in normal humans, vitamin E, contained in unsaturated vegetable fat, acts to prevent the formation of free radicals and serves as a built-in protection against accelerated aging."

By the way, vitamin E deficiency also causes the formation of a pigment, ceroid, which is thought to be part of aging.

Since our typical American diet is grossly deficient in vitamin E, supplementing it with extra vitamin E in capsule form would be one of the best things you could do for yourself to prevent premature aging, extend life, and stay younger longer. The best natural sources of vitamin E are whole grains, seeds, and nuts, and cold-pressed vegetable oils. Refined foods, such as white flour, white bread, or processed oils, do not contain enough vitamin E to keep you young, because most of the vitamin E in them has been removed or destroyed in processing.

Vitamin E in capsule form is sold in all health food stores and drug stores. Most doctors recommend doses up to 600 I.U. as perfectly safe. Older people can take twice as much. Those who suffer from serious diseases should consult their doctors regarding the proper dosage.

Another noted scientist who believes that vitamin E can help to control or even reverse the aging processes is Dr. Hans Selye, of the University of Montreal. Dr. Selye is the author of the famous stress theory: that all diseases, including premature aging, are caused by stresses which the weakened body is unable to counteract. Vitamin E is one of our basic anti-stress vitamins. It increases the body's resistance to stresses by improving circulation, strengthening the heart, preventing harmful oxidation of fats, and increasing the supply of oxygen to the tissues and cells. Dr. Selye tells how in animal studies he was able to cause all signs and symptoms of "old age" by deliberately withholding vitamin E from the test animals. Conversely, in the other group of test animals, life and youth were prolonged through the use of vitamin E.

Since, vitamin E is one of the truly miraculous, health-building, and health-restoring substances, and helps to save lives by favorably influencing such conditions as heart disease, diabetes, arthritis, arteriosclerosis, varicose veins, and ulcers, it must be considered to be one of the most important life prolongators and rejuvenators. Vitamin E is also a potent rejuvenator of male and female fertility and virility. It has a strong regenerative and stimulating effect on all sexual and reproductive functions. It can prevent miscarriages and spontaneous abortions; it increases fertility of both the male and female; it can restore virility in impotent men and banish frigidity in women. Although you may have heard repeatedly the official medical line that "there is absolutely no evidence" that vitamin E is a sex rejuvenator, there are dozens of reliable clinical studies from around the world which show that vitamin E indeed can do all of the things mentioned above. By improving and regenerating the functions of your sex glands, vitamin E can definitely help you to stay younger longer.

Vitamin A and cell oxygenation

It has been established by research that the oxygenation of the tissues is enhanced by a combination of vitamins E and A. Vitamin A increases the permeability of blood capillaries. The capillaries carry oxygen and other nutritive substances to every cell of your body. The more permeable these capillary walls, the more oxygen can be delivered to the cells. Thus, vitamin A is a third vitamin (in addition to E and C) that can improve cell oxygenation;

and efficient cell oxygenation is the ultimate secret of perpetual youth.

Vitamin A also helps keep your skin youthful at any age, by helping to prevent drying of the skin and keeping it free from blemishes.

Two scientists from Columbia University, Drs. H.C. Sherman and Oswald A. Roels, demonstrated that vitamin A helps to prevent premature aging and increases life expectancy. It regulates the stability of tissues in cell walls—cell membranes break down when there is a lack of vitamin A. Vitamin A is also essential for the health of all mucus linings and membranes in the body.

The best natural vegetable sources of vitamin A are carrots, tomatoes, and green leafy vegetables. Fish liver oils are the richest natural source. Vitamin A capsules are sold in all health food stores. Rejuvenative doses are 25,000 to 50,000 U.S.P. units a day. Large doses of vitamin A can be toxic when taken for prolonged periods of time. It would be wise, therefore, to make two-to three-week intervals every few months if you take doses larger than 50,000 units.

Lecithin

Lecithin is an organic phosphorized fat substance, the chief constituent of brain and nerve tissues. Close to 20 percent of brain substance is made up of lecithin. Lecithin is also present in abundance in the endocrine glands, especially the gonads—both male and female. Pituitary and pineal glands contain lecithin. The pineal gland is richer in lecithin than any other part of the body. Lecithin is also an essential component of semen, and a sufficient supply is necessary for normal semen production. Lecithin has been used successfully by some doctors to treat male sexual debility and glandular exhaustion. They claim that lecithin improves virility and prevents impotency.

Lecithin can also be a great life saver by helping to prevent heart disease caused by atherosclerosis. Lecithin can help dissolve cholesterol deposits in the arteries, thus lessening the chance of heart attack.

Dr. Lester M. Morrison, senior attending physician at Los Angeles County General Hospital, says that lecithin is "one of our most powerful weapons against disease." In the treatment of heart disease, Dr. Morrison "found lecithin to give the most rewarding results ..." He even found that lecithin can not only prevent atherosclerosis, but in many instances, reverse it, making old hardened arteries younger. This is significant, since many scientists believe that "you are as young as your arteries." If lecithin can help to keep your arteries from aging, it can help you to stay younger longer.

Lecithin is a truly miraculous food supplement. It is a rich source of many rejuvenative food elements, such as vitamins E, D, and K, essential fatty acids, and especially choline and inositol, two B-vitamins that are involved in helping to prevent the aging processes. Choline and inositol are perfect fat-dissolving agents.

Lecithin should be a part of every rejuvenation diet. It is sold in all health food stores in tablet, powder, or granular form. I recommend the granular form, which is also the most economical. Two to three teaspoonsful a day is the average dose, but some people take more.

Note: If large doses of lecithin are taken, calcium should be added to the diet (calcium lactate is available in health food stores) to balance the excess phosphorus obtained from the lecithin.

Rejuvenative herbs

Herbs have been used in every country and by every race for healing and rejuvenating purposes.

Damiana is mostly known and highly regarded as an aphrodisiac. It is used widely in Mexico and in most Central and South American countries. It is sold by every Mexican village or town herbalist.

There are many kinds of damiana. The kind most often used in Mexico is known botanically as *Turnera aphrodisiaca.* It grows in California, all over Mexico, and in Central and South America. Damiana grown in Baja California is considered to be the most potent. Damiana grows as a shrub or small tree, with small narrow leaves. The leaves are dried and used mostly as tea, which has a slightly bitter taste.

Damiana is an old remedy for sexual impotence. It is reported to strengthen and enhance the function of reproductive organs. It is known to be a tonic for the nerves and is used in cases of mental and physical exhaustion. This herb is also a stimulant to the kidneys and increases the flow of urine.

Damiana is prepared as most herb teas: 1 teaspoon of dried leaves to 1 cup of water. Pour boiling water over the leaves and let steep for 15 minutes. Strain and drink 1 cup twice a day.

Sarsaparilla is another well known rejuvenative herb. It is a tropical plant which grows mostly in Honduras, Mexico, Jamaica, and Equador, but also in China and Japan. The botanical name is *Smilax medica* or *Smilax regalii.* It is an evergreen shrub, and the root is the only part used for medicinal purposes.

Sarsaparilla is considered to be a powerful blood purifier and also is used for such conditions as chronic rheumatism, skin disorders, psoriasis, general weakness, and sexual impotence. It is considered to be a potent antidote for the toxic effects of any strong poison.

But, in terms of rejuvenation, the most important fact about sarsaparilla is that it is a potent natural source of male and female sex hormones, which are involved in keeping the body and mind young. American and Mexican scientists discovered—independently of each other—that sarsaparilla roots contain *testosterone,* a male sex hormone. And recently, it was discovered that sarsaparilla also contains *progesterone,* the female sex hormone. Even *cortin*—one of the adrenal hormones—was found in sarsaparilla.

In recent times, therefore, Mexican and South American pharmaceutical companies have been manufacturing male and female sex hormone tablets from natural hormones isolated from sarsaparilla.

It is generally considered that the strength of the

endocrine glands, and particularly the sex glands, and their ability to produce sufficient hormones, is directly related to the general vitality and healthy functioning of the body. Sexual virility largely determines a man's youthfulness, health, vitality, and longevity. Likewise, plentiful sex hormone production in the female makes her look, feel, and act young. The decline in sex hormone production results in gradual aging and decreased life span. Therefore, sarsaparilla can be listed as one of the most important of natural herbal rejuvenators. It can help to supply the missing hormones and bring the spark of youth back into your life.

Sarsaparilla roots (the red Honduras sarsaparilla is considered to be the most potent) are boiled in water for 15 to 30 minutes, and the decoction is drunk as a tea twice a day. Use 1 ounce of the root to 1 pint of water.

Perhaps this will be the proper place to give a few other herbal secrets, especially for female rejuvenation. The aging processes in the female are accelerated after menopause, when the glandular activity slows down and sex hormone deficiencies, especially the deficiency of estrogen, manifests itself. Many women drug themselves with synthetic estrogen to slow down the aging processes. This can be very dangerous as it is well known that taking this synthetic hormone can lead to the development of cancer. There are several sources of natural estrogen, which are totally harmless: licorice, unicorn roots, Mexican wild yam, false unicorn roots, black cohosh, and elder flowers. Using these herbs in the form of teas on a regular basis can help to compensate for diminished hormone supply due to menopause.

Importance of exercise

In my studies of various people around the world known for their exceptional health and long life in youthful vitality, I found that one factor in their lifestyles is common to them all: a vigorous life with lots of physical labor and exercise.

To see how important exercise is for your health and

for keeping you younger longer, read the special section on exercise in Chapter 2. After reading it, I am sure you will agree with me that exercise is even more important than good nutrition for your health and well-being, and you know how much I think of nutrition!

Relaxation and positive, health-oriented, youthful state of mind

The 166-year-old Russian centenarian, Shirali Mislimov, asked for his secrets of long life, summed them up better than any gerontology scientist could do. He said, in his poetic language of the Azerbaidzhan Mountains:

"I was never in a hurry in my life and I am in no hurry to die now. There are two sources of long life. One is a gift of nature, and the pure air and clear water of the mountains, the fruit of the earth, peace, rest, and the soft warm climate of the highlands. The second source is within us. He lives long who enjoys life and who bears no jealousy of others, whose heart harbors no malice or anger, who sings a lot and cries a little, who rises and retires with the sun, who likes to work and who knows how to rest."

And the famous and renowned Chinese professor and herbalist, Li Chung Yun, who lived to be 256 years old, when asked to what he attributed his long life, said:

"I attribute my long life to INWARD CALM."

I have found that all people who lived extraordinarily long lives in various parts of the world, in addition to all the other factors, such as sound nutrition of simple, unadulterated foods, systematic undereating or scanty eating, poison-free environment, and plenty of exercise, have possessed that unmistakable quality Professor Yun was talking about—INWARD CALM. They were all contented—happy with their lot whatever it was, didn't envy anyone—and they usually held important positions in the community and were respected by their families, neighbors, and the other villagers. This sense of importance, of being useful, having the respect and adoration of families and neighbors is, in my opinion, an extremely important factor in longevity.

Are you shortening or prolonging your life?

There are many ways of prolonging life and keeping younger longer as we have seen so far. By far the best method of prolonging life and looking and feeling young was expressed by Herbert Spencer, when he wrote:

"The whole secret of prolonging one's life consists in doing nothing to shorten it."

Expressing the same thought, Dr. A. Ochsner, noted authority on aging, wrote in the *Journal of American Geriatrics Society,* that premature senility can be controlled to a great extent by avoiding factors that accelerate aging.

But modern man seems to go out of his way, using his ingenuity and inventiveness, to ruin his health and shorten his life. He is the only creature that spoils his food before he eats it—by heating, frying, freezing, preserving, processing, and refining. He poisons his air and water supply. He depletes his soil by chemicals that grow nutritionally-inferior food which cannot sustain health. He ignores the basic law of all life—need for motion—and shortens his life by a sedentary way of living, without sufficient physical exertion. Relaxation and peace of mind are most important for health and long life, but his life is filled with continuous stresses because he is haunted by the insatiable drive for more material wealth and power. He digs his own grave with his knife and fork, eating denatured, overprocessed, nutritionless, and poisoned foods which contribute to most of our serious or fatal diseases such as cancer, arthritis, and heart disease.

Men, indeed, seems to do all he can to shorten his life!

Are you shortening your life?

I must admit that we are all subjected to certain health-destroying factors that we cannot avoid. In this age of universal chemical pollution, it is not easy to live so that our health will not be endangered. Smog is difficult to escape. Equally difficult to avoid are the thousands of health-destroying and life-shortening poisons in water and food. But a few things can be done to improve our individual lives and to protect our health to the greatest possible extent, even from health-destroying poisons in our environment. I have mentioned already vitamins C and E and garlic. In *How To Get Well* I list many more specific vitamins, minerals, and other supplements that can neutralize or minimize the harmful effects of environmental poisons.

Conclusion

Only *you* can determine if your lifestyle will make you older, wrinkled, and senile before your time, or if it will prevent premature aging and keep you younger longer. I have thousands of letters in my files from readers of my books and those for whom I have planned personalized nutritional programs—they all report miraculous changes in their lives after changing their diets and their living habits. This works by the simple natural law of cause and effect. You have been violating the basic laws of health, and you have been feeling and looking accordingly. You cannot fool Mother Nature. "Whatsoever ye sow, that also shall ye reap." Stop working *against nature,* and start working *with nature.* Give nature a chance! Your body has a remarkable regenerative capacity. Remove all the health-destroyers and life-shorteners from your life—smoking, drinking, white sugar and white flour, processed, refined, denatured and poisoned foods, drugs, and other chemicals—and follow the Optimum Diet described in Chapters 3 and 4. Make use of all the various health and rejuvenation secrets from around the world which you have learned about in this chapter and *you will be amazed at the results!*

Are you shortening your life and growing old prematurely?

You can change your life pattern and start growing younger—TODAY! Today is the beginning of the rest of your life. You may continue in the old rut, and grow older by the day—or you may begin a new way of life which will help you to grow younger in body, mind, and spirit. Not only will most of your present health problems be solved, but you will feel and act like a new person. You will enjoy peace, contentment, happiness, and joy in living as you never have before. It's up to you!

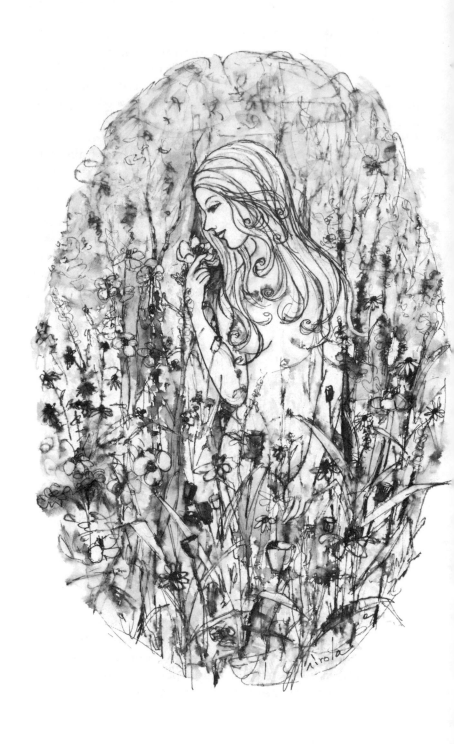

32

Looking Beautiful— Naturally!

Every woman wants to look beautiful, or at least look her best. Vanity? No, just a basic, natural instinct to attract a man through physical appearance. This feminine instinct is based on a primal, protogenic impulse of perpetuation and preservation of the species. As far back in human history as we can go, perhaps ever since woman first caught her own reflection in the still waters of the forest spring, she has used great ingenuity to improve her appearance. Historical and anthropological studies show that from the very dawn of the human race, in every culture and in every corner of the planet, women have devised countless ways to make themselves more beautiful and desirable by applying natural colors and scents, wearing elaborate jewelry and seductive clothing, designing attractive hairdos, etc., etc.

In our modern "age of enlightenment" the understanding of this natural woman's instinct has become clouded. We have seen many women ignore or thwart the instinct to make themselves physically more attractive. Indeed, some seem to do just the opposite: they walk around in drab garb, with uncombed and unkempt, stringy hair; the misconception being that "people should like me for my true self, not just superficial, transient physical beauty." They reject the natural instinct to attract others through physical beauty as animalistic. True, animals do live by instincts. Instincts control and direct their behavior. But although human beings are able to consciously control and temper their instincts, the wise ones do not ignore or work contrary to them, but use them as tools of the spirit, as aids in their striving for perfection. Our bodies are temples of the spirit. The temple, as the house of the spirit, must be kept not only clean and healthy, but also beautiful and attractive—the true and glowing reflection of the beautiful spirit, the divine spark, that dwells therein.

Thus, looking from such a holistic point of view, the natural instinct of keeping ourselves as physically attractive and aesthetically appealing as possible—this instinct is intrinsic to both women and men, incidentally— makes our attempts to improve our physical appearance by all available means not only an inherent right, but an obligation and responsibility.

Beauty from within

Although in this chapter we will deal with various natural homemade cosmetics that can be used externally to create, maintain, and enhance beauty, we must not forget that real, lasting beauty comes *from within.* Glowing good looks are, more than anything else, a reflection of inner vitality, vibrant health, and unclouded happiness. Optimum nutrition, adequate exercise, relaxation and a positive, cheerful disposition are the royal roads to health as well as to beauty. A healthy body and beautiful spirit are the best cosmetic "foundations" that I know of.

Sure, age will eventually take its toll on most of us. But, with proper care, there is no reason to look old and wrinkled in the prime of life—as many, unfortunately, do. With an adequate, nourishing diet, sufficient exercise, relaxation, and rest you can keep your body healthy and youthful throughout life. Your skin can remain elastic and wrinkle-free, your eyes can keep the luster of youth, your lips can be full, your chin tight, your complexion smooth and luscious.

A dream? No, countless women of history were known to retain their legendary beauty and youthfulness in spite of their advanced chronological age. Helen of Troy, even when she was approaching fifty, looked as young and beautiful as a girl of twenty. The clear, velvety, blemish-less, and lusciously fresh complexion of Cleopatra is well known. Ninon de Lenclos, the scintillating French woman, when well in her eighties, looked one third her age, still wooed by younger men. On the home plane, look at Gloria Swanson, the most beautiful movie queen of the early era of Hollywood. Today, at the age of 80, and recently remarried, Gloria looks attractive and lovely. Her complexion, her hair, her eyes, all glow with the freshness of youth. And her beauty is not skin deep, either. As a personal friend, I can assure you that her outwardly beautiful and youthful appearance reflects and matches her inward vitality, seemingly limitless energy, youthful enthusiasm, and the refinement and beauty of her spirit.

I could go on and fill pages of both famous and unknown women who maintained their youth and beauty into advanced age. How did they manage? A lucky roll of the genetic dice? Inherited gifts from perennially youthful ancestors? Yes, that may account for a few of these geriatric marvels. But very few. Most of them *worked hard* to sustain and preserve their youthfulness and femininity. First, they *realized the importance* of attractiveness and a youthful appearance. Then, they *studied the secrets* of vibrant health and extended youth. And, finally, they *methodically worked* and applied what they had learned towards this goal: to feel and look healthier, younger, and more beautiful. In addition to taking care of their beauty from within with an adequate diet, exercise, and sufficient rest and relaxation, and avoidance of such health and beauty destroyers as smoking, alcohol, overeating, and constipation (which we spoke of in preceding chapters) most women known for their legendary beauty have used and still use many natural beauty aids, such as aromatic facial baths, magic herbs, exotic oils, natural masks, cleansers, and beauty packs, to create and maintain loveliness.

Natural vs. synthetic beauty aids

Until fairly recently, women relied on their own ingenuity to concoct, produce, and blend their cosmetics. They used natural herbs from the field, garden flowers, barks and roots, fruits, berries, and even clays and muds from the earth as beauty aids. Then, the commercially-oriented chemical industry invaded the field. Now, the recent generations of women have lost the art and knowledge of making their own natural cosmetics since creams, lotions, and pomades are now so easily available from every store. But, synthetic cosmetics, with their artificial, chemical ingredients, coal-tar colorings and imitation scents, and toxic, even carcinogenic, additives, have brought nothing but disaster to most women's complexions and overall appearances. A young woman today has only to look at her mother's troubled hair and complexion and compare them with her grandmother's still smooth and fresh skin and shining hair to realize that toxic chemical concoctions are no match for time-tested natural beauty aids.

In this chapter, I will list some simple, basic, 100 percent natural cosmetics that can be made in your own kitchen. Most of the ingredients are easily available from your own refrigerator, or can be acquired from your corner drugstore, health food store, or supermarket. Many recipes were developed by beauty-conscious women in my own home. Some I picked up on my world-wide travels, especially in the Scandinavian countries, where women are known for their exceptional beauty. I have learned a lot from Swedish women who have used for centuries, and continue to use now, certain elements in their daily diet and beauty care which the latest scientific research has proven to be miraculous beauty aids. Many of the recipes and formulas have been devised by my friends and given to me to be used for the benefit of others. Other formulas come from the past and have been traditionally used in various parts of the world for centuries—beauty secrets passed from mother to daughter for countless generations.

Not every cosmetic, recipe, or formula is for you. Not every natural cosmetic aid will bring immediate and magic results. Experiment and select those that work best on your skin or hair. We are all very different in our individual needs. Our response to certain substances in herbs or other natural ingredients is individual. You may even be allergic to some of the ingredients—in that case, avoid them, or make substitutions. Some women are allergic to milk, egg yolks, or brewer's yeast. Learn to eliminate or adjust the ingredients to meet your own specific requirements.

Since all ingredients used in my recipes and formulas are 100 percent natural (and, thus, easily lose their freshness since no preservatives are used), you must prepare the smallest quantity possible, and store them in the refrigerator.

Here, then, are a few time-proven beauty aids which you can use to make yourself over. If used sensibly and with dedication, they can go far to ward off the unwelcome ravages of age and preserve and enhance your natural beauty.

And, please, don't feel guilty or vain when trying to improve your appearance and look more beautiful. The pursuit of beauty is as natural as the love of beauty. To make this world a more beautiful, delightful, and aesthetically enjoyable place in which to live, we can start with ourselves.

FORMULA F

5 tbsp. sesame oil
4 tbsp. avocado oil
3 tbsp. olive oil
2 tbsp. almond oil
a few drops of your favorite perfume

Pour all ingredients in an empty bottle, close the cap tightly, and shake well. Store in refrigerator.

Apply a few drops of this oil to your face, neck, hands, and arms, and massage it gently into your skin. Then dry off the excess with a soft tissue. This will remove all the impurities, dead skin cells, and the stale residues of old, dried-up cosmetics.

This natural cosmetic, mixed from the most beautifying oils known to man, will do wonders to your skin. It will make your skin moist and soft, young and beautiful. The oils used in this formula are all available from your health food store.

FORMULA F PLUS

2 tbsp. sesame oil
2 tbsp. avocado oil
1 tbsp. olive oil
1 tbsp. almond oil
10,000 I.U. vitamin E, mixed tocopherols
200,000 USP units vitamin A
a few drops of your favorite perfume

Pour the oils into an empty bottle or small jar. Take 10 gelatin capsules of vitamin E (1,000 I.U. each) and 8 capsules of vitamin A (25,000 units each). Puncture the capsules with a needle, or cut the ends off with scissors, and squeeze the contents into the bottle. Add a drop or two of your favorite perfume, close the cap tightly, and shake well. Store in refrigerator.

I composed this formula specifically for those who have badly deteriorated complexions and a prematurely aged skin, covered with wrinkles and blemishes. The healing and the beautifying oils of Formula F Plus, fortified with generous amounts of vitamins A and E, will feed your skin with the nutrients it needs and help to revitalize and restore its normal biological activity. Use this formula alternately with regular Formula F: one week use regular Formula F, the next week Formula F Plus, and so on.

The most effective way to use Formula F Plus is to take a few drops and massage gently into your face, neck, hands, and arms every night before going to bed and leave it on overnight. By morning it is usually totally absorbed into the skin.

You will be amazed at the rejuvenative effect Formula F Plus will have on your complexion if used regularly.

FORMULA F CREAM

½ cup sesame oil
¼ cup avocado oil
¼ cup almond oil
2 fresh egg yolks
1 tsp. apple cider vinegar
few drops of your favorite perfume

Place the eggs in a bowl and beat with a rotary beater until thick. Mix the oils in a cup and add slowly to the beaten eggs and continue beating. When smooth, add perfume and vinegar and beat a little more. Keep in a tightly covered jar, preferably in the refrigerator. This cream is excellent for dry, rough skin. It is rich in lecithin, vitamin A, and polyunsaturated oils. It will make your skin soft and moist.

MAYONNAISE FACIAL

½ cup sesame oil
½ cup olive oil
1 egg
2 tbsp. lemon juice or apple cider vinegar

Put sesame oil, egg, and lemon juice into the blender, cover, and run blender at the highest speed until thick. Add olive oil slowly while the motor is still running; continue blending until well mixed. Place in a jar and keep in refrigerator until needed. Homemade mayonnaise facial is great for an aging and parched complexion. Apply daily to face, neck, and hands, leaving on for 5 - 15 minutes, or longer, if possible. Rinse off with tepid water.

HONEY-EGG MASK

White of 1 egg
½ tsp. honey

Beat the egg white with honey and apply liberally to your face and neck. Leave it on for about 10 - 15 minutes, then wash off with clear, cold water. You may save what is left over for the next day if you keep it in a tightly closed jar in the refrigerator.

This simple beauty mask will startle you with its most amazing results. The albumin in the egg white is a natural astringent. It will "draw" your skin together and tighten it. Honey is a wonderful moisturizer and a softener. Together they work miracles on your skin.

CUCUMBER ASTRINGENT

1 cup fresh cucumber juice (make in your own juice extractor, or grate very fine and press through a cloth)
¼ tsp. honey

Pour ingredients into an empty bottle and shake well. Apply with a cotton pad to your face and neck and let it dry. Leave it on overnight, if desired, or use as a base under makeup. It will keep for a few days if stored in the refrigerator.

Cucumbers contain natural vegetable hormones which are very beneficial for your skin. Cucumber is also a natural, harmless skin tightener or astringent. It will do wonders for your wrinkles and lines.

CUCUMBER BEAUTY MASK

1 small cucumber
¼ cup skim milk
½ tsp. honey
1 tsp. crushed ice

Cut cucumber into 1 inch pieces and mix in an electric blender with skim milk, honey, and ice to the consistency of porridge. Blend for approximately three to five seconds at low speed, being careful not to let the blender run for so long that the formula becomes too liquid.

Apply generously all over face, neck, and hands. Lie down for ten or fifteen minutes of rest and relaxation, then rinse mask off with cold water.

HONEY LOTION

Dissolve 1 tablespoon of honey in 1 cup of cold water. Add ½ teaspoon lemon juice or apple cider vinegar.

Apply freely to your face, neck, and arms, especially after a bath when soap or shampoo was used. Leave it on and let dry. It will moisturize and soften your skin and help to restore the skin's natural acid mantle, which was disturbed by the bath. Honey is a natural *humectant,* or skin softener. Beauty-conscious women have used honey as a cosmetic for centuries.

SWEDISH FACIAL SAUNA

Swedish facial sauna is a very effective treatment for blackheads, pimples, acne, and other blemishes, and for the thorough cleansing of your face.

Take a tablespoon of your favorite herbs—peppermint, anise, camomile, or, as do the Swedish women, use pine needles or birch leaves. Those with acne or oily skin can use yarrow flowers. Put in a pot of water and bring to a rolling boil. Lower your head over the pot, cover it with a big bath towel, and steam your face for about 3 - 5 minutes. Turn your face so that every part of it, as well as your neck, will receive the benefit of this aromatic facial bath.

PAPAYA - MINT FACIAL

If you have been using commercial cosmetics, harsh soaps, and especially if you live in a polluted environment, your skin could be clogged with impurities, cosmetic residues, and hardened sebaceous matter. Your complexion cannot glow with freshness unless it is able to breathe. Pores choked with impurities become infected and diseased and can lead to skin irritation and blemishes.

One of the most effective ways to thoroughly cleanse your skin from all accumulated debris and give it a new life, is a papaya-mint facial.

Buy papaya-mint herb or tea bags at your health food store. Boil 2 cups of water in a stainless steel or glass pot. Place 2 papaya-mint tea bags or 1 tbsp. of loose herb in the pot of boiling water, remove the pot from the stove, and let stand for a few minutes.

Take three regular size white face cloths. Dip all three into the tea, wring them out just enough to prevent dripping, and apply, folded double, one cloth to the forehead, one over the face below the eyes (do not cover the eyes), and one over the neck. Arrange a comfortable reclining chair near the teapot, so you can continue with the treatment for at least fifteen minutes. As the cloths cool down, dip them again in the hot tea and re-apply. The cloths must be as hot as possible, but they should not burn the skin or be uncomfortable.

Remember, treatment must be extended to at least fifteen minutes to be effective. It can be used weekly on troubled complexion, or monthly as a "maintenance" treatment. Papaya-mint facial will rejuvenate, cleanse, and stimulate your skin to a new glowing youthfulness.

Note: Never use hot masks or hot facials if you have very fragile small blood capillaries which show as tiny hair-like red veins. The veins must be strengthened before hot compresses can be used.

CORN MILK FACIAL

Take 1 or 2 ears of corn. Try to get as fresh corn as possible, preferably right from your own garden. Remove husks and silk and cut off kernels with a sharp knife or a hand grater. Place the kernels in a blender and run it on high until you have a smooth corn milk.

Apply to the whole freshly cleaned face and throat area. Let dry, then apply a new layer, gently massaging it in. Keep re-applying for 15 - 20 minutes. Allow the last layer to dry completely. Rinse with warm, then cool water.

This corn facial is an excellent treatment for dry, tough skin and will produce a silky smooth complexion if used daily for one to two weeks.

AVOCADO RUB

Here is another simple treatment for dry skin. Take an avocado skin (after you used the insides for your salad) and rub your face, neck, and hands, with the inside part. Leave for a few minutes. Rinse with tepid water.

REJUVENATIVE YEAST MASK

First, scrub your face and neck thoroughly with a pure, acid-balanced soap and complexion brush.

Take 1 tablespoon of powdered brewer's yeast and mix with 2 tablespoons of warm water. Use only good quality bottled spring or mineral water. Make a paste thick enough so it won't drip from the face, adjusting the quantities of water or yeast. Apply the mixture to face and neck, patting gently with fingertips. Leave on for at least 15 to 20 minutes, even for 30 minutes, if possible. Remove with a washcloth and warm water.

This brewer's yeast mask is an excellent treatment to

rejuvenate aging skin and give it new life. It draws fresh blood to the skin and nourishes it as it draws and tightens it. It stimulates the circulation and improves the skin function, especially if skin is too oily. If your skin is dry, apply a thin coating of Formula F after the mask is removed.

FULLER'S EARTH MASK

Buy Fuller's Earth, a naturally occurring, clay-like substance, from your drugstore. Get one which is unbleached, if possible. Mix with fresh pulp of garden-ripe tomatoes into a smooth paste. Rub into the skin, avoiding the eye area, and leave until completely dried. Rinse with warm, then cold water. Blot dry.

This clay mask absorbs excess oils from the skin and stimulates the circulation, normalizing skin function.

For this mask you can also use various cosmetic or nutrtional clay products sold in health food stores.

MORE TREATMENTS FOR OILY SKIN

1. Wash face with pure soap and, after rinsing it well, use a solution of 8 parts water to 1 part apple cider vinegar, as a final rinse.

2. Rub face with a slice of raw potato. After 15 minutes, clean face with a dampened cotton square.

3. Rub face with a slice of fresh cucumber.

4. Rub face with fresh tomato. Leave on for 10 minutes. Wash off with cold water.

OATMEAL MASK

    1 cup milk
    4 tbsp. old-fashioned rolled oats
    1 tsp. of your favorite herbs; choose from elder flower,
        peppermint, papaya leaves, rosemary

Cook oats in milk to a soft porridge consistency. Place in blender, add herbs, and blend well. When still warm (but not burning hot) spread over the face and neck and leave for 20 minutes. Rinse with tepid water. Blot dry.

Oatmeal mask is a time-proven remedy for a blotchy,

aging skin. It is used by many women, especially in the Scandinavian countries and England. It has a remarkable ability to restore and rejuvenate an aging skin if used on an every-other-day basis for a few weeks.

NATURAL SKIN CLEANSERS

1. *Dry skin.* Take 1 cup blanched almonds. Grind to a fine powder in your seed grinder. Wet hands and face and apply almond meal to face and neck with wet hands, working up a lather. Rub with upwards motions. Rinse several times with tepid water.

2. *Normal skin.* Same as above, but use a mixture of blanched almonds and oatmeal, half and half.

3. *Oily skin.* a) Same as #1, but use mixture of 1/3 cup almonds, 1/3 cup oatmeal, and 1/3 cup raw bran. Pulverize all in a seed grinder. b) Yellow cornmeal powder or flour. Use as above.

YOGURT-BASED SKIN AIDS

MASK. Mix 1 tbsp. of plain yogurt, 2 tsp. of honey, and 1 fresh egg yolk. Apply the mixture to face and neck. Leave for 15 minutes. Rinse with warm water. For final rinse, add 1 tbsp. apple cider vinegar to 1 cup of water.

CLEANSER. Mix 1 tbsp. of plain yogurt with ½ tbsp. of almond butter (sold in health food stores). Apply to face and neck, rubbing gently upwards. An excellent pore cleanser.

FRECKLE CREAM

In case you think freckles are unsightly (most men don't think so), here is a perfectly natural, safe, and according to many reports, effective, way to bleach or remove light freckles, or tone down darker ones.

½ tsp. vitamin C powder
1 tbsp. plain yogurt
½ tsp. lemon juice
½ tsp. of freshly grated horseradish
1 tbsp. fine almond meal
½ tbsp. almond oil

Mix ingredients into a smooth cream. Use more yogurt if needed. Apply 2 - 3 times a day, leaving on for 10 - 15 minutes. Rinse with warm water. If your skin is too sensitive, once a day may be sufficient.

Plain lemon juice can also be used to bleach freckles. Pat on freckled areas with a cotton ball and leave overnight. Wash off in the morning. If skin is too sensitive, lemon juice can be diluted with distilled water.

HOT OIL HAIR TREATMENT

For dry, damaged, lifeless, straw-like hair, many women have used this oil treatment successfully:

Warm 2 tbsp. of olive oil over hot water. When oil is as hot as your fingers can stand, gently massage it into scalp, covering every part. Wring out a towel in hot water, and wrap around the head, turban style. When the towel cools, wet it again in hot water and repeat the process two or three times. When finished, wash hair thoroughly with an herbal shampoo, applying shampoo before water to cut the oil. Rinse, adding apple cider vinegar to last rinse water.

This oil treatment can be given 2 - 3 times a month if needed.

Castor oil or jojoba oil can be used instead of olive oil, which many hair experts believe will give even better results. Follow the same procedure as above.

EGG YOLK SHAMPOO

This is a time-proven natural shampoo, used in dozens of variations by women around the world. Here is my favorite:

    2 raw egg yolks
    1 cup warm water
    ½ tsp. lemon juice or apple cider vinegar

Beat the ingredients thoroughly. Pour over the head and carefully massage both scalp and hair for a few minutes. Place plastic bag over the scalp and wait for another five minutes. Rinse thoroughly with warm water. Do not use soap or shampoo for rinsing.

This marvelous shampoo not only cleanses your hair, but also feeds it and restores its natural luster.

OTHER TIPS FOR HEALTHIER HAIR

For dry shampoo. Use one of the following:
1. Finely ground cornmeal.
2. Orris powder (available through botanical supply houses).

Rub powder into hair and scalp, then brush out thoroughly with a fine, natural bristle brush. This is best done outdoors or in the bathtub.

Herbal rinse. Nettle leaves or raspberry leaves, made into a strong tea, can be used as a final rinse after shampoo. Both give body to the hair and aid in hair growth.

Falling hair. Make an herb tea of equal parts of rosemary and sage. Rub into scalp and hair. Blot away excess as this mixture can stain. Used over a period of time, these herbs will help strengthen the hair and prevent it from falling.

Graying hair. Boil two cups of water. Add ½ cup dried sage and steep for several hours. Strain. Pour through the hair several times. Do not rinse. Squeeze out excess and let dry. Other natural substances, taken internally, that help to restore color to the hair are: PABA, pantothenic acid, folic acid, brewer's yeast, and blackstrap molasses. Multiple mineral supplement, containing silicon, such as "Nature's Minerals" is also beneficial.

For blond hair. Camomile rinse is an excellent herbal treatment to bring out the natural blond tones in faded or dull blond hair. Boil a pint of water and add 1 cup of dried camomile flowers. Let steep for 30 minutes. Cool. After shampooing, pour camomile tea through the hair several times, catching the excess in a basin and reusing it. Squeeze out the excess and towel dry. Drying hair in the sun will enhance the effect.

Dandruff. Plain yogurt, massaged into the scalp and left on for 20 - 30 minutes before shampooing can help eliminate dandruff.

Sage tea is also good for dandruff.

Hair color. For a bright auburn tint, henna has been used as an effective and safe coloring since before Cleopatra's time. Henna and camomile, mixed half and half, will produce a reddish brown tone. On gray or white hair, henna will give a flaming orange color. Henna not only colors the hair safely, but actually improves the quality of the hair, without damaging it. Since henna color is so strong and its final tone will depend on the strength you use and the actual color of your hair, it is best to do a strand test before the final process.

Hair loss. Boil a quart of water and mix two heaping tablespoons of whole sea salt. Let cool. Rub a small amount into the scalp daily, preferably after shampooing.

Another traditional treatment for hair loss and baldness is as follows:

Dilute ½ ounce of pearl ash and 4 ounces of onion juice with 1 pint of water. Massage a small amount into the scalp daily.

Onion juice has been used in many cultures to help stimulate hair growth. Squeeze a small amount of onion juice with a garlic press and massage into the scalp just before retiring. Or you can simply cut a small onion in half and rub the scalp with it. Wear a night cap or curler bonnet, and shampoo with an herbal shampoo in the morning, using apple cider vinegar in the water for the last rinse.

Keep in mind, however, that the most important measure in preventing hair from falling out is feeding it properly from within. For specific vitamins and other hair nutrients, and treatments for baldness and hair loss see my book, *How To Get Well.*

Other useful beauty tips

HAND LOTION

1 tbsp. almond oil
1 tsp. liquid honey
¼ tsp. liquid lecithin
¼ tsp. apple cider vinegar
few drops of your favorite perfume or cologne

Blend ingredients into a smooth lotion. Apply a small quantity and rub in well, until hands are almost dry. Blot excess with a tissue.

SUN TAN LOTION

There are many commercial brands of suntan lotion, but the best of them all are those made with PABA, which is one of the B-complex vitamins. You can make your own, if you wish to play pharmacist, by mixing 5 percent PABA with 70 percent ethyl alcohol and 25 percent aloe vera gel. PABA tablets and aloe vera gel are sold in health food stores. Or you can simply buy a ready-made PABA suntan lotion which is also sold in health food stores.

KID GLOVE TREATMENT FOR HANDS

Here's a centuries-old practice to have nice, smooth, wrinkle-free hands, even at an advanced age.

Beat the following into a smooth lotion:

> 1 tbsp. sweet almond oil
> 2 egg yolks
> 1 tsp. rice flour
> ½ tsp. tincture of benzoin (sold at pharmacies)

Mix first three ingredients well before slowly adding liquid benzoin, as you continue beating. Add mineral water, if needed, to make right consistency.

Rub the lotion into your hands before retiring and put on white kid gloves, a size or two too large; leave gloves on all night. In the morning, rinse hands in warm water without using soap. The treatment should be repeated once a week as a preventative, and several times a week if hands are very dry with parchment-like and wrinkled skin.

NATURAL DEODORANTS

In our body-odor conscious culture, women (and men) buy billions of dollars worth of deodorants each year. Most of the commercially-available deodorants are made from strong irritating chemicals which are toxic. Furthermore, they suppress the body's normal perspiration, which can have far-reaching health damaging effects.

Perspiration in itself is practically odorless, certainly not offensive. The offensive odor comes from bacteria that grow in the moist, warm environment, especially when tight clothing made from synthetic fabric is worn.

Here are two natural, safe, non-toxic, inexpensive, and effective deodorants, both working on the same principle: altering the pH of the skin so that bacteria cannot grow. However, one works by increasing the pH, the other by decreasing it; in both cases, making the environment unsuitable for the growth of the odor-causing bacteria.

1. *Apple cider vinegar.* Use full strength under arms and on feet, once a day. For other areas, if needed, dilute with water—1 tbsp. per glass of water.
2. *Baking soda.* Mix 1 tsp. of regular baking soda powder in a cup of water, and rub solution under arms each morning.

EYE WASH

Eyebright, an herb that can be bought from most herb houses and some health food stores (or if you are familiar with it, you can pick it yourself), has been used for centuries to keep eyes bright, sparkling, and strong. Indeed, many herbalists claim that regular use of eyebright will prevent and even cure all kinds of eye and vision problems. The famed 17th Century English herbalist, Culpeper, wrote, "If this herb was but used as much as it is neglected, it would spoil the spectacle trade of England."

Place a teaspoonful of dried eyebright in a cup and fill it with boiling water. Let stand 15 minutes. Allow to cool. Strain very well through several layers of cheese cloth or a paper-type coffee strainer. Bathe eyes with the lotion as often as you can. You can use a special eye wash cup, which is sold in drugstores, or just splash the solution in with your fingers.

By the way, the same eyebright tea, sweetened with honey and drunk internally, is said to be good for a failing memory!

RED EYES

The best treatment for red, irritated eyes, is bathing them with the above-mentioned eyebright tea and taking vitamin B_2 internally, 100 - 200 mg. a day, along with 1 tablet of high-potency B-complex, and large doses of vitamin C with bioflavonoids.

CHAPPED LIPS

1 tbsp. beeswax
1 tbsp. olive or sweet almond oil

Place ingredients in a small dish and heat over boiling water, mixing well as they melt. Pour in a small pill or cream jar before it cools. Carry in your handbag and rub on your lips with your finger when needed.

33

Overweight: Must It Be A Lifetime Struggle?

By definition, a person who weighs 30 percent or more over ideal weight is obese. In practical terms, that means that if your ideal weight is 115, but you weigh 150, you are obese. Even if you are not that severely overweight, you still have a weight problem if you weigh 125 or more, when you should weigh only 115.

Let's face it—we are a nation of adipose (fat) people. According to experts' conservative estimates, about 1/3 of all Americans—75 million people!—are more or less overweight.

What's wrong with being overweight?

In this culture of ours, where slimness is so sought and praised, obesity is cosmetically and aesthetically undesirable. In addition, chronic overweight is a severe *medical* problem and can be a contributory cause of many disabilities, serious health complications, diseases, and premature death.

Here are a few of the health problems to which chronic overweight can contribute:

- High blood pressure
- Diabetes
- Heart disease
- Atherosclerosis and circulatory disorders
- Hardening of the arteries
- Osteoarthritis through an increased strain on joints
- Greater susceptibility to infectious diseases
- Personality problems
- Poor adjustment to hot weather or temperature changes

- Greater susceptibility to cancer (75% greater, according to a new study[1])
- Premature aging
- Premature death (50% greater mortality when 20% overweight[2])

Clearly, overweight shouldn't just be laughed off or dismissed with, "oh, well, some are skinny, and some are pleasantly plump." Medical evidence, as well as statistics from insurance companies, are convincing proof that obesity not only causes lots of health disorders and unhappiness, but also shortens the life span.

What causes overweight?

There are many contributing causes: emotional, glandular, metabolic, nutritional, and psychological.

Persons with a low metabolic rate, so-called "slow burners," can put weight on faster than those who are "fast burners." Thyroid insufficiency slows down the metabolism as well as physical activity—thus contributing to overweight.[3]

Emotional factors play an important part in overweight. People who feel lonely and unwanted, useless and hopeless, often eat a great deal because eating is one of their few pleasures. Women who are unhappy in marriage or bored with the dullness of everyday routines, overeat simply to calm their anxieties or relieve boredom. Worries, tensions, insecurity, jealousy, fears, hostility—all can trigger an uncontrolled desire for eating.

Some medical problems, such as liver or kidney damage, can be a cause of obesity. A damaged liver is unable to synthesize an adequate amount of energy-producing enzymes. Thus, excessive calories are not burned properly.[4] Hypoglycemia can also contribute to obesity. Frequent blood sugar fluctuations increase the craving for foods.[5]

Lack of exercise, is, of course, one of the prime causes of chronic overweight. To keep your weight at normal levels, you have to balance your calorie intake with calorie expenditure. If calorie intake is bigger than calorie expenditure, the excess calories will be stored in the body as fat. For example, there are 150 calories in a glass of beer, 100 calories in a portion of ice cream, 125 calories in one doughnut. If your body doesn't need the energy these calories provide, and if you don't want the beer and the doughnut to end up as fatty tissue, you will have to run for 10 minutes, swim for 20 minutes, or walk for 40 minutes in order to burn up the extra calories.

Overeating

All experts agree, however, that the number one cause of overweight is *overeating!*

But, what causes overeating? In addition to the contributing factors already mentioned, such as hypoglycemia, and emotional and psychological factors, the main cause of overeating is nutritional deficiencies. Paradoxically, overweight persons are *overfed but undernourished!*

Here's how that works. When you eat a diet of denatured, overprocessed, refined, frozen, overcooked, sugar-loaded, pre-packaged, man-made so-called foods (the kinds of "junk" foods most Americans eat today), although you are getting a lot of calories, you are not getting an adequate amount of vital nutrients that your body needs, because most of these nutrients have been refined out or destroyed in processing and manufacturing. Consequently, even though your stomach is full after a meal of such nutritionless foods, your body is still, nutritionally speaking, hungry. This hunger is expressed in a constant craving for something to eat. So you snack, you take a coke or a cup of coffee, eat sweets. Again, you are loading yourself with *empty* calories while your body is craving real nutrients: vitamins, minerals, trace elements. Such malnutrition by overeating of nutritionless foods sets up a pattern of constant craving for food and chronic overeating—and consequent obesity.

Your appetite is controlled by a mechanism in the brain called the appestat. Normally, the appestat creates the sensation of hunger only if there is the actual need for fuel for energy production. Many factors, however, can disrupt the work of the appestat. As mentioned before, negative emotions, insecurity, unhappiness, boredom, etc., can put the appestat out of order. Nutritional deficiencies can do the same.

The "fat cell" theory

Recent studies have demonstrated the danger of overfeeding infants. These studies showed that a too high caloric intake in infancy and early childhood can lead to the development of an excessive number of fat cells, which may be permanently fixed in number.[6, 7] These fat cells will be waiting to be filled throughout life. The increase in fat cells in early infancy may set the food thermostat (appestat) to a higher level. Thus, the appetite may be increased permanently.[8]

If the fat cell theory (actually an established fact in animal studies) is correct, it may explain, in part at least, why dieting to lose weight is so difficult for many, and especially for those whose obesity started in infancy or adolescence. The only way to diminish the number of fat cells in the body is by prolonged juice fasting, which I will describe later in the chapter.

The fat cell theory emphasizes the importance of *early prevention* of obesity. Mothers should be extremely cautious about allowing their babies to become "nice, cuddly, and plump," i.e., fat. Early infant overweight may set a pattern for a lifetime struggle with the obesity problem (see Chapter 15).

Dieting racket

Where there is a demand, there is always a quick supply, at least in our free-enterprise society. An estimated 75 million overweight Americans are desperate for a cure. And so we have a booming $10 billion-a-year weight control industry—a dieting racket which is a haven for rip-off artists and charlatans! Greedy doctors and enterprising businessmen prey on unhappy and desperate overweight Americans with an ever mushrooming number of dangerous diets, reducing spas, gadgets, and gimmicks for shedding fat.

The public's health has been put in jeopardy by what Dr. Paul A. Lessler, specialist in medical therapy for weight control calls "marginal doctors, quasi-nutritionists, big business, and food manufacturers." Tabloids and periodicals feature a "new, amazing, and revolutionary" reducing diet every week. No one seems to become suspicious of why we need a *new* diet every week: has last week's diet already failed? Although the press occasionally reports that certain diets have killed so and so many people, one can only shudder at the estimates of how many lives have been wrecked and serious health hazards suffered by millions of victims of all the health-damaging diets, drugs, and reducing rackets: amphetamines, wired jaws, bowel surgery, electroshocks, liquid protein, starvation, HCG shots ...

Have you noticed that all reducing diets, in addition to being billed as "new, amazing, and revolutionary," always emphasize the fact that they are "eat-all-you-want-and-reduce" diets?

As a joke, I once proposed a "Dr. Airola's *really new, revolutionary,* and *amazing* reducing diet: eat-LESS-and-reduce-all-you-want diet!"

The truth is, this is the only reducing diet that will work. Unfortunately, it would be difficult to get it published, since most periodicals are dependent on the food industry advertising, and nobody wants to hear about such a diet anyway. What obese people want is a diet which promises that they can eat all they want and still reduce!

I think it is time we wake up and look the scientific facts right in the face:

1. Reducing diets don't work! They do not affect the basic causes of overweight or overeating—they only take some weight off temporarily, which comes back as fast as it came off.
2. Most reducing diets are dangerous to the health. Liquid protein diets, or any high protein diet, are examples of how diets can cause severe health

problems and even death. Low- or no-carbohydrate diets are equally harmful. Severe restriction of carbohydrates with no restriction of fats and protein may take weight off effectively, but can have a disastrous effect, causing irrepairable damage to the brain, nervous system, and heart.

3. The medical racket by "fat doctors" of treating obesity with amphetamines, HCG injections, and other anti-obesity drugs (AOD's) is not sanctioned by the honest medical consensus, and may lead to drug addiction and serious health damage, such as high blood pressure, liver damage, paranoid psychoses and changes in libido.[2, 10]

The only safe way to reduce

The only safe and effective way you can *lose* weight and *keep your weight at normal levels* is by:

a) eating less;
b) making sure that what foods you do eat are nutritious and health-building;
c) changing your eating patterns; and
d) exercising more.

This common-sense approach to losing weight is slow but effective. The reason such a reducing program is not sold is that the only one who profits from it is *you.* The best news of all is that this program will not only take extra pounds off, but it will improve your health while doing so.

Here, in a nutshell, is what you do:

1. Go on a low-calorie Airola Optimum Diet as recommended in Chapters 3 and 4 of this book. Don't worry that the diet described in those chapters is recommended for pregnant and lactating women—it is an optimal diet for anyone! Follow the menu in Chapter 4, preferably making low-calorie choices from proposed selections. Do not avoid grains or seeds completey—you need them. However, the emphasis should be on raw and cooked vegetables and raw fruits, sprouts, lactic acid milk products (such as yogurt) and fruit and vegetable juices.

2. Eat 4 to 6 small meals a day in preference to 2 or 3 large meals. Studies show that while 2,000 calories eaten at one large meal may put on weight, the same 2,000 calories eaten in 4 - 5 small meals throughout the day can actually help to reduce. When small meals are eaten, most of the food is converted into energy. But when a large meal is eaten, the body's enzyme systems are overstimulated to the extent that much of the food cannot be utilized; neither is such a great amount of calories needed for energy at that time. Hence, a major portion of such a large meal is stored as fat.[9]

3. Avoid all white or brown sugar and all refined and denatured foods, especially white bread and everything else made with white flour. Eat only 100% natural, unprocessed, whole foods, as recommended in Chapters 3 and 4. On such a diet of natural high-fiber foods, bran is not necessary.

4. Avoid salt. Train your taste buds to enjoy the natural flavor of unsalted foods. An excess of salt in the diet will interfere with effective reducing.

5. Take the following vitamins and supplements daily:
    C—1,000 - 3,000 mg.
    Cod liver oil—2 tsp.
    B-complex, with B_{12}, high potency
    B_6—50 - 100 mg.
    Brewer's yeast powder—2 - 3 tbsp. or equivalent in tablets
    E—600 I.U.
    Inositol—500 mg.
    Choline—500 mg.
    Lecithin—2 tsp. of granules
    Kelp—3 - 5 tablets, or 1 tsp. of granules or powder (can be used as a salt substitute on foods)
    Calcium—500 mg.
    Magnesium—500 mg.
    "Nature's minerals," multiple mineral and trace element complex—5 tablets

All vitamins should be divided and taken with the major meals. The above dosage is for persons over 20.

Younger persons should take a half dose. Take your vitamins and food supplements *after meals* to minimize the appetite-stimulating effect of some vitamins, notably vitamins from the B-complex. Brewer's yeast should be taken 1 hour before meal on an empty stomach.

6. Drink lots of liquids: herb teas, fruit and vegetable juices, or plain water. The best herbs for reducing are: chickweed, Irish moss, sassafras, chaparral. The best fruit juices: lemon, grapefruit, pineapple, papaya. Dilute sweet juices with water, fifty-fifty; the sweeter the juice, the more water. The best vegetable juices are: cabbage, celery, and "green juice" (see Recipes & Directions).

7. And, finally, *exercise!*

Overweight and exercise

Since the difference between maintaining weight and putting on weight is the proper balancing between calorie intake and calorie expenditure, and since it is admittedly very difficult to *eat less,* and thus cut down on calorie intake, the logical course of action, then, is: increase the calorie expenditure. That is, get as much exercise as possible.

What kind of exercise is best for reducing? *Vigorous* exercise; exercise or other physical activity (such as heavy physical labor) that burns lots of calories: running, jogging, playing tennis, basketball, or other vigorous games, swimming, walking briskly. A combination of intermittent jogging and walking is best for most people, especially those who are not very young.

If you haven't jogged or run before, start slowly, and increase the time and distance gradually.

Here are a few other helpful tips on jogging:

- Do not, if possible, jog on a heavily trafficked street or road. The health hazard of pollution from cars may negate every good that jogging can accomplish. Jog in a park, or outside of the city, or on a back alley or dead end street.
- Always wear light- or bright-colored clothes, especially when dark, so motorists can spot you.

Many joggers have been killed by motor vehicles.

- When jogging at night, convince a friend to join you. There's safety in numbers.
- If tired, stop and rest. Jog and walk intermittently: jog until you are running out of breath, then walk for awhile. Do not press too hard. Have fun! Enjoy! Don't try to set a world record!

What about yoga and regular calisthenics? Every little bit helps. However, for maximum reducing, you need *vigorous,* perspiring, exhausting activity. The best time for some stretching exercises and calisthenics is just before your daily jogging routine.

For rainy days and for city-dwellers, a small trampoline-type rebounder (advertised in many health magazines) is a great exerciser. It is also good for those who can't do more strenuous running or jogging.

Juice fasting: the fastest way to reduce

The two most important requirements for any reducing system are: 1) it must be effective; 2) it must be 100% safe. The reducing program should not only be able to take pounds and inches off, but also be able to supply your body with the necessary nutrients to keep it in top health condition while and after you reduce. That's why my *juice fasting* program, which I introduced in the United States in 1969 with my book, *Health Secrets From Europe,* and then in 1971 with *How To Keep Slim, Healthy, and Young With Juice Fasting,* is the fastest and the safest way to lose weight, *while improving your health generally.*

Most reducing diets or programs will take pounds off, but only at the high price of ruining your health. Some reducing diets are so unhealthful, so health-damaging, that they actually cause weight loss by making you *sick!* High protein meat or egg diets, for example, cause such a severe auto-toxemia, acidosis, and metabolic or biochemical imbalance in the system, that if you continue for too long, they will eventually lead to serious disease, and even death. Even some reducing methods which use the word "fast," such as "protein-sparing fast," or a pure water fast, can be extremely harmful.

As I stated before, the only sensible and safe way to reduce is to eat less. But, here is the crux: "eat less" is easy to say, but ... oh, how difficult to practice! As many compulsive eaters will testify, eating less is more difficult than not eating at all! In my clinical experience, I found that it is much easier for most people to reduce weight by juice fasting than by cutting down on the amount of food.

One particular case from my earlier clinical experience has been etched permanently in my memory. I supervised hundreds of fasts in my clinic, but most were for therapeutic reasons. Miss L. came to me strictly for reducing. She had been working most of her life in the field of health and beauty. She operated a figure control salon in Los Angeles, and had helped countless women to better health and better figures through proper exercise plus a gym-type program of steambaths, swimming, and workouts! For many years, she was a wonderful example and advertisement for the effectiveness of her methods.

When she reached 45, her health and her looks started to deteriorate. She began putting on weight, and in spite of her rigid program of exercises, didn't seem to be able to control it. Also, the signs of premature aging began to appear. Her hair started to turn gray. Wrinkles appeared on her face. Her complexion began to deteriorate rapidly. Her skin was dry and lifeless. She felt exhausted most of the time, and lost interest in her work. She sold her business and tried to find new interests—without success.

In the meantime, she developed an uncontrollable appetite and was putting on weight rapidly. She tried some reducing diets, but none of them really worked on her—she kept getting fatter and fatter. She wanted to work with young people and applied for a job as a health, beauty, and personality counselor in a home for young girls, but she was turned down because of her "age and overweight." That incident was a great shock to her and a turning point in her life. She suddenly realized that she had to do something, and do it fast, if she didn't want to live the rest of her life, in her words, "as a fat, old, sick blob."

She had noticed with horror that people started to feel sorry for her. Her personality had changed. Her view on life was negative. She became critical of everyone and everything, and her temper was getting worse and worse. No wonder she had not many friends left.

There are hundreds of thousands of women who are in a similar situation. They blame their condition on the "change of life," and usually become resigned to the idea that they are becoming old and that nothing can be done about it. But, Miss L. was not ready to give up. She decided to pull herself out of her dismal condition. Although she had worked most of her life in the figure control and beauty field, she had never thought much about nutrition and what role it plays in health. However, when some friends showed her my books and the advertisement for our clinic, she decided to pay us a visit and give it a try.

Miss L. was 54 when she came under my care. She weighed 184 pounds, and looked like she was 60. She stayed for three months, fasted a total of 44 days, and lost 52 pounds. When she left the clinic, she weighed 132 pounds. From size 20, she was now size 12, and she had to shop for some new clothes before she could return to Los Angeles. But you should have seen the change in her looks and her personality. Instead of being the old, tired, apathetic, discouraged, and disillusioned woman of three months earlier, she now looked and behaved like a young woman of 40, filled with energy and enthusiasm, full of exciting plans for the future, determined to get that job she was refused! Her vitality and enthusiasm seemed limitless and the change in her appearance was nothing but miraculous.

One year had passed before I had the opportunity to see her again at one of my lectures in Los Angeles. She looked even better—slimmer, healthier, and younger, than when she left us.

"How have you managed to keep slim?" I asked. "I remember you had such a hard time staying away from food."

"How?" she laughed. "*You* should know. I just follow your advice. I fast one day each week and go on a 2-week juice fast every two or three months. Of course, I try to follow your diet, too!"

I am sure you have many questions in your mind already. Can anyone fast? How is juice fasting done? How long can I fast? How much weight can I lose?

Since, within the size and format of this book, it would be impossible to outline a complete fasting program in detail as it should be, I strongly suggest that if you are considering juice fasting, you should acquire my book, *How To Keep Slim, Healthy, and Young With Juice Fasting,* where all the phases of fasting, day by day, hour by hour, are described in detail. The book is sold in most health food stores or can be ordered by mail directly from the publishers: P.O. Box 22001, Phoenix, Az., 85028.

Here are the answers to some of your questions:

- Yes, anyone in good health can juice-fast for 10-14 days at a time, following the instructions in my book. Longer fasts should be supervised by a doctor or experienced professional.
- If you suffer from any health disorder, you should consult your doctor before undertaking a juice fast. A therapeutic fast should always be prescribed and supervised by a doctor.
- Fasting is not advisable during pregnancy or lactation, neither is it advisable for children, except for a day or two during an acute illness with fever.
- You lose about one pound a day on a fast for the first 20 days or so. After that about one half pound a day.
- If you follow all the instructions in the book, juice fasting is safe and will not only take weight off, but will have a health-improving, revitalizing, and rejuvenating effect on all the body functions.[11]
- Juice fasting is much easier and safer than a pure water fast. Juices supply vitamins, minerals, enzymes, and easily digestible fruit sugars which minimize the stress of fasting by providing an

alkaline balance and supporting the function of all vital organs.

- Will you feel hungry during the fast? For the first few days, yes. But, remember, juices will satisfy most of your hunger. After the third day, when the body begins to "feed on itself," the hunger will gradually disappear.

- It is important that the fast be **broken** correctly. Follow to the letter the instructions in the book regarding the breaking of the fast.

- After the fast, it will be easier to eat less since you will find smaller portions to be satisfying.

Importance of developing new eating patterns

Mental attitudes toward yourself and toward food and your eating patterns and habits must be changed before any dieting and reducing program can be effective and lasting. Here are some helpful tips:

1. Keep all food well out of sight. There is quite a bit of research evidence suggesting that individuals are more likely to overeat when food is physically visible and within easy reach. Likewise, don't store tempting foods in front in the refrigerator so that if you open the door they are staring you right in the face. You are less likely to snack on them if they are well hidden, or better yet, not even in the house. "Out of sight, out of mind" is a good rule to remember.

2. Serve small portions at a meal and keep the rest of the food in the kitchen, not on the table. You are more likely to take second or third helpings if the bowl of food is left on the table.

3. Eat slowly and chew well. Eating too fast causes the body to miss the important nerve signals of fullness and satisfaction from the stomach to the appestat. Dr. M.J. Mahoney, who studied the effects of fast eating says, "If you wolf your food down, you may overshoot your biological needs."[12] By chewing well, you also improve the digestibility and assimilability of the foods so that less

food will be needed to satisfy both hunger and the body's need for nutrients.

4. Stop eating at the very first sign of fullness or satisfaction—even if there is some food left on the plate. "A clean plate" is one of the worst eating habits and one of the prime contributing factors to overweight. It is better that the food go to *waste* than to *waist!*

Let your subconscious mind help you to slim down

Finally, you can program your subconscious mind to work towards a new and slimmer you by visualizing the figure and body you want to have and a daily positive confirmation that you are actually getting it.

Here is a very effective method I've devised (called SPM-Subconscious Programming Method) that has helped many people. Cut out the head of one of your own photographs and attach with tape or glue over the body of a picture (from a magazine or photo) that you would like yours to be. Try to find a scantily clad or nearly nude picture, so you can see the whole body. Each evening before you go to bed, stand in front of a full-length mirror in the nude and take a good, long, and honest look at yourself. Look at the composite picture for awhile, then again at your own body. Visualize how your whole life will change when your body will look like the one in the composite picture. Every night, as you go through this routine, make a determined decision and commitment: "that's the way I am going to look!"

Then, as you go to bed, relax and feel good about the fact that you are on the way to acquiring a new and beautiful figure. As you are slowly falling asleep, keep repeating, silently, the following words (which are a paraphrase on Dr. Emile Coué's famous words cited in Chapter 35):

"Every day, in every way, I'm getting slimmer, and slimmer, and slimmer."

Then, throughout the day, as you go about your work, or while driving the car, or on your daily walks, say *loudly* to yourself the same words: "Every day, in every way, I'm getting slimmer, and slimmer, and slimmer!" Say that at least five times a day, and I assure you that wonderful things will begin to happen. Your mental visualization of your ideal body and conscious positive affirmation of the fact that you are on the way to achieving that goal, will register as a working order and a goal on your subconscious mind which will "instruct" all the glands, organs, and processes of the body to initiate and eventually to accomplish that goal. Your eating habits, workings of your appestat, and all the glands, the digestive, and assimilative mechanisms, effectiveness of fat metabolism, your degree of will power, and desire to work toward the desired goal—all will be positively influenced and affected on a subconscious level by such programming of your mind. The power of the mind is limitless. It can accomplish wonders. I have seen remarkable wonders accomplished by a positive attitude and mind programming in hundreds of cases. The power of the mind is so great that the above-mentioned method *alone* can help you to lose weight. Imagine how successful you can be if you use it as an adjunct to all the other approaches to reducing recommended in this chapter!

Summary

As you may have observed, whether I discuss a minor illness, or a serious and fatal disease, I always recommend what I call a *TOTAL HOLISTIC APPROACH*— attacking the problem from all directions at the same time, and giving the body's own healing mechanism support with all possible means. The problem of overweight is no exception. It is, perhaps, for most people, one of the most difficult health problems to cope with. You may have to deal with the excessive number of fat cells developed in infancy. You may have genuine physical, metabolic, glandular, or hormonal derangements underlying your overweight problem. Maybe emotional and psychological factors are involved: depression, frustration, insecurity, guilt, boredom ... It is also possible that *all* or *most* of these contributing factors are involved to some extent in your case. This is why it is important that you read and study this chapter carefully and try to develop your own personalized reducing program where *all* of the suggested aids to reducing will be incorporated:

- Repeated short juice fasts, 7 to 14 days each.
- Low calorie menu of several meals of nutritious foods from the Optimum Diet in Chapter 4.
- New eating patterns which prevent overeating.
- Plenty of hard physical work or vigorous exercise to burn excess calories.
- Special vitamins and supplements that are known to improve your metabolism, help burn fat, and prevent overeating.
- Visualizing your goal and programming your subconscious mind to help achieve it.

If you are willing to try and undertake the above-mentioned TOTAL HOLISTIC APPROACH to reducing, I can assure you that the problem of overweight will not have to be a lifetime struggle, and that the suggested programs will help you to make your dream of a slimmer, healthier, and more beautiful you an accomplished reality.

34

Menopause: Dreadful Affliction or Glorious Experience?

Menopause, "the change of life," is, perhaps, the most dreaded time of a woman's life. Child-bearing ability ceases, and with that many women feel that they have lost their femininity and womanhood. In our youth-oriented culture, menopause is associated with a "beginning of the end" feeling—the end of youthful attractiveness and feminine sex appeal, and the beginning of the dreaded old age, with loss of attractiveness to the opposite sex. In America, where there is very little respect and honor for the old, the advent of menopause is often traumatic and depressing. Such a mental attitude only multiplies and magnifies the real or imagined physical discomforts associated with menopause.

Traditionally, the menopausal years have been associated with emotional instability and irritability, hot flashes, irrational behavior, diminished interest in sex (or excessive interest, in some cases!), disturbances in calcium and zinc metabolism, backache, pyorrhea, osteoporosis, and "menopausal arthritis"—to name a few common symptoms.

The purpose of this Chapter is to review the question of menopause in the light of the newest research and to help readers who are approaching menopause, as well as those already in menopause, to realize that most menopausal symptoms can be prevented or greatly minimized with proper understanding and nutritional means. Certainly, none of the traditional problems associated with menopause have to be experienced as early as they are by most women. Menopause, in fact, can be postponed for as long as 10 to 20 years. Moreover, the negative experiences of menopausal syndrome will be minimal, even non-existent, if one has led a health-building life and adhered to an Optimum Diet.

Why menopause?

Menopause is a perfectly normal, natural state, and should not be looked upon as some sort of disorder or ailment. It is a condition designed by nature whereby a female, past the age when a safe and healthy pregnancy and delivery can be assured, is deprived of further possibility of impregnation. The ovaries stop ovulation and become less active in producing sex hormones. So menstruation stops (which may take several months of more or less profuse bleeding, on and off), and, with it, the blood level of estrogen, and other female hormones, goes down. Most menopausal problems are due to this lowering of hormones in the body.

Now, most women confronted with the first distressing symptoms of menopause, such as hot flashes, run to their doctor, and the average doctor will immediately put them on estrogen therapy. If he is a conventional doctor, he will most likely prescribe a diethylstilbestrol-type synthetic estrogen. If the doctor is of the "new breed," and nature-oriented, he may prescribe a more "natural" form of estrogen, a so-called conjugated hormone naturally occurring in pregnant mare urine, usually Premarin. In whatever form, estrogen therapy is not only completely unnecessary, but is a very dangerous way of trying to interfere with a natural process in this period of a woman's life.

Here is what one concerned woman wrote to me recently:

"Dear Dr. Airola, I am 49 years old, and I must have reached the age of "change of life," since my menses have practically stopped—three or four months in between. I went to my gynecologist, and he immediately said that I must take estrogen. Since I have been health-oriented for many years, I am leery about taking drugs—so I went to another gynecologist. He also prescribed estrogen, the synthetic kind to boot. He said I must take it or I would have all kinds of problems and will be an old sick woman in no time at all. Now, tell me, Doctor, why do I have to have this drug? My mother, who was very healthy and lived to be 92, and my aunt, who lived to be 89, never took estrogen. And my mother looked very young and had a beautiful complexion at the age of 90! Why must I take estrogen?"

Why, indeed? During the thousands of years of present civilization, millions of women lived healthy and happy lives and aged gracefully, without taking estrogen injections. But, in this drug-oriented era, doctors as well as many women seem to be more concerned with the elimination of an unpleasant symptom than the health of the whole body. Women in our culture must assume some blame for the existing estrogen-therapy craze. Fearing the approach of old age, and trying desperately to stay young in our youth-worshipping society, they demand from their doctors supposedly rejuvenative estrogen therapy. And many doctors willingly oblige.

Danger of estrogen therapy

Here are two letters I received recently:

"Dear Doctor Airola, I took Premarin for 12 years, also 800 I.U. of vitamin E daily, plus all other vitamins. Three weeks ago my doctor told me, after taking a biopsy, that I have cancer of the uterus. I have to take 25 radiation treatments, a 4-week rest, and then have a complete hysterectomy. I am 60 years old. What should I do?"

"Dear Dr. Airola, I am 48 years old. In June of this year, I had to have a hysterectomy, because doctors found a fibroid tumor the size of a walnut. My problem is, I was put on estrogen therapy. I have heard lots of arguments for and against it, so I asked my doctor. He said, "nothing to worry about." He told me of all the dreadful ways I would suffer if I didn't take estrogen. This morning I read in the paper: 'Two studies link estrogen therapy to cancer.' I have a book by Robert A. Wilson, M.D., called *Feminine Forever,* which convinced me of the importance of estrogen therapy. Now I am very worried. What do you think I should do?"

The scientific studies referred to in this letter, linking estrogen therapy to cancer, were conducted recently and reported in the New England Journal of Medicine, a reputable medical journal.[1] One study was made at the University of Washington in Seattle, where the records of 317 patients with uterine cancer were compared with an equal number of patients with other types of cancer. The study found that women exposed to estrogen therapy had about five times greater risk of developing cancer of the uterine lining. The second study was carried out by the Kaiser Permanente Medical Center in Los Angeles, and Drs. Harry K. Ziel, and William D. Finkle, who conducted the study, have found that the cancer risk factor increased five to seven times in middle-aged women on estrogen therapy. The risk increased in proportion to the length of time the drug was used. For women who had used estrogen for seven or more years, the risk of developing cancer of the uterus was fourteen times higher than normal!

These studies, and many other reports from world-wide medical literature, suggest clearly that estrogen (whether in the form of the contraceptive pill or Premarin) is a definite contributing cause of uterine cancer. Doctors would do well to wake up from the "estrogen craze" and be more cautious in prescribing estrogen therapy as a standard treatment for menopausal syndrome.

Cancer is not the only condition you are inviting when taking estrogen medication. Studies at Oxford University by Dr. Joel Mann showed that women between the ages of 40 and 44 who took the birth control pill increased by five times their chances of dying from a heart attack.

How badly misused estrogen therapy is at present was pointed out by Dr. Sheldon H. Cherry, of Mount Sinai Medical School, in his book, *The Menopause Myth.* Dr. Cherry said that of the $80 million a year women spend on menopausal and post-menopausal pills and injections, only

20 percent may be justified.[2] Dr. Cherry adds: "The indiscriminate use of estrogen therapy by all women of climacteric age, irrespective of individual symptoms, as advocated by some, is not warranted; indeed, it may well be dangerous. There is good evidence that estrogen use may also cause an increase in blood clots in the legs and brain."[2]

"Fountain of youth" or fake?

Dr. Cherry is one of several scientists who are now discrediting estrogen-replacement therapy that is claimed to reverse the aging process and keep woman young. "Estrogen doesn't help wrinkles, doesn't keep women young, and doesn't prevent aging." Dr. Cherry said that the psychological symptoms—depression, anxiety, and irritability—connected with menopause are extensions of a previously existing disorder, and can't be helped or solved by an estrogen pill. "The vast majority of women need only education, reassurance, a healthy mental outlook, exercise, and good dietary habits as they pass through the menopausal phase of life," said Dr. Cherry.

A British study supports Dr. Cherry's view. In a six-month study, half of the women were given "natural" estrogen (Premarin-type), while the other half of the women received dummy pills—sugar pills coated with the same material as the estrogen pills. The women were monitored for such common symptoms of menopause as nervousness, depression, insomnia, dizziness, headaches, joint pain, and hot flashes. Doctors were surprised to discover at the end of the first half of the study that there was no significant difference between the response to estrogen and the placebo—both groups improved dramatically—except that hot flashes were not relieved as completely in the placebo group.[3] Thus, the conclusion was that the symptomatic relief effected by estrogen could be largely psychological. The British study also clearly established that so-called "natural" estrogen causes the same potentially dangerous increase in blood clotting as the synthetic variety.[3]

Vicious cycle

Estrogen medication, in addition to being linked to cancer, heart attacks, strokes, and blood clots, also causes a serious disorder in body chemistry, especially in its mineral balance. It raises the copper level and lowers the zinc level in the blood. Zinc deficiency can lead to depression and psychosis and the elevated copper contributes to the "blues" and moodiness associated with menopause. Thus, estrogen therapy is actually causing the symptoms it is supposed to correct! Estrogen therapy also increases the need for vitamin E, which is much greater anyway during menopause, in fact 10 to 50 times over that which is normally required.[4]

Research Continues

The studies to which I referred above, indicting estrogen therapy as a serious threat to health, have been recently challenged by some investigators. Lila Nachtigall, M.D., in *Nachtigall Report* (Putnam Company, 1978), cites a new study which showed no difference in the occurrence of cancer of the endometrium between the women on estrogen and the women who did not take estrogen. There are a number of conscientious physicians in this country, who do give estrogen (in a cycle with progesterone) to their patients.

The estrogen-replacement therapy is still a controversial issue. Although, in my opinion, the causative relationship between cancer, heart disease, stroke, etc., and estrogen therapy (as in contraceptives or estrogen-replacement therapy) is well established, the research in this area still continues, and whether a woman of menopausal age should take or reject hormone therapy must, therefore, be her own carefully considered decision.

As the research material reported in this chapter shows, the decision should not be difficult. Indictment against estrogen therapy is heavy and my guess is that the future research will only confirm the already known and/or suspected dangers of estrogen medication.

The holistic approach

Biological medicine considers menopause to be a normal, natural process, and under conditions of optimum health and a health-conducive lifestyle, it should be as painless and distress-free a change in a woman's life from one phase to another as her change at puberty. Healthy women in other cultures known for a more natural lifestyle do not take estrogen pills or injections, and yet do not experience any distressing symptoms of menopause. Furthermore, when a woman enjoys good health, her normally functioning adrenal glands produce a number of sex hormones which replace those from inactivated ovaries.[5] Consequently, a woman can go through this normal conclusion of the reproductive cycle without any physical discomforts if she is mentally, physically (nutritionally), and psychologically prepared to accept this phase of life as a natural biological process. She must not attempt to compete with young girls, but go through a normal process of gradual, graceful aging, thanking the Providence for the blessings, wisdom, and experience attained during a long and productive life. Happiness is, among other things, accepting each phase of our life cycle as we approach it, without looking back with regrets, remorse, or jealousy, but looking forward with expectations for the new adventures and increased knowledge and wisdom which each new phase will grant us.

Well, this all sounds rational and sensible enough, but through my life-long close association with, and study of, women, I know that you cannot expect them (nor men, for that matter) always to be rational and sensible. Marital unhappiness, unfulfilled dreams, fear of losing sex appeal and femininity, jealousy, vanity, and the daily look in the mirror and at the scale play havoc with emotions and rational thinking, and most women are ready to run, not walk, to the nearest doctor in the search of a "fountain of youth"—even if it is only in the form of an estrogen pill or injection.

I will attempt to show how you can turn the wheel of

life and reverse the aging processes without carcinogenic drugs and injections; how you can prevent and minimize the symptoms of menopausal syndrome; how you can actually postpone menopause for 10 or more years; and how you can, in fact, stop growing old and start growing younger—all this with perfectly natural, harmless, nutritional, herbal, and other biological means.

Optimum Nutrition—true Fountain of Youth

My study of the secrets of long life convinces me that the true Fountain of Youth springs from Optimum Nutrition and a health-building lifestyle, as I showed in Chapter 31. The ultimate secret of staying young is basically the secret of staying healthy. The best way to prevent or even avoid menopausal syndrome and remain younger longer is to build up a high level of health and resistance to disease and aging by proper diet, plenty of strenuous exercise, adequate rest and relaxation, and a positive mental attitude. Or, as Dr. Cherry, quoted earlier, expressed it, "Physical fitness comes closest to being the Fountain of Youth for the woman—and man—going through or past the change of life." He named nutrition, weight control, and physical exercise as most important factors in "physical fitness."

It is easy to advise Optimum Nutrition, but *what* is it? There are almost as many nutritional philosophies as there are nutritionists. Confusion in this area is rampant, compounded by hundreds of new fads, and books by "experts" published each year. On the basis of my own life-long studies of nutrition, I have concluded—and this conclusion is supported by a growing number of doctors and nutritionists around the world and recently by the U.S. Senate Select Committee on Nutrition—that the Optimum Diet with the greatest potential for preventing premature aging, including the traditional menopausal syndrome, as well as extending a youthful appearance and vitality far into old age, is the Optimum Nutrition Diet which is described in Chapters 3 and 4 of this book. It is basically a lacto-vegetarian diet with emphasis on seeds, grains and nuts, vegetables, and fruits, with specific supplementary foods and vitamins and minerals as mentioned in Chapter 31.

Hormone-vitamin interdependence

Hormones—even sex hormones—are made from the material supplied by food. Some vitamins, fatty acids, and minerals have a specific enhancing effect on the body's own hormone production. There is a constant interplay between vitamins and hormones and the deficiency of one may lead to the deficiency or imbalance in another.[7] For example: hormones from the pituitary gland—the master gland—regulate the absorption of nutrients from the food we eat, and pituitary dysfunction may lead to nutritional deficiencies; but dietary deficiencies or inadequacies may impair the pituitary function. A vicious cycle! A properly functioning thyroid gland is essential for normal sex hormone production. The thyroid secretes the hormone, thyroxin, which has a direct stimulating effect on the sex glands. An underactive thyroid leads to underactive, lazy sex glands and insufficient sex hormone output. Iodine (as in kelp) is essential to keep the thyroid glands secreting sufficient thyroxin. A malfunctioning parathyroid gland may lead to the derangement of calcium and vitamin D metabolism and utilization (which can be corrected by magnesium supplementation[8]). It is also known that the effectiveness of estrogenic hormones is increased by the simultaneous administration of vitamins B_6, E, and C. PABA and folic acid (which contains PABA) have the same effect. Thus, taking these vitamins at the time of menopause or post-menopausal period, when the body's estrogen output is drastically lowered, may improve and enhance the effectiveness of the endogenous estrogen without the need to resort to drugs.

One of my readers wrote to me:

"Two years ago, when I was 47, I found that I had reached the 'change of life' age with unmistakable symptoms of disrupted menstrual cycle and bothersome hot flashes. Hot flashes were unbearable and very frequent—at times every few minutes. I resisted the urge to run to my doctor and turned to the menopausal section of your book, *How To Get Well*.[9] You advised taking 1200 I.U. vitamin E and stated that it stimulates the production of estrogen. You also suggested PABA as being a natural substitute for estrogen, and pantothenic acid for delaying of menopause. So, I started taking 1200 I.U. of E per day, plus all the other vitamins you recommended, and drank licorice tea, which you advised. And, in less than a week, my hot flashes and other symptoms disappeared completely. Within a few months, my periods became normal, and now, two years later, I am still menstruating as regularly as ever. I feel like a young girl again. And my husband says these vitamins are doing something to me, and that I never was so sexy in my life. Thank you for writing that wonderful book."

A striking example of how vitamins can improve the body's own estrogen production and postpone menopause!

Vitamin E effect scientifically confirmed

Several clinical studies have confirmed the ability of vitamin E to alleviate the most distressing symptoms of menopause.

Dr. N.R. Kavinoky treated a group of menopausal patients with 10 to 25 I.U.of vitamin E daily. They were relieved of hot flashes and backaches. In another group of 79 patients, using larger doses of vitamin E—50 - 100 I.U. per day—Dr. Kavinoky reported even better results: fatigue, nervousness, restless sleep and insomnia, in addition to hot flashes, were reduced in more than half, and nearly all patients were relieved of dizziness, heart palpitations, and shortness of breath.[10]

Henry A. Gozen, M.D., reported on his vitamin E treatment of 66 patients with menopausal troubles. He said that vitamin E eliminated serious symptoms in 59 patients out of 66.[11] W.H. Perloff, M.D., reported on his treatment of 200 menopausal women with vitamin E doses of 75-150 I.U. daily: 26% were relieved of all symptoms, and another 26%

were improved. He believes that higher dosages of vitamin E might have relieved those who did not respond.

According to some studies, during menopause, the need for vitamin E soars to 10 to 50 times greater than that previously required.[4]

Vitamin and mineral supplements for menopause

Here is the list of specific supplements, vitamins, and minerals which you should take daily if you are approaching menopausal age, if you are in menopause right now, or for a post-menopausal supplementation (in addition to specific foods and food supplements recommended earlier):

E—up to 1200 I.U.

Vitamin E stimulates production of estrogen and helps alleviate hot flashes and other distressing symptoms of menopause.[4, 10, 12, 20] (Note: vitamin E seems to exert a normalizing effect on estrogen levels: increasing the hormone output in women who are deficient, and lowering it in those who are prone to an excess.)

B_6—up to 100 mg.

Vitamin B_6 enhances the effectiveness of estrogenic hormones and helps prevent "menopausal arthritis."[12] It also helps to control menstrual edema.[13]

PABA—up to 100 mg.

PABA is a natural substitute for estrogen; an estrogen synergist—it enhances the effect of estrogen.[7]

Folic acid—up to 5 mg.

Folic acid is similar to PABA in its action as an estrogen synergist.[7]

B_{12}—50 mcg.

Vitamin B_{12} is synergistic with folic acid and other B vitamins.

Pantothenic acid—up to 100 mg.

Pantothenic acid can help delay menopause.[9, 21]

A—25,000 units.

Vitamin A is essential for the healthy functioning of the sex glands.[9]

C—up to 3,000 mg.

Vitamin C is a detoxifier, rejuvenator, and a stimulant of thyroid and sex glands.[9, 21]

B-complex, high potency.

Vitamin B-complex formula can help enhance the effect of isolated B vitamins which are specific for menopause: PABA, folic acid, B_6, and pantothenic acid. B vitamins can boost thyroid gland and increase sexual vigor.[15]

Kelp—up to 5 tablets or 1 tsp. granules

Kelp improves the function of the thyroid gland, a primary sex gland stimulator, and can help prevent obesity often associated with menopause.[15]

Calcium-magnesium supplement.

At least 1,000 mg. of calcium daily is advisable to support parathyroid function.[8, 21]

Zinc—up to 30 mg.

Zinc is needed for reproductive hormone and enzyme production, for the formation of RNA and DNA, and for proper vitamin and mineral utilization, especially for the metabolism of vitamin A, and for synthesis of insulin and body protein.[9]

D—up to 1,000 units.

Vitamin D improves mineral metabolism and utilization. Most women, especially those who spend much of their time indoors, are deficient in vitamin D.[19]

Betaine Hydrochloride—1 tablet after each meal

Supplementary hydrochloric acid will improve mineral assimilation in older people who often have a low output of their own digestive acids.

A comprehensive trace-element formula with iron, copper, manganese, selenium, etc.—all youthifying factors.[15]

Whey powder—up to 2 tbsp.

The regular use of whey will help improve digestion and assimilation of foods and prevent intestinal putrefaction and constipation, which is often associated with menopause.

Specific herbs for menopause

Specific herbs helpful in postponing and/or alleviating the symptoms of menopause are: Mexican Wild Yam, Lady's slipper, liferoot, and passion flower. Black cohosh, Honduras sarsaparilla, false unicorn roots, elder, and licorice—all contain some natural estrogen and can be used as supplements to the body's own diminished hormone production during menopause or after hysterectomy.[9, 17] One herbalist recommends the following herb combination to combat the distressing symptoms of menopause: blessed thistle, squaw vine, raspberry leaves, golden seal, lobelia, gravelroot, gingeroot, cayenne, parsley, and marshmallow root.[18] Another herbal formula for hormonal imbalances produced by menopause includes: sarsaparilla, licorice, and blue vervain.

The best herbal combination for hot flashes is black cohosh, licorice root, sarsaparilla, blessed thistle, false unicorn roots, red raspberry leaves, elder, and squaw vine.

Another specific herb for menopause is Motherwort (Leonurus Cardiaca). It is used mostly for palpitations of the heart due to the endocrine or functional nervous disorders associated with menopause.[22] This herb increases menstrual flow, so it shouldn't be used by those who suffer from excessive flow.

Many herbs sold in health food stores today are either in capsule form, or in the form of dried herbs, prepackaged in cartons or bags. The best way to use herbs: take 1 tsp. of dried herbs or open and empty 2 - 3 capsules of powdered herbs into a cup and pour boiling water over it. Let stand for 10 - 15 minutes, strain, sweeten with honey, if desired, and drink. For therapeutic uses, take 2 - 3 cups a day, on an empty stomach.

A health-building lifestyle to keep you young

For the postponement of menopause and prevention of premature aging, a total health-building lifestyle is just as important as diet or specific supplements, vitamins, minerals, and herbs. One of the most important rejuvenative factors is vigorous exercise.[2] And, by exercise, I do not mean a few stretching or other motions in front of your T.V. set each morning. I mean daily strenuous, perspiring, outdoor exercise: brisk walking, jogging, swimming, horse or bicycle riding, tennis, and other games, or actual physical labor in garden or fields to keep your glands working at full steam.[6] (See more on importance of exercise in Chapter 2.)

Mental and emotional stresses and constant fears and worries not only can produce any ailment in the medical book, but will also age you before your time. Do not worry about getting old, just do something to postpone aging! You must also get sufficient sleep, rest, and relaxation—even develop the habit of taking an afternoon siesta.

An active sex life is important in keeping young. As I said in one of my books, *Rejuvenation Secrets From Around the World—That "Work,"*[6] "We do not stop sexual activity because we grow old—we grow old because we stop sexual activity." My research indicates that vibrant health, long life, and sexual virility go hand in hand. Sexual interest and activity keep your sex and adrenal glands producing hormones, and these hormones in turn will help to keep you young. Interest in sex should remain (although, of course, at a gradually diminishing level with age) as long as we live if the Optimum Diet with emphasis on the gland-stimulating vitamins, minerals, and herbs is maintained. Research shows that the sexual desire is not lessened by menopause; it often is increased. This may be due, in part, to the fact that (for many) menopause represents a liberation from the fear of pregnancy.

What a health-building lifestyle can do to improve the quality of your life, increase vitality and youthful energy, femininity, and sex appeal (and, conversely, what a health-destroying life style can accomplish) is dramatically illustrated by the following case from my files:

Case history of Mr. and Mrs. P.H.

A couple in their middle years came to me for nutritional advice. He was a balding, overweight man, looking to be around 60. She was the opposite: thin, emaciated, with a dull complexion, and thin, graying hair, appearing to be in her early 50's. I had my first surprise when I found that he was 46 and she was 39!

The couple told me that they were desperate for help. First, they had tried everything else: medical specialists, expensive tests, fancy clinics, a long line of drugs, psychiatrists, more medical specialists, more drugs— without receiving help, but actually getting worse. Then, in desperation, they came to me.

Here is their story in his words:

"We had pretty good health until a few years ago. Then something happened. My wife became tired all the time, lost all of her interest in life—just laid in bed all day, complaining of aches and pains. Doctors couldn't figure out what was wrong with her. Her menses stopped, so doctors gave her drugs and hormone shots, suspecting premature menopause. But nothing helped. I began putting on weight a few years ago. I am tired all the time, hardly able to move. I can't sleep. Our sex life is completely finished, too—I haven't touched my wife for a year. Not that she cares—she is so beat that sex is the furthest thing from her mind. I'm afraid of losing my job—I can't think straight, and I bark at everyone at work. After a few hours at the office, I am ready to quit and go home. Coffee is the only thing that keeps me going—I drink a cup about every half hour."

As he talked, they both chain-smoked. The interview revealed that the couple had been violating all the known rules of health for decades. Their lives centered around almost nightly parties where they drank lots of alcohol. Their diet consisted largely of coffee (at least 10 - 15 cups a day), frozen dinners, sweets, and party snacks at night. They hardly ever ate fresh vegetables or fruits, nor whole grain bread and cereals. Their physical exercise was limited to walking from the bed to the bar, and to and from the car. It is significant that *none of the doctors they consulted had ever asked them what they ate, or how they lived.*

When I suggested to them that their premature aging—her premature menopause, gray hair, rundown condition; his obesity, lack of vitality, sexual impotence—was brought about by their terrible living habits, their total disregard of all the elementary rules of health, they looked not only surprised, but disappointed. They expected that I would give them a bottle of vitamin pills which would miraculously wipe out all their problems and restore their health and vitality. Instead, I said that if they wanted their health and youth back, their libido and vitality restored, her menstrual cycle normalized and menopause postponed, they must stop smoking, stop drinking alcohol, soft drinks, and coffee, and stop eating nutritionless junk foods. They must give up all-night parties, and start a regular program of strenuous physical exercise beginning with long walks and swimming. I outlined nutritional and supplementary programs for them along the lines of diet and vitamins suggested in this book.

It was difficult to convince them to make such a drastic change in their lifestyle. It had never occurred to them—nor to the doctors they consulted—that their condition had anything to do with their way of living. But, they had no choice: life was so miserable that they were willing to try anything!

The first few weeks were dreadful. Without the stimulation of alcohol and coffee, (they weren't able to stop smoking for another 6 months) they could hardly drag their feet. But, month after month brought gradual improvement, and finally, after 6 months, they reported that my rejuvenation program "accomplished a miracle." They felt like two new people. All tiredness was gone, her hair began to turn dark, menstrual regularity was restored, and she was full of vitality and slept like a baby. He lost over 30 pounds, enjoyed his work at the office again, and their sex life was completely straightened out. I have never seen a happier or more enthusiastic couple!

Summary

Scientific studies and actual cases cited in this chapter show that:

- Menopause is a natural, normal process in a woman's life cycle, and it does not have to be associated with the pain and discomfort experienced by most women in Western cultures.

- The traditional menopausal syndrome of hot flashes, irritability, irrational behavior, and back pain are brought about by our denatured lifestyle, nutritional deficiencies, lack of exercise, and consequent lowered resistance, plus wrong psychological, social, and mental attitudes toward it. Women in more "primitive" (read: natural) cultures do not suffer from menopausal syndrome.

- Commonly employed hormone replacement therapy for menopausal and post-menopausal syndrome (or post-hysterectomy) can be extremely harmful and is scientifically proven to be causatively linked to increased risk of blood clots, heart disease, and cancer.

- Optimum nutrition, a health-building lifestyle, adequate exercise, rest, relaxation, a positive mental outlook, and specific vitamins, supplements, and herbs, mentioned in this chapter, can help to alleviate pain, hot flashes, and other distressing symptoms associated with menopause, and postpone the onset of menopause for as long as ten or more years. Such a holistic program will help prevent premature aging and assure painless, youthful vitality and optimum health at any age.

- The body's lowered output of estrogen associated with menopause can be partially offset by specific vitamins and herbs as outlined in this chapter. But, a proper mental attitude toward menopause is just as important as optimum nutrition, vitamins, supplements, and exercise. Think young! Don't look upon menopause as "the beginning of the end," the dreaded end of youthfulness, sex appeal, and femininity. Menopause is merely a time of maturation, when women's central focus shifts from the care of children and family to developing of her own interests and talents, increasing reflection and gaining wisdom. Menopause is a divinely-designed phase in woman's life, with a purpose of liberating her from her role as co-creator with God and giving her time for self-improvement, spiritual growth, and for further perfection of her human and divine characteristics. Properly understood, menopause, instead of being a dreadful affliction, can become a most glorious and fulfilling experience in woman's life!

35

The Completion of a Lifecycle: A New Birth

"Birth is not a beginning; death is not an end."
—*Chinese proverb.*

We started this book with birth—the beginning of a lifecycle. We will conclude it with the end of a lifecycle—death.

The approaching of old age and the realization of the inevitability of death can be a fearful and alarming experience for those who do not understand the immortal, everlasting nature of human life and the transiency of our brief encounter on this planet. If death would be an end to life, such an apprehension would be understandable. However, death is but a birth into a new life. We are immortal beings who lived in higher, spiritual realms before assuming physical bodies during this brief earthly experience, and we will return to the spirit world to continue our eternal life of spiritual growth and progression. Death is not an end. It is a beginning, a rebirth, a transformation from one form of life into another. Like the caterpillar changes from its confining life form into the less restricted and freer life of the butterfly, so we, at death, are freed and transformed into a higher form of life as spiritual beings.

We should look upon death with the same anticipation and sense of great accomplishment as the school graduate looks at the graduation ceremony. The schooling is over, the assignment and mission completed; we are finally ready to return to the Source, being reborn into the immortal spirit world from whence we came. Death is really the beginning of a new experience—the supreme adventure of humanity!

One of my favorite philosophers, Benjamin Franklin, expressed this sentiment eloquently:

"A man is not completely born until he is dead. Why then should we grieve that a new child is born among the immortals? We are immortal spirits. That bodies should be lent us while they afford us pleasure, assist us in acquiring knowledge, or in doing good to our fellow creatures is a kind of benevolent act of God. When they become unfit for these purposes and afford us pain instead of pleasure, instead of an aid become an encumbrance ... it is equally kind and benevolent that a *way* is provided by which we get rid of them. Death is that *way*."

To die is as natural as to be born. From this imperfect world of earthly existence, which is ridden with pain, sorrow, disappointments, and problems, we enter a new and perfect world of eternal happiness. In the words of Walt Whitman: "Nothing can happen more beautiful than death."

The Divine purpose of life

Although this book has devoted most of its pages to the physical aspects of woman's life—pregnancy, child-feeding and -rearing, nutrition, the biological approach to reproductive and other health disorders and problems, I would not wish to leave my readers with the impression that I consider the biological functions and pursuits of good nutrition and good health to be the sole purpose and goal in life. As worthwhile and as enjoyable as good health can be, it won't guarantee happiness and fulfillment. We have all seen people who are in perfect physical health, yet unhappy and miserable. On the other hand, I have known those who were afflicted with obvious misfortunes and ill health, yet they have overlooked or ignored their seeming burdens, and instead of falling into the trap of self-pity, have radiated joy and happiness, and shown love and concern for the welfare and happiness of others.

Improving one's health and building a strong, disease-free body can be a rewarding and joyous experience. But let us not consider the attaining of beautiful body, lovely figure or smooth complexion as a goal in itself. The body is a "temple" in which the spirit dwells and develops. It should, therefore, be kept healthy and clean. But, the ultimate goal and purpose of life is not just building and maintaining a healthy and disease-free "temple," but the development and perfection of the spirit that dwells therein.

The source of happiness

The true and lasting happiness comes from the realization of the divine origin and purpose of all life and from the directing of our own lives and channeling of all our energies towards the expression and exemplification of the Divine Plan in our daily lives. Supreme happiness can be experienced only by those who give happiness to others. We receive only in the measure in which we are willing and able to give.

This all sounds common sense and elementary. But many who reach old age and say, "God knows I 'gave' a lot in my lifetime, but now I am unloved, unneeded, forgotten, and alone. My children and grandchildren are grown up; they seldom, if ever, remember me. Even my attempts to demonstrate my love to them seem to be rejected."

Yes, in our youth-worshipping culture, old people are easily shuffled aside. What a loss to the intelligence pool of humanity that refuses to tap the accumulated knowledge and experience of the old and wise! But do not let this embitter you and tarnish the few remaining years of your life—years that should be most beautiful and fulfilling. There is more pleasure in loving than in being loved. You are not alone as long as you have wonderful memories of happy times while raising your family. Although your children and loved ones seem at the present to be engrossed in their pressured and competitive pursuits of worldly success, their love for you has not vanished. Just let them grow up a little and your need of appreciation for all the efforts made in their behalf will be more obvious to them. You may have gone to the other world by then, of course. But one is never dead or forgotten who has loved and who has been loved. One is never forgotten as long as there are those who remember him with fondness. One is never gone if one showed kindness, affection, unselfishness, patience, loyalty, friendliness, helpfulness, sympathy, and generosity. Any of the above acts have earned you a piece of immortality and eternal gratitude from those whose lives have been touched by yours.

This sounds like a sermon, I know. And, you may rightfully ask: "Who is he to speak on *this* subject with assumed authority? Isn't he a scientist, biochemist, nutritionist, and physician? What does he know about old age, spirituality, and death?

It is true that expertise in these areas cannot be earned within university walls. However, I may qualify to speak on aging and old age and the concerns associated with it, since I am myself a so-called "senior citizen." I have lived a long, busy, creative, productive, and eventful life. I have raised a happy family of five children, who are constantly adding to my increasing flock of grandchildren. I have achieved professional recognition in several fields associated with close human relationships. I have had my share of pain and suffering, spending almost ten years of my life in the midst of three devastating wars, beginning with World War I. I suffered several injuries and severe damage to my health during World War II. But, as I approach the zenith of my life, I have no bitterness nor regrets—nothing but appreciation for all the trials and triumphs, sorrows, pain, and disappointments, as well as the joys and happines that it was my lot to experience. I have no fear of approaching inevitable death. I have touched the lives of many with my work. I have had many friends who have enriched my life. I thank my Creator every day for the many blessings, joys, and opportunities for service and fulfillment I have been granted. When the day of moving into a new sphere of life comes, I will meet it with joy and anticipation, with peace and serenity, without a trace of loss or sorrow. I am not trying to fill this chapter on old age and death with abstract philosophical rhetoric.

I speak of my own personal experience. When I say that death is not an end, but a beginning of a new and more glorious life, I say this with a sincere and deep conviction of the truthfulness of the statement.

Rewarding golden years

The golden years of your life can be the most rewarding and fulfilling of all. Now you can have time to contemplate and center your attention on the real issues of life and its purpose. You can see things in the right perspective and place emphasis on the right priorities. With the right attitude and the understanding of the true purpose of life, old age can be an exciting period with new horizons of happiness. You now have more time to take care of your physical and spiritual needs. Give special attention to your diet. Don't overload your digestive system, which now has a diminished capacity to digest foods, with nutritionless, prepackaged, processed foods. You must exercise regularly! Just a walk, as long as possible, is the best form of exercise at this age. Do not allow yourself to become overweight or constipated—two dangerous, deadly afflictions of the old. Keep your hobbies and interests up. Do something creative and absorbing. By continuing to learn you will find that boredom and mental depression, two other common afflictions of the old, will vanish and a new universe of personal fulfillment and awareness will open up.

If your health is not at the point you wish it to be—and, let's be honest, whose is at an old age?!—don't become alarmed or dwell on it excessively. Accept some of the symptoms of natural aging gracefully and without complaint. This doesn't mean you should do nothing about the signs of illness. Of course you should do everything you can to keep yourself in as good a physical and mental health as possible, and if you notice a sign of serious illness, you should see your doctor. But don't be a hypochondriac as many older people tend to be. Don't worry exorbitantly about a spot here and a pimple there that you didn't have when you were younger. Don't dwell on or talk about disease constantly. Dwelling on, and worrying about, disease, will only make you worse! Develop a health-oriented attitude. *Think* health, *talk* health, *visualize* health—and better health will be your reward!

The holistic approach to total health

The 20th Century philosopher, William James, said, "The greatest discovery of our generation is that a human being *can* alter his life by altering his attitudes." And, I would add that it is the greatest discovery of *any* generation! One of the main causes of failure is the wrong attitude. With the wrong attitude, you can do everything right and fail, but with the right attitude, you can do everything wrong and still succeed. We must build success on attitude, not attitude on success! It is highly significant that God provided man with control over the power to shape his own thoughts and the privilege of fitting them into any pattern of his choice. A positive mental attitude is the starting point of all riches. And one of the best riches of all is abundant health.

A happy, peaceful, positive state of mind is the most powerful vaccination for the prevention of virtually any disease! And not for prevention only: for healing as well! A positive attitude, faith, belief in your body's own inherent power to heal itself, as well as reliance on the Greater Power for assistance, are the best medicines known to medical science.

Everyone has seen, heard, or read about miraculous healings performed by healers who use such unconventional modalities as the laying on of hands, holy waters, psychic surgery, or prayer. The implication is always that the healer possesses a great healing power. Actually, the great healing power that accomplishes such miraculous healing is within our own bodies; the healer merely helps to release it. Your body is equipped with the most powerful and the most effective healing system known to medical science. Your body is designed to be a self-cleansing, self-repairing, and self-healing mechanism. However, this healing power must be switched on by an act of faith before it can begin to work. Just as your room can be wired with electric power for brilliant light yet will remain in darkness until you switch the power on, so your own great healing capacity will remain untapped and unused, unless it is switched on by the act of faith. When Jesus walked this earth and healed the sick, he used this same power to accomplish his miracles. Everytime he was thanked for miraculous healing, he replied, to the effect: don't thank me—"Thy faith has made thee whole."

Faith is not only the greatest *healing* power, but the greatest power known to man, period. This was realized by one of the foremost scientists and Nobel Prize Laureat, Prof. Alexis Carrel, who wrote in his classic book, **Man the Unknown,** that "Prayer is the greatest power known to man." Prayer is an expression of faith. With faith *all* things are possible. Faith not only switches on the healing power within the body, but it releases all the vital energies that can potentiate any goal or accomplishment.

That a positive state of mind and the power of the subconscious can accomplish miraculous healings, was demonstrated on a large scale by the famous French physician, Dr. Emile Coue, in the beginning of this century. Dr. Coue achieved a world-wide reputation by curing thousands of people of every conceivable disease by a most unusual therapy. He sent patients back home, asking them to repeat aloud five times a day, the following words: "Every day, in every way, I am getting better, and better, and better!" To skeptics who laughed at such "nonsense," he said, "I don't care what you think, or even whether you believe it or not, just follow my prescription and you will be cured." And, sure enough, those who followed his advice saw to their amazement how every day, in every way, they *did* feel better, and better, and better; how their pains and ailments gradually disappeared; and how they eventually were totally cured. The loud repetition of the words had registered them on the subconscious mind, which "instructed" the healing powers within the body to initiate, and eventually to accomplish, the healing. The phenomenon of faith is actually a conviction on the intuitive, emotional level, as compared to mere belief, which is a conscious, intellectual process.

Relaxation, peace of mind, a positive outlook on life, a contented spirit, an absence of worries and fears, a cheerful disposition, unselfishness, love of mankind and faith in God—these are all powerful health-promoting factors without which optimum health cannot be achieved. And when health is lost, it cannot be restored **unless** the adequate nutritional and biological therapeutic program is "supplemented" with a good dose of "vitamin X": peace of mind, positive attitude, happy disposition, the will to live, and faith in God—the faith that Nature and God will do **their parts** in helping to restore health, if we do **our part.**

If it is His will ...

However, the divine plan does not include living on this planet Earth forever. We all reach a time in our lives when continued existence would be of no purpose. Thus, in the words of Benjamin Franklin, "God provides a way" by which the physical life is terminated and a rebirth into a higher, spiritual realm is accomplished. Death is but a new birth, a transformation from a lower form of physical existence into a higher consciousness of eternal spiritual progression.

If reading this chapter has helped you to realize the divine origin and purpose of your life and that old age and death are but essential, natural phases of this overall lifecycle, then nearing the completion of the earthly phase of this cycle can be looked upon with great anticipation, appreciation, and love for the grand and magnanimous plan our Creator has designed for our lives. As I stated in the first chapter of this book, the woman's role in this Divine plan is of decisive importance to the fate of humanity. If you have fulfilled your mission and exemplified your Divine purpose at its best throughout your life, you can approach death with the supreme joy of knowing that your Divine earthly experience is completed and you can now be reborn into the spirit world—a world without disease, sorrow, or pain—rewarded with joy, happiness, and peace of mind for all eternity.

Questions
&
Answers

Conception Without Menstruation

Q. I am twenty-six years old, and I haven't menstruated for the last four years. About two years ago, I became a vegetarian, and shortly thereafter, a pure fruitarian. I've just heard a lecture by a man whose book was instrumental in my becoming a fruitarian. He said that menstruation is a sign of poor health and body toxicity due to eating animal foods, grains, and cooked foods, and that truly healthy women on his diet do not menstruate—yet they ovulate normally, which is evidenced by the fact that they do become pregnant. Now I am worried. I have sexual intercourse quite regularly, but ever since my menses stopped four years ago, I haven't used any contraceptives. Could I become pregnant even though I do not menstruate?

A. Menstruation is a perfectly normal physiological function of all healthy women between the ages of puberty and menopause. After ovulation, if impregnation of the female egg did not occur, the special lining of the uterus, which was instituted as preparation for a possible pregnancy, is shed and passed out of the body via the vagina. The menstrual flow is the mixture of this uterine lining with vaginal mucus.

When a woman conceives, menstruation stops because ovulation stops. In most women, ovulation does not occur for several months after the birth of her baby. Sometimes, if the mother nurses her baby, the menstrual cycle does not resume until the baby is weaned. Ovulation and menstruation cease completely at menopause, usually between the ages of 45 and 55.

It is well known medically that menstruation is closely related to the general health status of the woman. Any severe disturbances in normal health, such as serious illness, glandular malfunction, especially within the endocrine system, hypoglycemia, malnutrition and severe nutritional deficiencies, and excessive mental or physical stress, can cause a cessation of menstruation. Even prolonged therapeutic fasting can have this effect. The medical consensus regarding the absence of menstruation is clear and simple: when the body is weakened for any reason and is incapable of bearing a child without a serious threat to the well-being of mother and/or baby, it is, by a wise act of nature, deprived of the ability to reproduce. This is a natural law aimed at preventing women with inferior health from conceiving and producing defective or imperfect offspring. Thus, the species is protected from physical degeneration.

However, the fanatic advocate of fruitarianism you refer to is not entirely wrong. In the overly toxic woman, menstruation can *also* serve as a means of voiding bodily impurities. Women with weakened kidneys or who are chronically constipated, often have heavier and more odorous menstruations. It has also been noticed that adherence to an optimum, health-promoting, cleansing diet, as recommended in Chapters 3 and 4 of this book, will often result in a reduced menstrual flow. I receive many letters from women who change to the Optimum Diet and report on many remarkable improvements in their health and well-being; one very common observation which makes so many women happy is that their previously bothersome, profuse, and/or painful menstrual periods become easy and painless and of shorter duration.

The report that non-menstruating women have been known to become pregnant may not necessarily be untrue, either. The wishful thinking of the man to whom you refer, and his desire to prove his theories led to his delusion and misjudgement of what actually may have taken place. Just think of your own situation. You haven't menstruated for four years, and you are having sexual intercourse regularly. Your absence of menstruation could have been caused by poor health, malnutrition, or a run-down condition. If you optimize your diet and maximize your health level, your ovulation may begin any time, let's say, next month. If you are active sexually and happen to have intercourse during the *very first* ovulation, you may become pregnant—*before* the first menstruation. Menstruation usually occurs about fourteen days after ovulation, but if you were already pregnant, it, of course, would not come at all. Also, because of the strain of delivery and lactation, you may not begin to menstruate for months, possibly a year, after giving birth. Under such circumstances, it would be easy to be deceived into the delusion that conception took place with a complete absence of the normal monthly cycle of ovulation and menstruation. Especially if you are a "true believer" with the zeal of a faddist!

So, to answer your direct question about the possibility of becoming pregnant in the absence of ovulation and menstruation, the answer is a definite *no,* except in the hypothetical circumstances described above. And since you can never know ahead of time when your ovulation will resume, you run the risk of becoming pregnant any month if you are active sexually.

Sex During Pregnancy

Q. My husband has a strong libido, but since I became pregnant three months ago, I do not feel as interested in sex, as before. I am willing to please my husband, though, if sex is OK now and would not hurt the baby. Is it harmful to have sex during pregnancy, and could intercourse hurt the baby?

A. No two women, neither two men, react exactly the same way to pregnancy. Some women, especially those who were bothered by the use of contraceptives, feel more free during pregnancy and enjoy sex even more. Some develop distaste for intercourse, possibly because of a conscious or unconscious fear of hurting the fetus. Men, too, vary in their attitude toward sex during pregnancy. Some find pregnant women beautiful and desirable; for some, her changing figure is a turn-off, sexually. They, too, are often afraid that vigorous intercourse may harm the baby.

It is important that during pregnancy a couple show a greater concern for each other and a consideration for each other's feelings. This is the time of life when a couple can grow closer together, bound by a new purpose in their lives, when their love for each other is given an opportunity to grow a new dimension and reach a higher plateau. Their sexual activity during pregnancy, must, therefore, be guided by the above-mentioned psychological considerations.

Strictly physically and medically speaking, here are some answers that most medical experts in our Western culture would agree with:

• Generally speaking, intercourse is permitted throughout pregnancy until the last few weeks, when— some doctors feel—vigorous sex might possibly cause premature rupture of the membranes.

• It is virtually impossible to harm the fetus in the uterus even by vigorous intercourse. The fetus is well protected by a bony pelvis and the womb where it floats in fluids. Even if you happen to feel the baby moving or kicking during intercourse, it may have nothing to do with your sexual activity.

• The answer to the question, "is it harmful to have an orgasm during pregnancy?" is *no.*

• As pregnancy progresses, it would be wise to use positions during intercourse that avoid undue pressure on the abdomen. For example, man approaching from the side or back, or woman-on-top position can be more comfortable.

• If the woman has a history of miscarriages, she must abstain from intercourse for the first three months of pregnancy, then follow her doctor's advice.

• Intercourse should be curtailed and your doctor consulted if:

    a) your "bag of waters" has broken

    b) you have vaginal bleeding, itching, or discharge

    c) you feel pain in the vagina or abdomen.

Baby's Teeth

Q. Today I noticed in my 8-month-old daughter her first brand new tooth coming in. Since I had such very bad teeth as a child and was so self conscious about it, what can I do to make sure that my daughter will have perfect teeth?

A. Most parents don't start thinking about their baby's teeth until the first one begins to emerge. But, according to Dr. Beryl Slome, of the University of North Carolina School of Dentistry, calcification, the process of laying down enamel on the tooth surface, begins in the fourth or fifth month of pregnancy. By the time a baby is born, not only are her so-called baby teeth completely formed, but also her permanent front teeth have started to form.

This shows you that to assure perfect teeth for your daughter, you should have started a careful "tooth-building program" during the early months of your pregnancy—preferably even before conception.

The program of optimum nutrition and special vitamins and mineral supplements, as advocated in Chapters 3 and 4 of this book, if started one year before conception and continued throughout pregnancy and lactation, will give you the best possible assurance that your child will have better teeth than you had. Of course, to make sure that all of your children have good dental health throughout life, they should be breast-fed, they must continue with optimal nutrition after they are weaned, avoid all refined sugar and sweets, drink 1 - 2 glasses of raw cow's or goat's milk a day, take mineral and vitamin supplements such as bone meal, brewer's yeast, kelp, dolomite, "Nature's Minerals," vitamin C, and cod liver oil for A and D (see Chapter 9 for dosages).

Premature Sexuality

Q. My daughter, who is nearing the age of fourteen, is developing an inferiority complex because she still hasn't started menstruating and her figure is still that of a child, while all of her girl friends in school look like bosomy grownups. I've tried to tell her not to worry, that nature will take its course in due time, but she is not convinced. Should we go to a doctor for hormone shots?

A. Please, don't be concerned, and try to convince your daughter not to be concerned, and just wait a little longer. Most importantly, do not give her hormones or drugs to speed up her physical development. She may suffer severe consequences from such treatment for the rest of her life. As you said, nature, indeed, will take its course, and she will soon catch up with her girlfriends.

Actually, you and your daughter should be happy for her prolonged "childhood." Early sexual maturity in girls is a relatively recent development, and an undesirable development at that. The female body is designed to mature slowly and today's early puberty is the result of our denatured diets, especially the excess of sugar and refined carbohydrates and sex-hormone (DES) contaminated meats, accompanied by a lack of exercise.

Studies made in the United States and Europe show that menarche (the beginning of menstruation) has been occurring at steadily earlier ages for the past century. While one hundred years ago the typical age of menarche was about fourteen to fifteen (and in Scandinavian countries as late as seventeen), today it is about twelve.[1] The average doctor will attribute this to "better nutrition" in affluent countries. This concept, however, is challenged by Otto Schaefer, M.D., who has studied this phenomenon extensively.[2] He has found that "primitive" natives in many countries, who enjoyed nearly perfect health on their "deficient" native diets, when exposed to the "better nutrition" of the Westerners, with processed, refined foods, and plenty of sugar, not only soon began to suffer from all the diseases of civilized man, such as diabetes, obesity, acne, gallbladder disorders, atherosclerosis, and tooth decay, but also within a couple of generations the girls developed a two-year advancement of the beginning of puberty. It would be difficult to argue that such pathological manifestations of a Westernized diet occur because of "better nutrition." Dr. Schaefer, on the basis of his extensive studies, concluded that "earlier puberty and more rapid growth are both closely linked to the epidemiology of civilization afflictions like diabetes, atherosclerotic cardiovascular disease, and obesity."[2] He also suggested that heavy sugar consumption in Western cultures speeds up growth and sexual development by overstimulating the endocrine and hormone systems. And, as I am sure you know, both growth and sexual development are regulated by hormones. Excessive sugar intake stimulates the production of the hormone insulin. Since there is a delicate balance and interrelationship between the function of all hormones, the overstimulation of any part of the hormonal system may upset the workings of hormones throughout the body, including the hormones involved in sexual maturity.

I mentioned earlier that a sedentary life and reduced physical activity in children is another factor involved in premature puberty. Studies show that the average age of the onset of menstruation for girls involved in school athletics is 13.58 years, while the average age for non-athletes is 12.23 years[3]—more than a year's difference! So, excessive sugar consumption, our overprocessed diets, hormone residues in meat and poultry, and lack of exercise are factors that are responsible for the earlier sexual maturity in our adolescents today.

With teenage pregnancies increasing each year (with over one million pregnancies a year—and at an earlier and earlier age) you should be happy that your daughter is maturing at a normal (rather than an accelerated) rate. "It is neither normal nor good for girls to begin menstruation as early as most do today."[4]

Plugged Duct

Q. I have a slight swelling with a red spot on my breast. It is very sore to the touch. I have a three-month-old baby whom I nurse. What is this, and what can be done for it?

A. You more than likely have a plugged duct. Flu-like symptoms may also be associated with this condition. According to the La Leche League International, the best treatment for this is complete bed rest for 24 to 48 hours, along with nursing as much as possible on the sore breast.

Also, a castor oil pack may be applied to the breast. This is done by saturating a cloth with castor oil and applying to the breast. Cover with plastic wrap, place soft dry towel and heating pad over this. It should remain on as much as possible between nursings. After a castor oil pack, wash breast carefully with warm water and soap before nursing. Care should be taken to prevent chilling the breast when removing the heating pad.

With the above-mentioned treatments, accompanied by adequate diet and extra vitamin C (2,000 to 3,000 mg. a day) the plugged duct condition should clear up in a few days. If swelling and soreness persists, you must see your doctor, as the symptoms may be indicative of a more serious problem.

Mother-Daughter Sex Talk

Q. I have two daughters, eight and ten. In our church, we are opposed to sex education in school. My mother never told me anything about sex or the function of sex organs. Somehow, I learned most from other girls—and boys! Now, I am wondering about my daughters: should I have a mother-daughter talk with them and explain the basic functions of the sex organs? Or should I just let them find out on their own?

A. Please, please! Have a "mother-daughter sex talk" with them, as soon as possible! Every time this topic of sex education comes up, I remember the tragic story told by Rev. Chad Varah explaining how he got involved in sexual counseling as a young priest in England, more than forty years ago: "I had to officiate at the funeral of a teen-age girl who had committed suicide when her menstrual periods started because she thought she had venereal disease."

Early sex education is especially important for girls so that they are well prepared for the physical and emotional changes that puberty involves. Personally, I believe that outside of the elementary reproductive function discussion in the school's biology class, sex education of children is the responsibility of parents. Father-son and mother-daughter frank, open, and factual talks, explaining the sexual differences, functions, and changes, as children grow up, should be done well before puberty. If you do not feel qualified to explain sexual functions, use a good home encyclopedia or home medical book. But, sex education of children is your—the parents'—responsibility! Don't shirk it and "just let them find out on their own." The most natural and least traumatic way for a young girl to learn intimate things about her body and the purpose and functions of her sex organs is from her mother.

Streak Ovaries

Q. I am eighteen years old, and have what my doctor diagnosed as "streak ovaries." My doctor prescribed the hormone, Premarin, which he said I must take daily for the rest of my life. I have been taking it for a year, but now I am worried since I read somewhere about the carcinogenic effect of the Pill, and other sex-hormone containing drugs. I would like to know:

1. What exactly are "streak ovaries"?
2. Are there natural substitutes for synthetic hormone drugs which are completely harmless?
3. Are there health risks involved if I continue taking Premarin?
4. Is there anything in the vitamin or natural food line I can take that will undo the possible damage caused by the drug?

A. "Streak ovaries" is a descriptive medical term for a condition where the ovaries have failed to develop and the area where the ovary should have normally developed is really only a fibrous band referred to as a streak.

Since, functionally speaking, you have no ovaries, you will have no ovulation or menstruation and you will be sterile for all of your life. Streak ovaries means that you have no ovarian tissue at all, so there is no point in trying to make the ovaries function by any kind of medical or alternative interference.

The reason your doctor insists that you take Premarin (a natural estrogen substitute made from the urine of pregnant mares) is that you do not have a sufficient level of estrogen supply in your body which would normally be produced by your ovaries. Although estrogen is produced in small quantities by the adrenal glands and other organs in your body, this limited supply is not sufficient to maintain normal female functions, such as the maintenance of female sex characteristics, the development of breasts, youthful, feminine figure, and the proper development and the function of the genital tract. Without sufficient female hormones, your breasts will not develop (and if they have already developed they will slowly decrease in size), the vagina will become very thin-walled, dry, and subject to infections as well as pain during intercourse, and the distribution of fat on your body will be abnormal. Without a substitute for what you would normally be receiving from your own ovaries, you not only will be unable to function as a normal female, but you will also age prematurely.

Now, to the risks connected with hormone drugs. You already know that by taking supplementary estrogen you do subject yourself to the increased risk of cancer, especially uterine cancer. Studies show that women on Premarin-type estrogen therapy had about five to twelve times greater risk of developing cancer of the uterine lining (see Chapter 25). Now some studies show that estrogen replacement therapy increases the incidence of blood clots in legs and brain, and increases the chances of heart attacks and breast cancer as well. Therefore, you have to weigh carefully and thoughtfully the pros and cons of estrogen medication. You must consider accepting a certain health risk which comes with estrogen medication against the overall long-term effect of severe estrogen deficiency that you would suffer from in your condition. If you allow your body to function without estrogen for any length of time, the changes that will occur in your body, inwardly and outwardly, would be very difficult, if not impossible, to reverse—even if you would decide to take the hormone in the future.

On the positive side, the risk of taking estrogen medication in your case would be relatively minor when compared to the effect of the birth control pill or the menopausal estrogen-replacement therapy. You see, in the above-mentioned cases, the estrogen is aded to the body's own normal supply—in your case the medication will be virtually the only source of hormone. But again, only you can make a decision and the choice. The reason I go into such detail in explaining all this is that I want you to make an intelligent choice, based on the thorough knowledge of the benefits and drawbacks of such medications.

As far as your other question is concerned:

1. There are natural estrogen-containing herbs and foods, such as licorice, Mexican wild yam, sarsaparilla, black cohosh, elder, and unicorn root, but their estrogen content is too small for your purpose, although they can be used during menopause or after a hysterectomy to supplement the body's own diminished production (see Chapters 23 and 24). Perhaps by using them regularly you can decrease the dosage of Premarin.

2. As far as nutritional protection against the possible damage caused by estrogen medication is concerned, the following vitamins and supplements (to be used in conjunction with optimum nutrition as described in Chapters 3 and 4) have a protective property against all cancers, including those caused by drugs: C, A, E, B-complex, B_{15}, brewer's yeast, selenium, lecithin, and kelp. For dosages, see Chapter 25. The same chapter also reports in detail why these supplements are effective protective factors against cancer.

Infertility

Q. My husband and I have been married for six years. At first we didn't want children and used contraception, but now we have been trying hard to have a child, but don't seem to be able. We have sex regularly, two - three times a week—still no pregnancy. My periods, though, are very irregular, and sometimes I do not menstruate for several months. What's wrong? What shall we do?

A. Today, a shocking 20 - 25 percent of American couples can't have children! Medically speaking, failure to conceive can be caused by total infertility or low sperm count in the male, or ovulation disorder or failure to ovulate in the female. The factors involved in these underlying causes of infertility can be many, both physical and emotional. Here are some suggestions that may help in your case:

1. First, your husband should go to a doctor and have the quality of his sperm checked. If the sperm count is low, it could be the result of a functional disorder such as caused by varicocele (varicose veins in the scrotum) or even such a thing as excessive heat in the scrotum. Sperm cannot be manufactured in excessive heat. Even heat from too hot showers, baths, or saunas, as well as tight fitting underwear or pants, or electric blankets at night, can be damaging to the sperm production. Suggest to your husband that he take cold showers several times a day, especially a few hours before sexual intercourse. Cold sitz-baths are also effective (see my *How to Get Well* book for instructions).

2. If your periods are irregular, that means your ovulation is irregular, too. You can only conceive during ovulation, which is usually about 14 days before menstruation (see Chapter 22). Try to have intercourse during the most fertile 2 or 3 days right before or at the time of ovulation.

3. To help normalize your menstrual cycle and to improve the chances of conception, take the following supplements daily:

Vitamin E—600 I.U.

Wheat germ—2 - 3 tablespoons; make sure it is fresh

Wheat germ oil—2 - 3 teaspoons; again, make sure it is fresh

Bioflavonoids—500 mg.

Vitamin C—1,000 mg.

B-complex tablets

Multi-mineral tablets, such as "Nature's Minerals"

Zinc—15 - 20 mg.

Cod liver oil—1 tablespoon

Your husband can benefit from taking these same supplements, too.

Bust Size and Firmness

Q. Is there anything one can do nutritionally or through natural therapy for small breasts? Or to keep breasts firm? I am 34 years old and very "flat"—I mean very, very! Short of silicon implants, what can I do?

A. First, I am very much against silicon implants—too little is known of their possible pathogenic effect.

Exercise of the pectoral muscles, with or without special exercisers, will cause the breasts to protrude further, although this will not actually increase the breast size itself. Research shows that women who live in dry, mountainous climates tend to have larger breasts than those from low, wet climates; and a cold climate causes breasts to remain firmer than a hot one. Massage, with or without vitamin E, tends to help breasts become firmer, due to the swelling caused by stimulation.

Dr. Melvin Page reports remarkable success with a pituitary hormone therapy. You can ask a nutritionally-oriented doctor about it. Reversing the gravitational pull by doing headstands regularly might be helpful for firmness. Some doctors administer female hormones on the premise that a low sex hormone output is responsible for small breasts, which are secondary female sex organs. Hormone therapy, is, however, not always successful. If you wish to consider it, make sure by proper tests that your hormone level is actually low; otherwise you may be increasing the risk of contracting cancer. This applies to the pituitary hormone treatment as well.

No doubt dietary heredity plays a role in breast development, and a general optimum diet should help in prevention of abnormally small or flabby, sagging busts in future generations.

Keep in mind that in most cases of underdeveloped breasts the condition is corrected by itself as soon as a woman becomes pregnant—nature's way to assure that the baby can be breast-fed.

Finally, if none of the tips for breast enlargement mentioned here work for you, think of all those of us—and we are legion—who think that small breasts are very beautiful!

However, if you insist on trying to enlarge your breasts, the following perfectly harmless natural supplements and herbs will help increase the estrogen levels in the body and may contribute to the development of larger breasts:

PABA (para-amino-benzoic acid)
Vitamin C
Vitamin E
Vitamin B$_6$
Folic acid
Glutamic acid
Licorice root, blue cohosh, unicorn roots, sarsaparilla, and Mexican wild yam.

Health food stores carry all of these. The above-mentioned herbs should not be used by pregnant women.

Poor Sexual Response

Q. I am in my early 60's and had a complete hysterectomy about twelve years ago because of a growth. I am in good health, take a full complement of vitamins, am happily married, and lead an active life. During the past five or six years, I have found that my sexual responses are very poor most of the time, and even when I feel aroused emotionally, there is never a vaginal flow at the time of intercourse. I use petroleum jelly, but this obviously is not ideal either for me or my husband. I find the petroleum jelly irritating, and wonder if anything else could be used instead.

Is the change that has taken place in me irreversible, or is there anything that could help at all? I've felt too inhibited to discuss this with my doctor, and would appreciate your advice.

A. It is rather common that with age, the vaginal lubrication is diminished. This is due to several factors, but low sex-hormone levels is the most likely factor in your case. At the end of the reproductive cycle, the hormone-producing glands, such as the ovaries, become inactive. Also, the lowered levels of other endocrine hormones, such as thyroid, pituitary, and adrenal hormones, can contribute to diminished sexual interest and/or response. Likewise, dietary lack of the following vitamins, or the body's inability to utilize them properly, can contribute to the symptoms you describe: vitamin B_6, vitamin E, vitamin D, and vitamin A. The lack of hydrochloric acid in older people is one of the common causes of mineral deficiencies, because without sufficient hydrochloric acid many important minerals cannot be properly assimilated. It is well-known that severe deficiencies of calcium and magnesium can result in shriveled sex glands, as well as other endocrine glands, and a consequent loss of sex interest. Needless to say, chronic fatigue, depression, boredom, and mental and physical stresses can drive away the ecstacy from the bedroom and contribute to vaginal dryness.

To answer your question whether your lack of sexual response is permanent, or if it can be corrected, I am inclined to believe that if you build up your physical and mental health to the optimum level, take specific vitamins and hormone-containing herbs recommended in Chapter 34, and will continue to show warmth, tenderness, and love towards your husband and meet without inhibitions his sexual and emotional needs, your body will respond with normalizing all its functions and secretions, including those in the vagina. Physiologically speaking, the vaginal dryness need not be associated with aging.

Preventing Hysterectomy

Q. What would you suggest as a preventative for a hysterectomy?

A. Hysterectomy is a surgical removal of the uterus, sometimes also the ovaries. It is not a condition or disease. To avoid a hysterectomy, you must avoid anything and everything that leads to a uterus so badly diseased that it must be removed.

Here are some of the causes that have been shown to be involved or linked to the pre-cancerous or cancerous development which is the most common reason for hysterectomies:

1. Prolonged use of birth control pills.

2. Prolonged use of any birth control device, such as I.U.D.'s, foams, diaphragms, etc.

3. Prolonged estrogen replacement therapy as treatment for menopause or post-menopause, even with such "natural" preparations as Premarin.

4. Untreated vaginal infections.

5. General lowered resistance to disease due to health-destroying mode of living, especially inadequate diet, smoking, lack of exercise and sufficient rest, emotional and physical stresses, etc.

The total avoidance of the above-mentioned contributing factors and the adherence to a health-building lifestyle and Optimum Diet as advocated in this book, will give you the best possible assurance in the future that a hysterectomy can be prevented.

Migraine Headaches

Q. Is there any solution to migraine headaches except to grin and bear it?

A. Although the exact cause of migraine headaches seems to be unknown, some research indicates that it is a basic inherited metabolic defect that makes a person prone to migraines.

In Great Britain, research has been done on the detection of a biochemical defect present in some migraine sufferers. There is an alteration in the body's final handling of certain foods which contain tyramine, phenylethylamine, and other amines.

Tyramine is present in cheese, wine, and citrus fruits. Phenylethylamine is present in chocolate and alcohol, especially in colored rum, rye, scotch, red wine, and beer. A migraine attack may develop up to 24 hours after ingestion of such items. There seems to be many trigger factors which can set off a migraine attack. Of course, not all the factors would apply to one sufferer. These trigger factors can be grouped under the following headings: dietary; hormonal; stress; weather; and low blood sugar. Stress covers both mental and physical strain, as well as the stress caused by drugs, chemicalized environment, etc.

Migraine sufferers should avoid foods mentioned above that contain the offensive amines. The diet should be predominantly alkaline, with emphasis on fruits and vegetables and sprouted seeds. Eat frequent small meals. Avoid overeating.

Plenty of exercise in fresh air is imperative. Deep breathing exercises are of specific importance. If constipated, the problem should be corrected, since constipation is one of the most common trigger factors. See Chapter 31 regarding an anti-constipation program.

The following supplements are suggested for daily use by migraine sufferers:

Niacin—up to 300 mg. (100 mg. 3 times daily)
B_{15}, calcium pangamate—150 mg.
B-complex, with B_{12}
Pantothenic acid—100 mg.
Magnesium—400 mg.
Brewer's yeast—2 tbsp.
Rutin—200 mg.
E—up to 1200 I.U.
Selenium—50 mcg.
B_6—50 mg.
C—2,000 mg.

Calcium—1,000 mg.
Garlic capsules or tablets—3
"Nature's Minerals"—5 tablets

Cellulite

Q. Would you have any suggestions or solutions to the fibrositis, or more commonly-called cellulite (orange-rind syndrome)? It seems to be prevalent in females only. I have it on the upper thigh, which seems to be the most common place. Medical doctors don't seem to know too much about the condition or its cause (or care to know about it, considering it to be of purely cosmetic significance). I am a natural food-oriented person, take ample vitamin supplements, and get plenty of exercise. My thighs are very unsightly, and I would appreciate any information or suggestions relating to this, particularly to the cause of the condition.

A. I think you are confusing fibrositis with cellulite. They are two different conditions. Fibrositis is an excessive growth of *fibrous* tissue, usually due to an injury or inflammation, such as that which takes place around the shoulder involved in bursitis, or in tennis elbow. Cellulite is an excessive growth of *fatty* tissue. Sometimes, both fibrositis and cellulite condition can occur simultaneously, however.

The exact cause of excessive cellulite buildup is not known, but most experts agree that the primary cause is excessive caloric intake, especially in the form of fatty foods, oils, and concentrated fats, and the consequent obesity. The secondary cause could be hormonal imbalances, especially the excess of female sex hormones. Thyroid insufficiency can also be involved.

In my experience, the most effective way to get rid of cellulite is by prolonged juice fasting therapy, combined with vigorous massage, strenuous exercise, and severe caloric restriction. When your caloric expenditure exceeds the calories supplied by the diet, your body will be forced to consume its own fat deposits. Naturally, all junk foods, especially those containing refined sugar and white flour, should be eliminated, as they are easily converted into fat in the body. Following the general reducing program recommended in Chapter 33 of this book will help more than anything else in solving your cellulite problem.

Broken Capillaries

Q. I have what I think are broken capillaries showing on the outsides of my thighs, behind my knees, and they are starting to appear around my ankles. I am 22, and very self-conscious about this. What causes this problem, and how can it be reversed?

A. I don't know if you can reverse it, but you certainly can prevent the worsening of the condition and the development of new blue webs on your body. Often this condition is associated with pregnancy, overweight, or nutritional deficiencies. Capillary fragility is usually associated with a bioflavonoid deficiency. Minerals and vitamins C and E are also involved, as well as choline.

I would advise an adequate nutritional support, such as my Optimum Diet (see Chapters 3 and 4), plus the following specific vitamin and mineral supplements daily:

Rutin—200 mg.
Bioflavonoids—300 mg.
Vitamin C—3,000 mg.
Vitamin E—600 I.U.
Lecithin—2 tsp. granules
Bone meal, raw—3 tablets
"Nature's Minerals"—5 tablets

Buckwheat, millet, sesame seeds, and vitamin C-rich fruits are good foods for your capillaries.

Gaining Weight

Q. Today people are becoming aware of excessive weight problems and possible dangers to health. But, very little is said about thin people. How can one gain weight?

A. The best foods to gain weight on are raw nuts and seeds, such as almonds, brazil nuts, peanuts, sesame seeds, pumpkin seeds (all finely ground before consuming) and cooked grains such as cooked cereals, breads, beans, corn tortillas. Old fashioned oatmeal is rather fattening, in my experience. Some of the above-mentioned "fattening" foods could be used at every meal, plus between meals as snacks. Eating a relatively large meal late in the evening will also help to put on weight. Also, eat 2 tbsp. of vegetable oil (olive or sesame seed oil) every day, or its equivalent in butter.

The above advice is given with a heavy heart, since I've met only two persons in the United States that were truly too thin and could benefit from gaining weight. My usual advice to those who think they are too thin is to thank the Lord for what is actually a blessing, not a problem. According to insurance companies' statistics, thin people not only have less degenerative diseases, but outlive fat people by ten or more years. As Dr. C.M. McCays, of Cornell University, who did extensive animal studies on relationship between overweight and premature death, put it, "The thin rats bury the fat rats."

Will Exercise Cause Weight Gain?

Q. I have great difficulty in keeping my weight down. I am always ten to fifteen pounds overweight. I have tried exercise, especially walking and jogging. But, now, I read that exercises only increase your appetite, so you eat more and get fatter. Is this true or false?

A. False. A recent study, conducted at the University of California at Irvine under the direction of Dr. Grant Gwinup and reported in the publication of the American Medical Association, showed that obese persons lose plenty of weight by exercise alone, without any dietary changes.[5] In this study, 11 obese women lost from 10 to 38 pounds, an average 22 pound loss, during the period of one year—on exercise alone. Dr. Gwinup said that brisk walks, preferably two to three hours, are the best form of exercise for reducing.

It stands to reason that a combination of exercise, which can take off a half a pound or more a week, with a low-calorie Optimum Diet, as described in Chapter 33, will bring the best results.

Bran and Weight Loss

Q. I have heard that wheat bran is helpful in weight loss, as it helps in quicker passing of food through the digestive tract—and, therefore, there is less calorie absorption. Is this correct? Would this and regular exercise help me to lose those extra pounds?

A. The answer to both of your questions is yes. Bran is practically 100 percent undigestible cellulose. It fills you up without supplying fat-producing calories. Also, it speeds up the elimination of food from the digestive tract, reducing the absorption of calories.

However, the problem of overweight is much more complicated than this, and should be approached from many different angles, which are described in detail in Chapter 33.

Bloodshot Eyes

Q. My eyes have been bloodshot for years. The doctor says I have perfect vision and have no eye problems. I have been on your Optimum Diet for over a year, and I take all the natural supplements, such as cod liver oil, brewer's yeast, etc., plus we bake all our own bread. I sleep eight hours a night and run two miles a day. My question is, if the eyes are the mirror of the state of the whole body, why won't mine clear up? Do some people have bloodshot eyes like others go bald, regardless? Do you think that my eyes will eventually clear up, or will I always have this characteristic? Many of my friends who are junk food eaters have very clear eyes. What can you advise?

A. As you speculate, some people have a predisposition for one thing, some for another. Although you are in good health *generally,* your eyes may be your weak area, so that even a "normal" amount of stress may affect them.

Bloodshot eyes usually are symptomatic of a B_2 deficiency. Brewer's yeast, which you take, does contain B_2, but not in sufficient amounts to correct a severe deficiency. Try a high-potency B-complex supplement which is 100 percent natural, 3 - 4 tablets a day. Also take an isolated B_2 supplement, a 100 mg. tablet twice a day for four weeks. Then reduce to 50 mg. a day for several more weeks. In addition, take 20,000 units of vitamin A, 600 I.U. of vitamin E, 1,000 mg. of vitamin C, 50 mg. of pantothenic acid, and 50 mg. of vitamin B_6 daily for at least several months, and continue with your cod liver oil and brewer's yeast powder, which you have mentioned. These supplements, in addition to an Optimum Diet and avoidance of excessive stress on your eyes, especially reading and TV watching, will, I am sure, clear your red eyes within a few weeks. If they don't clear up, they must be affected by some stubborn, chronic infectious condition, in which case you should see a doctor.

Gray Hair, Stress, Melanine, and Nutrition

Q. I read in a book (not yours) that melanine, the coloring matter in hair, is affected by stress. What exactly is melanine? And, where or in what foods, can melanine be found?

A. Melanine is the dark brown pigment that occurs in the skin, in the hair, and in other organs, such as the eyes, etc. It is not a nutrient, and cannot be obtained from foods—it is manufactured by the body for its own needs. The thought that severe mental stress can affect the color of the hair is medically substantiated. There are recorded cases where severe traumatic mental shock resulted in a rapid graying of the hair. I am sure you are aware of the fact that severe and prolonged mental stress can contribute to the development of virtually every disease in the medical book.

Graying of the hair is also definitely related to nutritional deficiencies. There are many recorded cases of excellent results of hair recoloring through improved nutrition. There are also many failures. You must realize that nutrition is a two-phase process. One, the quality of your nutritional intake; two, your body's ability to assimilate ingested nutrients. You may take all the nutrients that are needed for hair health, but if your assimilation is defective, your hair will not be receiving them.

Nutritionally speaking, foods rich in B-vitamins, such as brewer's yeast, nuts, grains, fresh wheat germ, lecithin, etc., are extremely important for the health of the hair. Russian studies also show that vitamins A, C, and E play important roles in restoring hair color. Minerals are not to be overlooked in a hair recoloring program, especially zinc, copper, calcium, magnesium, and silicon. Isolated B-vitamins that are effective in restoring natural color to gray hair are PABA, pantothenic acid, folic acid, biotin, B_6, inositol, choline, and niacin. Blackstrap molasses contains important nutritive elements needed for maintaining hair color.

There are many herbs which have been traditionally used for the maintenance of healthy hair, such as horsetail, nettles, parsley, kelp, onions, and cayenne pepper—all taken internally. But, sage and nettles, together or separately, steeped in boiling water for several hours, can be used for a hair rinse (see Chapter 32 for additional information on hair rinses).

Keep in mind, however, that hair recoloring is a very slow process. It usually takes six to twelve months of persistent and uninterrupted supplementation and dietary regime to accomplish visible results. A holistic approach is best even in regard to the health of the hair. The hair is a part of the whole body and reflects the health status of the entire system. And, since every nutrient influences the total health, the Optimum Diet, which supplies an adequate amount of all important nutrients for the maintenance of general health, is imperative for healthy and natural colored hair as well.

Mood-Altering Drugs

Q. After my divorce three years ago, my doctor prescribed Valium because of my anxieties and depression. Since then, I've heard that Valium can be addictive. Several times I've tried to stop taking it, but I get severe withdrawal reaction: I become depressed to the point of despondency. Although my doctor says that Valium is not physically addictive, I am beginning to wonder. Am I hooked on it, and must I take it for the rest of my life? What should I do?

A. Addiction to legally-prescribed drugs is a growing health problem in America—especially among women. American doctors write more than 75 million prescriptions a year for tranquilizers, including more than 50 million prescriptions for Valium alone. Other close chemical relatives to Valium are Librium, Serax, Tranxene, and Dalmane. Miltown and Equanil are other commonly-prescribed tranquilizers.

Addiction to tranquilizers is largely a female problem. More than two thirds of all the prescriptions for mood-altering drugs are written to women. The National Institute on Drug Abuse estimates that 32 million American women, or 42 percent of all adult women, have used tranquilizers, compared to only 19 million, or 27 percent, of the men. It is estimated that between 5 and 6 million women have been taking prescription drugs long enough to begin the addiction process.

Yes, mood-altering drugs can be addictive, *if taken for a prolonged time.* The body gradually builds up a tolerance to them. As a result, the user must increase the dose to get the same effect. Also, most tranquilizers and sedatives produce a "rebound effect" when they wear off, which means that the feelings of anxiety or depression that the drug was supposed to relieve can come back stronger than ever. In addition, the increased doses of mood-altering drugs can be toxic. Gradually-built-up toxic levels can cause such symptoms as drowsiness, poor muscular coordination, inability to concentrate, irritability, and even such physical symptoms as nausea, skin eruptions, edema, and menstrual irregularities.

The problem is compounded when tranquilizers are taken in combination with alcohol. Alcohol magnifies the effect of drugs on both mind and body. A recent national monitoring program revealed about a thousand accidental deaths within a year involving mood-altering prescription drugs, usually taken in combination with alcohol.

Unlike alcoholism, which has long been recognized as a disease, and unlike the drug addiction to such illicit "street drugs" as heroin or cocaine, the abuse of legally-prescribed mood-altering drugs has received little attention from medical, scientific, or law-enforcement sources. In fact, in the American culture, the use of prescription drugs and alcohol are as socially acceptable as coffee or tea. But, as Muriel Nellis, head of the federally-funded study of the impact of drugs and alcohol put it, "Women throughout the nation are in dreadful trouble because of overused combinations of prescription drugs and alcohol."[6]

To answer your direct question: you may be addicted to Valium already *if you have taken it for three years.* But, the sooner you stop taking the drug, the sooner you'll break the dependence and prevent even greater damage to your mind and body that the drug would eventually cause. You may experience the more or less severe symptoms of withdrawal. These can be minimized by taking large amounts of vitamin C (which is an effective detoxifier), magnesium, calcium (tranquilizers usually cause severe magnesium and calcium deficiencies), high-potency B-complex and brewer's yeast (which will help to stabilize your nervous system), and vitamin A (which is also usually depleted by drugs). Optimum nutrition as described in this book, and sufficient rest, relaxation, and daily vigorous exercise are also important in effective breaking of drug dependence and building of optimal physical and mental health.

Vegetarian Mother's Breast Milk

Q. I read in my local paper recently that the breast milk of vegetarian mothers was found to contain dangerous amounts of PCB and pesticide residues. The tone of the article was that nursing mothers would be better off eating meat. Is this true?

A. The contrary is true. In a French study in 1974, it was found that vegetarian women had 50 to 60 percent less PCB and pesticide residues in their milk than the French women who ate meat. Also, a recent extensive American study by the prestigious U.S. Environmental Defense Fund, showed the same preliminary results. Although the study is not yet concluded, and the data is still being tabulated, the existing data indicates that the breast milk of vegetarian women contains one-third to two-thirds less PCB's and pesticide residues than that of their meat-eating counterparts. The vegetarian women who took part in the recent American study were not necessarily eating an "organic food" diet.[7]

Abortion - Health Risks

Q. I have what is called an unwanted pregnancy, and I am considering an abortion. What health risks are involved?

A. First, the moral, religious, and psychological ramifications of abortion must be taken into careful consideration by each individual who considers abortion.

I believe in the sanctity of life and the importance of motherhood. I realize that there are circumstances which might cause a woman to consider an abortion as a medical and/or socio-medical necessity. When the health or life of a woman is threatened by pregnancy, her physician might be considering the termination of the pregnancy as an alternative. There are also pregnancies that result from violent crimes of rape.

If you are considering an abortion, you should carefully evaluate the risks involved and the consequences of it. I suggest you consider the following advice carefully:

1. Do not rush "below the border" to a quack who may cripple you for life or even kill you, neither run to an illegal abortionist in your home town. Abortion is, as any surgery, a severe shock to the body, and health risks exist. Once experiencing abortion, the body will be less likely to carry a pregnancy to full term. Thus, miscarriages are frequent in those who have undergone previous surgical abortions.

2. Do not make any hasty decisions on your own. Consult your family doctor or pediatrition. Also, discuss the issue with your closest friends and loved ones: the father of the baby, your parents, your minister, your teacher. When an unwanted pregnancy is discovered, or a medical problem in a pregnancy arises, the state of shock and despair makes it impossible to make a clear, logical and sensible decision without the help of very close and dear friends who are vitally concerned with your welfare and the welfare of your child.

Don't forget that you are within your rights to ask questions of your doctor, for the decision ultimately rests with you.

Children's Sleepwear

Q. I've read about possible harmfulness of children's sleepwear that has been treated with fire-retardant chemicals, especially with *TRIS*. I am very concerned now, and would like to know where I can buy children's clothes that are from natural, not synthetic, fabrics, and are free from dangerous chemicals. Also, can the flame-retardant be washed out of the fabric?

A. As late as 1972, over 50 percent of the children's sleepwear on the market was made from cotton; most of the remainder was cotton/polyester blends. Today, over 90 percent is made from synthetic fibers. This is deplorable, since synthetic fabrics are not only uncomfortable and "sweaty" (they don't breathe), but are also unhealthy. Many children have allergic reactions to synthetic fabrics and if a child has eczema or other skin disorders the condition if often aggravated by synthetic materials.

Regarding the flame-retardant fabrics: in 1972, the government passed a law, the Flammable Fabrics Act, which essentially prohibited the sale of untreated cotton sleepwear. Consequently, all manufacturers started treating fabrics chemically to make them flame-retardant. TRIS is one of the most commonly-used chemicals for this purpose. However, after studies by Dr. Bruce Ames, of the University of California, which showed that TRIS is a potent mutagen and possible carcinogen, and studies by the National Cancer Institute, which showed that TRIS is a definite carcinogen, were made public, the government finally banned its use in children's sleepwear (after TRIS had been used for five years). However, since some courts overruled the ban, TRIS is still being used, although on a smaller scale. Now manufacturers use "naturally" flame-retardant fabrics such as modacrylic, vinyon, or matrix—all synthetics.

I wish I could give you more satisfactory advice on how to avoid the use of synthetic and chemically-treated fabrics in your children's sleepwear than suggesting that you buy pure cotton fabrics and do your own sewing. Be careful when you buy fabrics, however, as even fabrics are often treated with fire-retardant chemicals—read the labels on the side of the bolts. The other choice is to buy untreated cotton in other countries if you happen to be traveling, or let your children sleep in cotton underwear, regular, or thermal.

Regarding the possibility of washing the flame-retardant chemical out of sleepwear: according to manufacturers' specifications, the flame-retarding characteristics last through 50 washings. However, the toxicity diminished with time. Anyone who buys flame-retardant sleepwear, should wash it at least three times prior to wearing.

What: A Bonnet On It?

Q. I have just returned from Europe where, I noticed, most babies and small children wear bonnets, or some other headcovering, when outside. In America, this custom would seem so old-fashioned. It occurred to me that perhaps the baby bonnet has a certain health significance. What is your opinion?

A. An important health significance, indeed!

America is going through a fashion craze—a hatless attire—that is causing far-reaching health problems in men and women, but especially in young children. For thousands of years, people of all races, nations, and tribes, anywhere on this planet, in cold, temperate, or tropical climates, traditionally covered their heads. In civilized countries, the type of covering varied with the fashions, but head coverings were never completely discarded until just the last two or three decades. My preliminary research into this phenomenon (and my research is still continuing) shows that the health-damaging consequences of this "hatless fashion craze," if it continues, can be nothing less than disastrous.

Here are a few reasons for such a gloomy pronouncement:

It is estimated that more than half of the body's heat is lost through the head. Especially in very cold weather, the heat quickly dissipates from the head, sapping the vital energies and depleting the body of life forces, causing severe stress on all organs and impairing all body functions. Not to mention the fact that the epidemics of colds, flus, sinusitis, tonsillitis, earaches, headaches, head colds, and rheumatic and arthritic conditions are often directly related to the exposure of the uncovered head to extremely cold temperatures.

Therefore, it really shakes my faith in the professed intelligence of Homo sapiens when I see men and women on the streets of our cities, walking or riding bikes, in sub-zero weather, wrapped in heavy coats and furs, with thick boots and heavy gloves—but *BARE HEADED!* Middle-aged and old men can be seen walking around, obviously cold, with coat collars turned up—*but without hats, snow falling on their bald heads!* At the other end of the spectrum, sunstroke and heatstroke are caused by exposure of the uncovered head to the intense heat and damaging rays of the sun.

The brain, vital glands, and nerve centers in the head can function at optimal efficiency only in the presence of constant temperatures. Too hot or too cold temperatures can affect brain function negatively. This must be one of the biological reasons for heavy hair growth on the head. Hair alone, however, cannot offer sufficient protection against temperature extremes, so hats are important even if you have a thick head of hair.

For babies and small children, uncovered heads may mean not only chronic earaches, colds, and infections during infancy and childhood, but eventual susceptibility to many of the chronic diseases in adulthood.

Yes, I am all for the baby bonnet! A wise mother should always have her baby's head covered when he is outside, and even inside when room temperatures are rather cold, or there is a draft. Do not let your baby's brains be cooked in the summer and frozen in the winter only because the current fashion does not call for a bonnet!

I know that my comments regarding the hatless fashion craze and its far-reaching ill effects on health may appear far-fetched and exaggerated. I do not anticipate an immediate acceptance of my contentions—it took at least ten years for most of my previous pioneering ideas to be widely accepted and recognized. My "hat theory" is not likely to be an exception. However, my research is turning up more and more evidence that it is not just a theory, but a workable hypothesis that has great scientific validity.

Early Pregnancy Test

Q. I've heard that there is now an easy, do-it-yourself pregnancy test, which can accurately detect pregnancy as early as nine days after a missed menstrual period. Is this true? If so, where can I get it and how do I use it correctly?

A. Yes, the EPT (Early Pregnancy Test) Kit was developed by a Dutch researcher in 1970, and is now available in the United States. It is sold without a prescription in most drug stores. The kit is inexpensive (around $10.00) and consists of a test tube, which contains chemicals that should detect a pregnancy hormone (HCG) in a woman's urine; a dropper; a vial with purified water; and a test tube holder with mirror.

To be effective, the test must be made no earlier than nine days after the menstrual period was due. The test is made by placing the purified water and three drops of urine in the tube, shaking the test tube for ten seconds, then letting the tube stand in the holder for two hours. If a dark brown ring forms in the bottom of the tube, as seen in the mirror, you can be 97 percent sure you are pregnant. If there no pregnancy, only a yellow-red deposit will be seen.

The early detection of pregnancy is of utmost importance in today's stress- pollution- and poison-filled world. The first days and weeks of pregnancy are crucial for the fetal development. Most birth defects are caused by a pregnant woman being subjected to the harmful effects of such agents as alcohol, smoking, drugs, X-rays, and environmental and household chemicals during the first 60 days of pregnancy. If an expectant mother detects pregnancy as early as nine days after the first missed menstrual period, she can take steps to avoid these environmental and other hazards and help prevent birth defects, as well as intrauterine death or miscarriage.

Pap Test: Dubious Validity

Q. My gynecologist surprised me during my last visit by telling me that medical opinion regarding the effectiveness and necessity of the Pap smear is in the process of a change, and that it is not necessary for me to have the test every year—a three-to-five-year interval is sufficient. All I've ever heard before was that yearly tests are an absolute must. Is there any substance to my gynecologist's attitude?

A. American woman have been urged since the early 1950's to have an annual Pap (named for its inventor, Dr. George Papanicolaou) smear as a screening test for cervical cancer. The need and wisdom of that recommendation has now been challenged, and both the American Cancer Society and the National Cancer Institute have subtly changed their recommendations, although *so* subtly that the majority of the American women are not aware of the policy change; your gynecologist apparently is.

About half the adult women in the U.S. have an annual Pap smear. The cost of mass annual screening, including office visit charges for women seeing their gynecologist solely for the annual test, runs into the millions. Now both Canadian and American studies show that "the results do not warrant the cost." American public health researcher Anne-Marie Foltz of New York University, and epidemiologist Jennifer Kelsey of Yale

University, charge that the Pap test became a yearly medical routine before its merits were established. The critics of the Pap test say that (1) the test is relatively inaccurate, (2) it's true efficacy is dubious. Although proponents of the test claim that it has helped reduce the incidence of invasive cervical cancer, they have no evidence to link the reduction with the test. Other factors, such as the increased number of hysterectomies, in which the cervix is almost always removed, may account for the decreased incidence. The possibility of an erroneous reading of the test—due either to the physician's taking an inadequate smear or the laboratory's misinterpreting it, may be over 30 percent. It is well known that many needless hysterectomies are performed on the basis of erroneous diagnosis.

Here are the current recommendations by Canadian and American authorities:

Canada: The first Pap test should be given at the age of 18 if the woman has had sexual relations. If the test is negative, another test should be administered after a year. If that, too, is negative, she should have the test every three years until the age of 35, then once every five years to age 60, and if the test is still negative, there is a need for further tests.

The National Cancer Institute (as advised by Dr. Margaret Sloan, of the NCI division of cancer control): The first Pap test should be given at age 20 or at the beginning of sexual activity. After two or three negative yearly tests, continue with tests at a three-to-five-year interval.

The American Cancer Society: While until two years ago it recommended annual Pap tests, it now advises "periodic" or "regular" testing.[8]

Dr. Emerson Day, Medical Director of the Cancer Prevention Center in Chicago, agrees with the current policy of the National Cancer Institute and the Canadian medical authorities. He says that the chances of discovering cancer of the uterus are not much different than if the test is done every two or three years. Basing his conclusion on findings in thousands of women who were tested during the past 25 years, he said, "I don't believe we need to repeat the Pap test each year.!"[9]

Fasting During Pregnancy

Q. I have read several of your health books; my favorite one is *Juice Fasting*. I have been on a juice fast many times with successful results. Each time has been for the losing of weight. I am getting closer and closer to my goal all the time. I now wish to go on another fast, but I think I may be pregnant. I am twenty-four years old and very healthy. I've fasted for as long as twenty-five days with no trouble. Please tell me: is it safe to fast during pregnancy?

A. I am delighted to hear that you enjoy juice fasting and are getting excellent results. But, as great as fasting is, it is *not* recommended during pregnancy or lactation. The biochemical changes in the body during fasting may affect the fetus unfavorably. Toxins released during fasting can reach the fetus through placenta. During lactation, fasting may result in diminished breast milk supply, or may affect the quality of the breast milk.

Baby's Weight Gain

Q. What is the ideal weight gain for a healthy baby? My baby seems much smaller than my best friend's baby (born at the same time) who is bottle-fed. I breast-feed my baby, and she seems to be healthy and happy, but I wonder if she should be gaining more.

A. For most babies, the ideal weight gain is two pounds a month, or one-half pound a week, during the first six months of life. For the second half of the baby's first year, weight gain should drop to one pound a month.

If your baby "seems healthy and happy," don't worry about slight differences in weight gain. After all, the above-quoted numbers are only the *average* weight gain— and you know your baby is anything but average! Your best friend's baby is bottle-fed and probably overweight; the truth is, most bottle-fed babies are overweight! And, overweight babies are not healthy. Not only do they have more trouble with diaper rash and diarrhea, and a higher number of respiratory infections than slim babies, but they will most likely suffer from obesity for the rest of their lives.

Age Spots

Q. My hands are covered with age spots, or what some people call liver spots. What causes them, and what can I do to get rid of these unattractive spots?

A. I wish I had a workable answer to this one. I do know that if you adhere to an optimum nutrition and a health-promoting lifestyle, your skin will stay younger longer and the unsightly brown age spots will be prevented until a very old age. But, once you've got them, I know of nothing that can effectively get rid of them. Oh, I've read and heard about all kinds of "age spot removers," but I've never seen any of them work. One popular health writer, now in his eighties, suggests the spots can be cleared up by an adequate intake of B_2 (riboflavin). Yet, he himself is covered by them. Maybe his intake of B_2 is not adequate! Other writers advise using vitamin E, castor oil, lemon juice, or herbs. But, frankly, I've never known of anything that will remove age spots completely, although in Chapter 32, I do list some homemade cosmetics that can help to lighten them or prevent their growth. An Optimum Diet is still the best preventative. I have seen many very old but healthy people on an Optimum Diet who do not have any age spots at all.

Medically known as *chloasma,* the unsightly light brown or dark brown spots, mostly appearing on hands, neck, arms, and shoulders, occur most often in older people and, although the exact cause or mechanics of their development is not known, medical opinion is that they are totally harmless and a part of normal aging processes of the skin. They are most likely caused by a disorder in the melanin (skin pigmentation) mechanism related to the general aging process. The actual biochemical mechanics may be as follows: The Chronic adrenal exhaustion, which results in abnormally low levels of cortisone in the bloodstream, causes overproduction of Melanin Stimulating Hormone (MSH)—and MSH triggers the production of the melanin, resulting in the familiar brown spots. By adhering to optimum nutrition as described in this book, and taking plenty of brewer's yeast, vitamins C, A, E, and B-complex, and possibly by using raw adrenal protomorphogens (ask your doctor), you will help to prevent age spots, and if you already have some, inhibit their increase in numbers. In my own experience, vitamin E, by improving oxygenation of the tissues, is an important factor in slowing down the formation of brown spots.

Iron Supplements

Q. I know that iron-deficiency anemia is common among women, mostly because of blood loss through menstruation. I've been taking iron pills for several years, but I've recently heard that iron pills can be toxic and dangerous. Is this true? If so, how can I get sufficient iron without taking pills?

A. It has long been known that iron supplements (especially ferrous sulfate) can be quite harmful. They tremendously increase the need for oxygen and pantothenic acid and destroy vitamin A, C, and E in the body (see references in Chapters 13 and 30). They can also cause liver damage. Iron salts are especially dangerous during pregnancy, when, by interfering with the oxygen supply to the fetus, they can cause miscarriages, premature births, birth defects, or cause the baby to be susceptible to anemia and jaundice.[10]

Very recently, a report from doctors at the Östersund Hospital in Sweden showed that too much supplementary iron in pill form or in food (as in so-called enriched bread, from where Swedes obtain 42 percent and Americans 25 percent of their dietary iron) may trigger a serious and often fatal hereditary illness, called hemochromatosis. It is an iron storage disorder which causes its victims to absorb and store too much iron. Possible complications of hemochromatosis are liver disease, diabetes, impotency, sterility, heart failure, or even sudden death.[11]

Supplementary iron is assimilated and metabolized only to a very small degree: some doctors estimate that only 5 to 10 percent of it is absorbed. The best way to make sure that you are getting enough life-giving iron is to eat iron-containing natural foods. Iron can be properly assimilated only if there is a sufficient amount of gastric juices, particularly hydrochloric acid. Some people are anemic in spite of plentiful iron in their diets because they lack sufficient hydrochloric acid in their stomachs. This is especially true with older people. Therefore, the iron-containing fruits, which contain their own enzymes and acids needed for iron digestion and assimilation, are the most reliable sources of dietary iron.

The best natural sources of iron are: apricots, peaches, bananas, black strap molasses, prunes, raisins, brewer's yeast, whole grain cereals, turnip greens, beets, beet tops, alfalfa, sunflower seeds, sesame seeds, whole rye, dry beans, lentils, kelp, dulse, liver, and egg yolks.

Also, keep in mind that vitamin C (up to 500 mg. daily) aids in the absorption of dietary and supplementary iron, while coffee and tea interfere with iron absorption.[12]

Can Sterilization Be Reversed?

Q. I was married at twenty to a divorced man much older than myself. We both decided that we did not want children, so I submitted to a tubal ligation. My husband died of a heart attack six years later. Now I am remarried and my new husband wants children desperately. To tell the truth, I want children, too, and regret my earlier decision to be sterilized. Can sterilization be reversed? Where should I go for information?

A. According to Victor Gomel, M.D., Associate Professor, Obstetrics and Gynecology, University of British Columbia, and Alvin M. Siegler, M.D., Clinical Professor, Obstetrics and Gynecology, Downstate Medical Center, Brooklyn, N.Y., chances of successful reversal of female sterilization, although somewhat improved since the introduction of microsurgery (performed under intensive magnification), are still very small. As of June, 1978, only about 150 such successful operations have been reported, world-wide. The success depends to a large degree on how the original sterilization operation was performed. If a considerable portion of the Fallopian tubes was removed, if there was excessive burning (surgical cauterization), if tubes were severed at the ends (near the ovaries), or if there is excessive scarring from infection or venereal disease, the odds for successful reversal are not very favorable. The "clip" method of sterilization, which only destroys about three-eights of an inch of tube, especially if the tubes have been excised near the middle, offers the best restorative odds.[13]

You should consult the doctor who performed the sterilization operation, find out what method was used, and ask his opinion as to the chances of successful reversal in your case. If he feels the odds are good, ask to be referred to a surgeon who specializes in microsurgery, and who has much experience in successful reversal of female sterilization.

Crib Deaths

Q. Is it true that crib death is caused by pasteurized milk, as was suggested in a magazine article I've just read?

A. Crib deaths, sudden unexpected deaths of apparently healthy babies, also referred to as the Sudden Infant Death Syndrome (SIDS), are responsible for an estimated 20,000 to 25,000 fatalities a year. The victims are mostly between the ages of two to four months and about 70 percent of them are boys. In the typical case, the baby is put to bed at night, seemingly in good health, and is found dead the next morning.

In spite of the tremendous amount of research into this strange syndrome, the cause of crib deaths is still a mystery. There are many theories, of course. Pasteurized milk has been suspected by many investigators. Bernard A. Bellew, M.D., wrote that "there is the disturbing possibility, if not probability, that 'unexplained crib deaths' may be due to an infant diet limited to artificial bottle feeding with corn syrup formulas prepared from heat-treated milks such as reconstituted non-fat dry milk solids, evaporated milks, and even soy milks and pasteurized milk."[14] Allergies, smothering, underdeveloped parathyroid glands—all have been blamed, but all have been disputed or disproven. Adelle Davis strongly suspected the deficiency of vitamin E in the infant diet, and referred to animal experiments where sudden deaths of vitamin E-deficient baby pigs was very similar to crib deaths in humans.[15] Vitamin E deficiency, as a possible cause of crib deaths, was also suggested in the *New Zealand Journal of Medicine.*[16]

"Sudden, massive and overwhelming infections" are suggested by the Boston Children's Medical Center as the most suspected cause at present,[17] although autopsies do not show any infection except a mild inflammation of the heart muscle.

Recently, a brand new theory was developed by the leading sleep expert, Dr. Christian Guilleminault, of Stanford University, California. He says that the baby's sleep patterns could be the missing link in the mystery crib deaths. In the deep dream stage of sleep known as REM (Rapid Eye Movement), the brain doesn't work as well as normal in controlling proper oxygen supply, thus, causing oxygen deficiency. The autopsies of victims of crib deaths reveal definite symptoms of oxygen deficiency. "It seems significant," the Stanford researcher says, "that the highest risk period is between two and four months, when babies are first learning to sleep for hours on end and developing REM sleep."[18]

A leading SIDS researcher and pathologist, Dr. Richard Naeye, of Pennsylvania State University College of Medicine, says that there is sound evidence that SIDS victims had slight anatomical abnormalities affecting the brain or breathing system.

A deficiency of selenium has also been implicated as a possible cause of crib death. The *Medical World News* (Feb. 2, 1973) reported that human milk contains as much as 6 times the amount of vitamin E of cow's milk, and has about twice as much selenium. Autopsies have shown that crib death victims were found to have significantly lower levels of vitamins E and selenium in the liver than were found in normal infants. Note that infant males, who require more selenium than females, are more often the victims of crib death.

Results of recent research, reported in the *Journal of International Academy of Preventive Medicine,* suggest that yet another nutritional deficiency may be involved in crib deaths—thiamine B_1 deficiency.[19] This is in agreement with clinical work by Dr. Derrick Lonsdale which showed that thiamine supplements in the diet of infants who were considered at risk of SIDS can prevent this syndrome.[20]

Perhaps the most important research on the causes of SIDS, this tragic syndrome, was done by Drs. Archie Kalokerinos and Glen Dettman, of Australia. Their studies show that crib deaths are "quite positively related to ascorbate deficiency" (vitamin C deficiency). "Such factors as minor infections, a polluted atmosphere (by smokers, sprays, etc.) food, drugs, trace element deficiencies, endotoxins, injuries, immunological insults, and physical stresses may be contributing factors, but only because they all increase the utilization of ascorbate and cause acute vitamin C deficiency."[21]

Independently of the Australian research, a prominent American doctor, Frederick Klenner, M.D., of the Annie Penn Memorial Hospital, Reidsville, North Carolina, came to the same conclusion regarding the connection between SIDS and vitamin C deficiency. He wrote in the *Journal of Preventive Medicine:* "In February, 1948, I published my first paper on the use of massive doses of vitamin C in treating virus pathology. By February 1960, some 25 scientific papers later, I realized that every head cold must be considered as a probable source of brain pathology. Many have died, especially children, following the sudden development of cerebral manifestations secondary to even a slight head cold and/or chest cold. These insidious cerebral happenings are responsible for the so-called crib deaths attributed to suffocation ... These infants and children who have been put to bed apparently well, except for an insignificant nasal congestion, will demonstrate bilateral pneumonitis at autopsy. Adequate vitamin C, taken daily, will eliminate this syndrome ... The information relative to crib syndrome is backed up case histories at Annie Penn Memorial Hospital, Reidsville, North Carolina. I have seen children dead in less than two hours after hospital admission, having received no treatment, simply because the attending physicians were not impressed with their illness. A few grams of ascorbic acid, given by needle while they waited for laboratory procedures or examination to fit their schedule, could have saved their lives. I know this to be a fact because I have been in similar situations and by routinely employing ascorbic acid, have seen death take a holiday."[22]

Recently, raw honey has been linked to crib deaths.[23] Although the medical evidence of the relationship is inconclusive, the world's largest honey-producing co-operative, the Sioux Honey Association, warned that there is the "possibility of a risk factor" in feeding infants less than 26 weeks of age raw honey as well as other raw agricultural products. The recent research has indicated that many cases of crib death may be undetected botulism poisoning, caused by botulism spores found in raw honey as well as other raw agricultural products, such as fruits and vegetables. (As I mentioned in Chapter 7, the young infant's digestive system is incapable of digesting any other form of sugar except lactose, or milk sugar. Therefore, honey, syrup, or sugar (sucrose) should never be used as sweeteners in the infant's diet.)

As you can see, much research on SIDS, this strange and mysterious syndrome, has been done, and research continues. The vitamin C connection seems quite convincing, as do some other studies especially related to nutritional deficiencies. However, I cannot say with absolute scientific certainty that the SIDS mystery is finally solved. In the meantime, it is comforting to know that this affliction, claiming one of every 350 babies born each year in the United States, is rare in infants receiving mother's milk exclusively. Dr. Kalokerinos said, "Breast milk provides infants with protection against infections and, therefore, reduces the chance of crib deaths."[21] The nursing mother, however, must see that her diet is adequate in all the nutritive factors, including vitamin C, which are needed for infant's maximum protection.

Cosmetic Plastic Surgery

Q. What do you think of plastic surgery? I am only 38 years old and have been eating health foods for six years. Yet, my fact is covered with wrinkles, especially around the eyes and on the forehead, and I am becoming despondent. Most of my friends of the same age have baby-smooth faces!

A. I believe that everyone should try to look his or her best. Vanity? Possibly. But I think a tasteful attire, neatness, personal hygiene, and attractive grooming, as well as cosmetic assistance in looking one's best, can help to make our co-existence on this crowded planet aesthetically more pleasant, and physically and psychologically more enjoyable. By all means, if a face lift will make you happier, have one. I don't think there is much danger or health hazard involved with it, if you make sure that:

(1) You deal with a very reputable, honest, and highly-recommended plastic surgeon.

(2) You are in top health condition.

(3) You prepare your body before surgery with optimum nutrition and adequate vitamin and mineral supplements which will help to counteract the stress of the surgery and/or the possible medication which will be connected with it—as well as continue with such supportive nutritional and supplementary program after the surgery.

Mastectomy—Then What?

Q. I never thought it would happen to me, but it did. I had a mastectomy of the left breast recently and, needless to say, I am still in a trauma. I am only thirty six. Before I left the hospital, my doctor discussed various ways to improve my "appearance." Because of my relatively young age and other physical factors, he seemed to think that I could be a good candidate for reconstruction of the breast by plastic surgery, rather than choosing the more common alternative of wearing a prosthesis, or false breast. What is your opinion of breast reconstruction? Is it safe?

A. Losing a breast through cancer is a tragedy a woman does not care to think of. It is something she feels could never happen to her. But chances of contracting breast cancer—and possible mastectomy—are increasing at an alarming rate. Statistically, one woman in twenty will have a mastectomy during her lifetime.

Mastectomy, a socially-acceptable clinical term for breast amputation, is a surgeon's last resort in the attempt to arrest the spread of breast cancer. The surgical profession has recently been accused of performing too many needless mastectomies. Four out of five breast swellings or lumps are caused by things other than cancer. Therefore, a 100 percent reliable diagnosis, preferably corroborated by several medical experts, especially those not financially connected to the case, is imperative. Also, new surgical techniques are now developing which do not involve removal of the whole breast. Make sure these options are considered as well.

However, in your case it's too late. The breast is gone—now what? Reconstruction of the breast by plastic surgery has been attempted in the recent past, but not with general success, and is presently frowned upon by many medical authorities. Suture complications are common and the aesthetic results are often less than satisfactory. Also, any additional surgery, especially as serious and complex as reconstruction of the whole breast, would add more stress to your body, which may have an unfavorable effect on your general health. You will be safer, especially in view of protecting your right breast, with an artifical breast, which can now be found in any shape or size from firms who specialize in prostheses, or even from some better department stores. There is a fair selection of artifical breasts on the market, including those made from lamb's wool or foam, as well as skin-like silicone forms bearing a nipple, and fluid-filled shapes. Prostheses are tax deductible as a medical expense. You may like to discuss with your doctor the type of prosthesis you should choose, but the sales personnel are usually very helpful and experienced.

I suggest you study carefully Chapter 25 in this book, which may help you to save your remaining breast. It is now scientifically established that diet is related to breast cancer, both causatively and preventively.

Finally, cheer up! Although I know how traumatic a mastectomy can be, it's not the end—in fact, it may have prevented an untimely end. As one of my acquaintances, a nun who had a mastectomy, recently said, "being without a breast is less of a nuisance than losing a leg, or an arm. For me it has been a reprieve on a death sentence." You may have been given an important lesson. Learn from it! If you do, you may be able to enjoy your life now more than ever.

Poisons in Mother's Milk

Q. I've just read in my newspaper a report on a study which found that samples of mother's milk were found to contain such large amounts of DDT, PCB, PBB, and other environmental poisons and agricultural chlorinated hydrocarbons, many of which are carcinogenic, that the study concluded it is safer for a baby to be formula-fed. The formulas, especially if made from skimmed milk and vegetable oils, had a much lesser amount of toxic chemicals than mother's milk. I am nursing my baby at present, and am really worried about this report and about the future health of my baby. Should I continue nursing, or would you advise switching to formula feeding?

A. The presence of DDT in human milk was first discovered almost 30 years ago. As our environment has become more and more polluted, the number of undesirable chemicals in breast milk has multiplied. This is one of the most tragic consequences of the insane reliance by our agricultural and food processing industries, as well as by our profit-hungry society generally, on toxic insecticides and herbicides.

Yes, the various contaminants and pollutants, eaten, drunk, and breathed by a nursing mother will contaminate her milk. And, yes, they are not "good" for the baby, to say the least. The large quantities of chlorinated hydrocarbons and other toxic contaminants in breast milk can definitely be harmful for the baby. The situation is disheartening, indeed.

But, what are the alternatives? If you switch your baby to formula, he will still get a goodly concentration of the same contaminants from cow's milk, along with residues of drugs and hormones now commonly used in the dairy industry. Add to this the residues of detergents from milking machines and several new chemicals which are added during packaging and distributing processes. Soy-milk based formulas are also loaded with pesticide residues as well as spoilage retardants.

To completely avoid poisons today is practically impossible. Our total environment—air, water, household items, clothing, food, cosmetics—is contaminated by dangerous pollutants that our greedy chemical industry has poured out in the name of progress. Trying to raise a child under such conditions is upsetting and frustrating for a conscientious, loving, and responsible parent. Yet, life must go on. We must keep trying. We cannot change the course of the mad chemical race overnight. When the education and awareness begins to motivate the public to refuse buying or using contaminated foods or water, the attitudes and production methods of the agricultural and food manufacturing industries will change—this is the only language they understand. As long as the public is buying the poisonous and nutritionless junk they produce, they will keep producing it.

Now, what should you do about breast feeding?

As I said, the alternative—bottle feeding—is just as bad, as far as contaminants are concerned. Actually worse, because breast milk contains protective factors, such as anti-toxins, immunoglobulins, and antibodies that formulas do not. Since the nutritional quality of breast milk is far superior to any artificial formula, and since breast-fed babies are healthier and have a better resistance to disease and toxins in their environment, mother's milk is still, by far, the better choice of the two alternatives.

You can do several things to minimize the quantity of contaminants in your milk:

1. *Stay on a vegetarian diet.* The 1977 Environmental Defense Fund Study showed that the breast milk of vegetarian mothers contained one-half to two-thirds less the amount of pesticide residues than the milk of the average meat-eating American woman. Earlier British and French studies came to the same conclusion. Meat today is one of the most concentrated sources of contaminants. Most of these toxins are fat-soluble and are stored in animal fat; and meat is up to 40 percent fat. The Optimum Diet, as recommended in Chapters 3 and 4 of this book, will have the least level of contaminants of any diet.

2. Use brewer's yeast powder as one of the prime supplements in your diet. It is one of the few foods left which is virtually free from contaminants.

3. Try to get organically-grown vegetables and fruits if at all possible. Most better health food stores today sell organic produce. Scrub all fruits and vegetables thoroughly with biodegradable soap, then rinse well.

4. Use low-fat dairy products, such as homemade cottage cheese, and skimmed milk. Most contaminants are in the fat part of the milk.

5. Use pure bottled spring water or distilled water since most of the regular tap water is now contaminated with all kinds of agricultural chemicals, in addition to cancer-causing artificial fluorides and chlorine.

Finally, remember that in addition to the nutritional and protective benefits of mother's milk mentioned earlier, the emotional benefits derived from the nursing contact, both for mother and child, as well as the important psychological and physiological bonding between them (on which I elaborated in Chapters 7 and 8), make breast feeding still the much preferred alternative, even in this badly polluted world of ours.

Nursing as Birth Control

Q. My first baby was bottle-fed. Yes, I know how much you disapprove of it, but I was young and inexperienced, and I let my pediatrician talk me into it. I became pregnant three months after the birth of my first baby. My second child was breast-fed. In fact, I continued to nurse her 'til she was over a year old, although after the first six months she ate some other foods as well. Although my husband and I had frequent intercourse during that whole year, and we didn't use any birth control because of our religious beliefs, I didn't become pregnant until a year and a half after the birth of the second child—I didn't even menstruate for the first seven months. Now I've heard that nursing a baby prevents pregnancies and that it is as good a birth control as any. Is it true? It seemed to work that way in my case.

A. The birth control effect, or rather the "birth-spacing" effect, of breast feeding has been understood and recognized by women in many cultures throughout human history. But only recently has actual medical credence been given to this ancient belief. Dr. Derrick B. Jelliffe of the University of California at Los Angeles, is the first medical scientist to study the subject, and his conclusions are that breast feeding is *better* protection from pregnancy than any existing contraception devices or programs. However, there is a catch to it! Mother's breast must be available for nursing twenty-four hours a day.

Here's how it works. Breast feeding causes a secretion of a milk-stimulating hormone; this hormone, in turn, also produces a state of infertility. There must be a certain level of the hormone in the body, however, before it can have a sterilizing effect. In the U.S., breast feeding is customarily confined to the daytime hours—and this is not enough to produce sufficient quantities of the hormone needed for a constant state of infertility.

This explains why your menstrual periods didn't reappear until the baby was put on a mixed food diet. And, why after the first birth, when the baby was bottle-fed, you became pregnant so fast.

Although modern studies have confirmed the ancient belief that breast feeding has, indeed, a birth control or birth-spacing effect, it will work as such only if you feed your baby frequently throughout the twenty-four hour period, including those middle-of-the-night snacks.

Coffee During Pregnancy

Q. I am not a heavy coffee drinker: maybe two or three cups a day, especially in the morning. We have just found out that I am pregnant. A health-faddist friend of mine tells me that coffee can harm my unborn baby. Is that true? What if I drink just one or two cups a day?

A. Numerous animal studies have shown that caffeine is a teratogen (a substance that causes physical defects in developing embryos). It also increases the risk of infertility, miscarriages, and premature births. Coffee drinking or consumption of the numerous other caffeine-containing beverages and foods such as cola drinks, tea, and chocolate, and many over-the-counter drugs, can cause serious damage to the unborn baby and contribute to birth defects. This is especially true during the first sixty days of pregnancy.

Impressed by mounting evidence that caffeine interferes with the normal reproductive processes, Dr. Bengt A. Kihlman, Professor of Biochemical Cytogenetics at the famous Uppsala University in Sweden, stated recently: "A heavy consumption of coffee during the early states of pregnancy should be avoided." At a recent FDA hearing in Washington, Michael Jacobson, Executive Director of the Center for Science in Public Interest, testified on the hazards of consuming caffeine during pregnancy, recommending that pregnant women eliminate caffeine from their diets completely. He suggested that a warning label should be required on all foods and drugs that contain caffeine, so that pregnant women avoid caffeine as they would other drugs.[24]

Cooking Oil Hazard

Q. I know that you do not recommend using vegetable oils for frying, cooking, or baking, but I don't seem to be able to do without them. What should I use instead of oils? And, are some oils safer than others if I still choose to use them?

A. Studies have shown that when vegetable oils are heated to a high temperature of 350 - 400°F, as happens in frying or baking, they become carcinogenic. The saturated fats (such as butter or animal fats) are not as vulnerable to damage by heat as unsaturated vegetable oils are. The moral: do not use vegetable oils for frying or baking. If you insist on using fat for frying or baking, use butter (see Recipes & Directions on how to fry without, or with very little, fat).

There is another hazard involved with cooking oils: the residues of dangerous pesticides. This is especially true with cottonseed oil and soybean oil. One of the most commonly-used pesticides in agriculture is DBCP (dibromochloropropane). Although used extensively on most food crops for two decades, it is now largely banned because it was found to cause sterility in males. In addition, it is a powerful carcinogen (cancer-producing agent), as well as a mutagen—it damages the genetic code; this damage can be passed on to untold generations. DBCP can also damage the liver, kidneys, and cornea of the eye. Because of all this, the government suspended DBCP use for most food crops, but still permits its use on cotton, soybeans, citrus, and grapes. Cottonseed oil is most likely to contain large residues of DBCP because cotton crops are considered non-food crops and are sprayed extensively. Cottonseed oil, however, is a common ingredient in many vegetable oil compounds and margarines sold in super-markets. It is also included in a surprising number of breads, crackers, and cookies, including some "natural" brands.

The safest vegetable oils to use are olive oil and sesame seed oil. These two oils also are most likely to be genuinely cold-pressed, and are most resistant to rancidity. Use them sparingly (1 tbsp. a day per person) and only in the natural raw state, as in salad dressings.

Herbicides and Birth Defects

Q. I am pregnant with my second child. We live in Phoenix, in a subdivision next to a large farming area, which is constantly sprayed from an airplane. I feel ill every time the spraying is done. Often, the wind carries a cloud of spray mist right over our house. I am concerned with my health as well as that of my future baby. Can these sprays hurt my baby or cause birth defects?

A. I've just returned from a nation-wide lecture tour of Australia. Here's what I read in a Melbourne newspaper on the day of my departure. "Victoria (province) considers moves for a total ban on the controversial herbicides 2,4-D and 2,4,5-T. The action followed a report that four mothers gave birth to children with major birth defects after fields near their homes were sprayed with 2,4-D. Seven other women living near the sprayed fields miscarried."

Your neighborhood should organize and launch a strong protest with your local pesticide board and Environmental Protection Agency. Unfortunately, many government agencies are more concerned with the economic welfare of farmers than with public health. If I were in your situation, I would immediately move as far away from that neighborhood as possible.

Fetal Alcohol Syndrome

Q. My sister is seventeen, unmarried, and pregnant. I am concerned because she drinks beer and wine, and smokes. She realizes that smoking may be harmful for the unborn baby, and considers stopping. But, she claims beer and wine in moderation are OK. Can you give me some "ammunition" which I can use to convince her that alcohol can also harm her baby?

A. A team of doctors from the University of Washington, at Seattle, which included Dr. David Smith, Professor of Pediatrics at the University, and Drs. Ann Pytkowicz Streissguth, James Hanson, and Kenneth Jones, made a thorough study of the effects of alcohol on the fetus of the drinking pregnant woman. They were the first scientists to identify what is now known as the "fetal alcohol syndrome." Studies clearly indicate that every drink a pregnant woman takes hits her fetus "like a chemical sledgehammer." Dr. Smith said, "It still is widely believed that moderate drinking is safe for pregnant women. We now know clearly that alcohol is the most common teratogen (an agent that causes birth defects). We would advise any woman considering pregnancy, or who already is pregnant, to avoid alcohol altogether."

Doctors studied eight children of an alcoholic mother and discovered that four of them had the same malformations: small eyes with short eye slits; smaller than normal mid-face area; flat facial contours; and smaller heads, indicating smaller brains. The average IQ of the children with fetal alcohol syndrome ranges from 60 to 70, with some as low as 30.

At first it was believed that only heavy drinkers have children with fetal alcohol syndrome. The latest studies, however, show that even occasional binge drinking can cause malformations and birth defects. Also, it makes no difference if you drink wine, beer, or hard liquor—the alcohol is the damaging agent. The extent of damage is related to dose, naturally. A heavy drinker has a 30 - 50 percent chance of producing a malformed baby.

(Regarding the effect of smoking on the unborn baby, please read Chapter 28 in this book.)

Smoking and The Pill: A Deadly Combination

Q. My young granddaughter is on birth control pills and smokes cigarettes at the rate of a pack a day. My attempts to inform her regarding this deadly combination fall on deaf ears. Her response: "Oh, Grandma, how would you know!?" Can you help me get the message across to her?

A. In addition to what is already written in Chapters 22 and 28 on the health hazards of the Pill, especially in combination with smoking, here are some further indictments:

Recent studies by Dr. Anrudh K. Jain, of the Population Council, England, demonstrate that the Pill and cigarette smoking damage health "synergistically"—that is, the total health-damaging effect associated with the combination of these two factors is many times more severe than would result from each factor acting independently.

Here are the shocking statistics:

The incidence of death from heart attack in women between the ages of 40 and 44:

Those who neither smoke nor take
the Pill .... 7 per 100,000
Non-smokers on the Pill .... 10 per 100,000
Smokers not on the Pill .... 16 per 100,000
Smokers who use the Pill .... 59 per 100,000
Heavy smokers (over 15 cigarettes a day)
on the Pill .... 83 per 100,000

You can also tell your granddaughter that the deadly combination of smoking and the Pill increase her chances of developing cancer in about the same proportion as in regard to death from heart attack. (See Chapter 28.)

Herbs During Pregnancy and Lactation

Q. I have heard that it is dangerous to drink certain herb teas during pregnancy. Is this true? If so, which herbs should I avoid? I love herb teas and would like to know which I can use safely during pregnancy and lactation.

A. Most herbs have medicinal properties. Therefore, they should be used only in the treatment of illness—specific herbs for specific conditions as recommended in many chapters of this book and in my book, *How To Get Well.* Especially during pregnancy and lactation, you must avoid medicinal herbs which may affect the unborn or nursing infant unfavorably. This warning is especially true in regard to the herbs mentioned in this book for the treatment of menstrual and other reproductive disorders.

Here are some of the herbs that you should avoid during pregnancy (most of these are *abortifacients,* i.e., they may induce abortion): black cohosh, blue cohosh, golden seal, cinnamon, false hellebore, tansy, pennyroyal, cotton root, cramp bark, and wild yam.

Good herbs to use during pregnancy are: raspberry leaves, squaw vine, peppermint, camomile, filaree, hardhack, and dandelion. For morning sickness during the early stages of pregnancy, teas made from sundew or peach leaves are effective.

Good herbs to use during lactation (they stimulate and increase milk production) are: oat straw, borage, fennel seed, alfalfa, blessed thistle, comfrey, caraway, rosemary leaves, and milkworth. Periwinkle can be used to discourage overabundant milk production.

Other herbs that can be used for specific reproductive problems such as menstrual disorders, menopause, birth control, infertility, as well as in the treatment of female and children's diseases, are listed in various chapters of this book.

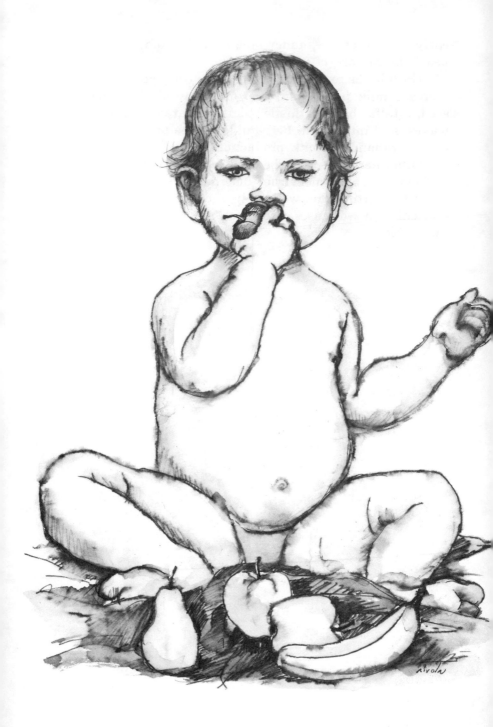

Recipes
&
Directions

FRUIT SALAD A LA AIROLA

1 bowl fresh fruits, organically grown if possible
1 handful raw nuts and/or sunflower seeds
3 - 4 soaked prunes or handful of raisins, unsulphured
3 tbsp. cottage cheese, preferably homemade, unsalted
1 tbsp. raw wheat germ (only if you can get it 100% fresh)
3 tbsp. yogurt
2 tsp. natural, unpasteurized honey
1 tsp. fresh lemon juice

Wash and dry all fruits carefully. Use any available fruits and berries, but try to get at least three or four different kinds. Peaches, grapes, pears, papaya, bananas, strawberries, and fresh pineapple are particularly good for producing a delightful bouquet of rich, penetrating flavors. A variety of colors will make the salad festive and attractive to the eye.

Chop or slice bigger fruits, but leave grapes and berries whole. Place them in a large bowl and add prunes and nuts (nuts and sunflower seeds could be crushed). Make a dressing with 1 teaspoon of honey (or more if most of the fruits used are sour), 1 teaspoon of lemon juice, and 2 tablespoons of water. Pour over the fruit, add wheat germ, and toss well. Mix cottage cheese, yogurt, and 1 teaspoon of honey in a separate cup until it is fairly smooth in texture, and pour it on top of the salad. Sprinkle with nuts and sunflower seeds. Serve at once.

This is not only a most delicious dish but it is the most nutritious and perfectly balanced meal I know of. It is a storehouse of high-grade proteins and all the essential vitamins, minerals, fatty acids, and enzymes you need for optimum health.

FORMULA P AND L
(Green Juice Cocktail)

1 cup any available garden greens: parsley, lettuce, kale, turnip tops, wheat grass, comfrey, alfalfa—any or all.
A small quantity of such strong-tasting greens as watercress, mint, radish tops, chives, etc., can be used. Even wild greens such as dandelion or common nettle are excellent in small quantities.
2 stalks celery
1 glass freshly-made carrot and beet juice
(80% carrot - 20% beets)

Pour carrot and beet juice in your electric blender and switch on low. Feed greens into the blender slowly. When all greens are in, switch on high and liquify well. You may add a pinch of kelp powder and/or other natural herbs or flavorings, if you wish.

Drink slowly, salivate well. Green juice cocktail is best taken ½ to 1 hour before lunch or dinner. Two to three ounces is sufficient, but a full 6-oz. glass is okay if taken 1 hour before a meal.

This is an excellent supplementary drink during pregnancy

and lactation. It is loaded with chlorophyll, vitamins, minerals, trace elements, enzymes, and other vital nutrients. Lactating mothers will find that it will aid in breast-milk production, especially if plenty of fresh alfalfa is used. Alfalfa is an excellent stimulant for the milk-producing glands.

Note: avoid such oxalic acid rich greens as spinach and rubarb, and use only *small* quantities of cabbage-family greens, such as broccoli, Swiss chard, kale, etc., when making green juice cocktail.

VEGETABLE BROTH

2 large potatoes, chopped or sliced to approximately
    half-inch pieces
1 cup carrots, shredded or sliced
1 cup celery, chopped or shredded, leaves and all
1 cup any other available vegetable:
    beet tops, turnip tops, parsley, or a little of everything.
    (Note: avoid oxalic acid-rich greens—See Formula P&L)
    However, broth can be made with only potatoes, carrots
    and celery.
Garlic, onion, and/or any of the natural herb spices

Place all vegetables in a pot and add 1½ quarts of water. Do not use aluminum utensils. Cover and cook slowly for about 30 minutes. Strain, cool until just warm, and serve. If not used immediately, keep in refrigerator and reheat before serving.

Vegetable broth is an alkaline, cleansing, mineral-rich drink which is used by biological clinics during juice fasting, especially in the treatment of rheumatic diseases. Lactating mothers can also use this broth to stimulate breast milk production.

EXCELSIOR

1 cup of vegetable broth (see recipe for Vegetable Broth)
1 tbsp. whole flaxseed
1 tbsp. wheat bran

Soak flaxseed and wheat bran in vegetable broth overnight. In the morning, warm it up, stir well, and drink—seeds and all. Do not chew the seeds, swallow them whole. Excelsior is especially beneficial for people with constipation problems. It helps to restore normal peristaltic rhythm. When used during fasting, excelsior must be strained.

SPLIT PEA SOUP

1 cup dried split peas
3 cups water
½ cup chopped onions
1 small carrot, diced
1 stalk celery, diced
1 tsp. sea salt
1 bay leaf

Wash peas, add vegetables, and cover with water. Bring to a boil. Reduce heat, add bay leaf, and simmer for 1½ hours, or until peas are tender. Add sea salt and your favorite herb seasonings. Remove bay leaf. Puree in blender or serve as is. Makes 4 - 6 servings.

AIROLA SOUPER SOUP

Have you ever wished to be an expert soup maker—to be able to make every kind of delicious vegetable soup without failure? Here is my "discovery" which will transform you into an instant gourmet chef, to the delight of your hungry family. You can sit back and enjoy the appreciative superlatives that will be sure to come your way.

Take *any or all* vegetables you happen to have in your refrigerator or in your own backyard garden. You can make this soup with as few as *one* vegetable, or as many as *several dozen.* Place vegetables in a pot and cover with water. Do not use aluminum utensils. Bring to a boil and simmer for 15 - 25 minutes, until vegetables are done. Do not overcook; vegetables must not be mushy. The length of cooking time depends on the vegetables. Such vegetables as rutabagas and carrots require longer cooking time. If fast-cooking leafy vegetables are mixed with slow-cooking vegetables, add them near the end of the cooking time. Season to taste with sea salt and your favorite herbs such as dried parsley leaves, dill weed, tarragon leaves, paprika, cayenne, celery seed, bay leaf, garlic and/or onion powder, or other favorites. Note: do not use black or white pepper. You may use vegetized seasonings or other ready-made seasonings. If you use bay leaf, do not crush the leaves, but use them whole, and remove after serving. Bay leaves are toxic, and should never be crushed or left in the soup.

If you prefer, you may mash vegetables with a potato masher, or place soup in the blender, making into a puree before serving.

Now, obviously, you have known all this before—so where is my "discovery?" Here: As I said earlier, use any vegetables you happen to have on hand. *Whatever vegetable happens to be the predominant contributor to the flavor gives the soup its name!* If the predominant ingredient is potatoes, you created Potato Soup; if the predominant ingredient is onions, you created Onion Soup; if you used mostly carrots in your soup—it is Carrot Soup; if zucchinis predominate it is Zucchini Soup, etc., etc. Your imagination is the limit! You can now create any vegetable soup you wish—all from one simple Souper Soup recipe!

AIROLA SALAD

Here is a completely new variety of vegetable salad. It differs from the conventional vegetable salad in two distinctive ways:
1. It is "chunky"; it has no soft, leafy vegetables, such as lettuce, parsley, cabbage, spinach, or mustard greens.

2. It is "hot"; it has a distinct Mexican flavor, being spiced with chili (cayenne pepper), and lime or lemon.

Use the following fresh vegetables: avocadoes, carrots, tomatoes, green peppers, cucumbers, red onions, celery stalks, radishes and Jerusalem artichokes. If any of the above are not available, use what you can get. Tomatoes, cucumbers, green peppers, celery, and onions are the basic ingredients.

Chop all vegetables into about 1 inch pieces. Carrots can be sliced into ¼-inch thick slices. Do not peel cucumbers or Jerusalem artichokes.

Place all chopped vegetables in a bowl and add the following ingredients to taste: sea water or sea salt (available in health food stores), cayenne pepper or chili, paprika, lime or lemon juice. Add some water, stir briskly, and serve.

It is important to have lots of lime and lemon juice,—at least the juice of ½ lime or ¼ lemon for each serving. That means if you make a salad for four persons, use 1 lemon or 2 limes. It is best to eat the Airola Salad with a spoon, being sure to consume all the dressing. This salad should be eaten as a meal in itself. Eat slowly and chew well. It is very filling and satisfying—and fantabulously delicious!

MILLET CEREAL

1 cup hulled millet
3 cups water
½ cup powdered skim milk

Method 1: Rinse millet in warm water and drain. Heat mixture of water, powdered skim milk, and millet to boiling. Simmer for 10 minutes, stirring occasionally to prevent sticking and burning. Remove from heat, cover, and let stand for a half an hour or more. Serve with milk, honey, oil, or butter—or homemade applesauce—and treat yourself to the *most nutritious cereal in the world!*

Method 2: Here's another, even better, way to make millet cereal (or any other cereal, for that matter). Place all ingredients in a pan with a tight cover. Use ovenproof utensils: pyrex, earthenware, or stainless steel, if possible. Place in the oven turned to 200° and leave for 3-4 hours. The cereal can be left in the oven longer if necessary, but it should be ready to eat after about 3 hours. To speed the process, the cereal can be heated to the boiling point before putting into the oven.

This cooking method is superior because of the low temperature, which makes the nutrients—especially the proteins—of millet or other grains more easily assimilable.

Millet is a truly wonderful, complete food. It can rightfully be called the king of all cereals, possibly sharing this distinction with buckwheat. It is high in complete proteins and low in starches. It is very easily digested and never causes gas and fermentation in the stomach as some other highly starchy cooked cereals often do. Famed nutritionist Dr. Harvey Kellogg said that millet is the only cereal that can sustain or support human life when used as the *sole item in the diet.* Besides complete proteins, millet is rich in vitamins, minerals, and important trace elements, such as molybdenum and lecithin.

Method 3: First bring millet, water, and powdered skim milk to a boil on the stove. Pour mixture into a crockpot, and cook on low for 3 - 4 hours.

KASHA
(Buckwheat cereal)

1 cup whole buckwheat grains
2 to 2½ cups water

Bring water to a boil. Stir the buckwheat into the boiling water and let boil for 2 to 3 minutes. Turn heat to low and simmer for 15 to 20 minutes, stirring occasionally. If seasoning is desired, use a very little sea salt. When all the water is absorbed, take from the stove and let stand, covered, for another 15 minutes. Kasha must never be mushy. Serve hot with sunflower seed oil, olive oil, sesame seed oil, or butter.

Kasha is a favorite cereal in Russia and many other Eastern European countries. It has an unusual, mellow flavor, and is extremely nutritious. It contains complete proteins of high biological value, equal in quality to animal proteins, as shown in recent studies.

This is a quick way to prepare kasha if you do not have much time. For those who do have the time, the oven or crockpot methods, as described in the recipe for millet cereal, are preferable.

WAERLAND FIVE-GRAIN KRUSKA
(for four persons)

1 tbsp. whole wheat
1 tbsp. whole rye
1 tbsp. whole barley
1 tbsp. whole millet
1 tbsp. whole oats
2 tbsp. wheat bran
2 tbsp. unsulphured raisins
1 - 1½ cups water

Grind the 5 grains coarsely in your grinder. Place all ingredients in a pot. Boil for 5 - 10 minutes, then wrap the pot in a blanket or newspapers and let it stand for a few hours. Experiment with the amount of water used—kruska must not be mushy, but should have the consistency of a very thick porridge. Serve hot with sweet milk and homemade applesauce or stewed fruits.

Kruska is an extremely nutritious dish and should be eaten as a meal in itself.

POTATO CEREAL

2 large raw potatoes
2 tbsp. whole wheat flour
1 tbsp. wheat bran
4 cups water

Heat water to boiling. Add flour and bran and simmer for 2 to 3 minutes. Place a fine shredder over pan and quickly shred potatoes directly into pan. Stir vigorously. Remove from the stove and let stand for a few minutes. Serve hot with milk, butter, or cream; sprinkle wheat germ on top, if desired. Make sure the wheat germ is fresh, not rancid.

This is an alkaline and exceptionally nutritious cereal. It is especially good for people suffering from rheumatic diseases, in which case wheat flour should be excluded and only the bran used.

MOLINO CEREAL

1 cup water
1 tbsp. coarse whole wheat flour
2 tbsp. wheat bran
2 tbsp. whole flaxseed
2 - 3 chopped figs or soaked prunes
1 tbsp. unsulphured raisins

Place all ingredients in a pan and boil for 5 minutes, stirring occasionally to prevent burning. Serve immediately with sweet milk, a little honey, or homemade applesauce.

This cereal is beneficial for people with weak digestion, diverticulosis and a tendency toward constipation.

HOMEMADE COTTAGE CHEESE
(Quark)

Take homemade soured milk and warm it to about 110°F, by placing the container in warm water. When the milk has curdled, place a clean linen cloth or cheesecloth over a deep strainer and pour the curdled milk over it. Wait until all liquid whey has seeped through the strainer. What remains in the strainer is fresh, wholesome, and delicious homemade cottage cheese. If the cheese is too hard, add a little sweet or sour cream, and stir. The higher the temperature, the harder the cheese, and vice versa. Raw homemade cottage cheese (quark) can be made by straining soured milk through a fine cheesecloth, without warming it up first.

By the way, don't throw the whey away—it is an exceptionally nutritious and rejuvenating drink.

HOMEMADE KEFIR

To make your own kefir, you will need kefir grains. There is a mail order company, R.A. J. Biological Laboratory, 35 Park Ave., Blue Point, Long Island, New York, which sells kefir grains by mail. The kefir grains will last indefinitely; there is never any need to reorder. Merely follow the instructions which will come with the grains.

Place 1 tablespoon of kefir grains in a glass of milk, stir, and allow to stand at room temperature overnight. When the milk coagulates, it is ready for use. Strain and save the grains for the next batch. Kefir is a true "elixir of youth," used by centenarians in Bulgaria, Russia, and Caucasus as an essential part of their daily diet.

Freeze-dried kefir culture, sold in health food stores, can also be used in making kefir.

HOMEMADE YOGURT

Take a bottle of skim milk and heat it almost to boiling, then cool to room temperature. Add 2 to 3 tablespoons of yogurt, which can be bought in a grocery store or health shop. Stir well. Pour into a wide-mouthed thermos bottle. Cover and let stand overnight. In 5 to 8 hours it will be solid and ready to serve. If you do not have a thermos jar, use an ordinary glass jar and place it in a pan of warm water over an electric burner switched on "warm" for 4 to 5 hours, then switch to off until milk is solid.

Use 2 to 3 spoonfuls of your fresh, homemade yogurt as a culture for the next batch.

If you prefer, you can use a convenient automatic yogurt maker which can be bought in health food stores.

HOMEMADE SOURED MILK

Use only unpasteurized, raw milk. Place a bottle of milk in a pan filled with warm water, and warm it to about body temperature. Fill a cup or a deep plate, stir in a tablespoon of yogurt, cover with a paper towel (to keep dust off) and keep in a warm place—for example, near the stove, radiator, or wherever there is a constant warm temperature. The milk will coagulate in approximately 24 hours.

Use 1 or 2 spoonfuls of soured milk as a culture for your next batch (use yogurt or commercial buttermilk only as a starting culture for the first batch).

AIROLA SHAKE

¼ tbsp. brewer's yeast powder or flakes
¼ tsp. calcium lactate or bone meal powder
1 tbsp. flax seed, sesame seed, chia seed, or sunflower seeds
1 tbsp. wheat bran or rice polishings or wheat germ (if you

can get it fresh)
1 tsp. powdered lecithin or lecithin granules
1 tsp. honey
1 tsp. bee pollen
1½ cup certified, raw milk
1 raw egg yolk, if desired
1 banana, or 1 tbsp. carob powder (use either or both,
    depending on flavor preference)

Grind sesame, or flax, or chia, or sunflower seeds together with bran, rice polishings, or wheat germ in an electric seed grinder. If you use wheat germ, make sure it is 100% fresh, non-rancid.

Place all ingredients in blender, and run on high until mixture is smooth—approximately 15 seconds. Add more milk if needed.

Makes one large glass of super-nutritious and rejuvenating drink. In my Optimum Diet, this shake can be used as a replacement for either breakfast or lunch. You can take your regular vitamin supplements with it.

For people on the go (as many are these days), a liquid breakfast, made quickly in your blender, may be the answer to being sure of getting adequate nutrition in spite of a busy lifestyle.

YOGURT MASH

½ banana
3 tbsp. fresh papaya
2 tbsp. yogurt
Few drops lemon or lime juice

Mash the ingredients with a fork or potato masher. Feed to your baby with a teaspoon or let older infants eat by themselves.

WHOLE WHEAT BREAD

4 - 5 cups whole wheat flour, freshly ground
2 cups warm water
2 tbsp. or 2 packages active dry yeast
¼ cup honey
2 tsp. salt (optional)

Dissolve honey in 1 cup of warm water. Sprinkle yeast over it and stir gently. Let mixture stand for 10 minutes. Pour the contents into mixing bowl, add the remaining water and 2 cups of flour. Mix and beat well with an electric mixer. Cover and let stand for 15 minutes. Add remaining flour and knead well. Dough should be moist but not sticky. Cover, put in warm place, and let it rise to double in size. Knead again, shape into loaves and put in buttered and floured pans. Let rise once more until almost doubled in size. Bake for 45 minutes at 350° F. Makes 2 loaves.

SOURDOUGH RYE BREAD

(Black Bread, Russian Style)

8 cups freshly-ground whole rye flour
3 cups warm water
½ cup sourdough culture

Mix 7 cups of flour with water and sourdough culture. Cover and let stand in a warm place for 12 to 18 hours. Add remaining flour and mix well. Place in buttered and floured pans. Let rise in a warm place for approximately 1 - 2 hours, or until the loaf has risen noticeably. Preheat oven and bake at 350° - 400° F for 1 hour or more, if needed. Always save ½ cup of dough as a culture for the next baking. Keep the culture in your refrigerator. For the initial baking, it will be necessary to obtain a sourdough culture from a friend or from a commercial baker. This recipe makes a 2-pound loaf.

Note: The culture, if stored in a tight container without air (preferably in a plastic container, or plastic bag, as glass may break when the culture expands), can be potent for several weeks. If, after prolonged storage, a mold or discoloration appears (as a result of oxidation) remove the affected parts and use the fresher parts from the center.

Finally, sourdough bread baking is a delicate art. If you do not succeed at first, don't give up—keep experimenting until you bake a sublimely delicious loaf that will not only fill your house with Old-Country aroma, but will delight your family and justify the Biblical reference to bread as the "Staff of Life."

BUCKWHEAT PANCAKES

1 cup whole raw buckwheat
½ cup rolled oats or fresh wheat germ which is not over
   10 days old
2 eggs
2 cups buttermilk, yogurt, or kefir
pinch of sea salt

Place whole buckwheat and oats or fresh wheat germ in blender or seed grinder and grind well until a fine flour is obtained. Mix flour in a medium-sized bowl with remaining ingredients and blend well. If batter is too thick, add fresh milk. Fry on a lightly-buttered griddle on low heat.

Serve with butter, vegetable oil, or homemade applesauce. Makes 6 delicious medium-sized pancakes.

BRAN MUFFINS

6 tbsp. butter
¾ cup honey

1 egg
1 cup buttermilk
1 cup bran
2 cups whole wheat flour
1½ tsp. baking soda
¼ tsp. sea salt
½ tsp. allspice
¾ cup unsulphured raisins

Cream butter and honey. Add egg, buttermilk, and bran, and mix well. Sift together the whole wheat flour, baking soda, allspice, and sea salt. Add this to liquid ingredients with the raisins, and mix just until blended. Fill buttered muffin tins 2/3 full. Bake at 350° F for 20-25 minutes. Makes 1½ dozen.

CORN MEAL MUFFINS

2 cups yellow corn meal
2 cups whole wheat flour
1/3 cup non-fat dry milk
1½ cups lukewarm water
2 eggs, beaten
1 tbsp. active dry yeast
2 - 3 tbsp. honey
1 tsp. sea salt
¼ cup lukewarm water

Dissolve yeast in ¼ cup lukewarm water. Add honey, beaten eggs, salt, and the remaining 1½ cups water. Combine corn meal with wheat flour and non-fat dry milk and add to the liquid mixture. Stir until blended well. Fill buttered muffin cups ½ full and allow to rise in a warm place for 15 minutes. Bake at 400° F for 20 - 25 minutes. Makes 1½ dozen.

HOMEMADE OATMEAL RAISIN COOKIES

½ cup raisins
½ cup hot water
½ cup butter
¾ cup honey
2 eggs
2 cups rolled oats
2 cups whole wheat flour
1 tsp. vanilla extract
2 tsp. baking powder
1 tsp. ground cinnamon

Soak raisins in the ½ cup hot water for 20 - 30 minutes. Cream honey and butter. Add eggs, vanilla, and the water the raisins were soaked in. Sift dry ingredients together, and add to the liquid ingredients. Add raisins and rolled oats. Drop by rounded spoonfuls 2 inches apart on a buttered baking sheet. Bake at 400° F for 8 - 10 minutes. Makes 4 - 5 dozen.

HOMEMADE ICE CREAM

2½ cups raw sweet cream
2 large eggs, separated
½ cup raw honey
1 tsp. pure vanilla extract

Separate eggs. Beat egg yolks and honey together. Add the cream and vanilla and stir well. Place in quart container and freeze. When solidly frozen, remove from container and put in a mixing bowl. Mix until smooth, adding beaten egg whites as you mix. Replace in container and refreeze.

"Ice cream" can also be made by substituting yogurt for cream. For flavors other than vanilla, add carob flour (for "chocolate" ice cream), or chopped fruits or berries for fruit-flavored ice cream.

DATE BARS

2 cups chopped, pitted dates
1 cup water
½ cup honey
1 tsp. vanilla extract
2 eggs, separated
2 cups rolled oats
1½ cups whole wheat flour
½ cup butter
½ tsp. baking soda

Cream honey and butter together. Add 2 egg yolks, vanilla, and water. Mix thoroughly. Add flour, baking soda, dates, and rolled oats. Beat egg whites until stiff and fold into the batter. Pour into a 9 x 13 inch buttered baking pan. Bake at 350° F for 30 - 40 minutes. Cool and cut into squares.

CAROB SESAME BALLS

½ cup honey
½ cup soft butter
1 tsp. vanilla extract
¾ cup non-fat dry milk
¼ cup carob powder
½ cup hulled sesame seeds

Cream honey and butter together. Add vanilla. Combine non-fat dry milk and carob powder and add to the butter and honey mixture. Mix well. Shape into ½ inch balls and roll in sesame seeds. Chill in the refrigerator. Makes 2 dozen.

HOMEMADE OATMEAL CAROB COOKIES

1½ cup rolled oats
¼ cup melted butter
¼ cup carob chips
2 tbsp. liquid honey
1 egg

Place rolled oats in blender and run for 10 - 15 seconds. Mix oat flour and carob chips with butter, honey and egg and drop by spoon on buttered cookie sheet. Bake at 350° for 10 minutes. Since some carob chips contain sugar, try to find those that do not, or replace carob chips with freshly chopped nuts or raisins, or make oatmeal cookies without any of them.

DRY FRUIT MIX

¼ pound dried apricots
¼ pound prunes
½ pound pitted dates
¼ pound unsulphured raisins
¼ pound dried figs
Sunflower seeds and hulled sesame seeds

Put fruits through a food chopper, alterating fruits to mix them. Form ½ inch balls and roll in hulled sunflower or sesame seeds.

Freshly chopped nuts and sunflower seeds can be added to this fruit mix, if desired. This is a high energy, filling snack and should be used in moderation between meals.

HALVAH

1 cup hulled sesame seeds
2 tsp. honey, preferably coagulated solid honey

Grind sesame seeds in a small electric seed grinder. Pour sesame meal into a larger cup and knead honey into the meal with a large spoon until honey is well mixed in and the halvah acquires the consistency of a hard dough. Serve it as is, or make small balls and roll them in whole sesame seeds or sunflower seeds. This is an excellent, nutritious, and delicious candy, loved by children and grownups alike.

HOMEMADE APPLESAUCE

Any kind of apples may be used, but organically-grown sour apples such as Pippins, Roman Beauty, Jonathan, Northern Spy, Granny's, etc., are preferable.

Wash apples well and remove stems. Cut into approximately 1-inch pieces. NOTE: Do not peel or remove core or seeds—use the whole apple. Place in a pan, and add one inch of water (only enough water to cover the bottom and prevent burning; glass, earthenware, or stainless steel utensils are best—**do not** use aluminum).

Cover and bring to a boil. Simmer until apples are soft. Mash with potato masher or place in a blender if finer texture is desired. Do not use sugar or honey, but pectin may be added if desired. When sauce is cooled, place in jars and refrigerate. Keeps for approximately 1 week.

HOMEMADE SAUERKRAUT

Cut white cabbage heads into narrow strips with a large knife or grater, and place in a small wooden barrel or a large earthenware pot. A large stainless steel pail or a glass container could possibly be used, but under no circumstances use an aluminum utensil.

When the layer of cabbage is about 4 to 6 inches deep, sprinkle with a few juniper berries, cummin seeds, and/or black currant leaves—use your favorite or whatever you have available. A few strips of carrots, green peppers, and onions can also be used. Add a little sea salt—not more than 2 ounces total for each 25 pounds of cabbage. Continue making layers of grated cabbage and spices until the container is filled. Each layer should be pressed and pounded very hard with your fists or a piece of wood so that there will be no air left and the cabbage will be saturated with its own juice.

When the container is full, cover the cabbage with a clean cheesecloth, place a wooden or slate board over it, and on the top place a clean heavy stone. Let stand for 10 days to 2 weeks—longer if the temperature is below 70° F. Now and then remove the foam and possible mildew from the top, from the stone, and from the barrel edges. The cheesecloth, board, and stone should occasionally be removed, washed well with warm water and then cold water, and replaced. When the sauerkraut is ready for use, it can be left in the barrel, which now should be stored in a cold place, or preferably put into glass jars and kept in the refrigerator.

Sauerkraut is best eaten *raw*—both from the point of taste and for its health-giving value. Drink the sauerkraut juice, too. It is an extremely beneficial and wonderfully nutritious drink.

HOMEMADE PICKLED VEGETABLES

Use the same method as described in the recipe for Sauerkraut to make health-giving lactic acid vegetables. Beets, carrots, green and red peppers, beet tops, and celery are particularly adapted for pickling.

HOMEMADE SOUR PICKLES

Use only small, fresh, hard cucumbers. Place them in cold water overnight, then remove and dry well.

Place cucumbers in a wooden barrel or a large earthenware or glass container. Put a few leaves of black currants or cherries, caraway or mustard seeds, and dill branches in with the cucumbers.

Boil a sufficient amount of salt water, using about 4 ounces of sea salt for 5 quarts of water. Let the water cool down, then pour it over the cucumbers. Cover with a cheesecloth, place a wooden board over it, and on the top a clean heavy stone. There should be enough salt water to cover the board. Keep the container in a warm place for about 1 week, then move to a cooler place. Pickles are ready for eating in about 10 days to 2 weeks—longer if the temperature is cold. Every 5 days or so, remove the stone and the covers and wash them well, first in warm water, then in cold water, and replace them. Keep the top of the water clear of foam and mildew. When pickles are ready for eating they can be placed in glass jars and kept in the refrigerator.

HOW TO MAKE SPROUTS

First, make sure that the seeds or grains you buy for sprouting are packaged for food. Under no circumstances use seeds that are sold for planting; they more likely than not contain mercury compounds or other toxic chemicals. Play it safe and buy your seeds and sprouting grains at your health food store.

The seeds most commonly used for sprouting are: alfalfa, mung beans, soybeans, and wheat.

There are many different methods of sprouting seeds. Slow germinating seeds, such as wheat or soybeans, can be soaked in water for two days (changing water twice a day) then spread thinly on a plate or paper towel for 2 or 3 days, rinsing them under running water three times a day to prevent molding. If you prefer, you may use one of the very convenient sprouting kits sold in health food stores, with enclosed directions.

Here's my own way of sprouting seeds: place 1 tablespoon of alfalfa seeds in a quart jar and fill with water. Let soak overnight. Rinse seeds well the following morning and place them back in the glass jar without water, covering the jar with a cheesecloth held on by a rubber band. Keep rinsing the seeds 3 or 4 times a day. In 2 or 3 days, alfalfa sprouts are ready for eating. When seeds are fully sprouted, that is, the sprouts are 1 to 2 inches long, place the top on the jar and keep them in the refrigerator if they are not eaten right away. *Always rinse sprouts before eating.* Sprouts can be eaten as they are or mixed with salads or other foods. They can also be ground up in a drink, preferably with vegetable juices.

HOW TO SAUTE WITH WATER

Fill a cast-iron or other heavy skillet with water, ¼ to ½ inch deep. Heat the water to a boil. Add vegetables (or mushrooms or any other foods you wish to "fry") and saute as in oil, adding more water if necessary, and stirring until the vegetables are done. A small amount of oil or butter can be added, if desired.

This method should be experimented with as some vegetables contain more water, and some take longer to cook than others.

I have developed this Water Sautéing Method to eliminate cooking foods in oils, which become damaged by high heat. Oils heated to temperatures of 350° - 400° F, as happens in frying or baking, become not only difficult to digest, but also harmful, even carcinogenic. If a small amount of oil is added during water sauteing, it floats on top of the water, never reaching temperatures higher than that of boiling water, which is 212° F.

HOW TO DO DRY BRUSH MASSAGE
A simple but miraculous health and rejuvenation treatment.

I am going to tell you about a simple technique, which will cost you very little, which will take only 5 to 10 minutes a day to perform, but which will give a million dollars worth of benefits in terms of better health, better looks, and longer life. I have tested it for 30 years on myself and thousands of patients and students. The technique is called *dry brush massage.* It is described in several of my earlier books and I have received numerous glowing reports of great benefits derived by those who incorporate this simple procedure into their daily routine. It is of specific importance to those who are bedridden or convalescing after an illness.

How do you do a dry brush massage?

First, you have to get a suitable brush. The best brush for a massage is a natural bristle brush about the size of your hand, or larger if you can get it. Unfortunately, it is more and more difficult to find a natural bristle brush, especially in the United States. The brush should have a long handle so you can reach all parts of your body. If you cannot find a natural bristle brush right away, but are anxious to begin the dry brush program immediately, the following can be quite satisfactory:
- A regular, inexpensive natural plant-fiber vegetable brush which you can get at any drug store or hardware store.
- A coarse bath glove of twisted hog's hair.
- A loofah mitt (a coarse natural sponge).

Warning: Do not use nylon or synthetic fiber brushes—they are too sharp and may damage the skin.

Another tip: It is advisable to start out with a less harsh brush, and brush gently at first until your skin is "seasoned," then begin using a coarser brush.

Starting with the soles of your feet, brush vigorously, making rotary motions, and massage every part of your body. Brush in this order: first feet and legs, then hands and arms, back, abdomen, chest, and neck. Use as much pressure with the brush as you can comfortably stand. Sensitivity of the skin varies, of course, with every individual. Some can stand much harder brushing than others. Also, the various parts of the body differ in sensitivity. The face, the inner part of the thighs, the abdomen, and the chest are the most sensitive parts.

Brush until your skin becomes rosy, warm, and glowing. Five to ten minutes is the average time, although some people like to brush longer. But do not scrub all your skin off! Everything is best in moderation, including your dry brush massage.

The best time for dry brush massage is upon arising in the morning and again before going to bed.

Massage followed by shower

After dry brush massage, it is advisable to take a shower or rub down with a sponge or wet towel to wash away dead skin particles. Brushing loosens up copious amounts of dead layers of skin that you can see as a dust on your body.

There are two ways to go about taking a shower. One is the alternating hot-and-cold shower, followed by dry brush massage. First, take a hot shower for 3 minutes or so, until you feel warmed up, then take a cold shower for about 10 to 20 seconds. Repeat this 3 times, always finishing with cold—as cold as you can stand. After this hot-and-cold shower, rub yourself dry with a coarse towel and then give yourself a brush massage that will warm you up thoroughly.

The other way, which is most suitable for relatively healthy people, is to take the dry brush massage first and finish with an alternating hot-and-cold shower. Of course, if you cannot tolerate the hot-and-cold shower, you can have a warm shower only. But the alternating hot-and-cold shower has an exceedingly beneficial and stimulating effect on all the vital functions of your body, particularly on the glandular system, and has a rejuvenating effect on your skin. The combination of the dry brush massage and a hot-and-cold shower is an excellent way to start and finish your day.

Why dry brush massage is so beneficial

The number one cause of all so-called degenerative diseases and premature aging is to be found in the derangement of cell metabolism and in slowed-down cell regeneration. This derangement is caused mainly by the accumulation of waste products in the tissues which interferes with the nourishment and oxygenation of the cells.

Normally, under ideal circumstances, your body cleanses itself automatically without any conscious effort on your part. It is an ingeniously designed self-cleansing, self-protecting, and self-healing mechanism. Self-cleansing work is performed by a large group of specially-designed organs, glands, and transportation systems: the alimentary canal, kidneys, liver, lungs, skin, lymphatic system, and mucous membrane of various body cavities. But your largest eliminative organ is the skin.

It is estimated that one-third of all body impurities are excreted through the skin. Doctors often refer to the skin as the "third kidney"—and very appropriately so. Hundreds of thousands of very tiny sweat glands act not only as the regulators of body temperature, but also as small kidneys—detoxifying organs—ready to cleanse the blood and free the system from health-threatening poisons. The chemical analysis of sweat shows that it has almost the same constituents as urine. Uric acid, the main metabolic waste product, and a normal component of urine, is found in large amounts in perspiration. If the skin becomes inactive and its pores choked with millions of dead cells, uric acid and other impurities will remain in the body.

The other eliminative organs, mainly the liver and kidneys, will have to increase their labor of detoxification because of the inactive skin, with the result that they will be overworked and eventually weakened or diseased. Toxins and wastes will then be deposited in the tissues. Thus, you must realize the great importance of always keeping your skin in perfect working condition.

The eliminative capacity of the skin is demonstrated by the fact that more than one pound of waste products is discharged through the skin every day. This explains why man became aware of the healing effect of sweating very early in history. The Finnish sauna and the Turkish, Russian, and Roman baths have been used for healing purposes for thousands of years. The famous Seventeenth Century Dutch physician, Sylvius, said, "One-third of all diseases can be cured by sweating."

In addition to its eliminative work, the skin has many other vital functions. The body actually breathes through the skin, absorbing oxygen and exhaling carbon dioxide which is formed in the tissues. Also, certain nutrients are absorbed into the body through the skin. Russian scientific studies show that minerals from the sea water and sea air are absorbed through the skin. Other scientific studies have demonstrated that the skin is capable of assimilating various vitamins, minerals, and even proteins applied directly to the skin. It has long been known, too, that by a mysterious chemical process, vitamin D is manufactured on the skin by the influence of the sun's rays on the oils produced by the skin glands. Subsequently, vitamin D is absorbed into the system through the skin.

As you can see, your skin is a living, vital organ with a multiplicity of important functions. The tragedy is that the skin of modern man is the most neglected and mistreated organ. In our sheltered, air-conditioned existence, the skin is seldom exposed to life-giving fresh air or to stimulating temperature changes. How many times this week have you worked or exercised outdoors hard enough to cause profuse perspiration? Dry brush massage will give your skin the stimulation, exercise, and cleansing of which it may be deprived by a sedentary way of life.

Here is an impressive list of benefits you will derive from regular dry brush massage:

1. It will effectively remove the dead layers of skin and other impurities and keep pores open.
2. It will stimulate and increase blood circulation in all underlying organs and tissues, and especially in the small blood capillaries of you skin.
3. It will revitalize and increase the eliminative capacity of your skin and help to throw toxins out of the system.
4. It will stimulate the hormone- and oil-producing glands.
5. It will have a powerful rejuvenating influence on the nervous system by stimulating nerve endings in the skin.
6. It will help prevent colds, especially when used in combination with hot-and-cold showers.

7. It will contribute to a healthier muscle tone and a better distribution of fat deposits.

8. It will rejuvenate the complexion and make it look younger.

9. It will make you feel better all over.

10. It will improve your health generally, and help prevent premature aging.

Since dry brush massage also happens to be one of the most *pleasant* and enjoyable do-it-yourself health measures, don't you think that the above list is impressive enough to convince you to give this million-dollar health and beauty secret an honest try? I am quite confident that once you try it, you will be "sold on it" for the rest of your life!

Some important tips on dry brush massage

1. Every two weeks or so wash your brush with soap and water and dry it in the sun or in a warm place. Your brush will rapidly be filled with impurities and should be washed regularly.

2. For hygienic reasons, use separate brushes for each member of the family.

3. Avoid brushing the parts of your skin that are irritated, infected, or damaged in any way.

4. The scalp should be brushed, too. For scalp brushing, a good natural bristle brush is a must—no substitute will do. Scalp brushing will stimulate hair growth by increasing blood circulation, and will keep scalp free from dandruff, stale oils, and other impurities.

5. The facial skin of most people is too sensitive for brushing; therefore, it is better to leave it alone.

6. If you don't have a brush with an extended handle, ask your husband to help you with the brushing. Brush massage is doubly enjoyable when somebody else gives it to you. A mutual morning and evening brush massage session may even add a new dimension to your marriage!

7. If your skin is dry and shows the signs of premature aging, an excellent way to improve the quality of your skin and the looks of your complexion is to rub or massage your whole body with a nourishing oil immediately after dry brushing. I particularly recommend the following oils: sesame oil, olive oil, avocado oil, almond oil. Or better still, use my *FORMULA F-PLUS* (see Chapter 32).

HOW TO TAKE A SITZ BATH

There are three kinds of sitz baths: the hot sitz bath, the cold sitz bath, and the alternating hot-and-cold sitz bath.

The hot sitz bath is beneficial for relieving pain and inflammation in the reproductive organs and other organs of the pelvic region. The water should be as hot as can be borne comfortably and the duration of the bath should be 10 to 15 minutes.

The cold sitz bath has a stimulating and invigorating effect on the reproductive organs and the spine. It is popularly called a "youth bath," because of its rejuvenative effect as the result of increasing blood circulation to the vital centers. The temperature of the water should be 50° - 65° F, and the duration of the bath from 3 to 5 minute. After the bath, rub yourself warm with a coarse bath towel.

The alternating hot-and-cold sitz bath has great therapeutic value in most internal disorders. Not only are organs and glands of the pelvic region stimulated and revitalized, but practically all body functions are beneficially affected. This bath is especially beneficial for all who have lowered vitality.

For the alternating hot-and-cold sitz bath, two tubs are required: one containing hot, and the other cold, water. For a do-it-yourself sitz bath, some large metal or plastic household tubs (like a baby bath, for example) can be used. The temperature of the hot water should be about 98° - 100° F and the cold water should be about 50° - 65° F. Sit in hot water first for 5 minutes, then switch to cold water for 5 to 10 seconds. Repeat twice.

For the hot *or* cold sitz baths, you can use the regular tub in your bathroom. Fill the tub with water about 8 inches deep, or a little less than half-full. Sit in the tub with your knees drawn up (use a little box or stool) so that only the "sitz" is covered by the water. If a cold sitz bath is given to a person in very weak condition, it is advisable to place the feet in a small tub or pan filled with warm water.

A sitz bath can be taken 2 or 3 times a week.

HOW TO TAKE AN ENEMA

Enemas should be taken during therapeutic or cleansing fasting mentioned in several chapters of this book.

To take an enema, you must have an enema can or bag with a rubber hose and a nozzle, which can be obtained at any drug store.

Fill the enema bag with lukewarm water—about 99° F. Add a few drops of fresh lemon juice or a cup of camomile tea if desired, but you may use just plain water. For a do-it-yourself enema, 1 pint to 1 quart of water is sufficient.

The best position for taking an enema is on your knees, head down to the floor, with the enema bag hanging 2½ to 3 feet above the anus in order to get sufficient pressure in the flow of water. The flow can be regulated by squeezing the tube with the fingers; some enema bags have a special clamp to regulate the flow. Before inserting the nozzle into the anus make sure there is no air left in the tube; let the water run for a moment. Use some vaseline or other lubricant on the nozzle to make insertion easier. If you feel discomfort or pain when the water is running in, stop the flow for a while and take a few deep breaths; then continue until the bag is empty.

If you can retain the water for a while and do not feel forced to empty the bowels at once, you may lie down for a few minutes and let the water do its dissolving and washing work before letting it out. First lie on the back for a minute, then on the right side, then on the stomach, and then on the left side. While you are doing this, gently massage your stomach with your hands. Then go to the toilet and let the water run out. Stay long enough to make sure that the bowels are empty.

An enema should be taken at least once each fasting day. The best time is the first thing in the morning. After the fast is broken, enemas should be continued until the bowels begin to move naturally. This usually takes 2 or 3 days. As soon as normal peristalsis is established, enemas should be discontinued.

Here are some points to watch:

- Make sure that the enema water is not too cold or too hot; it should be of body temperature or slightly above.
- Keep the equipment clean; wash it with soap and water. If several people are using the same equipment, disinfect the nozzle with rubbing alcohol, then rinse with water.

HOW TO USE HERBS AND HERB TEAS

Herbs have been used as healing agents since the beginning of time by every race upon the earth. Primitive people in every corner of this planet possessed remarkable knowledge of the medicinal value of certain roots, barks, seeds, and plants that grew in their environment. This knowledge was handed down from one generation to the next.

Later, when the primitive medicine man was replaced by modern medical doctors, almost 90 percent of the medical pharmacopoeia that doctors used was made up of botanical medicines: herbs, roots, etc. The oldest medical literature, such as **Papyrus Ebers** (Second Century B.C.), **Atherva Veda,** and all the records of Persian, Roman, Hebrew, Chinese, and Egyptian medicine, shows that herbal medicine was in highest regard and used extensively to treat practically every ill known to man. As late as in the 1800's, fully 80 percent of medicines available to doctors were plant derivatives.

Although with the advance of chemical science, doctors of today have all but forgotten the healing treasures of nature, in many parts of the world herbs are still used as remedial agents. In Mexico, botanical medicine was highly advanced during the Mayan, Incan, and Aztec cultures and has survived until present times. It is not an exaggeration to say that more herbs than chemical drugs are used in Mexico today for healing purposes, judging by the amount of herbs sold in numerous herbal shops and stands on every market in every village, town, and city. In Indian, China, Central and South America, Africa, and the Pacific Islands, herbs are still widely used—the art of botanical medicine having been carefully preserved by skillful herbalists.

Even modern Twentieth Century medical science, after being contemptuous of herbal medicine for decades, is now turning "back to nature" and is engaged in world-wide research of old-time herbal remedies. Some of our largest pharmaceutical companies are testing thousands of herbs and plants in hopes of isolating the supposedly active medicinal ingredient and put it in tablet form. Some of today's most commonly-used tranquilizers are made from a plant called snakeroot (Rauwolfia). A commonly-used heart medicine, digitalis, is made from the leaves of the plant called foxglove. In Mexico, testosterone tablets (male sex hormone) are now manufactured by a leading drug company from sarsaparilla root. Chemists from all major drug companies are studying old books on herbs in hopes of finding effective and harmless medicines to replace some of the harmful and ineffective chemicals in modern drugstores. Even the National Cancer Institute is now seriously investigating natural plant treatments for cancer. Several universities, notably the University of Arizona, California College of Medical Evangelists, Utah University, and others, backed by government and private grants, are engaged in a search of medicinal plants that can be used in the treatment of a mushrooming list of diseases that chemical drugs have been powerless against: cancer, arthritis, multiple sclerosis, psoriasis, heart disease, etc.

Medical science is now confirming what the Bible told us from the beginning and what "primitive" people around the world know all along—that man's best medicine is close to him and all around him, in the plant kingdom. There is not a single disease in man that does not have a corresponding remedy or cure in some herb, root, bark, or other botanical medicine. As it is said, "for every disease there is a cure," and this cure was given to man by a wise and loving Creator right in his close environ-ment—in the plant kingdom. It behooves us to learn about and use these God-given herbal remedies to cure our ills.

Most herbs are available in health food stores. They are also sold through the mail by numerous herb houses. Look in the Yellow Pages of your telephone directory for one nearest you. They also usually advertise in health magazines.

Some of the useful herbs may grow in your own environment: dandelion, birch leaves, camomile, common nettle, alfalfa, peppermint, comfrey, rose hips, raspberry leaves, chaparral, eucalyptus leaves, juniper berries, parsley—to name a few. These herbs can be picked and dried for future use. They should be picked early in the summer, preferably when the plant is in full bloom; berries and fruits are picked at the peak of ripeness. Herbs should then be dried outside in the shade, in a well-ventilated area. When they are thoroughly dry, keep them in tightly closed glass jars or in heavy brown paper bags. The same applies to barks and roots, although they require a much longer time for drying.

How to prepare herbs for use

The most common way to use herbs, especially leaves, blossoms, and small plants, is in the form of *teas,* or what are professionally called *infusions.*

Here's how you make herb tea: take 1 tsp. of dried herbs to a cup of water, or 1 ounce of the herb to 1 pint of water if a larger quantity is desired. Boil the water. Place herbs in a cup or container and pour the boiling water over the herb. Cover and let steep for 3 to 5 minutes. After that, stir, let settle, strain, and let cool down to drinking temperature—never drink the tea boiling hot! There is no wisdom in curing acne and dying of stomach cancer, which drinking boiling hot liquids surely can cause! Tea may be sweetened with a little natural honey. *NOTE: Infusions* or ***herb teas*** should never be boiled!

Another way to use herbs is in the form of a ***decoction.*** Decoctions are made by boiling herbs in water for a considerable length of time. Hard materials, such as roots, barks, seeds, etc., are normally prepared as decoctions, since it would require a longer time to extract the active ingredients from them.

Here's how to make decoctions: place 1 ounce of roots, bark, or seeds in 1½ pints of cold water. Cover and boil for ½ hour. Let stand and steep for another ½ hour. Then strain, cool, and drink, or store in glass jar in the refrigerator for future use. While teas should be made fresh every day, decoctions can be stored for about 1 week.

Some herbs are used in the form of ***tinctures.*** Tinctures are herb extractions made with the help of pure or diluted spirits of alcohol, or brandy or vodka. The main reasons for making tinctures are that the medicinal property of some herbs is destroyed by the use of heat, and some herbs will not yield the active ingredient to water alone.

Tinctures are made in the following way: 1 ounce of ***powdered*** herb is mixed with 12 ounces of pure spirits diluted with 4 ounces of water. Vodka or brandy do not require water and can be used straight. The mixture is allowed to stand for 10 to 14 days; the bottle should be shaken every day. After that, the contents are strained through a fine flannel, the sediments discarded, and the clear tincture is bottled for future use.

Poultices are another way to use herbs. There are two ways in which poultices are usually applied:

1. Fresh whole leaves—usually large leaves of such plants as comfrey, cabbage, raspberries, or nettles—are placed directly on the affected part, such as the joints or abdomen, in layers of several leaves over each other, then covered with a piece of cloth and finally wrapped with a large towel or blanket. Such a poultice "draws" the disease out of the affected part and soothes the pain.

2. Fresh leaves or plants are crushed and heated in a little water (sometimes in castor oil), then spread as hot as can be tolerated directly on the affected parts and covered with cloth. A plastic sheet is placed over the cloth, then a towel, and on top of all, an electric heating pad. The poultice should be left on for ½ to 1 hour. The medicinal property of the herb in combination with heat has a powerful healing effect, especially in rheumatic and arthritic conditions. Dried herbs can also be used for such a poultice if fresh herbs are not available.

References

Chapter 1
The Fulfilling Role of Motherhood

1. Clymer, R. Swinburne, *Prenatal Culture: Creating the Perfect Baby,* Philosophical Publishing Co., Quakertown, PA., 1950.
2. Randolph, B.P., *Race Regeneration,* Philosophical Publishing Co., Quakertown, PA.

Chapter 2
Preparing for Pregnancy

1. Airola, Paavo, *Are You Confused?,* 9th edition, 1978, and *Health Secrets From Europe,* Health Plus Publishers, P.O. Box 22001, Phoenix, AZ., 85028.
2. Price, Weston, *Nutrition and Physical Degeneration,* Price-Pottinger Foundation, Santa Monica, CA.
3. Report in *Datamation* Magazine, October, 1977. Also, *Arizona Republic,* Nov. 4, 1977.
4. Thurston, Emory W., *Nutrition for Tots to Teens,* Argold Press, Inc., Encino, CA., 1976.
5. Larson, Gena, *Better Foods for Better Babies,* P.O. Box 582, Leeds, Utah, 84746.
6. Ott, John, *Health and Light: The Effects of Natural and Artificial Light on Man and Other Living Things,* Davin-Adair Co., 1973.
7. *Canadian Medical Association Journal,* Oct. 23, 1965.
8. Airola, Paavo, *Rejuvenation Secrets From Around the World—That "Work,"* Health Plus Publishers, P.O. Box 22001, Phoenix, AZ., 85028, 3rd edition, 1977.

Chapter 3
Optimum Nutrition for Mother-To-Be

1. Schweigart, H.A., Prof., Dr. Med., *Eiweis, Fette, Harzinfarkt,* Verlag H.H. Zanner, Munchen, Germany.
2. Passwater, Richard, *Supernutrition for Healthy Hearts,* The Dial Press, N.Y., 1977.
3. Brackbill, Yvonne, "Obstetrical Medication and Infant Behavior," *Handbook of Infant Development,* ed. J.D. Osofsky, John Wiley & Sons, 1978.
4. Gennser, Gerhard, et al., "Maternal Smoking and Fetal Breathing Movements," *American Journal of Obstetrics and Gynecology,* Vol. 123, No. 8, 1975.

5. Airola, Paavo, *How To Get Well,* Health Plus Publishers, P.O. Box 22001, Phoenix, AZ., 12th edition, 1978.

6. Ivy, A.C., *Gastroenterology,* March, 1955.

7. Airola, Paavo, *Are You Confused?,* Health Plus Publishers, P.O. Box 22001, Phoenix, AZ., 85028, 9th edition, 1978.

8. Williams, Roger J., *Nutrition Against Disease,* Pitman Publishing Corporation, N.Y., 1971.

9. Airola, Paavo, *Rejuvenation Secrets From Around The World—That "Work,"* Health Plus Publishers, P.O. Box 22001, Phoenix, AZ., 85028, 3rd edition, 1977.

10. Taub, Harold J., "We May Have the Answer to Breast Cancer," *Let's Live,* June, 1976.

11. Airola, Paavo, "The Folly of the High-Protein Diet" (fully documented and referenced), *Hypoglycemia: A Better Approach,* Health Plus Publishers, P.O. Box 22001, Phoenix, AZ., 85028, 4th edition, 1978.

12. *A Bircher-Benner Way to Positive Health and Vitality,* Bircher-Benner Verlag, Zurich, Switzerland. Also: *Der Wendepunkt,* Vol. 52, p. 443, 1975.

13. *Resolution #80,* International Society for Research on Diseases of Civilization and Environment, Belgium.

14. *Dietary Goals for the United States,* prepared by the staff of the Select Committee on Nutrition and Human Needs, United States Senate, Washington, D.C., 1977.

15. Gerber, Donald A., Report in *New York Times,* April 7, 1965.

16. Bernstein, D.S., and Wachman, A., Department of Nutrition, Harvard University, "Diet and Osteoporosis," *Lancet,* Vol. 7549, p. 958, 1968.

17. Vascular Research Laboratory Report in *American Medical Association News Release,* June 21, 1965.

18. Thomas, W.A., et al., *American Journal of Cardiology,* Jan. 1960, Also, *AMA News Release,* June 21, 1965.

19. Visek, Willard, "Report on Cornell University Research," *Los Angeles Times,* March 29, 1973.

20. Issels, Josef, "Nutritional Protection Against Cancer," *Tidscrift For Halsa,* No. 2, 3, and 4, 1972, Stockholm, Sweden.

21. Jones, Kenneth L., et al., *Lancet,* June 9, 1973, pp. 1267-1271.

22. Newton, Niles, and Modahl, Charlotte, "Pregnancy: The Closest Human Relationship," *Human Nature,* March, 1978.

23. Pantel, Robert, et al., *Taking Care of Your Child: A Parent's Guide to Medical Care,* Addison-Wesley Publishing Co., Inc. Reading, Mass.

24. Lindberg, W.O., *American Journal of Clinical Nutrition.*

Chapter 5
Understanding Your Pregnancy

1. Newton, Niles, and Modahl, Charlotte, "Pregnancy: The Closest Human Relationship," *Human Nature,* March, 1978.

2. Gennser, et al., *American Journal of Obstetrics and Gynecology,* Vol. 127, No. 8, 1975.

3. Jones, Kenneth L., et al., *The Lancet,* June, 1973.

4. O'Rahilly R., and Gardner, E., "The Timing and Sequence of Events in the Development of the Human Nervous System During the Embryonic Period Proper," Z. Anat. Entwickl. Gesch. 134:1, 1971.

5. Winick, M., and Nobel A., *Journal of Nutrition,* 89:300, 1966.

6. Pitkin, Roy M., Editor, "Nutrition in Pregnancy," *Dietetic Currents,* Vol. 4, No. 1, Jan.-Feb., 1977.

7. Zucker, T.A., *American Journal of Clinical Nutrition,* 6, 65, 1958.

8. Davis, Adelle, *Let's Get Well,* New American Library, Inc., N.Y., N.Y., 1972.

9. *Recommended Dietary Allowances,* Seventh Revised Edition, Food and Nutrition Board, National Research Council, National Academy of Science, Washington, D.C., 1968.

10. *Recommended Dietary Allowances,* Eighth Revised Edition, Food and Nutrition Board, National Research Council, National Academy of Science, Washington, D.C., 1974.

11. King, J., "Protein Metabolism During Pregnancy," *Clin. in Perinatol.,* 2:243, 1975.

12. Sontag, Lester W., "Implications of Fetal Behavior and Environment for Adult Personalities," *Annals, New York Academy of Sciences,* Vol. 134, 1966, pp. 782-786.

13. Newton, Niles, "Emotions of Pregnancy," *Clinical Obstetrics and Gynecology,* Vol. 6, 1963.

14. Larson, Gena, *Better Foods for Better Babies,* P.O. Box 582, Leeds, Utah, 84746.

15. Rorvik, David M., with Landrum B. Shettles, M.D., Ph.D., *Your Baby's Sex: Now You Can Choose,* 1970.

Chapter 6
Natural Childbirth

1. Read, Grantly Dick, *Childbirth Without Fear: The Principles and Practice of Natural Childbirth,* Harper and Brothers, N.Y., revised edition, 1953.

2. Tanzer, Deborah, *Why Natural Childbirth?,* Doubleday Co., Inc., Garden City, N.Y., 1972.

3. Velvovsky, I., *Painless Childbirth Through Psychoprophylaxis,* Foreign Languages Publishing House, Moscow, 1960.

4. Lamaze, Fernand, *Painless Childbirth,* Simon & Schuster, Inc., N.Y., 1976.

5. Chabon, Irwin, *Awake and Aware,* Dell Publishing Co., Inc., N.Y. 1970.

6. Bradley, Robert A., *Husband-Coached Childbirth,* Harper & Row, N.Y., 1965.

7. Meerlo, Joost, "The Psychological Role of the Father," *Child and Family,* Vol. 7, No. 2, Spring, 1968.

8. "Home Birth vs. Hospital Birth," *Mothering,* Vol. VII, Spring, 1978.

9. Maynard, Fredelle, "Home Births vs. Hospital Births," *Woman's Day,* June 28, 1977.

10. *Consumer Reports, The Medicine Show,* Consumers Union, Mount Vernon, N.Y., 1970.

11. Hoffeld, D.R., et al., "Effect of Tranquilizing Drugs During Pregnancy and Activity of Offspring," *Nature,* 218:357 - 58, 1968.

12. Yuncker, Barbara, "Peril to Fetus in Sweets," *New York Post,* April 17, 1971.

13. Herron, J.R., *Bulletin of Maternal Welfare,* 2:9, 1956.

14. Buxton, C. Lee, *A Study of Psychophysical Methods for Relief of Childbirth Pain,* W.B. Saunders Co., Philadelphia, PA., 1962.

15. Hellman, Louis M., et al., *Williams Obstetrics,* 14th ed., Appleton-

Century-Crafts, N.Y., 1971, p. 459.
16. Windle, William F., "Brain Damage by Asphyxia at Birth," *Scientific American,* Vol. 221, No. 4, October, 1969.
17. Borgstedt, A.D., and Rosen, M.G., *American Journal of Diseases of Children,* 115:21-24, 1968.
18. Langmuir, Alexander, Editorial, *New England Journal of Medicine,* Vol. 284, No. 16, April 22, 1971.
19. Milinaire, Caterine, *Birth,* Harmony Books, N.Y., N.Y., 1974.
20. Borbach, Arthur, *Pregnancy, Birth, & The Newborn Baby,* The Boston Children's Medical Center, Delacorte Press/Seymour Lawrence, Boston, 1972, p. 180.
21. Montagu, Ashley, *Life Before Birth,* New American Library, Inc., N.Y., 1964, 5th printing, 51-53.
22. Archavsky, J.A. (original text in Russian), *Vopr. Pediatri,* 20:45, 1953.
23. Baum, J.D., and Scopes, J.W., *Inst. Ch. Health,* Hammersmith Hospital, London, (September, 1968).

Chapter 7
Infant Feeding

1. Fomon, Samuel J., *Infant Nutrition,* Second edition, W.B. Saunders Co., Philadelphia, PA., 1974.
2. Newton, Niles, *Family Book of Child Care,* Harper and Row, New York, 1957.
3. Ritchie, J.H., et al., *New England Journal of Medicine,* 279:1185, Nov. 28, 1968.
4. Josephs, Hugh, "Iron Absorption in Human Physiology," *Blood,* 13:1-54, 1958.
5. Wilson, John E., et al., "Sensitization to Cow's Milk May Cause One Form of Iron-Deficiency Anemia," *Journal of Pediatrics,* 60:5, 787-99.
6. Freedman, S.S., "Milk Allergy in Atopic Eczema," *American Journal of Diseases of Childhood,* 102 (1961) :76.
7. Grulee, C.G., and Sanford, N.H., "The Influence of Breast and Artificial Feeding on Infantile Eczema," *Journal of Pediatrics,* 9 (1936) :223.
8. Gerrard, John W., "Allergy in Infancy," *Ped. Annals,* October, 1974.
9. Backman, K.D., and Dees, S.C., "Milk Allergy: Observations on Incidence and Symptoms of Allergy to Milk in Allergic Infants," *Pediatrics,* 2 (1957) :400.
10. Fruthaler, G.J., "Can Allergy Be Prevented?", *So. Med. J.,* 58:836, 1965.
11. Soloman, J.B., *Fetal and Neonatal Immunology,* North Hollywood Publishing Co., 1971, pp. 118-21.
12. Hanson, L.A., and Winberg, J., "Breast Milk and Defense Against Infections in the Newborn," *Arch. of Diseases in Childhood,* 47:845, 1972.
13. Seligman, Jean, "The Tanka Syndrome," *Newsweek,* Sept. 12, 1977.
14. Larson, Gena, *Better Food For Better Babies,* P.O. Box 582, Leeds, Utah, 84746.
15. Myres, A.W., "Infant Overfeeding," *Nutrition Today,* 9:36, 1974.
16. Taitz, L., "Infantile Overnutrition Among Artificially-Fed Infants in the Sheffield Region," *British Medical Journal,* 1:315, 1971.
17. World Health Organization, Report of Twenty-Seventh World Health Assembly, Resolution, May 18, 1974.

18. Michael, J.G., et al., "The Antimicrobial Activity of Human Colostrum Antibody in the Newborn," *Journal of Infectious Diseases,* 124:445-8.
19. Thurston, Emory W., *Nutrition For Tots and Teens,* Argold Press, Inc., Encino, CA., 1976.
20. Gyorgy, Paul, "Trends and Advances in Infant Nutrition," *W. Va. Medical Journal,* 53:121, 1957.
21. Hill, L.F., et al., Report of the Committee on Nutrition of the American Academy of Pediatrics on "The Feeding of Solid Foods to Infants," *Pediatrics,* 21:685, 1958.
22. Taitz, L., Infantile Overnutrition Among Artificially-Fed Infants," *British Medical Journal,* 1:315, 1971.
23. Myres, A.W., "Infant Overfeeding," *Nutrition Today,* 9:36, 1974.
24. Yomans, John B., "The Changing Face of Nutritional Disease in America," *Journal of the American Medical Association,* 189:672, 1964.
25. Brobeck, J.R., ed., *Best & Taylor's Physiological Basis of Medical Practice,* 9th edition, Williams & Wilkins, Baltimore, MD., 1973, pp. 2-37.
26. Torress-Pinedo, et al., "Studies on Infant Diarrhea III," *Pediatrics,* 42:303-311.
27. Chaney-Ross, *Nutrition,* 7th Edition, Houghton Mifflin Co., Boston, 1966, p. 385.
28. Fomon, S.J., et al., "Excretion of Fat by Normal Infants Fed Various Milks and Formulas," *American Journal of Clinical Nutrition,* 23:1299.
29. Hogan, A.G., *Nutrition Abstracts Review,* 19:750, 1950.
30. Haemel, Helmut, "Human Normal and Abnormal Gastrointestinal Flora," *American Journal of Clinical Nutrition,* 23:1433-49.
31. Bullen, J.U., et al., "Iron-Binding Proteins in Milk and Resistance to E. Coli," *British Medical Journal,* 1:69-75.
32. *Science,* April 5, 1974.

Chapter 8
Solid Foods: When, What Kind, How Much

1. Fruthaler, G.J., "Can Allergy Be Prevented?", *So. Med. Journal,* 58:836, 1965.
2. Kimball, E. Robbins, Paper presented at La Leche League International Convention, 1964.
3. Gyorgy, Paul, "Trends and Advances in Infant Nutrition," *W. Va. Medical Journal,* 53:121, 1957.
4. Tschetter, Paul, *La Leche League News,* May/June, 1965.
5. Hill, L.F., et al., Report of the Committee on Nutrition of the American Academy of Pediatrics on "The Feeding of Solid Foods to Infants," *Pediatrics,* 21:685, 1958.
6. Yomans, John B., "The Changing Face of Nutritional Disease in America," *Journal of the American Medical Association,* 189:672, 1964.
7. Forbes, Gilbert B., Editorial, *Journal of Pediatrics,* 51:496, 1958.
8. Airola, Paavo, *How To Get Well,* Health Plus Publishers, P.O. Box 22001, Phoenix, AZ., 85028, 12th edition, 1978.
9. Airola, Paavo, *Are You Confused?,* Health Plus Publishers, P.O. Box 22001, Phoenix, AZ., 85028, 9th edition, 1978.

Chapter 10
The Development of Character

1. *The Bookshelf Plan of Child Development*, The Mother's Department, The University Society, Inc., 1963.
2. Flinders, Neil J., "Principles of Parenting," *The Ensign*, April, 1975.
3. Airola, Paavo, "Nutrition Forum," *Let's Live*, January, 1977.

Chapter 11
Love and Sexual Behavior: Emerging Womanhood

1. Gerson, A., *Psychology Reports*, February, 1976.
2. Dodson, F., *How To Parent*, Signet, The New American Library, N.Y., 1970.
3. "The Parent Gap," *Newsweek*, September 22, 1975.
4. Cronley, Connie, *"Blackboard Jungle Updated,"* TWA Ambassador, Sept., 1978.
5. Skolnick, A., *Intimate Environment*, Little, Brown & Co., Boston, 1973.

Chapter 12
Allergies

1. Kimball, E. Robbins, Paper presented at La Leche League International Convention, 1964. (See LLL *Information Sheet No. 16*).
2. Gerrard, John W., "Allergy in Infancy," *Ped. Annals*, October, 1974.
3. Backman, K.D., and Dees, S.C., "Milk Allergy: Observations on Incidence and Symptoms of Allergy to Milk in Allergic Infants," *Pediatrics*, 20 (1957) :400.
4. Freedman, S.S., "Milk Allergy in Atopic Eczema," *American Journal of Diseases in Childhood*, 102 (1961) :76.
5. Grulee, C.G., M.D., and Sanford, H.N., M.D., "The Influence of Breast and Artificial Feeding on Infantile Eczema," *J. Pediatrics*, 9 (1936) :223.
6. Fallstrom, S.P., Winberg, J., and Anderson, H.J., "Cow's Milk Induced Malabsorption as a Precursor of Gluten Intolerance," *Acta Paediatrica Scand.*, 54 (1965) :101.
7. Frier, S., "Paediatric Gastrointestinal Allergy," *Clinical Allergy*, 3 (1973) :597.
8. Brobeck, J.R., ed., *Best & Taylor's Physiological Basis of Medical Practice*, 9th edition, Williams & Wilkins, Baltimore, MD., 1973, pp. 2-37.
9. Fomon, Samuel J., *Infant Nutrition*, 2nd edition, W.B. Saunders, Philadelphia, PA., 1974, p. 370.
10. Fruthaler, G.J., "Can Allergy Be Prevented?", *So. Medical Journal*, 58 (1965) :836.
11. Johnstone, Douglas E., "Office Management of Food Allergy in Children," *Annals of Allergy*, 30 (1972) :173.

Chapter 13
Infant Anemia

1. "Anemia," La Leche League International, Inc., *Information Sheet No. 24*, September, 1974.

2. Josephs, Hugh, "Iron Absorption in Human Physiology," *Blood,* 13:1-54, 1958.
3. Friedman, L., et al., *Journal of Nutrition,* 65:143, 1958.
4. Priev, I.G., "Effect of Bottle Feeding on Copper and Iron Metabolism in Infants During the First Year of Life," *Fed. Proc., Pt. II,* 24:T614, 1965.
5. Ritchie, J.H., et al., *New England Journal of Medicine,* 279:1185, 1968.
6. Thurston, E.W., *Nutrition for Tots and Teens,* Argold Press, Inc. Encino, CA., 1976.
7. Bullen, J.J., et al., *British Medical Journal,* 1:69, 1972.
8. Davis, Adelle, *Let's Have Healthy Children,* New American Library, Inc., N.Y., N.Y., 1972.
9. Meyer, Herman F., *Infant Foods and Feeding Practices,* Chas. Thomas Publishers, Springfield, Ill., 1960.
10. Wilson, John E., et al., "Sensitization to Cow's Milk May Cause One Form of Iron-Deficiency Anemia," *Journal of Pediatrics,* 60:5, 787-99.
11. Harfouche, Jamal K., *Growth and Illness Patterns of Lebanese Infants,* Published in Beirut, 1966, p. 198.
12. Aitken, F.C., et al., *Nutrition Abstracts Review,* 30:341, 1960.
13. Finch, Clement A., "Iron Metabolism," *Nutrition Today,* Summer, 1969.
14. Kimball, E.R., Paper presented at La Leche League International Convention, 1964, *LLL Information Sheet No. 203.*
15. Albritton, E.C., *Standard Values in Blood,* W.B. Saunders Co., Philadelphia, PA., 1952.
16. Davison, W.C., and Levinthal, J., *The Complete Pediatrician,* 8th Revised Edition, Duke Press, 1961.
17. Tedeschi, C.G., et al., *American Journal of Obstetrics and Gynecology,* 71:16, 1956.

Chapter 14
The Hyperactive Child

1. Feingold, Ben F., *Why Your Child is Hyperactive,* Random House, Inc., N.Y., N.Y., 1975.
2. Pfeiffer, Carl C., *Zinc and Other Micronutrients,* Keats Publishing Co., New Canaan, Conn., 1978.
3. Yudkin, John, *Sweet and Dangerous,* Bantam Books, Inc., N.Y., N.Y., 1973.
4. Cheraskin, Em., et al., *Psychodietetics,* Stein and Day, N.Y., N.Y., 1974.
5. Ott, John, et al., *Academic Therapy,* Fall, 1974.
6. Preston, Harley, J., et al., "Hyperkinesis and Food Additives: Testing the Feingold Hypothesis," *Pediatrics,* 61:818-828, June, 1978.
7. Conners, C. Keith, et al., "Food Additives and Hyperkinesis," *Pediatrics,* 58:154-166, August, 1976.
8. Williams, J. Ivan, et al., "Relative Effect of Drugs and Diet on Hyperactive Behavior," *Pediatrics,* 61:811-817, June, 1978.

Chapter 15
Infant Obesity

1. Fomon, S., *Infant Nutrition,* p. 79, 1974.
2. Knittle, J., and Ginsberg-Fellner, F., *Diabetes,* 21:754, 1972.

3. Hirsch, J., and Knittle, J., *Federation Proceedings*, 29:1516, 1970.
4. Rodin, Judith, "The Puzzle of Obesity," *Human Nature*, Feb., 1978.
5. Asher, P., *Arch. Diseases of Childhood*, 44:672, 1966.

Chapter 16
Colic

1. *Pregnancy, Birth, and the Newborn Baby*, The Boston Children's Medical Center, Boston, 1972.
2. Thurston, Emory, *Nutrition for Tots and Teens*, Argold Press, Inc., Encino, CA., 1976.
3. Smith, Lendon H., *The Children's Doctor*, Prentice-Hall, Inc., Englewood Cliffs, N.J.
4. *White Paper on Infant Feeding*, Center for Science in the Public Interest, Washington, D.C., 1974.
5. Miller, T., *Journal of Bacteriology*, 98:949, 1969.
6. Gyorgy, P., *American Journal of Clinical Nutrition*, 24:970, 1971.
7. Hentges, D., *Journal of Bacteriology*, 93:2029, 1967.
8. Bullen, J., et al., *British Medical Journal*, 1:69, 1972.

Chapter 17
Acne

1. Bosco, Dominick, "The Case Against the Pill," *Prevention*, March, 1976.
2. Hawaii Permanente Medical Group, Inc., Kaiser Medical Center, *Report*, April, 1976.
3. *Medical Tribune*, June, 1976, pp. 41, 51.
4. Wright, Jonathan V., "A Case of Menstrual Upset with Acne and Depression," *Prevention*, September, 1976.
5. Michaelsson, Gerd, et al., *Archives of Dermatology*, January, 1977.
6. *The Natural Way to A Healthy Skin*, Rodale Books, Inc., Emmaus, PA.
7. Airola, Paavo, *The Miracle of Garlic*, Health Plus Publishers, P.O. Box 22001, Phoenix, AZ., 85028, 1978.
8. Plewig, G., et al., *Archives of Dermatology*, March, 1970.
9. Airola, Paavo, *How To Keep Slim, Healthy, and Young with Juice Fasting*, Health Plus Publishers, P.O. Box 22001, Phoenix, AZ., 85028, 9th edition, 1978.
10. Bricklin, Mark, *The Practical Encyclopedia of Natural Healing*, Rodale Press, Inc., Emmaus, PA., 1976.

Chapter 19
The Circumcision Decision

1. Aitken-Swan, and Baird, *British Journal of Cancer*, 19:217, 1965.
2. Khanolkar, *Acta Un. Int. Cancer*, 6:881, 1950.
3. Preston, *Journal of American Medical Association*, 213:1853, 1970.
4. Leith, *Australian Pediatric Journal*, 6:59, 1970.
5. Prensky, J., *Mothering*, Vol. II, 1977, p. 29.
6. King, Howard S., and Feinbloom, Richard I., in *Pregnancy, Birth and the Newborn Baby*, The Boston Children's Medical Center, Delacorte Press/Seymour Lawrence, 1972.
7. Topp, Sylvia, *Mothering*, Vol. VI, 1978.
8. Will, *No. Carolina Medical Journal*, 29:103, 1968.

Chapter 20
Immunizations: A New Look

1. Gordon, Douglas, *Health, Sickness, and Society,* University Queensland Press, 1976.
2. Stewart, Gordon T., *British Medical Journal,* Jan. 31, 1976.
3. Dettman, Glen, Communication to *Mordialloc-Chelsea News,* May 18, 1977.
4. Dettman, Glen C., "Immunization: Is It Now a Health Hazard?", paper presented at the combined seminar, 1974, at the University of Hong Kong.
5. Kalokerinos, Archie, and Dettman, Glen, "Science Friction," *Cosmos,* Vol. 5, No. 1.
6. Bechamp, A., *The Blood and Its Third Anatomical Element,* John Onsley, London, 1912.
7. "Life, Death, and Medicine," *Scientific American,* 1973.
8. Powles, D., *National Times,* Nov. 12, 1973.
9. The *Journal of the American Medical Association,* January 23, 1978.
10. The *Journal of the American Medical Association,* March, 1975.
11. Reprint from Congressional Record on Compulsory Vaccination, available from Health Research, P.O. Box 70, Mokelumne Hill, CA.
12. Cooke, Robert, "Rubella Vaccine: A Doubtful Program," *Let's Live,* November, 1971.
13. Kalokerinos, Archie, and Dettman, Glen, "Does Rubella Vaccine Protect," *Australasian Nurses Journal,* May, 1978, p. 4.
14. Allan, B., *Australian Journal of Med. Tech.,* Vol. 4, Nov. 1973, p. 26-27.
15. Mendelsohn, R., *The People's Doctor, A Medical Newsletter for Consumers,* Vol. 2, No. 4, April, 1978.
16. Honorof, Ida, *Leaves of Healing,* Vol. 1, No. 4, June 19, 1977.
17. *Modern Medicine,* Australia, March 9, 1973, and August 6, 1973.
18. *National Health Federation Bulletin,* Nov., 1969.
19. *Morbidity and Mortality Weekly Report, U.S.A.,* Vol. 26, No. 29, July 22, 1977, Center for Disease Control.
20. Giles, P.F.H., *Australian and New Zealand Journal of Obstetrics and Gynecology,* 13:77, 1973.
21. Krugman, S., *Journal of Pediatrics,* 78:1, 1971.
22. Hannisian, A.S., et al., *Modern Medicine,* Jan. 7, 1974, p. 43.
23. Salk, Jonas, and Salk, Darrell, *Science Abstracts,* Vol. 195, April 4, 1977.
24. Fox, Rosemary, *British Medical Journal,* Feb., 1976.
25. *Sunday Telegraph,* October 21, 1973.
26. Miller, et al., *British Medical Journal,* Vol. 2, 210-213, 1967.
27. Mendelsohn, Robert, "Ask The Doctor," *San Francisco Chronicle,* May 22, 1978.
28. Fredericks, Carlton, "Hotline," *Prevention,* September, 1976.
29. Honorof, Ida, "The Untold Dangers," *Vegetarian World,* No. 11, 1977.
30. Nittler, Alan H., "Immunizations," *Let's Live,* Nov., 1974.
31. Wilson, Sir Graham, *The Hazards of Immunization,* Athlone Press, University of London, 1967.
32. Douglas, Hume E., *Bechamp on Pasteur,* 3rd edition, C.W. Daniel Co., Ltd., Essex, U.K., 1947.

33. Burnet, Sir MacFarlane, "Influenza—The Disease," *Medical Journal of Australia,* 1:6, 1973.
34. Rimland, Bernard, *Science News,* Vol. 114, August 12, 1978, p. 99.
35. Kalokerinos, A., "Australian Aborginal Health and Vitamin C," *Australian Nurses Journal,* December, 1977.
36. Stone, Irwin, *The Healing Factor: Vitamin C,* Grosset & Dunlap, N.Y., 1972.
37. Sandine, W., Communication to Dr. Glen C. Dettman, referred personally to the author.
38. Airola, Paavo, *The Miracle of Garlic,* Health Plus Publishers, P.O. Box 22001, Phoenix, AZ., 85028, 1978.
39. "Drug Warnings and Precautions," *International Medical Digest,* July, 1969.
40. Pauling, Linus, *The Journal of the Australian College of Biomedical Scientists,* July 6, 1973.
41. Klenner, F., *The Journal of the International Academy of Preventive Medicine,* Vol. 1, No. 1, 1974.
42. Bricklin, Alice, *Mother Love, The Book of Natural Child Rearing,* Running Press, Philadelphia, PA., 1975.
43. Prensky, Joyce "Simple Home Remedies," *Mothering,* Vol. 1, 1976.

Chapter 21

Other Health Problems in Childhood

1. Airola, Paavo, *How To Get Well,* Health Plus Publishers, P.O. Box 22001, Phoenix, AZ., 85028, 12th edition, 1978.
2. Pauling, Linus, *Vitamin C and the Common Cold,* W.H. Freeman & Co., San Francisco, 1970.
3. Airola, Paavo, *The Miracle of Garlic,* Health Plus Publishers, P.O. Box 22001, Phoenix, AZ., 85028, 1978.
4. *Lancet,* June 22, 1968.
5. The *Journal of the American Medical Association,* Vol. 145, No. 3, 1951.
6. Gross, P., et al., *New York State Journal of Medicine,* 50:2683, 1950.
7. Davis, Adelle, *Let's Get Well,* New American Library, Inc., N.Y., N.Y., 1972.
8. Clark, Michael, "Natural Treatment for Eczema," *Prevention,* October, 1973.
9. Mességué, Maurico, *Of Men and Plants,* Macmillan Co., 1973.
10. Wilson, Janney Carole, "Childhood Sleep Disorders," *Bestways,* September, 1978.
11. Smith, Lendon H., *Improving Your Child's Behavior Chemistry,* Prentice-Hall, N.Y., 1976.
12. Olness, Karen, *Clinical Pediatrics,* March, 1975.
13. Clymer, R.S., *Prenatal Culture: Creating the Perfect Baby,* The Philosophical Publishing Co., Quakertown, PA., 1950.
14. Clymer, R.S., *The Mystery of Sex* and *Race Regeneration,* The Philosophical Publishing Company, Quakertown, PA., 1950.
15. Randolph, B.P., *The Immortality of Love,* Beverly Hall Corporation, Quakertown, PA., 1978.
16. Poesnecker, G.E., *Creative Sex,* Clymer Health Clinic Publication, Quakertown, PA., 1976.
17. Ricchio, Paul P., from Doctor Ricchio's correspondence to the author.

Chapter 22
Birth Control: Natural and Unnatural

1. "The Menace of the Pill and the Help You Can Get From Vitamins," *Today's Living*, July, 1975.
2. Okie, Susan, "Women Abandon Pill for Less Hazardous Birth Control Methods," *Arizona Republic*, August 5, 1975.
3. Fredericks, Carlton, "Hotline to Health," *Prevention*, Feb., 1974.
4. Bricklin, Mark, "Nutrition and Personal Appearance," *Prevention*, July, 1975.
5. Greenwald, Judith, "Rating the Latest Methods of Birth Control," *Harper's Bazaar*, March, 1975.
6. Airola, Paavo, *Sex and Nutrition*, Award Books, N.Y., 1970.
7. Fredericks, Carlton, "Hotline to Health," *Prevention*, May, 1973.
8. Klein, Jill, *"B_6 and a Woman's Femininity,"* Prevention, Aug., 1975.
9. DeVries, Julian, "Contraceptive Pill Criticized," *Arizona Republic*, Aug. 7, 1975.
10. "Vitamin A, The Pill, and Liver Cancer," *Today's Living*, July, 1975.
11. *Medical Tribune Report*, Feb. 5, 1968.
12. "The Pill: A New Warning," *Time*, Sept. 8, 1975.
13. *Journal of the American Medical Association*, Feb. 28, 1966.
14. "B_{12} Levels Change in Women on the Pill," *Prevention*, July, 1975.
15. *Lancet*, May 24, 1975.
16. Janerich, D.T., et al., *New England Journal of Medicine*, Oct. 3, 1974.
17. *Lancet*, August 31, 1974.
18. *Let's Live*, September, 1975, page 78.
19. Long, Howard, "Commentary," *Bestways*, July, 1975.
20. Hirsch, Roseann, "Zinc: Mini Nutrient, Maxi Importance," *Bestways*, August, 1974.
21. Kremer, William F., and Kremer, Laura, *The Doctors' Metabolic Dictionary*, Rutlege Books, 1975.
22. Honorof, Ida, *A Report to the Consumer*, Vol. VIII, No. 170, March, 1978.
23. *Nature*, Dec. 12, 1966.
24. "Medical World News," report in *Forum*, Oct., 1976.
25. Klenner, Fred, M.D., *The Key to Good Health: Vitamin C*, Graphic Arts Research Foundation, Chicago, Ill., 1969.
26. Lacey, Louise, *Lunaception: A Feminine Odyssey Into Fertility and Contraception*, Coward, McCann, and Geoghegan, N.Y., 1975.
27. Rorvik, David, "What's Better Than the Pill, Vasectomy, Celibacy, and Rhythm?", *Esquire*, January, 1975.
38. Lucas, R., *Common and Uncommon Uses of Herbs for Healthful Living*, Parker Publishing Co., N.Y., 1970.
29. Vogel, V., *American Indian Medicine*, Ballantine Books, N.Y., 1970.
30. DeMeo, James, "Herbal-Oral Contraceptives," *Mothering*, Vol. 5, 1977.
31. Himes, N., *Medical History of Contraception*, Schocken Books, N.Y., 1970.
32. Billings, J., M.D., *The Essence of the Ovulation Method*, Melbourne, 1972.
33. Nofziger, Margaret, *A Cooperative Method of Natural Birth Control*, The Book Publishing Co., Tenn., 1976.
34. Jackson, Leah, "Natural Birth Control: Seeing the Forest and the Trees," *East-West Journal*, Aug. 15, 1975.

Chapter 23
Ilolistic Approach to Menstrual Problems

1. Hoffman, Jay, Ph.D., *Hunza: Fifteen Secrets of the World's Healthiest and Oldest Living People,* Professional Press Publishing Association, Escondido, CA., 1968.
2. Airola, Paavo, *How To Get Well,* Health Plus Publishers, P.O. Box 22001, Phoenix, AZ., 85028, 12th edition, 1978.
3. Airola, Paavo, *Are You Confused?,* Health Plus Publishers, P.O. Box 22001, Phoenix, AZ., 85028, 9th edition, 1978.
4. Airola, Paavo, *Hypoglycemia: A Better Approach,* Health Plus Publishers, P.O. Box 22001, Phoenix, AZ., 85028, 4th edition, 1978.
5. Clark, Linda, "Ginseng, Fact or Fancy?", *Let's Live,* Sept., 1971.
6. Davis, Adelle, *Let's Get Well,* New American Library, N.Y., 1972.
7. "Bioflavonoids: Mother Nature's Answer to Female Problems," *Prevention,* October, 1974.
8. Lucas, Richard, *Common and Uncommon Uses of Herbs,* Parker Publishing Co., N.Y., 1970.
9. Kadans, Joseph, *Encyclopedia of Medicinal Herbs,* Parker Publishing Co., N.Y., 1970.
10. Ellis, John M., *The Doctor Who Looked At Hands,* Vantage Press, N.Y., 1966.
11. Airola, Paavo, *Sex and Nutrition,* Award Books, N.Y., 1970.
12. Passwater, Richard, Ph.D., "Vitamin E Deficiencies," *Prevention,* April, 1974.
13. Griffin, LaDean, *Is Any Sick Among You?,* Bi-World Publishers, Provo, Utah, 1974.
14. Fredericks, Carlton, "Hotline," *Prevention,* November, 1974.
15. Cheraskin, E., M.D., and Ringsdorf, W., M.D., *Psychodietetics,* Stein and Day, N.Y., 1974.
16. Hutchens, Alma, *Indian Herbology of North America,* Merco, Ontario, 1974.
17. Murray, Judith, "Disorder of Menstruation," *Mothering,* Vol. 5, 1978.
18. Christopher, John, *The Healthview Newsletter,* No. 18, 1978.

Chapter 24
Vaginitis: A Natural Approach

1. Airola, Paavo, *Sex and Nutrition,* Award Books, N.Y., 1970.
2. Wright, Joyce, M.D., "No. 1 Vaginitis Problem Today," *Sexology,* December, 1974.
3. *Forum,* January, 1975, p. 22.
4. Airola, Paavo, *How To Get Well,* Health Plus Publishers, P.O. Box 22001, Phoenix, AZ., 85028, 12th edition, 1978.
5. Davis, Adelle, *Let's Get Well,* New American Library, N.Y., 1972, p. 249.
6. Klenner and Bartz, *The Key to Good Health: Vitamin C,* Graphic Aids Research, Chicago, 1969.
7. Ant, M., *Annals of the New York Academy of Sciences,* No. 52, p. 374, 1949.
8. Shute, E.V., *Canadian Medical Association Journal,* No. 82, p. 72, 1960.
9. Airola, Paavo, *The Miracle of Garlic,* Health Plus Publishers, P.O.

Box 22001, Phoenix, AZ., 85028, 1978.
10. Green, H.N., et al., *British Medical Journal*, No. 2, p. 595, 1931.
11. Nittler, Alan, M.D., *Let's Live*, March, 1974, p. 109.
12. Nittler, Alan, M.D., *Let's Live*, June, 1974, p. 14.
13. Homola, Samuel, *Dr. Homola's Natural Home Remedies*, Prentice-Hall, N.Y., N.Y., 1973.
14. Griffin, LaDean, *Is Any Sick Among You?*, Bi-World Publishing Co., Provo, Utah, 1974.
15. Wigmore, Ann., N.D., Hippocrates Health Institute, Boston, Mass.
16. Kadans, Joseph, *Encyclopedia of Medicinal Herbs*, Parker Publishing Co., N.Y., 1970.
17. Kloss, Hutchens, Griffin, Kadans, and others.
18. Kabnick, Stuart, "Cabasil: Forms and Indications for Use," available from him at Broad-Locust Building, Philadelphia, PA.
19. Boston Women's Collective, *Our Bodies, Ourselves*.
20. Hutchens, Alma, *Indian Herbology of North America*, Merco, Ontario, 1974.
21. Schoenfield, Eugene, M.D., "Dr. Hippocrates," *L.A. Star*, No. 4, 1975.
22. "Feminine Hygiene: A Dangerous Myth," *Prevention*, Jan., 1977.
23. Gerber, Michael L., M.D., Personal Correspondence to the author, 1979.

Chapter 25

Breast Cancer Can Be Prevented

1. Annual Reports of the American Cancer Society and National Cancer Institute.
2. Newton, Niles, *The Family Book of Child Care*, Harper and Row, N.Y., 1957.
3. Homburger, F., and Fishman, W.H., *The Physiopathology of Cancer*, Paul B. Hoeber, N.Y., 1970.
4. Knight, G.F., Martin, Coda W., et al., "Possible Cancer Hazards of Feeding Diethylstilbestrol to Cattle," evidence presented at Congressional Hearings on Food Additives, 1957-58, pp. 283-5.
5. Taub, Harold, J., "We May Have the Answer to Breast Cancer," *Let's Live*, June, 1976.
6. Airola, Paavo, *Cancer: Causes, Prevention, and Treatment—The Total Approach*, Health Plus Publishers, P.O. Box 22001, Phoenix, AZ., 85028, 6th edition, 1977.
7. Airola, Paavo, "A Case for Freshness," *Let's Live*, October, 1977.
8. Airola, Paavo, *Are You Confused?*, Health Plus Publishers, P.O. Box 22001, Phoenix, AZ., 85028, 9th edition, 1978. See also: "A Case For Freshness," *Let's Live*, Oct., 1977.
9. Shamberger, Raymond, *Journal of the National Cancer Institute*, May, 1971.
10. Boynton, Herbert H., "Mighty Multi-Purpose Nutrient—Selenium," *Let's Live*, August, 1976.
11. *Journal of the American Medical Association*, August 14, 1954.
12. Larson, Gena, "Is There an Anti-Cancer Food?", *Prevention*, April, 1972.
13. Shamberger, Raymond J., *Journal of National Cancer Institute*, May, 1971.
14. "Vitamin A Fights Cancer," *Prevention*, April, 1972.
15. Adamstone, F.B., *American Journal on Cancer*, 28, 540, 1936.

16. Issels, Josef, *Cancer: A Second Opinion*, Hodder and Stoughton, London, 1975.

17. Warburg, Otto, "Concerning the Ultimate Cause and the Contributing Causes of Cancer," address delivered at a meeting of Nobel Prize Winners in Lindau, Germany, July, 1966.

18. Fredericks, Carlton, *Breast Cancer: A Nutritional Approach*, Grosset and Dunlap, 1977.

19. *Dietary Goals for the United States*, prepared by the staff of the Select Committee on Nutrition and Human Needs, United States Senate, U.S. Government Printing Office, February, 1977.

20. Seligman, Jean, "The Tanka Syndrome," *Newsweek*, Sept. 12, 1977.

21. Brody, Jane E., *You Can Fight Cancer and Win*, Quadrangle, The New York Times Book Co., N.Y., 1976.

22. Upton, Arthur C., M.D., Director, National Cancer Institute, Washington, D.C.

23. Lindberg, W.O., *American Journal of Clinical Nutrition*, 6, 1958.

24. Seeger, P.G., German Medical Journal, *Hippokrates*, Vol. 13, 1951.

25. Hueper, Wilhelm C., "Lung Cancer: Danger in the Air," *Newsweek*, Jan. 11, 1960.

26. Taylor, Alfred, *Proceedings of the Society for Experimental Biology and Medicine*, Vol. 119, p. 252, 1965.

27. Yiamouyiannis, John A., *National Health Federation Bulletin*, July-August, 1975, and September, 1975.

28. Garten, Max, *Civilized Diseases and Their Circumvention*, Maxmillion World Publishers, San Jose, CA., 1978.

29. Lewis, Howard R., and Martha E., *Psychosomatics*, Viking Press, Inc., N.Y., N.Y.

30. LeShan, Lawrence, "Cancer and Personality: A Critical Review," *Journal of the National Cancer Institute*, Jan., 1959.

31. From a speech delivered at the Special Conference on Breast X-rays, sponsored by the National Institutes of Health, September 14, 1977, Washington, D.C.

32. Stiller, Richard, "Selenium: Can It Protect Against Breast Cancer?", *Family Circle*, June 14, 1978.

33. Turner, James S., *The Chemical Feast*, Grossman Publishers, N.Y., 1970.

34. Lewis, Howard R., and Martha E., *Psychosomatics*, Viking Press, Inc., N.Y., N.Y.

35. LeShan, Lawrence, "Cancer and Personality: A Critical Review," *Journal of the National Cancer Institute*, January, 1959.

Chapter 26

Varicose Veins:
Prevention and Treatment

1. Dodd, H., *Lancet*, 2:809, 1964.

2. Burkitt, D.P., et al., *Lancet*, July 24, 1976.

3. Nittler, Alan, H., *Let's Live*, March, 1974, and August, 1974.

4. Passwater, Richard A., *Prevention*, March, 1976.

5. Lofgren, Eric P., and Lofgren, Karl A., *Geriatrics*, September, 1975.

6. Taub, Harold J., "How Women Should Use Vitamin E," *Let's Live*, May, 1976.

7. "Four Ways Women Can Prevent Varicose Veins," *National Enquirer*, August 22, 1978.

Chapter 27
What Every Woman Should Know About Sexually-Transmitted Diseases

1. *Family Health Guide and Medical Encyclopedia,* Editor James A. Maxwell, The Reader's Digest Association, Inc., Pleasantville, N.Y., 1976.
2. Rodgers, Joann, "The Dark Side of Intimacy," *Ladies' Home Journal,* Vol. XCIII, No. 10, October, 1976.

Chapter 28
What Smoking Does to Women

1. *National Study on Smoking Among Teenagers and Women,* American Cancer Society Report, 1976.
2. Report by Arthur C. Upton, M.D., Director, National Cancer Institute.
3. Field, Sydney S., *The Reader's Digest,* February, 1976.
4. Jick, Hershel, et al., *Lancet,* June, 1977.
5. Gennzer, Gerhard, Marshal, Karel, and Brantmark, Bo, "Maternal Smoking and Fetal Breathing Movements," *American Journal of Obstetrics and Gynecology,* Vol. 123, No. 8, 1975.
6. Brackbill, Yvonne, "Obstetrical Medication and Infant Behavior," *Handbook of Infant Development,* ed., J.D. Osofsky, John Wiley & Sons, 1978.
7. *Journal of the American Medical Association,* June 30, 1978.
8. "Smoking, A Big Killer of Women," *Sunday Telegraph,* Oct. 22, 1978.

Chapter 29
Depression: A New Epidemic

1. Kushner, Ross, "Depression: How To Cure It," *Forum,* 1977.
2. Kline, Nathan S., *Medical Tribune,* February 11, 1976.
3. Kline, Nathan S., *Journal of the American Medical Association,* March 11, 1974.
4. Weissman, Myrna M., Report at a National Association Mental Health Meeting in Washington, D.C., October, 1975.
5. Feltman, John, *Prevention,* July, 1976.
6. Watson, George, *Nutrition and Your Mind,* Harper and Row, N.Y., 1975.
7. Flack, Frederic, *The Secret Strength of Depression,* Lippincott, N.Y., 1974.
8. *British Medical Journal,* February 21, 1976.
9. *Lancet,* November 8, 1975.
10. *Lancet,* September 13, 1975.
11. Davis, Adelle, *Let's Get Well,* New American Library, Inc., N.Y., 1972.

Chapter 30
What Women Should Know About Anemia

1. **Herbert V.,** *American Journal of Clinical Nutrition,* 12:17, 1963.
2. Davis, Adelle, *Let's Get Well,* New American Library, Inc., N.Y., 1972.
3. Marvin, H.N., et al., *Proceedings of the Society for Experimental*

Biology and Medicine, 105:473, 1960.

4. Bishop, E.H., et al., *Journal of American Medical Association,* 178:812, 1961.
5. Horwitt, M.K., et al., *Journal of American Dietetic Association,* 38:231, 1961.
6. Hodges, R.E., et al., *American Journal of Clinical Nutrition,* 11:180, 1962.
7. Hines, J.D., et al., *American Journal of Clinical Nutrition,* 14:137, 1964.
8. Deaton, John G., *Prevention,* July, 1972.
9. Valberg, L.S., et al., *British Journal of Nutrition,* 15:473, 1961.
10. McCurdy, P.R., *Journal of American Society,* Vol. 21, February, 1973.

Chapter 31
How to Stay Younger Longer

1. Airola, Paavo, *Rejuvenation Secrets From Around the World—That "Work,"* Health Plus Publishers, P.O. Box 22001, Phoenix, AZ., 85028, 3rd edition, 1977.
2. Smolyanski, B.L., *Fed. Proc.,* 22:T1173, 1963.
3. Klenner, F.R., *Tri-State Medical Journal,* February 1959, February, 1960.
4. *Journal of the American Medical Association,* Vol. 235, No. 2, January 12, 1976.
5. Visek, Willard, "Report on Cornell University Research," *Los Angeles Times,* March 28, 1973.
6. Thomas, W.A., et al., *American Journal of Cardiology,* Jan., 1960; and *AMA News Release,* June 21, 1965.
7. Gerber, Donald A., report in *New York Times,* April 7, 1965.
8. Bernstein, D.S., and Wachman, A., *Lancet,* Vol. 7549, 1968.
9. Airola, Paavo, *The Miracle of Garlic,* Health Plus Publishers, P.O. Box 22001, Phoenix, AZ., 85028, 1978.

Chapter 33
Overweight: Must It Be A Lifetime Struggle?

1. Study at Medical College of University of Wisconsin, *Natural Health World and the Naturopath,* Vol. 17, No. 6, June, 1978.
2. Wolfe, Sidney, "The New Drop-Dead Diets," *Mother Jones,* June, 1978.
3. Watson, George, *Nutrition and Your Mind,* Harper and Row, N.Y., 1975.
4. Zelman, S., *Archives of Internal Medicine,* 90:141, 1952.
5. Airola, Paavo, *Hypoglycemia: A Better Approach,* Health Plus Publishers, P.O. Box 22001, Phoenix, AZ., 85028, 4th edition, 1978.
6. Knittle, J., and Ginsberg-Fellner, F., *Diabetes,* 21:754, 1972.
7. Hirsch J., and Knittle J., *Federation Proceedings,* 29:1516, 1970.
8. Feinbloom, Richard, "Obesity," *Pregnancy, Birth, and the Newborn Baby,* The Boston Children's Medical Center, Delacorte Press, Seymour Lawrence, Boston, 1972.
9. Gwinup, G., et al., *American Journal of Clinical Nutrition,* 13:209, 1963.

10. Editorial, *Journal of the American Medical Association*, 173: 1141, 1960.
11. Airola, Paavo, *How To Keep Slim, Healthy and Young With Juice Fasting*, Health Plus Publishers, P.O. Box 22001, Phoenix, AZ., 85028. 9th edition, 1978.
12. Mahoney, M.J., and Mahoney, Kathryn, *Permanent Weight Control*, W.W. Norton & Co., Inc., 1976.

Chapter 34
Menopause: Dreadful Affliction or Glorious Experience

1. *New England Journal of Medicine*, Dec. 4, 1975.
2. Cherry, Sheldon, H., *The Menopause Myth*, Ballantine Books, 1975.
3. *British Medical Journal*, October 18, 1975.
4. Fuhr, R., et al., *Annals of New York Academy of Science*, 52, 63, 1949.
5. Selye, H., *The Stress of Life*, McGraw-Hill, N.Y., N.Y., 1956.
6. Airola, Paavo, *Rejuvenation Secrets From Around the World—That "Work"*, Health Plus Publishers, P.O. Box 22001, Phoenix, AZ., 85028, 3rd edition, 1977.
7. Fredericks, Carlton, "Hotline to Health," *Prevention*, July, 1973.
8. *Lancet*, April 14, 1973.
9. Airola, Paavo, *How To Get Well*, Health Plus Publishers, P.O. Box 22001, Phoenix, AZ., 85028, 12th edition, 1978.
10. *Annals of Western Medicine and Surgery*, Vol. 4, pp. 27-32, 1950.
11. *New York State Journal of Medicine*, May 15, 1952.
12. Klein, Jill, "B_6 and Woman's Femininity," *Prevention*, Aug., 1973.
13. Ellis, John M., and Presley, James, *Vitamin B_6: The Doctor's Report*, Harper and Row, N.Y., 1973.
14. Gasmami, N.M., *The Journal of Chronic Diseases*, Vol. 16, No. 363.
15. Wade, Carlson, *Nature's Cures*, Award Books, N.Y., 1972.
16. Lucas, Richard, *Common and Uncommon Uses of Herbs*, Parker Publishing Co., N.Y., 1970.
17. Hutchens, Alma, *Indian Herbology In North America*, Merco, Ontario, Canada, 1973.
18. Malmstrom, Stan, *Herbal Remedies II*, Family Press, Salt Lake City, Utah, 1975.
19. Smith, R.W,. et al., *American Journal of Clinical Nutrition*, 14:98, 1964.
20. Finkler, R.S., *Journal of Clinical Endocrinology*, 9:89, 1949.
21. Davis, Adelle, *Let's Get Well*, New American Library, Inc., N.Y., 1972.
22. Murray, Judith, "Female Remedies," *Mothering*, Vol. 5, 1978.

Questions & Answers

1. Dann, T.C., and Roberts, D.F., *British Medical Journal*, August 4, 1973.
2. Schaefer, Otto, *Nutrition Today*, November-December, 1971.
3. Malina, Robert M., *Medicine and Science in Sports*, Vol. 5, No. 1, 1973.
4. Jennings, Joan, "Children, Sugar, and Premature Sexuality," *Prevention*, October, 1975.

5. *International Medicine,* May, 1975.
6. Rensberger, Boyce, "How Unsuspecting Women Get Hooked on Drugs," *Woman's Day,* September 1, 1978.
7. *Natural Life Magazine,* No. 15, Sept.-Oct., 1978, p. 43.
8. *Time,* November 19, 1978.
9. *Chicago Sun-Times,* March 9, 1978.
10. Davis, Adelle, *Let's Get Well,* New American Library, Inc., N.Y., 1972.
11. "Bread and Iron," *Time,* May 22, 1978.
12. Airola, Paavo, *How To Get Well,* Health Plus Publishers, P.O. Box 22001, Phoenix, AZ., 85028, 12th edition, 1978, p. 278.
13. Rockmore, Milton, "Can Vasectomies, Sterilizations Be Reversed?", *The Arizona Republic,* June 7, 1978.
14. Bellew, Bernard A., and Joeva Galas Bellew, "Processed Milks Linked to Unexplained Crib Deaths," *Let's Live,* August, 1974.
15. Davis, Adelle, *Let's Have Healthy Children,* New American Library, Inc., N.Y., 1972.
16. The *New Zealand Journal of Medicine,* January, 1970.
17. *Pregnancy, Birth, and the Newborn Baby,* Delacorte Press, Bantam, 1972.
18. "Sleep May Be Missing Link in Mystery Crib Death," The *STAR,* May 23, 1978.
19. Whaley, A.M., *Journal of the International Academy of Preventive Medicine,* Dec., 1976.
20. Lonsdale, Derrick, *Pediatric Research,* Vol. II, No. 4, 1977.
21. Kalokerinos, Archie, and Dettman, Glen, "The Sudden Infant Death Syndrome," *Australasian Nurses Journal,* March, 1978.
22. Klenner, F., *The Journal of Preventive Medicine,* Vol. 1, No. 1, Spring, 1974.
23. *New York Times,* July 7, 1978.
24. *New Directions for Women,* Autumn, 1978.

COMPOSITION OF FOODS
100 grams, edible portion

(dash (—) denotes lack of reliable data for a constituent believed to be present in measurable amount)

FOOD	CALORIES	PROTEINS grams	FATS grams	CARBOHYDRATES grams	CALCIUM mg.	PHOSPHORUS mg.	MAGNESIUM mg.	IRON mg.	SODIUM mg.	POTASSIUM mg.	VITAMIN A VALUE IU	B_1 mg.	B_2 mg.	NIACIN mg.	VITAMIN C mg.
ACEROLA cherry, raw	28	.4	.3	6.8	12	11	—	.2	8	83	—	.02	.06	0.4	1,300
ACEROLA JUICE, raw	23	.4	.3	4.8	10	9	—	.5	3	—	—	.02	.06	.4	1,600
ALMONDS, dried	598	18.6	54.2	19.5	234	504	270	4.7	4	773	0	.24	.92	3.5	trace
APPLES, freshly harvested	58	.2	.6	14.5	7	10	8	.3	1	110	90	.03	.02	.4	7-20
APPLE JUICE, canned or bottled	47	.1	trace	11.9	6	9	4	.6	1	101	—	.01	.02	.1	1
APRICOTS, raw	51	1.0	.2	12.8	17	23	12	.5	1	281	2,700	0.3	.04	.6	10
APRICOTS, dried, uncooked	260	5.0	.5	66.5	67	108	62	5.5	26	979	10,900	.01	.16	3.3	12
ARTICHOKES, globe or French, raw	9-47	2.9	0.2	10.6	51	88	—	1.3	43	430	160	.08	.05	1.0	12
cooked	8-44	2.8	.1	9.6	51	68	—	1.1	30	301	150	.07	.04	.7	8
ARTICHOKES, Jerusalem, raw	7-75	2.3	.2	16.7	14	78	11	3.4	—	—	20	.2	.06	1.3	4
ASPARAGUS, raw spears	26	2.5	.2	5.0	22	62	20	1.0	2	278	900	.18	.20	1.5	33
cooked spears	20	2.2	.2	3.6	21	50	14	.6	1	183	900	.16	.18	1.4	26
AVOCADOS, raw	167	2.1	16.4	6.3	10	42	45	.6	4	604	290	.11	.20	1.6	14
BANANAS, common, raw	85	1.1	.2	22.2	8	26	33	.7	1	370	190	.05	.06	.7	10
BARLEY, pearled, light	349	8.2	1.0	78.8	16	189	37	2.0	3	160	0	.12	.05	3.1	0

BEANS, common white, cooked	118	7.8	.6	21.2	50	148	37	2.7	7	416	0	.14	.07	.7	0
red, cooked	347	7.8	.5	21.4	38	140		2.7	3	340	trace	.11	.06	.7	
pinto, raw	349	22.9	1.2	63.7	135	457	46	6.4	10	984		.84	.21	2.2	
lima, immature cooked	123	8.4	.5	22.1	52	142	48	2.8	2	650	290	.24	.12	1.4	29
lima, mature, cooked	138	8.2	.6	25.6	29	154		3.1	2	612		.13	.06	.7	
mung, sprouted, raw	38	3.8	.2	6.6	19	64	32	1.3	5	223	20	.13	.13	.8	19
green, raw	32	1.9	.2	7.1	56	44	21	.8	7	243	600	.8	.11	.5	19
green, cooked	25	1.6	.2	5.4	50	37	25	.6	4	151	540	.07	.09	.5	12
BEETS, red, raw	43	1.6	.1	9.9	16	33	15	.7	60	335	20	.03	.05	.4	10
red, cooked	32	1.1	.1	7.2	14	23		.5	43	208	20	.03	.04	.3	6
BEET GREENS, raw	24	2.2	.3	4.6	119	40	106	3.3	130	570	6,100	.10	.22	.4	30
cooked	18	1.7	.2	3.3	99	25		1.9	76	332	5,000	.07	.15	.3	15
BLACKBERRIES, raw	58	1.2	.9	12.9	32	19	30	.9	1	170	200	.03	.04	.4	21
BLUEBERRIES, raw	62	.7	.5	15.3	15	13	6	1.0	1	81	100	.03	.06	.5	14
BRAZIL NUTS, raw	654	14.3	66.9	10.9	186	693	225	3.4	1	715	trace	.96	.12	1.6	
BROCCOLI, raw spears	32	3.6	.3	5.9	103	78	24	1.1	15	382	2,500	.10	.23	.9	113
cooked	26	3.1	.3	4.5	88	62	21	.8	10	267	2,500	.09	.20	.8	90
BRUSSELS SPROUTS, raw	45	4.9	.4	8.3	36	80	29	1.5	14	390	550	.10	.16	.9	102
cooked	36	4.2	.4	6.4	32	72	21	1.1	10	273	520	.08	.14	.8	87
BUCKWHEAT, whole grain	335	11.7	2.4	72.9	114	282	229	3.1		448	0	.60		4.4	0
BUTTER, salted	716	.6	81.	.4	20	16	2	0	987	23	3,300				0
unsalted	720	.6	82.	.4	20	16		0	8	9	3,350			0	
BUTTERMILK, cultured, from skim milk	36	3.6	.1	5.1	121	95	14	trace	130	140	trace	0.4	.18	.1	1
CABBAGE, white, raw	24	1.3	.2	5.4	49	29	13	.4	20	233	130	.05	.05	.3	47
red, raw	31	2.0	.2	6.9	42	35		.8	26	268	40	.09	.06	.4	61
savoy, raw	24	2.4	.2	4.6	67	54		.9	22	269	200	.05	.08	.3	55
CAROB FLOUR	180	4.5	1.4	80.7	352	81									
CARROTS, raw	42	1.1	.2	9.7	37	36	23	.7	47	341	11,000	.06	.05	.6	8
CASHEW NUTS	561	17.2	45.7	29.3	38	373	267	3.8	15	464	100	.43	.25	1.8	
CAULIFLOWER, raw	27	2.7	.2	5.2	25	56	24	1.1	13	295	60	.11	.10	.7	78
cooked	22	2.3	.2	4.1	21	42		.7	9	206	60	.09	.08	.6	55
CELERY, raw	17	.9	.1	3.9	39	28	22	.3	126	341	240	.03	.03	.3	9
CHARD, Swiss, raw	25	2.4	0.3	4.6	88	39	65	3.2	147	550	6,500	.06	.17	.5	32
cooked	18	1.8	.2	3.3	73	24		1.8	86	321	5,400	.04	.11	.4	16

FOOD	CALORIES	PROTEINS grams	FATS grams	CARBOHYDRATES grams	CALCIUM mg.	PHOSPHORUS mg.	MAGNESIUM mg.	IRON mg.	SODIUM mg.	POTASSIUM mg.	VITAMIN A VALUE IU	B1 mg.	B2 mg.	NIACIN mg.	VITAMIN C mg.
CHEESE, Blue or Roquefort	368	21.5	30.5	2.0	315	339	48	.5	700	82	1,240	.03	.61	1.2	
Cheddar	398	25.0	32.2	2.1	750	478	45	1.0	229	85	1,310	.03	.46	.1	
Cottage, creamed	106	13.6	4.2	2.9	94	152	—	.3	290	72	170	.03	.25	.1	
Cottage, uncreamed	86	17.0	.3	2.7	90	175	—	.4	710	104	10	.03	.28	.1	
Swiss	370	27.5	28.0	1.7	925	563	—	.9		—	1,140	.01	.40	.1	
Brick	370	22.2	30.5	1.9	730	455	—	.9		—	1,240	—	.45	.1	
CHERRIES, sour, red, raw	58	1.2	.3	14.3	29	19	14	.4	2	191	1,000	.05	.06	.4	10
sweet, raw	70	1.3	.3	17.4	22	19	9	.4	2	191	110	.05	.06	.4	10
frozen, sour, red	55	1.0	.4	13.4	13	22	10	.7	2	188	1,000	.04	.07	.3	5
CHESTNUTS, fresh	194	2.9	1.5	42.1	27	88	41	1.7	6	454	—	.22	.22	.6	—
COCONUT MEAT, fresh	346	3.5	35.3	9.4	13	95	46	1.7	23	256	0	.05	.02	.5	3
dried	662	7.2	64.9	23.0	26	187	90	3.3	—	588	0	.06	.04	.6	0
COCONUT WATER, from green coconuts	22	.3	.2	4.7	20	13	28	.3	25	147	0	trace	trace	.1	2
COLLARDS, raw, leaves	45	4.8	0.8	7.5	250	82	57	1.5	—	450	9,300	0.16	.31	1.7	152
cooked	33	3.6	.7	5.1	188	52	38	.8	1	262	7,800	.11	.20	1.2	76
CORN, whole-grain, dried, raw	348	8.9	3.9	72.0	22	268	147	2.1	trace	284	490	.37	.12	2.2	
SWEET, on-the-cob, raw	96	3.5	1.0	22.0	3	111	48	.7	trace	280	400	.15	.12	1.7	12
cooked on the cob	91	3.3	1.0	21.0	3	89	19	.6	1	196	400	.12	.10	1.4	9
flour	368	7.8	2.6	76.8	6	164	106	1.8		—	340	.20	.06	1.4	
bread, whole-grain	207	7.4	7.2	29.1	120	211	—	1.1	628	157	150	.13	.19	.6	1
CRANBERRIES, raw	46	.4	.7	10.8	14	10	8	.5	2	82	40	.03	.02	.1	11
CUCUMBERS, raw	15	.9	.1	3.4	25	27	11	1.1	6	160	250	.03	.04	.2	11

CURRANTS, black, raw	54	1.7	.1	13.1	60	40	15	1.1	3	372	230	.05	.05	.3	200
DANDELION GREENS, raw	45	2.7	.7	9.2	187	66	36	3.1	76	397	14,000	.19	.26	—	35
DATES	274	2.2	.5	72.9	59	63	58	3.0	1	648	50	.09	.10	2.2	0
EGGS, whole, raw	163	12.9	11.5	.9	54	205	11	2.3	122	129	1,180	.11	.30	.1	0
yolks, raw	348	16.0	30.6	.6	141	569	16	5.5	52	98	3,400	.22	.44	.1	0
cooked, whole	163	12.9	11.5	.9	54	205	—	2.3	122	129	1,180	.09	.28	.1	0
EGGPLANT, cooked	19	1.0	.2	4.1	11	21	—	.6	1	150	10	.05	.04	.5	3
ELDERBERRIES, raw	72	2.6	.5	16.4	38	28	—	1.6	—	300	600	.07	.06	.5	36
ENDIVE, raw	20	1.7	.1	4.1	181	54	10	1.7	14	294	3,300	.07	.14	.5	10
FIGS, raw	80	1.2	.3	20.3	35	22	20	.6	2	194	80	.06	.05	.4	2
dried	274	4.3	1.3	69.1	126	77	71	3.0	34	640	80	.10	.10	.7	0
FILBERTS (hazelnuts)	634	12.6	62.4	16.7	209	337	184	3.4	2	704	—	.46	.08	.9	trace
GARLIC, raw	137	6.2	.2	30.8	29	202	36	1.5	19	529	trace	.25	—	.5	15
GOOSENBERRIES, raw	39	0.8	.2	9.7	18	15	9	0.5	1	155	290	—	.02	—	33
GRAPEFRUIT, raw	41	.5	.1	10.6	16	16	12	.4	1	135	80	.04	.02	.2	38
juice	39	.5	.1	9.2	9	15	12	.2	1	162	80	.04	.03	.2	38
GRAPES, raw	69	1.3	1.0	15.7	16	12	13	.4	3	158	100	.05	.02	.3	4
juice, bottled	66	.2	trace	16.6	11	12	13	.3	2	116	—	.04	.05	.2	trace
GUAVAS, whole, raw	62	.8	.6	15.	23	42	13	.9	4	289	280	.05	.04	1.2	242
HONEY	304	.3	0	82.3	5	6	3	.5	5	51	0	trace	—	.3	1
HORSERADISH, raw	87	3.2	.3	19.7	140	64	34	1.4	8	564	—	.07	—	—	81
KALE, leaves, raw	53	6.0	.8	9.0	249	93	37	2.7	75	378	10,000	.17	.26	2.1	186
cooked	39	4.5	.7	6.1	187	58	—	1.6	43	221	8,300	.10	.18	1.6	93
KELP, raw	—	5.0	1.1	—	1,093	240	740	3.7	3,007	5,273	—	—	—	—	5-140
KOHLRABI, raw	29	2.0	.1	6.6	41	51	37	.5	8	372	20	.06	.04	.3	66
KUMQUATS, raw	65	.9	.1	17.1	63	23	—	.4	7	236	600	.08	.10	—	36
LEMONS, peeled, raw	27	1.1	.3	8.2	26	16	10	.6	2	138	20	.04	.02	.1	53
LEMON JUICE, raw	25	.5	.2	8.0	7	10	8	.2	1	141	20	.03	.01	.1	46
LENTILS, dry, cooked	106	7.8	trace	19.3	25	119	80	2.1	—	249	20	.07	.06	.6	0
LETTUCE, raw, romaine	18	1.3	.3	3.5	68	25	11	1.4	9	264	1,900	.05	.08	.4	18
Iceberg, New York	13	.9	.1	2.9	20	22	18	.5	9	175	330	.06	.06	.3	6
MANGOS, raw	66	.7	.4	16.8	10	13	—	.4	7	189	4,800	.05	.05	1.1	35

FOOD	CALORIES	PROTEINS grams	FATS grams	CARBOHYDRATES grams	CALCIUM mg.	PHOSPHORUS mg.	MAGNESIUM mg.	IRON mg.	SODIUM mg.	POTASSIUM mg.	VITAMIN A VALUE IU	B1 mg.	B2 mg.	NIACIN mg.	VITAMIN C mg.
MILK, cow's, whole	65	3.5	3.5	4.9	118	93	13	trace	50	144	140	.03	.17	.1	1
skim	36	3.6	.1	5.1	121	95	14	trace	52	145	trace	.04	.18	.1	1
dry, whole	502	26.4	27.5	38.2	909	708	98	.5	405	1,330	1,130	.29	1.46	.7	6
dry, skim non-instant	363	35.9	.8	52.3	1,308	1,016	143	.6	532	1,745	30	.35	1.80	.9	7
MILK, goat's, raw	67	3.2	4.0	4.6	129	106	17	.1	34	180	160	.04	.11	.3	1
MILLET, whole-grain	327	9.9	2.9	72.9	20	311	162	6.8	—	430	0	.73	.38	2.3	0
MOLASSES, blackstrap	213	—	—	55	684	84	258	16.1	96	2,927	—	.11	.19	2.0	—
MUSHROOMS, cultivated, raw	28	2.7	.3	4.4	6	116	13	.8	15	414	trace	.10	.46	4.2	3
MUSKMELONS, raw, cantaloupe	30	.7	.1	7.5	14	16	16	.4	12	251	3,400	.04	.03	.6	33
honeydew	33	.8	.3	7.7	14	16	—	.4	12	251	40	.04	.03	.6	23
MUSTARD GREENS, raw	31	3.0	.5	5.6	183	50	27	3.0	32	377	7,000	.11	.22	.8	97
NECTARINES, raw	64	.6	trace	17.1	4	24	13	.5	6	294	1,650	—	—	—	13
OATMEAL or rolled oats, dry	390	14.2	7.2	68.2	53	405	144	4.5	2	352	0	.60	.14	1.0	0
cooked	55	2.0	1.0	9.7	9	57	21	.6	—	61	0	.08	.02	.1	0
OKRA, raw	36	2.4	.3	7.6	92	51	41	.6	3	249	520	.17	.21	1.0	31
ONIONS, mature, raw	38	1.5	.1	8.7	27	36	12	.5	10	157	40	.03	.04	.2	10
green, bulb & top	36	1.5	.2	8.2	51	39	—	1.0	5	237	2,000	.05	.05	.4	32
ORANGES, peeled, raw	49	1.0	.2	12.2	41	20	11	.4	1	200	200	.10	.04	.4	50
ORANGE JUICE, raw	45	.7	.2	10.2	11	17	11	.2	1	200	200	.09	.03	.4	50
PAPAYA, raw	39	.6	.1	10.0	20	16	—	.3	3	234	1,750	.04	.04	.3	56
PARSLEY, raw	44	3.6	.6	8.5	203	63	41	6.2	45	727	8,500	.12	.26	1.2	172
PARSNIPS, raw	76	1.7	.5	17.5	50	77	32	.7	12	541	30	.07	.08	.1	10
PEACHES, raw	38	.6	.1	9.7	9	19	10	.5	1	202	1,330	.02	.05	1.0	7
PEANUTS, raw, with skins	564	26.0	47.5	18.6	69	401	206	2.1	5	674	—	1.14	.13	17.2	0

Food															
PEARS, raw	61	.7	.4	15.3	8	11	7	.3	2	130	20	.02	.04	.1	4
PEAS, raw, from pods	53	3.4	.2	12.0	62	90	35	.7	—	170	680	.28	.12	—	21
green, cooked	71	5.4	.4	12.1	23	99	—	1.8	1	196	540	.28	.11	2.3	20
split, cooked	115	8.0	.3	20.8	11	89	—	1.7	13	296	40	.15	.09	.9	—
PECANS	687	9.2	71.2	14.6	73	289	142	2.4	trace	603	130	.86	.13	.9	2
PEPPERS, raw, sweet, green	22	1.2	.2	4.8	9	22	18	.7	13	213	420	.08	.08	.5	128
raw, red	31	1.4	.3	7.1	13	30	—	.6	—	—	4,450	.08	.08	.5	204
PERSIMMONS, raw	127	.8	.4	33.5	27	26	8	2.5	1	310	—	—	—	—	66
PINEAPPLE, raw	52	0.4	0.2	13.7	17	8	13	0.5	1	146	70	.09	.03	.2	17
juice, canned, unsweetened	55	.4	.1	13.5	15	9	12	.3	1	149	50	.05	.02	.2	9
PLUMS, prune-type, raw	75	.8	.2	19.7	12	18	9	.5	1	170	300	.03	.03	.5	4
POTATOES, raw	76	2.1	.1	17.1	7	53	34	.6	3	407	trace	.10	.04	1.5	20
baked in skin	93	2.6	.1	21.1	9	65	—	.7	4	503	trace	.10	.04	1.7	20
boiled in skin	76	2.1	.1	17.1	7	53	—	.6	3	407	trace	.09	.04	1.5	16
PUMPKIN, raw	26	1.0	.1	6.5	21	44	12	.8	1	340	1,600	.05	.11	.6	9
PUMPKIN SEEDS, dry	553	29.0	46.7	15.0	51	1,144	—	11.2	—	—	70	.24	.19	2.4	—
RADISHES, raw	17	1.0	.1	3.6	30	31	15	1.0	18	322	10	.03	.03	.3	26
RAISINS, natural, uncooked	289	2.5	.2	77.4	62	101	35	3.5	27	763	20	.11	.08	.5	1
RASPBERRIES, raw, black	73	1.5	1.4	15.7	30	22	30	0.9	1	199	trace	.03	.09	0.9	18
red	57	1.2	.5	13.6	22	22	20	0.9	1	168	130	.03	.09	0.9	25
RICE, brown, cooked	119	2.5	.6	25.5	12	73	29	.5	3	70	0	.09	.02	1.4	0
RICE BRAN	276	13.3	15.8	50.8	76	1,386	—	19.4	trace	1,495	0	2.26	.25	29.8	0
RICE POLISHINGS	265	12.1	12.8	57.7	69	1,106	—	16.1	trace	714	0	1.84	.18	28.2	0
RUTABAGAS, raw	46	1.1	.1	11.0	66	39	15	.4	5	239	580	.07	.07	1.1	43
cooked	35	.9	.1	8.2	59	31	—	.3	4	167	550	.06	.06	.8	26
RYE, whole-grain	334	12.1	1.7	73.4	38	376	115	3.7	1	467	0	.43	.22	1.6	0
flour, dark	327	16.3	2.6	68.1	54	536	73	4.5	1	860	0	.61	.22	2.7	0
SAUERKRAUT, solids and liquid	18	1.0	.2	4.0	36	18	—	.5	—	140	50	.03	.04	.2	14
SESAME SEEDS, dry, whole	563	18.6	49.1	21.6	1,160	616	181	10.5	60	725	30	.98	.24	5.4	0
SOYBEANS, dry, raw	403	34.1	17.7	33.5	226	554	265	8.4	5	1,677	80	1.10	.31	2.2	—
cooked	130	11.0	5.7	10.8	73	179	—	2.7	2	540	30	.21	.09	.6	0
sprouted, raw	46	6.2	1.4	5.3	48	67	—	1.0	—	—	80	.23	.20	.8	13
sprouted, cooked	38	5.3	1.4	3.7	43	50	—	.7	—	—	80	.16	.15	.7	4

SOYBEAN CURD (TOFU)	72	7.8	4.2	2.4	128	126	111	1.9	7	42	0	.06	.03	.1	—
SOYBEAN FLOUR, full-fat	421	36.7	20.3	30.4	199	558	247	8.4	1	1,660	110	.85	.31	2.1	0
SOYBEAN MILK, powder	429	41.8	20.3	28.0	278	—	300	—	—	—	—	—	—	—	—
SPINACH, raw	26	3.2	.3	4.3	93	51	88	3.1	71	470	8,100	.10	.20	.6	51
cooked	23	3.0	.3	3.6	93	38	65	2.2	50	324	8,000	.07	.14	.5	28
SQUASH, summer, all varieties, raw	19	1.1	.1	4.2	28	29	16	0.4	1	202	410	.05	.09	1.0	22
cooked	14	.9	—	3.1	25	25	16	0.4	1	141	370	.05	.08	.8	10
winter, raw	50	1.4	.3	12.4	22	38	17	.6	1	369	3,700	.05	.11	.6	13
cooked (baked)	63	1.8	.4	15.4	28	48	17	.8	1	461	4,200	.05	.13	.7	13
STRAWBERRIES, raw	37	.7	.5	8.4	21	21	12	1.0	1	164	60	.03	.07	.6	59
SUNFLOWER SEED KERNELS, dry	560	24.0	47.3	19.9	120	837	38	7.1	30	920	50	1.96	.23	5.4	—
TOMATOES, ripe, raw	22	1.1	.2	4.7	13	27	14	.5	3	244	900	.06	.04	.7	23
TOMATO JUICE, canned	19	.9	—	4.3	7	18	10	.9	200	227	800	.05	.03	.8	16
TURNIPS, raw	30	1.0	.2	6.6	39	30	20	.5	49	268	trace	.04	.07	.6	36
cooked	23	.8	.2	4.9	35	24	—	.4	34	188	trace	.04	.05	.3	22
TURNIP GREENS, raw	28	3.0	.3	5.0	246	58	58	1.8	—	—	7,600	.21	.39	.8	139
WALNUTS, black	628	20.5	59.3	14.8	trace	570	190	6.0	3	460	300	.22	.11	.7	—
English	651	14.8	64.0	15.8	99	380	131	3.1	2	450	30	.33	.13	.9	2
WATERCRESS, raw	19	2.2	.3	3.0	151	54	20	1.7	52	282	4,900	.08	.16	.9	79
WATERMELON, raw	26	.5	.2	6.4	7	10	8	.5	1	100	590	.03	.03	.2	7
WHEAT, whole-grain, spring	330	14.0	2.2	69.1	36	383	160	3.1	3	370	—	.57	.12	4.3	0
winter	330	12.3	1.8	71.7	46	354	160	3.4	3	370	—	.52	.12	4.3	0
WHEAT BRAN	213	16.0	4.6	61.9	119	1,276	490	14.9	9	1,121	0	.72	.35	21.0	0
WHEAT GERM, raw	363	26.6	10.9	46.7	72	1,118	336	9.4	3	827	0	2.01	.68	4.2	0
WHEY, powder	349	12.9	1.1	73.5	646	589	130	1.4	—	—	50	.50	2.51	.8	—
YAM, tuber, raw	101	2.1	.2	23.2	20	69	31	.6	—	600	trace	.10	.04	.5	9
YEAST, brewer's debittered	283	38.8	1.0	38.4	210	1,753	231	17.3	121	1,894	trace	15.61	4.28	37.9	trace
torula	277	38.6	1.0	37.0	424	1,713	165	19.3	15	2,046	trace	14.01	5.06	44.4	trace
YOGURT, from whole milk	62	3.0	3.4	4.9	111	87	12	trace	47	132	140	.03	.16	.1	1
from skimmed milk	50	3.4	1.7	5.2	120	94	13	trace	51	143	70	.04	.18	.1	1

SOURCES: Agriculture Handbook No. 8, U.S. Dept. Agric. Washington, D.C.; Home and Garden Bulletin No. 72.

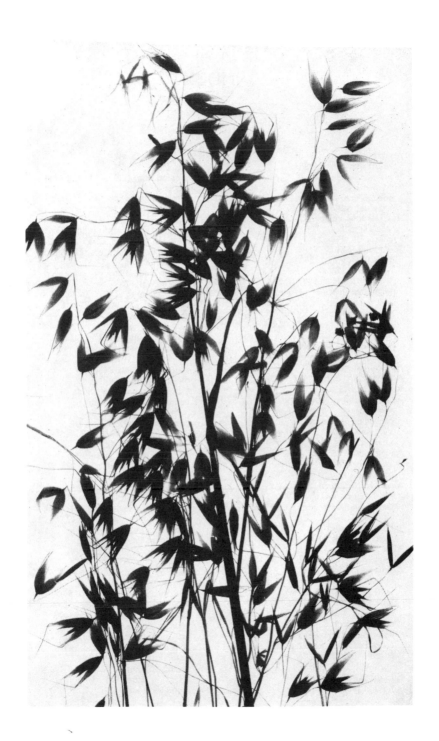

INDEX

W

X

Y

Z

ABOUT THE AUTHOR

Paavo Airola, Ph.D., N.D., is an internationally-recognized nutritionist, naturopathic physician, educator, and award-winning author. Raised and educated in Europe, he studied biochemistry, nutrition, and natural healing in biological medical centers of Sweden, Germany, and Switzerland. He lectures extensively world-wide, both to professionals and laymen, holding yearly educational seminars for physicians. He has been a visiting lecturer at many universities and medical schools, including the Stanford University Medical School.

Dr. Paavo Airola is the author of thirteen widely-read books, notably his two international best-sellers, *How To Get Well,* and *Are You Confused?* The American Academy of Public Affairs issued Dr. Airola the Award of Merit for his book on arthritis.

How To Get Well, the comprehensive Handbook of Natural Healing, is the most authoritative and practical manual on biological medicine in print. It is used as a textbook in several universities and medical schools, and regarded as a reliable reference manual, the "Bible of Natural Healing," by doctors, researchers, nutritionists, and students of health and holistic healing. Dr. Airola's book, *Hypoglycemia: A Better Approach,* has revolutionized the therapeutic concept of this insidious, complex, and devastating affliction.

Dr. Airola's newest monumental work, *Everywoman's Book,* is a great new contribution in the field of holistic medicine. It not only confirms Dr. Airola's unchallenged leadership in the field of nutrition and holistic healing, but demonstrates his genius as an original thinker, philosopher, and profound humanitarian.

Dr. Airola is President of the International Academy of Biological Medicine; a member of the International Naturopathic Association; and a member of the International Society for Research on Civilization Diseases and Environment, the prestigious Forum for world-wide research founded by Dr. Albert Schweitzer. Dr. Airola is listed in the *Directory of International Biography,* in *The Blue Book, The Men of Achievement, Who's Who in American Art,* and *Who's Who in the West.*

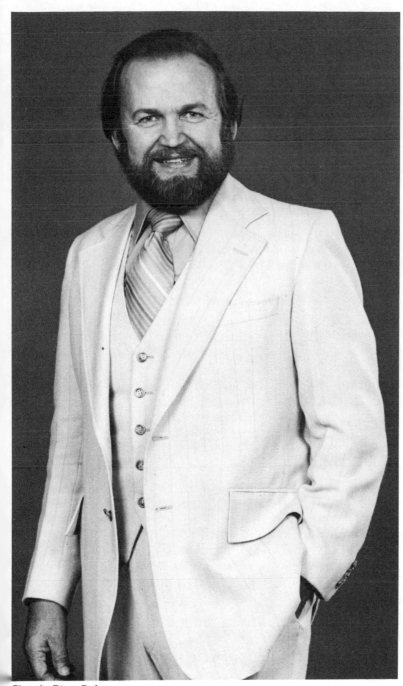

Photo by Diane Padys

Open Mar–Nov, New Year.
Rooms 10 double, 1 single. No telephone. 2 self-catering cottages.
Facilities Drawing room, lounge/bar, restaurant. No background music. 28-acre grounds on loch: private beach, fishing, boating; mountain bikes available. Pony-trekking, golf, stalking nearby. Only restaurant suitable for &.
Location From A82 S of Fort William take Corran ferry, then A861 to Strontian.
Restrictions No smoking: restaurant, bedrooms. Dogs by arrangement; not in public rooms.
Credit cards MasterCard, Visa.
Terms [2001] Room: single £48–£90, double £64–£130. Breakfast £8.50–£12.50. Set dinner (2 to 4 courses) £20.50–£29.50. Discounts for 3 or more nights. New Year package.

SWINTON Scottish Borders   **Map 5:E3**

The Wheatsheaf at Swinton   *Tel* 01890-860257
Main Street   *Fax* 01890-860688
Swinton, nr Duns TD11 3JJ   *Email* reception@wheatsheaf-swinton.co.uk
                                   Website www.wheatsheaf-swinton.co.uk

An old stone-built inn, on the green of a pretty village in the rolling countryside of the Merse, near the Berwickshire coast and the river Tweed. It is now a restaurant/pub-with-rooms, 'pleasant and civilised', 'extremely well-run' by owner/chef Alan Reid and his wife, Julie. It has won many commendations for its food – described by Alan Reid as 'modern Scottish with French influence'. This is served informally in the bar, which has a daily-changing blackboard menu, and in the restaurant, which specialises in Scottish game and seafood. The seasonal menu includes, eg, timbale of salmon, prawns and spinach with a dill and saffron dressing; roast loin of venison in a juniper and quince sauce; steamed lemon sponge pudding with crème fraîche and citrus zest. The conservatory is now part of the restaurant, and there is a lounge on the ground floor. The bedrooms are simple but comfortable; those by the road can get traffic noise. All have bathroom or shower *en suite*. Service is 'helpful, unhurried and genuinely welcoming', and breakfast includes freshly squeezed orange juice, smoked salmon with scrambled egg, grilled kippers, or a grilled vegetarian dish. There are good packed lunches. Local attractions include Paxton House, Abbotsford (home of Sir Walter Scott) and Mellerstain, a fine Adam house. (Good Pub Guide*, and others*)

Open All year, except Christmas, New Year, last 2 weeks Jan. Restaurant closed Sun evening/Mon.
Rooms 7 double.
Facilities Lounge bar, public bar, 2 dining rooms; boot room, drying room. No background music. 1-acre garden: patio, children's play area. River Tweed 4 miles: fishing; golf nearby. Unsuitable for &.
Location Centre of village 10 miles SW of Berwick-upon-Tweed; on road to Kelso (12 miles). 2 rooms get traffic noise. Parking. Train: Berwick; taxi.
Restrictions No smoking: restaurant, bedrooms. No dogs in public rooms.
Credit cards MasterCard, Visa.
Terms B&B: £42–£70. Alc lunch £15–£18; set dinner £28. 2-night breaks.

TALISKER Highland   Map 5:C1

Talisker House   *Tel* 01478-640245
Talisker   *Fax* 01478-640214
Isle of Skye IV47 8SF   *Email* jon_and_ros.wathen@virgin.net
                                         Website www.talisker.co.uk

Dramatically set beneath the imposing Preshal Mhor on the spectacular west coast of Skye, this Wolsey Lodge is a pretty whitewashed
Georgian house. Built in the 1720s as the dower house of the MacLeod
family, it was visited by Johnson and Boswell on their tour of the
Hebrides in 1773. It is now the family home of the 'helpful hosts', Jon
and Ros Wathen. The 'interesting building' has 'superb plasterwork'.
The setting, in a large garden with tall trees, is 'magically beautiful',
said one fan. There are fine views from the large bedrooms. 'Excellent
home-cooked food' – the Wathens describe this as 'modern Australian
eclectic' – is generally served communally, though two tables at dinner are just for two. A sample no-choice menu includes fish soup with
rouille; sweet chilli-roast chicken with lemongrass and risotto; glazed
Talisker apples with cinnamon ice cream. Some ingredients are home-
grown; ice creams and bread are home-made. Picnic lunches are good,
and the 'excellent' cooked breakfast comes with home-made preserves, on tables set with silver jugs. There are fine views from the
large bedrooms, where lavender bags on the pillows 'guarantee sweet
dreams'. Talisker Bay has safe swimming, and a sandy beach at low
tide. The nearby distillery produces a classic single malt. (*JM*)

Open April–end Oct.
Rooms 4 double. No telephone/TV. 1 suitable for &.
Facilities Drawing room, dining room. No background music. 5-acre grounds:
formal garden, croquet lawn. 10-min walk to Talisker Bay: sandy beach at low
tide; swimming.
Location W coast of Skye. Turn left off A863 from Sligachan on to B8009 to
Carbost. Veer left at top of village. Follow signs to Talisker (4 miles).
Restrictions No smoking. No children under 12. No dogs in house.
Credit cards MasterCard, Visa.
Terms [2001] B&B £43. Single supplement £14. Packed lunch £5. Set
dinner £25.

TANGASDALE Western Isles   Map 5:A1

The Isle of Barra Hotel   `BUDGET`   *Tel* 01871-810383
Tangasdale Beach   *Fax* 01871-810385
Isle of Barra HS9 5XW   *Email* barrahotel@aol.com
                                         Website www.isleofbarra.com/iob

'We cannot praise it too highly,' writes one satisfied visitor this year
to Diane Worthington's purpose-built hotel on this little island, just
four miles by eight. 'It is extremely well run, the owners are solicitous,
staff are welcoming, and the views are superb.' The setting is spectacular, overlooking Halaman Bay and the Atlantic, and with panoramic
views of Ben Tangaval. Arrival is by a small plane which lands on a
cockleshell beach or, more prosaically, by ferry from Oban. The

cocktail bar has seashell pictures; the restaurant has views over the sea. 'The food is excellent.' Neil MacDougall's four-course menus offer plenty of choice, and include Traigh Mhor cockles in garlic butter; spicy chicken wings; grilled Hebridean turbot; sirloin steak au poivre; brandy basket with vanilla ice cream and butterscotch sauce; there is always a vegetarian dish, eg, vegetable risotto. The '70s-style bedrooms are functional and not especially large, but they are clean, with comfortable beds and plenty of hot water. Coach parties are often accommodated. Activities include walking, bicycling, wild flower-spotting, seal watching, golf, fishing, and scuba diving; ancient Kisimul Castle, on a rocky outcrop in the bay, is worth a visit. (*Anne P Heaton*)

Open End Mar–early Oct, New Year.
Rooms 30 double. No telephone.
Facilities Residents' lounge, cocktail bar, public bar (live music occasionally), restaurant. Walking, fishing, sea angling, scuba diving; golf nearby. Unsuitable for &.
Location W side of island. Ferry, 4 times a week, from Oban to Castlebay, or British Airways Express daily flight from Glasgow. Bus from ferry and airport.
Restrictions No smoking: restaurant, lounge. No dogs in public rooms.
Credit cards MasterCard, Visa.
Terms B&B £32–£47; D,B&B £48–£62. Set dinner £21.95. 7 nights for the price of 6. Child in parents' room: under 2, free; 2–5, £5; 6–12, £10. *V*

TARBERT Western Isles   **Map 5:B1**

Leachin House   *Tel/Fax* 01859-502157
Tarbert   *Email* leachin.house@virgin.net
Isle of Harris HS3 3AH   *Website* www.leachin-house.com

'We could find no fault with this unexpected gem,' write visitors to Linda and Diarmuid Evelyn Wood's small stone inn, a Wolsey Lodge. Its name, pronounced Lee-ak-in, means 'house among the rocks'. Dramatically situated, it stands alone on the shores of West Loch, looking across to Ben Luskentyre, Taransay and the Atlantic ocean beyond, with Gilleval Glas rising to 1,500 feet behind. Its somewhat austere exterior contrasts with a comfortable interior: 'The spacious entrance hall is light and welcoming, and there is an interesting collection of family heirlooms, pictures and ship models' (reflecting the host's early career at sea). 'The welcome is superb.' 'The food is excellent and beautifully served' – communally, though the Woods don't dine with you – in the dining room, which still has the original 100-year-old hand-painted French wallpaper. No liquor licence, but a carafe of wine comes with the 'wonderful' no-choice set dinner (Linda Wood 'willingly provides an alternative if there's something you don't like') and 'a further carafe is offered with the cheese course'. A typical menu: scallops in vermouth; filet of local venison with sloe berry sauce; raspberry syllabub. The complimentary decanter of sherry in the bedroom is appreciated, too. Morning coffee and afternoon tea are included in the price, and breakfasts are huge. Bedrooms are spacious, with interesting old furniture; some have a loch view. Tarbert village (population 400) is a mile away. Local attractions include beaches, seals and otters, mountain walks, and wonderful wild scenery. Fishing and sea trips can be arranged, and bicycles hired. 'Mr Wood has time to talk about the islands, on which he is most knowledgeable.' Rugged, treeless Harris is a paradise for walkers and naturalists: orchids in April and May, and in June and July the hills are dotted with wild flowers. (*J Jewitt, PW Taylor*)

Open All year, except Christmas/New Year.
Rooms 3 double. 1 with facilities *en suite*, 1 with private bathroom. No telephone.
Facilities Drawing room, dining room. No background music. ½-acre garden. Sea 60 yds: safe bathing; fishing, walking nearby. Unsuitable for &.
Location 1 mile W of Tarbert on A859. Signposted on loch side. Bus from Tarbert/Stornoway.
Restrictions No smoking. No children under 10. Dogs by arrangement, not in house.
Credit cards MasterCard, Visa.
Terms [2001] B&B £45; D,B&B £75. 1-night bookings occasionally refused. 5-day breaks. ***V*** (Nov–Feb, as alternative to house discounts)

THURSO Highland *See SHORTLIST*   **Map 5:B2**

TIGHNABRUAICH Argyll and Bute   **Map 5:D1**

Royal Hotel   *Tel* 01700-811239
Shore Road   *Fax* 01700-811300
Tighnabruaich PA21 2BE
                              Email info@royalhotel.org.uk
                              Website www.royalhotel.org.uk

Traditional hotel in small garden, on shores of Kyles of Bute in charming unspoilt village. Owners, Roger (the chef) and Bea McKie, are refurbishing. Bold colours, local paintings and sculptures, books, family memorabilia in public rooms. 11 bedrooms: best ones are elegant, with Edwardian furniture, sea views, thoughtful touches. Lounge, restaurant, brasserie/bar; jazz, classical background music. Good 'modern Scottish' food, using local ingredients (venison, scallops, lobster, etc). No smoking: restaurant, bedrooms. Unsuitable for &. Dogs by arrangement. Closed Christmas. MasterCard, Visa accepted. B&B £33.50–£47; D,B&B £65–£100. Set dinner £22.95–£28.95 [2001]. 1-night bookings sometimes refused. New Year package with Scottish music, piper, fireworks, More reports, please. ***V***

TIMSGARRY Western Isles   **Map 5:B1**

Baile-na-Cille   **BUDGET**   *Tel* 01851-672242
Timsgarry, Uig   *Fax* 01851-672241
Isle of Lewis HS2 9JD
                              Email randjgollin@compuserve.com
                              Website www.njoi.co.uk/links/bailenacille

❧ *César award in 1990*

'An incomparable setting. Enough natural beauty and wildlife to keep you entranced for days,' says a visitor in 2001 to Richard and Joanna

Gollin's seaside guest house, in an old manse and converted cowshed. They have been 22 years at this 'Shangri-La of the Outer Hebrides'. 'Way further than the back of beyond', it stands gloriously on a sunny bank amid sheep and rabbits, facing a long white beach. Fastidious adults may feel out of their element – some of the accommodation is a bit basic, one visitor wrote of 'homely food, served like school dinners', and the style is splendidly eccentric. Mrs Gollin is often away, in Florida, where she runs a helicopter business, but Richard Gollin 'offers a cheery welcome to children, dogs and grannies', and many eulogies came this year: 'He was very good with our sons, taking them on boat-trips, etc.' 'Perfect in every way – the site, the welcome, the proprietor and his staff, the food, the wine, the rooms.' 'Our stay was nothing less than splendid.' 'Richard Gollin and his library are mines of local information. We liked the way he discussed evening meals in advance.' Local trout, salmon and venison are used; oxtail soup is a new dish this year. Dinners are communal: no choice, but vegetarians are catered for. No wine list: bottles come at two prices (£8.50 and £12.50). Breakfast includes black pudding and 'superb' local pork sausages. In summer, cricket is sometimes played on the beach until late. And there are 'loads of books, games and movies' for rainy days. Some simple but well-appointed bedrooms are in the main house. The rooms in the cowshed are cheaper. But all rooms now have facilities *en suite*. Upkeep may not always be perfect, but prices have remained unchanged for five years. (*Sir John Johnson; Anne P Heaton, MC; also Roger and Mary Hughes, and others*)

Open 1 Mar–7 Oct.
Rooms 10 double, 2 in annexe. Some on ground floor. No telephone/TV.
Facilities 3 lounges (1 with TV, 1 with music), dining room, conservatory; games room, drying room. No background music. 3-acre grounds: walled garden, tennis, children's play area, beach (dinghy, windsurfer, fishing rods available). Beaches, safe bathing, fishing, sailing nearby. Unsuitable for &.
Location 34 miles W of Stornoway. By air: Glasgow/Inverness to Stornoway; ferry from Ullapool. A858 to Garynahine, B8011 towards Uig; at Timsgarry shop (brown sign) turn right to shore. Post bus from Stornoway twice daily.
Restriction No smoking: dining room, bedrooms.
Credit cards MasterCard, Visa.
Terms B&B £24–£39; D,B&B £48–£63. Snack lunch £2–£10. Set dinner £24. Child in bunk room: B&B £14. Weekly rates.

TIRORAN Argyll and Bute   **Map 5:D1**

Tiroran House   *Tel* 01681-705232
Tiroran, Isle of Mull   *Fax* 01681-705240
PA69 6ES   *Email* colin@tiroran.freeserve.co.uk
                                  Website www.tiroran.com

'A wonderful place to stay – a lovely house, beautiful gardens, a magnificent view, good food, excellent rooms, and very friendly hosts.' Unequivocal praise for Colin and Jane Tindal's 150-year-old white-fronted house, a Wolsey Lodge member, in secluded grounds with a burn and waterfalls running down to Loch Scridain. 'We cannot speak too highly of the personal care and attention the Tindals show their guests. It really is like staying in a comfortable country house. The sitting rooms are cosy, but not too smart.' The two young assistants are 'friendly and efficient'. The six bedrooms are well decorated; the bathrooms are simple. The host looks after the lovely grounds. Using local ingredients, his wife cooks 'delicious food'. There is choice only in the second of five (including Scottish cheeses) courses, which might include spinach, garlic and tomato soup; Mull scallops, prawn tails and sole with Chardonnay sauce; roast lamb with orange, port and rosemary; chocolate mousse cake with Tia Maria. 'The wines on the modest list are refreshingly reasonably priced.' Meals are served in a small

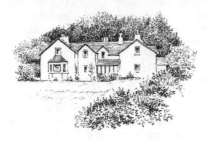

dining room or the adjoining sunroom. There are log fires in the lounges. No bar, but a restricted liquor licence. In the grounds are two self-catering cottages. A good base for visiting Iona and Staffa, or climbing Ben More, the island's only Munro. (*Prof. John Hearle, Colin Pearson, Roger Hughes*)

Open Late Mar–end Oct. Lunch not served.
Rooms 6 double. 2 on ground floor. 2 self-catering cottages. No telephone.
Facilities 2 lounges (1 with classical background music at night), dining room with sunroom. 16-acre grounds: river, path to seashore.
Location From car ferry at Craignure or Fishnish, take A849 towards Iona ferry. Right on B8035 towards Gruline. After 4 miles along sea loch, turn left at converted church. Tiroran is 1 mile further, on minor road.
Restrictions No smoking. Not really suitable for children under 12. Dogs by arrangement, not in house.
Credit cards MasterCard, Visa.
Terms B&B £49–£60; D,B&B £74–£85. Set dinner £26. 1-night bookings refused high season.

ULLAPOOL Highland   **Map 5:B2**

Altnaharrie Inn   *Tel* 01854-633230
Ullapool IV26 2SS
🔱 *César award in 1987*

The remote location, and the reverence with which Gunn Eriksen's cooking is regarded, make visiting *Altnaharrie* a pilgrimage of a gastronomic kind. In a secluded and beautiful setting on the southern shores of Loch Broom, this restaurant-with-rooms cannot be reached by road; guests leave cars in Ullapool, and make the ten-minute crossing by launch. This is the only place in Scotland with two *Michelin* stars, awarded for the inventive and 'superb' cooking of Norwegian-born Gunn Eriksen. That she is seldom seen adds to the mystique of the place, as does the fact that there is no menu; her husband, Fred Brown, recites each dish and, at the end, the names of up to 20 makes of cheese. He is front-of-house, and the staff are discreet. The 'Scandinavian beauty' of the decor is admired. The bedrooms in the main building, an old drover's house, are small; the ones in cottages in the grounds are larger. They are decorated simply, 'with exquisite colour and beauty, splendid warmth'. They have a king-size bed; plenty of towels in the bathroom. No radio or TV; lots of books. The decor of the two lounges is admired, too: flagstone floors, rugs, candles and lamps, log fire, comfortable sofas and chairs. Meals are served at polished antique wooden tables with elegant china and cutlery. Specialities include warm salad of lobster and caviar, and champagne sauce; squab and foie gras with cake of chicken livers. Ground elder fried in batter was found 'singular but delicious' by one couple. No choice until dessert; preferences are discussed at the time of booking. The wine list is 'extensive and sensibly priced'. No mains electricity supply: the generator is turned off late at night, hence the torch by the bed. The experience is found eccentric by some readers, 'heavenly' by others; all agree on the excellence of the food. There is limited walking from the house, up a steep track; further afield are heather-clad hills. Stout footwear is recommended. Plenty of wildlife: golden eagles, seals, otters, etc. More reports, please.

Open Most of the year (please telephone).
Rooms 8 double. 3 in 2 separate buildings. No telephone/TV, etc.
Facilities 2 lounges, dining room. No background music. 2-acre garden on loch: stream, pond, pebble beach, safe (cold) bathing; trout/salmon fishing by arrangement. Unsuitable for &.
Location On S shore of Loch Broom, reached by private launch (telephone from Ullapool). Free safe parking in Ullapool. Bus from Inverness to Ullapool.
Restrictions No smoking. No children under 8. No dogs: public rooms, main house bedrooms.
Credit cards Amex, MasterCard, Visa.
Terms [2001] D,B&B £165–£245. Set 5-course dinner £70. 1-night bookings occasionally refused Sat.

The Sheiling **BUDGET**   *Tel/Fax* 01854-612947
Garve Road, Ullapool IV26 2SX

'We buy the *Guide* to discover this sort of place,' a regular correspondent wrote this year of this small guest house. 'For a family activity holiday, this must be among the best in Scotland. The views are magnificent, the rooms are beautiful, the sitting room is comfortable on a rainy day.' Designed and built by its owners, Duncan and Mhairi MacKenzie, in 1989; the house looks across Loch Broom to the mountains beyond. 'Despite atrocious weather, we had a most enjoyable stay. We felt part of the household.' Charged only the basic B&B rate, they were showered with extras: a glass of wine or sherry most evenings, ice cream, home-made sloe gin', and, 'most hospitable of all, Duncan took me and my son up to Loch Achall and gave us a two-hour introduction to trout fishing'. The MacKenzies have rights on what they claim is the best wild brown-trout fishing to be had in the north of Scotland; most is free to *Sheiling* residents only, and a boat is kept for the use of guests. Fishermen of all degrees of experience and physical fitness are catered for. A log cabin in the grounds contains a self-service laundry, drying room, rod room and sauna. The bedrooms have light pine furniture, good beds, a good bathroom, loch views. The much-admired breakfast is served in a pleasant two-level room with a view of the loch. It includes a wide variety of teas, yogurts, etc, smoked haddock, home-made venison sausages with leeks and peaches. No dinners, but Ullapool, though small, is well provided with eating places. (*Canon and Mrs Michael Bourdeaux*)

Open All year, except Christmas, New Year.
Rooms 1 suite, 5 double. 2 on ground floor. No telephone. 2 have TV.
Facilities Lounge with TV, breakfast room. No background music. Log cabin: laundry, drying room, sauna, shower, rod room, motorcycle store. 1½-acre grounds: lochside patio. Trout fishing free to guests.
Location On A832, south side of village.
Restrictions No smoking. Guide dogs only.
Credit cards None accepted.
Terms B&B £24–£27.

WESTRAY Orkney   **Map 5:A3**

Cleaton House   BUDGET   *Tel* 01857-677508
Pierowall   *Fax* 01857-677442
Westray KW17 2DB   *Email* cleaton@orkney.com

Built in 1850 as a mansion for the Laird of Cleat, Malcolm Stout's small hotel is a 'haven of comfort', set in solitude on a promontory looking towards the little island of Papa Westray. 'A gem.' It is 'well furnished, welcoming and well run', say visitors, who find it 'good value for money'. The decor is simple, and the 'large and comfortable' bedrooms have views across the island and the sea; two have an antique four-poster. Mr Stout, a 'superb host', will meet guests at the ferry or the airstrip. A native of Westray, one of the most northerly Orkney isles, he has an endless supply of local knowledge, and a library of Orcadian books to go with the traditional local strawback chairs in the lounge. Lorna Reid's 'excellent cooking' uses local produce – notably fish, seafood and North Ronaldsay lamb – in a simple but imaginative way: dishes like twice-baked Orkney cheese soufflé; lobster and smoked salmon with a green pepper vinaigrette; saddle of venison; sticky toffee pudding. With coffee you get 'peedie fours'. The hotel also acts as an inn for locals, and serves good bar snacks. The island offers tranquillity, miles of sandy beaches, wonderful walking – Mr Stout will deliver guests to distant parts of the island in his Range Rover, so that they can make their way back on foot. It has the second largest breeding seabird colony in the UK (puffins between May and August), daylight until midnight in summer, free golf at the local course; also trout fishing, and day-trips to Papa Westray (via 'the world's shortest scheduled flight – 90 seconds'). More reports, please.

Open All year, except Christmas.
Rooms 5 double (1 family room), 1 single. 1 suite and a room equipped for ♿ planned for 2002.
Facilities Ramp. Lounge, bar (Scottish/folk background music; Scottish dancing fortnightly), restaurant. 1½-acre garden: *pétanque*; sea ¼ mile.
Location 2 miles SE of Pierowall village. Ferry/small plane from Kirkwall; they will meet.
Restrictions No smoking: restaurant, bedrooms. No dogs in public rooms.

Credit cards MasterCard, Visa.
Terms B&B £25–£50; D,B&B £45–£75. Set dinner £25. 2/3-night packages
Oct–end Apr. *V*

WICK Highland   Map 5:B3

Bilbster House   NEW/BUDGET   *Tel/Fax* 01955-621212
Bilbster, nr Wick   *Email* ianstewart@bilbster.freeserve.co.uk
Caithness KW1 5TB   *Website* www.accommodationbilbster.com

*Handsome listed 17th-century manor house, 'exceptionally well fur-
nished; very welcoming', run by Ian Stewart as unpretentious B&B
('we do not offer hotel standards,' he writes). 5 miles NW of Wick just
off A882. 'A good resting place in area with dearth of recommendable
accommodation,' says nominator. 3 large bedrooms, no telephone/
TV; 2 have facilities* en suite. *Open all year (by arrangement Oct–
Easter). Lounge, library, dining room; 5½-acre garden. No smoking.
Unsuitable for &. Credit cards not accepted. B&B £17.50–£18.50.*
(Alan Green)

****

Traveller's tale Hotel in London. The bedroom was unaccept-
able in terms of decor and condition of carpets and other items.
The headboard of the double bed was grimy with ingrained
grease from the heads of previous guests. In a number of places
the wallpaper was grubby. The chairs were well past their best.
The carpet was, frankly, disgusting. There was grime on the
wallpaper in the bathroom.

****

Traveller's tale Hotel in Wiltshire. On entering our small
'suite' we were taken aback by a roar resembling Niagara Falls,
coming from the bathroom. The porter accompanying us
expressed concern at this noise, which he said he had never
heard before. He went to investigate, and returned to say it was
a staff member using her bathroom immediately overhead.
Subsequently it emerged that this was a regular occurrence.
When we entered our bedroom we were struck by an electrical
whine coming from beneath its window. Reception expressed
baffled wonder that there could be such a noise, and concluded
that it came from the laundry room, where the tumble dryer was
in action from 9 am to 11 pm. I asked, without much hope, if
another room was available, but was told by the cheery receptionist that there was one unbooked room, but it was small and
unpleasant; he was sure we would not like it. We concluded that
a concern for the peace and quiet of the hotel's guests was not
one of its merits. We wrote a restrained letter of complaint, and
received a reply which expressed perfunctory regret, offered a
self-justificatory and inaccurate account of events, said no one
had complained before about noise from the water system and
laundry, and concluded with the suggestion that next time we
might try a monastery.

****

Wales

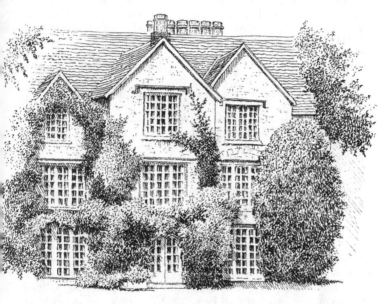

Llanwenarth House, Abergavenny

Few of our Welsh hotels are conventional purpose-built places, either in a town or by the sea. Our readers and inspectors often look beyond the Brecon Beacons to buildings of character, many of them converted rectories, manor houses and farmhouses. Many of these are run in warm personal style by Welsh (or sometimes English) families, some of whom are new to the hotel trade. Two of our new entries are at Mumbles, on the coast that Dylan Thomas loved, while old favourites include a number in or near the Snowdonia National Park. Cardiff is represented only in the Shortlist. Several hotels in this chapter are new to the Guide this year. Two are at Mumbles, south-west of Swansea, on the coast that Dylan Thomas loved. Another, with eight rooms, overlooks an 'idyllic' beach at Broadhaven, Pembrokeshire, and is thought to be ideal for children. A fourth, returning to our pages, is a converted 17th-century farmhouse above the river Wye, a mile from Tintern Abbey.

Some of our most admired Welsh hotels lie below the Brecon Beacons. Others are in or near the Snowdonia National Park, with glorious views. Two of these are rather special – Brian and Jane Pullee's 'unique old inn' at Nantgwynant with its 'wonderful evenings in the residents' bar'; and the famous Italianate fantasy village at Portmeirion, 'truly magical'. City hotels, on the other hand, are seldom favoured; neither Cardiff nor Swansea has any main entry.

So what is a typical good Welsh hotel? Few of those chosen by readers are conventional, purpose-built places, either in a town or by the sea. Many are converted rectories, manors or farmhouses, but fewer than in Ireland or England are former stately homes. Many are expertly run in a warm personal style by Welsh (or sometimes English) families, some of whom are new to the hotel trade.

The cooking, usually rather good, makes plentiful use of local produce, such as Welsh venison, lamb and black beef. That renowned Welsh vegetable, the leek, appears on many menus, often in soups. Some hotels provide Welsh laverbread, too, and just a few offer old Welsh recipes, such as Brythill y Cig Moch (trout fillet wrapped in bacon). Michelin bestows a star for cuisine on two places in Wales – at Llyswen and Llansanffraid – and both are in this chapter.

ABERGAVENNY Monmouthshire   Map 3:D4

 Llanwenarth House   *Tel* 01873-830289
Govilon, nr Abergavenny NP7 9SF   Fax 01873-832199

César award: Welsh country house of the year

Plenty more enthusiasm for Bruce and Amanda Weatherill's guest house in their family home, 'not grand but cosy'. 'We thoroughly enjoyed it. A country house atmosphere; owners helpful, sociable but not intrusive. Delightfully eccentric. Marvellous food and wines.' 'A special place with amazing personality; outstanding value.' 'You really feel like a private visitor (no keys to rooms).' Built of grey limestone, the 16th-century manor house stands above the Usk valley in the Brecon Beacons National Park. It is filled with 'decades worth of personal belongings, lovingly acquired' and dogs ('well behaved and beautiful'). Mrs Weatherill provides 'first-rate home cooking', in 'sophisticated surroundings'; her husband, waiting at table, 'gives a lengthy description of each ingredient' – most soft fruits and many vegetables are home-grown, as is the lamb. Vegetarians are well catered for. Oeufs en cocotte; halibut 'with a divine sauce', have been enjoyed; desserts include chocolate, orange and rum mousse; grapefruit and lime soufflé. Guests generally dine together at one large table, but there are smaller tables too. 'Superb breakfasts' include kippers, home-made jams, home-laid eggs, honey from hives in the orchard. There is usually a log fire in the Georgian drawing room. But the size of the rooms can make them difficult to heat in deep winter. Most bedrooms are big, and most have views of the lovely scenery. The large grounds, with two huge copper beeches, horses and chickens, are bordered by a canal where boats may be hired. Good walking nearby in the Welsh hills, where you can climb Sugar Loaf Mountain; or you can explore Blaenavon, now a World Heritage Site, and the castles of the Welsh Marches. Plenty of sporting activities are available (see below). But the place 'would not suit anti-hunting types', warns one report. (*Michael and Wendy Dods, JA McKinnell, EM Arnold, JH, Prof. Wolfgang Stroebe, and others*)

Open Mar–Jan; Christmas, New Year by arrangement. No lunches. Dining room opened 5/6 nights a week, depending on guests' requirements.
Rooms 5 double, 1 on ground floor. No telephone.
Facilities Drawing room, dining room. No background music. 2-acre gardens in 10-acre farm: canal (boat hire); stabling for visiting horses. Fishing, golf, pony-trekking, shooting nearby.
Location From junction of A40/A465/A4042, take A465 towards Merthyr Tydfil for 3½ miles. At roundabout take 1st exit to Govilon; the house's ½-mile drive is 150 yards on right. Train: Abergavenny, 4½ miles; then local bus/taxi.
Restrictions No smoking: dining room, bedrooms. No children under 10. No dogs in public rooms.
Credit cards None accepted.
Terms B&B double £82–£86; single occupancy £20 discount. Set dinner £26. Reductions for longer stays. 1-night bookings sometimes refused bank holidays.

ABERSOCH Gwynedd   **Map 3:B2**

Porth Tocyn Hotel	*Tel* 01758-713303
Bwlch Tocyn	*Fax* 01758-713538
Abersoch LL53 7BU	*Email* porthtocyn.hotel@virgin.net
	Website www.porth-tocyn-hotel.co.uk

❦ *César award in 1984*

'One of the nicest hotels we have stayed in, jolly good value'; 'superb food'; 'splendid, with fine views'. Lots more praise this year for the family-friendly *Porth Tocyn,* set peacefully above a popular yachting village, in full sight of Snowdonia and Cardigan Bay. The Fletcher-Brewers have owned and run it for more than 50 years: the 'exuberant', 'incredibly hard-working' Nick Fletcher-Brewer 'seems to be everywhere, helping out, chatting with guests'. His idiosyncratic style is a key feature of the hotel. 'He appears to revel in his repartee and his gong-sounding ritual at 7.30 pm.' 'The friendly atmosphere set by the staff soon affects the guests, who gather in the comfortable chintz-covered armchairs by the fire.' Lounges are traditional, with country antiques and fresh flowers, and there's a small children's sitting room with games, TV, video, etc. The bedrooms are cottagey rather than luxurious; many are connected for use by a family. Some walls are thin. Small children can have high tea separately, but older ones are now allowed at dinner if their parents wish. The cooking, by Louise Fletcher-Brewer and David Carney, is always liked: 'Imaginative and served in generous quantities; the fish dishes are especially good.' A three-course menu, with plenty of choice, might include clam chowder with truffle oil; roast duck breast with wild mushroom risotto; Jamaican rum pie. 'Outstanding fudge and petits fours after dinner.' Light weekday lunches are informally served; the Sunday buffet lunch is 'gargantuan'. So it seems are the breakfasts: 'They set you up until dinner time.' The owners write that this year the hotel's outside has been repainted, new showers and tiles put in bathrooms, some antique furniture restored. 'Though our ground-floor bedrooms were not designed for wheelchair users, we do attract quite a few disabled guests.' (*Richard Creed, David and Patricia Hawkins, BB, and others*)

Open Mar–early Nov.
Rooms 14 double, 3 single. 3 on ground floor.
Facilities 5 sitting rooms, children's room, bar, restaurant. No background music. 25-acre grounds: gardens, swimming pool (heated May–Sept), tennis. Beach, bathing, sailing, fishing, golf, riding, clay-pigeon shooting nearby.
Location 2 miles S of Abersoch, through hamlets of Sarnbach and Bwlch Tocyn. Follow brown signs.
Restrictions No smoking: restaurant, bedrooms. No small children at dinner (high teas until 6.15 pm). No dogs in public rooms.
Credit cards MasterCard, Visa.
Terms [2001] B&B: single £52.50–£68.50, double £70–£128. Cooked breakfast £5.25. Set Sun lunch £18, dinner (2 to 4 courses) £29.50–£32. Child in parents' room: free. 3- to 7-day breaks. 1-night bookings sometimes refused.

ABERYSTWYTH Ceredigion *See SHORTLIST*   **Map 3:C3**

BEAUMARIS Anglesey   **Map 3:A3**

Ye Olde Bulls Head   NEW   *Tel* 01248-810329
Castle Street   *Fax* 01248-811294
Beaumaris LL58 8AP
           Email info@bullsheadinn.co.uk
           Website www.bullsheadinn.co.uk

Beaumaris, a resort on the Menai Strait, has medieval origins and is 'a fun place to explore'. One of its historic buildings is this 'wonderfully atmospheric' old inn (1492), Grade II listed, near the castle. Dickens and Samuel Johnson stayed here, and three reports now restore it to the *Guide*. 'It *feels* like a Dickensian inn, with a charming 19th-century roadhouse ambience. You enter through the pub. The restaurant was one of the best we have been to in the UK.' 'Food very good; lovely fires, well tended; pleasant, comfy sitting room. Staff were efficient and charming without exception: one of the chefs carried my bags to the car.' The owners, Keith Rothwell and David Robertson (he is also manager), are 'doing the place up', after a period when housekeeping was sharply criticised by one reader. The bedrooms, named for Dickensian characters, are beamed and cottagey; some have a brass bed or a four-poster. All were refurbished in 2001. The rambling bar, popular with locals, is full of mementos of the inn's past, including a rare 17th-century brass water clock, some antique weapons, and the town's oak ducking seat. 'In great contrast', a new upstairs brasserie, with 'bright and clean modern design', serves 'old-fashioned pub food', while in the main restaurant, Ernst Van Halderen provides a large, elaborate menu of French-influenced dishes, eg, terrine of chicken and trumpet mushrooms with quince jelly; venison with fresh fig confit; rhubarb sponge with fudge ice cream. Local ingredients are used imaginatively. Good breakfasts, too. The large lounge has a log fire; there is a pretty courtyard. Beaumaris Castle, built by Edward I, has unique concentric fortifications. Two National Trust properties, Plas Newydd and Penrhyn Castle, are nearby; so is Bodnant Garden. (*HT Madoc-Jones, Lucy and Jim Bowers, Stephen Duckworth; also* Good Pub Guide)

Open All year, except 2 days over Christmas.
Rooms 13 double. 2 on ground floor.
Facilities Lounge, bar, brasserie (background music), restaurant. Sea nearby.
Location Main street (rooms double-glazed). Parking for 10 cars. Train: Bangor, 7 miles.
Restrictions No smoking: restaurant, bedrooms. No children under 7 in restaurant. No dogs.
Credit cards Amex, MasterCard, Visa.
Terms B&B: single £60–£70, double £87–£100. Bar meals. Full alc: brasserie £17, restaurant £37.

BETTWS GWERFYL GOCH Denbighshire   **Map 3:B4**

The Old Rectory   `BUDGET`   *Tel* 01490-460387
Bettws Gwerfyl Goch
nr Corwen LL21 9PU

'A comfortable private house where you stay as guests of Frank and Lesley Hart. Wonderful food, simple but imaginative.' 'Evenings by the inglenook fire with our dear and caring hosts. Superb breakfasts.' This 'homely old house', an 18th-century rectory, with modern additions, stands in a big garden ('a tour of it is an education in botany') on the edge of the Snowdonia National Park. The idiosyncratic style is liked by many readers: no television in the house; no smoking anywhere. The Harts are ex-teachers, 'knowledgeable about all things'. 'We expect guests to join in, and talk to us and each other, not hide in their rooms,' they write. They create an ambience 'of great peace'. Mrs Hart's 'marvellous home-made bread and delicious sweets' were again admired this year, and the vegetables that come with the 'plentiful' main dishes. Dinner, which must be booked the day before, is generally served round one long table, but anyone wishing to eat alone can do so in the conservatory, which also serves as a breakfast room. No licence: guests bring their own drink (no corkage is charged). A light supper is also available. There are open fires in the dining room and lounge, lots of books, a grand piano which guests may play. The snug bedrooms are provided with flowers and home-made biscuits. This year, a balcony has been added to the best bedroom, and ponds with waterfalls (and frogs and toads) have been created in the grounds, home to owls, badgers and Britain's rarest mammal, the pine marten. Frank Hart is an experienced hill-walker and can suggest walks in the area. Caernarvon and Conwy castles are within easy reach. (*Mr and Mrs W Mullins, Jim and Lucy Bowers, K and JW*)

Open 24 Mar–7 Jan.
Rooms 3 double. No telephone/TV.
Facilities Lounge (classical music/radio on request), dining room, conservatory/breakfast room. 1¼-acre garden. Fishing nearby, river, walks. Unsuitable for ♿.

Location NW of Corwen. A5 to Maerdy (4½ miles). Right after *Goat Inn*. After 1½ miles left at crossroads in centre of Bettws Gwerfyl Goch. *Old Rectory* 400 yds on left, behind high wall.
Restrictions No smoking. No dogs in house.
Credit cards None accepted.
Terms (*Not VAT-rated*) Double room: B&B £58–£68; D,B&B £94–£104. Packed lunches available. Supper £9, dinner £14–£18. Child in parents' room: under 3, free; 3–10, 50% of adult rate. Christmas package. *V*

BODUAN Gwynedd   Map 3:B2

The Old Rectory   *Tel/Fax* 01758-721519
Boduan
nr Pwllheli LL53 6DT

In a village amid woodlands on the beautiful Lleyn peninsula, this yellow 18th-century rectory has a 'lovely setting' – a big garden with lawns, a paddock and mature trees. It is now a guest house, owned and run in personal style by Roger and Gabrielle Pollard. 'Many of our guests leave us as friends,' they write, and recent visitors add: 'They made us very welcome in their beautiful and comfortable home. The public rooms are elegantly furnished, the bedrooms are well equipped.' Family photographs and antiques fill the house; there's a tall carved pine fireplace in the drawing room. An evening meal, with 'good home cooking' by Mrs Pollard, is served by arrangement, using local fish, meat and game. Dishes include duck terrine with apricot, apple and pistachio; fried guineafowl with red wine sauce; lemon ice-cream cake with hot gin blueberries. The short wine list starts at £9.95 a bottle. All bedrooms have recently been redecorated, and a self-catering cottage is new this year. Nearby are three golf courses, and miles of footpaths; also splendid beaches. Well placed for visiting Snowdonia; several castles, including Harlech and Caernarfon, are within an hour's drive. (*AE, and others*)

Open All year, except Christmas week.
Rooms 4 double. No telephone. Also self-catering cottage.
Facilities Drawing room (classical background music 'as appropriate'), dining room. 3½-acre grounds. Off-road driving, clay-pigeon shooting, archery, golf, go-carting, sailing, riding, sandy beaches nearby. Unsuitable for &.
Location 4 miles NW of Pwllheli off A497, opposite church. Train: Pwllheli; bus/taxi.
Restrictions No smoking. Small dogs by arrangement; not in public rooms.
Credit cards None accepted.
Terms B&B £35–£45; D,B&B £60–£70. Set dinner £25. 10% reduction for 3 or more nights. 1-night bookings refused bank holidays. *V*

BRECHFA Carmarthenshire   Map 3:D2

Tŷ Mawr   *Tel* 01267-202332
Brechfa SA32 7RA   *Fax* 01267-202437
                                       Email tymawr@tymawrcountryhotel.co.uk
                                       Website www.tymawrcountryhotel.co.uk

In a lovely setting beside the river Marlais, on the edge of Brechfa forest, this 15th/16th-century white-fronted farmhouse is owned and run as a small restaurant-with-rooms by Roger and Veronica Weston, 'a most pleasant couple, very solicitous'. It was liked again, with caveats, this year. The garden and terrace are said to need attention. One couple thought it 'unsophisticated, more like a pub-with-rooms, but food was above average'. Another found the food very good, but portions much too large. Mrs Weston's meals, served in the Gothic-style candlelit restaurant, offer plenty of choice, eg, Camembert soufflé; lamb with garlic and rosemary sauce; strawberry cream meringue; 'excellent Welsh cheeses' – and a vodka-laced sorbet between courses. *Tŷ Mawr* has its own 'charming' bakery and shop, and its 'delicious organic bread' is served with every meal, while 'scrumptious biscuits' are in the bedrooms. These, though not large, are well lit, with good storage space. 'Pretty flowered wallpaper gives a mid-Victorian feel.' Other features include low ceilings and stone walls, oak beams, tiled floors, deep floral armchairs, outsize fabric daffodils and a log fire in the large sitting room. There is a flowery terrace, with tables and chairs, looking over the garden and orchard. Breakfast was again admired this year, but the 'lavish buffet' may be absent if residents are too few, and one reader disliked the bacon. Sunday lunch is a speciality. Nearby are the nature reserve at Dinas, the new National Botanic Gardens of Wales, and Kidwelly, Carreg Cennen and Llansteffan castles. 'The roads around us are all virtually traffic-free,' say the Westons. (*Michael and Anne Forrest, HT Madoc-Jones, and others*)

Open All year, except Christmas.
Rooms 1 family, 4 double. No telephone.
Facilities Lounge, bar, 2 dining rooms (varied background music). 1-acre garden, river. Golf, fishing, riding, walking nearby; beach 12 miles. Unsuitable for &.
Location Centre of village (quiet road). 14 miles NE of Carmarthen (daily bus).
Restrictions Smoking in bar only. Dogs by arrangement; not in public rooms.
Credit cards MasterCard, Visa.
Terms B&B £42–£52; D,B&B £50–£76. Set dinner £25. Winter packages. *V*

BRECON Powys   **Map 3:D3**

Penpont   BUDGET   *Tel* 01874-636202
nr Brecon LD3 8EU   *Email* penpont@globalnomad.co.uk
                                        Website www.penpont.com

Set splendidly below the Brecon Beacons, by the rapid river Usk, this mellow stone house was built in 1666 by Daniel Williams, an ancestor of the present owners, Gavin and Davina Hogg. The ambience is 'warmly informal'. Guests can use the large oak-panelled sitting room lined with books and furnished with new sofas. In it are works by local artist Robert Macdonald. The Tapestry Room has its original 17th-century wall hangings. The large bedrooms (not all have facilities *en suite*) are furnished simply 'and with great charm'. Children are welcomed. Breakfast, served in a large room, is 'adequate', with a good choice of hot items. Dinner for a group can be provided by

arrangement, otherwise there are several good pubs within easy driving distance. Around is a working estate, with 40 acres of parkland
and some unusual old buildings, including a chapel, dovecote, and
stables. There is also a 'millennium maze' in the shape of a green man.
The area is rich in wildlife, and is ideal for walkers and birdwatchers.
Penpont is quite close to Dan-yr-Ogof caves and Big Pit; historic
Tretower Court and Caerphilly Castle are within easy reach. More
reports welcome.

Open All year, except Christmas, New Year.
Rooms 2 family (bathrooms across landing), 2 double. 2 with radio; no tele-
phone/TV. 6-bedroomed flat, sleeps 14.
Facilities Drawing room, dining room. No background music. 40-acre
grounds: maze, tennis, swings, river: 2 miles of fly-fishing. Walking, climbing
nearby. Unsuitable for &.
Location 4 miles W of Brecon, on A40 Brecon–Llandovery. Look for hang-
ing sign.
Restrictions No smoking in bedrooms. No dogs.
Credit cards None accepted.
Terms B&B £30–£40. Set dinner (by arrangement, groups only) £20. Child in
parents' room: 50% of adult rate. 1-night bookings sometimes refused.

BROADHAVEN Pembrokeshire	**Map 3:D1**

The Druidstone NEW	*Tel* 01437-781221
nr Broadhaven	*Fax* 01437-781133
Haverfordwest SA62 3NE	*Email* jane@druidstone.co.uk
	Website www.druidstone.uk

'My favourite of all time. I go with my young son every year.' A correspondent writes rapturously about this small holiday hotel on the
Pembrokeshire coast, west of Haverfordwest. 'From its magnificent
setting on the cliffs, it looks over the sea. Below lies one of the best
beaches in Britain, a vast curve of smooth sand that stretches to rocky
outcrops with caves and rock pools. Here, we play games, build elaborate sandcastles, and go crabbing. This, the only building overlooking the bay, is the family home of Rod, Jane and Angus Bell, who
create a relaxed atmosphere plus a real sense of comfort. Staff are
friendly: but nobody wishes you a "nice day", because they've been
on a hotel management course. Inside the late 19th-century stone
house are worn antique furniture, wooden floors, rugs, plenty of paintings. Both the cellar bar and the dining room open on to a terrace and
garden facing the sea. In the dining room, the cooking is of a high standard, but most of our suppers we took in the bar, which serves hearty
soups, stews and salads. My favourite dinner was in the old kitchen,
with its Raeburn cooker – a whole sea bass which I'd almost seen
being caught. All the parents are eager to supervise the delicious
children's teas, held here. Children and pets are welcomed, and
families return year after year to enjoy the simple pleasures of a beach
holiday. There are daily horse rides along the beach at low tide; and
windsurfing, sailing and birdwatching locally.' Jane Bell calls her
cooking 'instinctive': try her 'Mexican fruity little number'; leek and
tofu pancake with smoked cheese; duck breast with mulled strawberries

and raspberries; passion fruit and citrus soufflé. Not for all comers (no private bathrooms). (*Michelle de Larrabeiti*)

Open Probably all year (check website for closures).
Rooms 1 suite, 6 double, 2 single. No private facilities (3 shared bathrooms); no telephone/TV. Also 5 cottages, 2 suitable for ♿.
Facilities Sitting room, bar (background 'quality' CDs; occasional live music), TV room, restaurant; conference/function facilities. 20-acre grounds. Sandy beach, safe bathing 200 yds. Civil wedding licence.
Location 5 miles W of Haverfordwest by B4341. In Broadhaven, turn right at sea. 1½ miles further, turn left at sign for Druidstone Haven. Puffin bus in summer.
Restrictions No smoking: restaurant, farmhouse kitchen. No dogs in restaurant.
Credit cards Amex, MasterCard, Visa.
Terms B&B: single £35, double £70–£80, suite £120. Bar meals. Full alc £22. Children charged according to accommodation and age (under-3s free in parents' room). Courses, conferences. Christmas package. 1-night bookings refused Sat.

CAERNARFON Gwynedd *See SHORTLIST*   **Map 3:A1**

CAERSWS Powys   **Map 3:C3**

Maesmawr Hall   *Tel* 01686-688255
Caersws, nr Newtown   *Fax* 01686-688410
SY17 5SF   *Email* reception@maesmawr.co.uk
    Website www.maesmawr.co.uk

'The owners and staff are friendly and efficient, the food is beautifully cooked, our room was large and comfortable.' New praise this year for a 16th-century half-timbered hunting lodge, set amid the hills of mid-Wales, near a village in the Severn valley, and reached up a long tree-lined drive through mature gardens. Its lounge has wood panelling, oak beams and an open log fire. Its owners, Isabel and Alan Hunt and Marilyn and John Pemberton (he is the chef), have carefully modernised and are steadily refurbishing. They are 'always visible and friendly' and are 'proud of what they do'. The flexibility over food is also liked: dishes are available as bar snacks or room-service meals. The set-price menu offers plenty of choice, eg, warm chicken and smoked bacon salad; fried Welsh lamb on a courgette couscous; lemon mousse torte. The fresh vegetables are 'outstanding', and the wines are varied and fairly priced. The best bedrooms, with 'generous towels, good linens', are in the main house; some have a sloping ceiling and a four-poster: sloping floors, too, and many steps, which might not suit the less mobile. Newer rooms are in the coach house across the lawn (some are a bit small). Breakfast includes fresh fruit salad, hot dishes

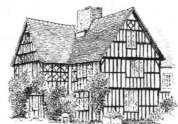

cooked to order. One snag: 'The only residents' lounge is combined with the bar.' 'With Carno and Newtown nearby, this is something of a staff hotel for Laura Ashley, and many of the fabrics hail from those factories.' The hotel also courts the function/conference trade. It offers fishing on the river Severn, and can arrange rough shooting. There is good walking in the Montgomeryshire hills and the Shropshire Mynd. Powis and Montgomery castles are nearby. (*AJ Gillingwater*)

Open All year, except 24 Dec–2 Jan.
Rooms 16 double, 1 single. 6 in coach house, some on ground floor.
Facilities Lounge/bar, restaurant; 'easy listening' background music; function room with bar and dance floor. 4-acre gardens. River Severn, fishing 250 yds; pony-trekking, golf nearby. Unsuitable for &. Civil wedding licence.
Location 6 miles W of Newtown. Off A489 1 mile before Caersws (300-yd drive on right). Train: Caersws, 1 mile.
Restrictions No smoking: restaurant, some bedrooms. Dogs in annexe only, not in public rooms.
Credit cards Amex, MasterCard, Visa.
Terms B&B: single from £60, double from £80; D,B&B (min. 2 nights): £57.50–£65. Set lunch £14.50, dinner £25. Child in parents' room: B&B £5–£15. Weekly rates. *V*

## CAPEL GARMON Conwy								Map 3:A3

Tan-y-Foel							*Tel* 01690-710507
Capel Garmon							*Fax* 01690-710681
nr Betws-y-Coed LL26 0RE				*Email* enquiries@tyfhotel.co.uk
									Website www.tyfhotel.co.uk

Reached up a stony track, the Pitman family's old stone house stands peacefully in wooded grounds above the lush Conwy valley, in the Snowdonia National Park: the views are superb towards the sea and the mountains. A welcome new report this year: 'It is very well furnished, with innovative modern design in the lounge and breakfast rooms. We felt that the precision and perfection gave a somewhat impersonal feeling. But the food was first rate, notably the local lamb and beef. Breakfasts were good and the portions large.' Janet Pitman's much-admired cooking has been called 'definitely *nouvelle*, beautifully presented', with Mediterranean and oriental influences and use of organic meat and vegetables. On the short menu, enterprising dishes might include cappuccino of chicken livers with roasted artichoke; steamed char sui marinated fillet of salmon with a julienne of organic vegetables and Szechwan pepper sauce. The wine list is wide-ranging. The bedrooms are decorated in vibrant colours and lavish fabrics. Some have a king-size or four-poster bed; they are supplied with chocolates and other extras, and have a good-size bathroom. Breakfast is 'every bit as good as dinner'. Guests are asked not to arrive before 3.30 pm or later than 9.30 pm. Conwy Castle and Bodnant Garden are not far off. (*David and Patricia Hawkins*)

Open Jan–Dec; closed Christmas. Limited opening Dec, Jan, Feb. Restaurant closed lunchtime; dinner must be booked.
Rooms 7 double. 2, with own entrance, adjoining main house.
Facilities Lounge, breakfast room, restaurant. No background music. 8-acre grounds. Unsuitable for &.

Location 1½ miles E of Betws-y-Coed towards Llanrwst. Take 2nd right to
Capel Garmon/Nebo off A470. 1½ miles up hill; sign on left.
Restrictions No smoking. No children under 7. No dogs.
Credit cards All major cards accepted.
Terms B&B: single £70–£90, double £99–£150; D,B&B double £168–£208.
Set dinner £39. Winter/summer breaks. 1-night bookings often refused, espe-
cially bank holidays.

CARDIFF *See SHORTLIST*   **Map 3:E4**

CLYTHA Monmouthshire   **Map 3:E4**

Clytha Arms   `BUDGET`   *Tel* 01873-840206
Clytha, nr Abergavenny   *Fax* 01873-840209
NP7 9BW   *Email* one.bev@lineone.net
                      Website website. lineone.net/~one.bev

6 miles SE of Abergavenny, off A40, on B4598 (old road to Raglan):
converted dower house, owned and run as informal country pub, very
lively, by Beverley and Andrew Canning (he and daughter, Sarah, are
chefs). Eager service by cheerful young staff. Very good breakfasts,
using local ingredients (including wild boar sausages). Good, imagi-
native dinners in no-smoking restaurant (eg, oysters in beer batter
with Thai sauce; roast squab with port and whimberries); wide range
of bar snacks; real ale. Lounge. No background music. Four pleasant
smoke-free bedrooms, some large (one with four-poster). 2-acre gar-
dens. Fishing in river Usk 2 miles. Closed 25 Dec; restaurant closed
Sun night/Mon. Unsuitable for &. No dogs. All major credit cards
accepted. B&B: single £45–£65, double £60–£80. Set meals £15.95;
full alc £30. More reports, please.

CRICKHOWELL Powys   **Map 3:D4**

The Bear   *Tel* 01873-810408
High St, Crickhowell   *Fax* 01873-811696
NP8 1BW   *Email* bearhotel@aol.com
                      Website www.bearhotel.co.uk

A 'super old coaching inn', large and creeper-clad, 'very well run' by
its enthusiastic owners, Judith Hindmarsh and her son, Stephen. 'We
are not a hotel in the grand manner,' they write. They and their staff
'are all cheerful and efficient'. Dating back to 1432, *The Bear* stands
in the centre of a charming market town below the Brecon Beacons. It
has a cobbled forecourt and an inner courtyard; in summer everywhere
is colourful with flowery hanging baskets and tubs. Some bedrooms
have a four-poster, some a spa bath. Some are in a building in the style
of a Tudor manor house – each room leads off a balcony. Room 36 is
'spacious with chintzy decor and a pleasant sitting area with a bay
window looking over the very pretty small garden'. The suite is in a
cottage. Lighting may be dim. The popular bar serves snacks, or more
elaborate dishes like linguine with crabmeat and coriander. One

dining room has oak beams, stone walls, a flagstone floor; another is intimate, with candles, fresh flowers and lace tablecloths. 'A positive army of friendly staff served excellent food', eg, boudin of guineafowl with wild mushrooms; venison with spiced pears and red cabbage. Wines are competitively priced, and many are available by the glass. The 'calmly civilised lounge', heavily beamed, has rugs on a parquet floor, bentwood armchairs, cushioned settles, a log fire, an antique dresser, and a view of the market square. In summer, meals are served under a pergola. The cooked breakfast 'is very generous', but 'the toast is not special'. 'Well-behaved dogs are welcomed, much to the dismay of our own dogs,' write the Hindmarshes. Langorse Lake is nearby, with sailing, water sports and wildlife; or you can be strenuous up in the Brecon Beacons (see below). (Good Pub Guide, *LW, and others*)

Open All year.
Rooms 1 suite, 34 double. 13 in courtyard. 4 on ground floor.
Facilities 2 lounges, 2 bars, 3 dining rooms. No background music. Courtyard, garden. Climbing, gliding, golf, fishing, caving, pony-trekking nearby.
Location Central (quietest bedrooms at rear). Train: Abergavenny, 6 miles.
Restriction No dogs in dining rooms.
Credit cards Amex, MasterCard, Visa.
Terms B&B: single £52–£98, double £68–£126; D,B&B £25 added per person. Full alc £30.

EGLWYSFACH Powys   **Map 3:C3**

Ynyshir Hall   *Tel* 01654-781209
Eglwysfach   *Fax* 01654-781366
nr Machynlleth SY20 8TA   *Email* info@ynyshir-hall.co.uk
                                   Website www.ynyshir-hall.co.uk

❧ *César award in 1997*

'A lovely hotel, one of our favourites.' 'A very special place. Top marks on all counts.' 'Everything is perfection.' 'The Reens, natural hosts, generate a tremendous warmth amongst their guests – a very happy atmosphere.' High praise again this year for Rob and Joan Reen's smart white Georgian longhouse. It stands in wide landscaped gardens on the shore of the Dyfi estuary, surrounded by the RSPB's large and 'fantastic' Ynyshir bird reserve (lots of red kites). 'It is stunning, luxurious, wonderfully restored, in superb grounds. Our bedroom and bathroom, with clouds on the ceiling, made us feel like royalty. Prices are high, but worth it.' 'The bar has just been redecorated, and looks fabulous.' Rob Reen, a professional painter, has created a 'stunning decor'. Bedrooms, named after great artists, glow with vibrant colours, lots of blues and apricots, coordinated with Welsh pottery, antiques, rich fabrics and bright rugs. But they vary in size and outlook. 'Ours had good reading lights, a decanter of sherry, dramatic paintings. The large marble-floored bathroom had huge bathrobes.' The new chef, Les Rennie (formerly at *Cliveden*, Taplow, *qv*), 'produces stunning food', says a visitor this year – cèpe risotto; tortellini of prawn; roast saddle of Welsh venison; roast duck with an intense flavour; superb cheeses; excellent wines. The dishes are light; herbs and spices create great contrasts.' 'Presentation is artistic.' Lavish breakfasts include 'very good fresh porridge; fruit compote with Greek yogurt'. The two-roomed studio suite, with a tiny kitchen, 'would be ideal for a family'. You can visit the Centre for Alternative Technology ('very green') just north of Machynlleth. Harlech, Powys and Chirk castles are not far off. (*Padi and John Howard, Gordon Hands*)

Open All year, except Jan.
Rooms 4 suites (1 on ground floor), 6 double. 2 in studio annexe.
Facilities Drawing room, bar lounge, breakfast room, restaurant (piped harp/classical music sometimes at night). 14-acre gardens in 365-acre bird reserve: croquet, putting. Beaches, sailing, river and sea fishing, riding, pony-trekking, golf nearby. Civil wedding licence.
Location Just W of A487, 6 miles SW of Machynlleth, 11 miles NE of Aberystwyth. Train: Machynlleth; taxi.
Restrictions Smoking in bar lounge only. No children under 9. Dogs by arrangement, in 1 bedroom only, not in public areas.
Credit cards All major cards accepted.
Terms B&B: single £85–£150, double £120–£180, suite £150–£205. Set lunch £22, dinner £38. Christmas, New Year packages. 1-night bookings sometimes refused high-season weekends. ***V***

GARTHMYL Powys   **Map 3:C4**

Garthmyl Hall   *Tel* 01686-640550
Garthmyl   *Fax* 01686-640609
nr Montgomery SY15 6RS

🍷 *César award in 2000*

'It has mild eccentricity plus considerable comfort,' runs a new eulogy this year for this lovely late-Georgian house, now a country hotel of 'unintimidating charm'. It stands in the rolling countryside of the Welsh Marches, amid wild and formal gardens and fields. 'The grounds are lovely and the house is delightful – elegant, beautifully furnished.' The 'hard-working and enthusiastic' owners, Nancy and Tim Morrow, 'are always around if you want something, but are not intrusive.' They write: 'We aim to offer the relaxed informality of a country home', and one couple adds: 'The gracious living (drinks in the library) made us feel we were in a 1930s novel. The food was excellent.' Others have admired the 'marvellous' stone-floored hallway and sandstone staircase, and the bedrooms. The luxury ones are 'large, light and airy'. 'Ours had a beautiful antique French painted bed, a Victorian writing table, flowers, chocolates, bottled water, a lovely bathroom.' The huge main reception room has an ornate gilded ceiling and a log fire; there is a cosy library. The 'beautiful dining room' has green walls, intricate carvings, and plants and flowers giving a country feel (but its lighting may be a bit dim for some). Local ingredients are used in the three-course dinner menu, served at 8 pm (no choice, preferences discussed in advance), eg, scallops with a Thai herb salad; Welsh Black beef with salsa verde; tarte Tatin. A 'fresh and plentiful' breakfast is served in a room where checked tablecloths give a café feel. 'We had wonderful scrambled eggs from the hens that scratch about outside.' The busy main road 'can be audible'. The interesting old town of Montgomery is nearby; or you can visit Powis Castle, Berriew village with black-and-white houses and peacock topiary. (*Sir Timothy Harford, J and JW*)

Open All year. Dining room closed midday and Sun/Mon.
Rooms 8 double, 1 single. TV on request.
Facilities Drawing room, morning room with informal bar, library with TV, dining room (background music if requested); function facilities. 14-acre grounds: 5-acre gardens, croquet, 9-acre fields. River Severn ½ mile, fishing. Unsuitable for &. Civil wedding licence.
Location On A483 halfway between Welshpool and Newtown. Train: Welshpool; then bus to village.
Restrictions Smoking in library only. No dogs.
Credit cards Amex, MasterCard, Visa.
Terms B&B: single £45–£80, double £60–£105. Child in parents' room: £15. Picnic lunch by arrangement. Set dinner £21.50.

KNIGHTON Powys   **Map 3:C4**

Milebrook House   *Tel* 01547-528632
Milebrook   *Fax* 01547-520509
Knighton LD7 1LT   *Website* www.milebrookhouse.co.uk

'Superb: excellent, spacious room, food marvellous, and a friendly welcome.' 'We enjoyed it so much.' More plaudits this year for this small hotel, where Beryl and Rodney Marsden are the 'hard-working and genial hosts'. It is a grey 18th-century house near the English border, on the river Teme outside Knighton. 'It has good gardens running down to a stream, and a rustic feel despite the main road in front'; rear rooms are quietest, including four luxurious new ones with thick carpets, a blue-tiled bathroom. The restaurant is popular with locals, and the food is 'simple but interesting, and beautifully cooked'. The *prix-fixe* menu might include herring fillets with juniper berries; pancake stuffed with ham and mushrooms; bruschetta with olive pesto; Herefordshire beef with blue cheese. Many vegetables are from the garden. 'The tables are a bit close, but the company was good, so why worry?' A disabled guest found the hotel very comfortable. But one couple thought the dining room chairs hard. In the grounds are a formal garden, a croquet lawn, a pond, meadows with wild flowers and a riverside walk. The hotel has a mile-long stretch of the Teme for trout fishing, and Rodney Marsden is happy to advise on birdwatching. Some of the best stretches of Offa's Dyke Path are near by, and Knighton has a heritage centre for the dyke. (*M and NJ Gibson, Stephen Potts, John and Joan Wyatt, JM*)

Open All year. Restaurant closed Mon midday.
Rooms 10 double. 2 on ground floor.
Facilities Ramps. Lounge, bar, restaurant. No background music. 3½-acre grounds on river: croquet, fishing. Golf nearby.
Location 2 miles E of Knighton on A4113 (rooms double-glazed). Train: Knighton.
Restrictions No smoking: restaurant, lounge, bedrooms. No children under 8. No dogs.

Credit cards Diners, MasterCard, Visa.
Terms [2001] B&B £38.90–£56.60. Set lunch £12.50, dinner £21; full alc £33.
Special breaks. Christmas, New Year packages.

LLANDDEINIOLEN Gwynedd   **Map 3:A3**

Ty'n Rhos   *Tel* 01248-670489
Seion, Llanddeiniolen   *Fax* 01248-670079
nr Caernarfon LL55 3AE   *Email* enquiries@tynrhos.co.uk
                                              Website www.tynrhos.co.uk

The 'scenic location, with a not-to-be-believed view from our room with its three large windows' was enjoyed this year, at Nigel Hughes and Lynda Kettle's converted farmhouse. It stands in large grounds on the wide plain between Snowdonia and the sea. The decor is cosy rather than smart: squashy sofas and chairs, books and games and a wood-burning stove in the large lounge; wicker chairs in the conservatory; pine furniture and fresh flowers in the bedrooms. One room on the ground floor is 'large and lovely, with pretty blue wallpaper, picture windows with a sliding door on to the patio, large comfortable armchairs, good beds, an excellent bathroom'. Three rooms are in converted farm buildings. 'The staff are helpful, the house is cosy and warm.' Linda Kettle herself is now chef, doing 'modern British' cooking, eg, leek and goat's cheese tart; confit of Welsh duck with lentils, garlic and a sherry sauce; steamed marmalade pudding. Residents are encouraged to take the no-choice dinner menu at £19.50, which is included in the half-board rate. The more expensive *carte* has variety and more ambitious dishes. Again this year, s vice was found to be 'disorganised' at busy times, particularly in the owners' absence. Breakfast is 'excellent value'. It includes fresh orange juice, kedgeree, kippers; home-made preserves. 'No small butter and jam packs,' says Linda Kettle. A conference and business centre, and a new dining room, have been added this year. Beyond the garden are fields with sheep and cattle, and two small lakes with ducks, coots and moorhens. Nearby attractions: Caernarfon and Penrhyn castles, Bodnant Garden, narrow-gauge railways. (*Claire Lavery*)

Open All year, except Christmas. Restaurant closed Sun evening to non-residents.
Rooms 11 double, 3 single. 3 in cottage. 1, on ground floor, designed for &.
Facilities Ramp. Lounge, bar, restaurant, conservatory; conference/meeting room. 70-acre pastureland, 1-acre garden: croquet, carp lake. Sea 9 miles.
Location 6 miles NE of Caernarfon. From Llandudno take A55 to Bangor, left on to A5. Immediately turn right on to B4366. House signposted after 5 miles.
Restrictions Smoking in lounge only. No children under 6. No dogs in house.
Credit cards Amex, MasterCard, Visa.
Terms B&B: single £55, double £80–£110; D,B&B: single £74.50, double £119–£149. Set lunch £12.95, dinner £19.50; full alc £30.

Please don't hesitate to write again about an old favourite. Too many people feel that if they have written once, years ago, there is no need to report on a revisit.

LLANDEILO Carmarthenshire   **Map 3:D3**

The Cawdor Arms	*Tel* 01558-823500
72 Rhosmaen Street	*Fax* 01558-822399
Llandeilo SA19 6EN	*Email* cawdor.arms@btinternet.com
	Website www.cawdor-arms.co.uk

Liked again in 2001 ('really smart, warm and comfortable'), this
Georgian inn 'has the feel of a large country house hotel', but is in the
main street of a small market town. The owners are English: John
Silver, former nuclear engineer, and his wife Sylvia, former teacher.
An inspector found the hotel 'agreeable, with a friendly atmosphere';
this year, one report tells of amateurish service, another of a 'gracious'
reception. The Silvers have re-created the aura of late Victorian
Britain: warm wallpaper, large fireplaces and substantial furniture
mark the public rooms. And if they have shown restraint on Victorian
clutter, they have let themselves go on Victorian sentimentality: teddy
bears in pinafores and bonnets outside bedroom doors, a rocking sheep
on the landing. Bedrooms, too, have a late Victorian feel: 'Ours,
Charlotte's Room, with dusky blue wallpaper, was comfortably furnished and looked over a garden. Bedside lighting was good. The service at dinner, by Mrs Silver and her staff, was friendly. In the large,
handsome dining room, the food was beautifully presented.' The
Silvers' daughter, Jane, is now chef, offering such dishes as duck confit with red cabbage sauerkraut; pork with twice-baked thyme soufflé.
We'd welcome reports on her work. 'Mr Silver, in an attractive vari-
coloured waistcoat, served us a good Merlot. Dinner, and breakfast
too, came with a selection of delicious home-made breads. Our only
criticism: background music, a sort of bluesy jazz, in the evenings.'

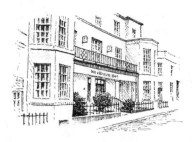

The hotel welcomes children,
and has plenty of books for
them. Special events include
'Murder Mystery' evenings
and also weekend painting
courses. Public areas have
been 'boldly decorated'. 'An
interesting experience, very
Welsh despite the owners
being very English.' (*DT,
APW, and others*)

Open All year.
Rooms 15 double, 2 single.
Facilities Lounge (live piano or tapes, evenings), bar, breakfast room, restau-
rant. Courtyard. Fishing (river Towy) nearby. Unsuitable for &.
Location Centre of town (front rooms double-glazed). Parking.
Restrictions No smoking: restaurant, some bedrooms.
Credit cards Amex, MasterCard, Visa.
Terms B&B: single £45–£60, double £60–£80; D,B&B: single £65–£80,
double £100–£120. Set lunch £14.50, dinner £24. Child in parents' room: £15;
babies free. Weekend programmes: painting, 'Murder Mysteries', etc.
Christmas package.

LLANDRILLO Denbighshire   Map 3:B4

Tyddyn Llan   *Tel* 01490-440264
Llandrillo   *Fax* 01490-440414
nr Corwen LL21 0ST   *Email* tyddynllanhotel@compuserve.com
                            Website tyddynllan.co.uk

❧ César award in 1989

'Service and welcome were friendly, my room was large and comfortable, dinner was delicious.' An inspector's verdict in 2001 on Peter and Bridget Kindred's grey stone Georgian mansion, set amid lovely country in the Vale of Edeyrnion – 'a beautifully restored house in a wonderful, quiet location'. The public rooms are 'strikingly and pleasantly decorated', with antiques and period furniture, and clever use of colour. The bedrooms are pretty and well lit. The Kindreds 'know how to create the atmosphere of a family home', but 'though friendly when you meet them, they keep a low profile', and this has led some readers to find the welcome rather cool. In the restaurant, service 'is attentive', and the food 'very good'. There is a new chef again this year, Matthew Haines, whose 'modern British' cooking includes dishes such as goat's cheese soufflé; Welsh lamb cooked in Moroccan spices, with couscous; 'perfect' crème brûlée. This year, a sorbet was 'wittily presented', and 'my vegetarian concoction was delicious'. There is a simple lunch menu. Wines are 'interesting and fairly priced'. Salads are picked from the neo-Elizabethan herb garden, and jellies are made from the owners' quinces and crab apples. Peter Kindred, whose own work hangs in the dining room, runs painting weekends between March and June. Wine tastings and gourmet dinners are held. There's good walking in the nearby Berwyn mountains; Chirk Castle and Erddig House are within a half-hour drive. The hotel has a four-mile stretch of the river Dee, with fishing, mostly for grayling.

Open All year, except 2 weeks Jan.
Rooms 10 double.
Facilities 3 lounges, bar, restaurant; classical background music. 4-acre grounds: water garden, croquet. River fishing (ghillie available), riding, golf, sailing, walking nearby. Only restaurant suitable for &. Civil wedding licence.
Location From A5 W of Corwen take B4401 to Llandrillo. Train: Wrexham; taxi/bus.
Restrictions No smoking in restaurant. No dogs in public rooms.
Credit cards All major cards accepted.
Terms B&B: single £67.50–£85, double £105–£140; D,B&B: single £95–£112.50, double £160–£195. Full alc: lunch £28, dinner £38.50. Special interest weekends, painting courses, in low season. Christmas, New Year house parties. ***V***

The ***V*** sign at the end of an entry indicates a hotel that has agreed to take part in our Voucher scheme and to give *Guide* readers a 25 per cent discount on their room rates, subject to the conditions explained in *How to read the entries*, and listed on the back of the vouchers.

LLANDUDNO Conwy   Map 3:A3

Bodysgallen Hall   *Tel* 01492-584466
Llanrhos   *Fax* 01492-582519
Llandudno LL30 1RS   *Email* info@bodysgallen.com
                                            Website www.bodysgallen.com

♥ *César award in 1988*

Set on a hillside in a large park outside the resort, with fine views of
Snowdonia, this is a Relais & Châteaux member, judged 'truly excellent' by recent visitors, and well managed by Matthew Johnson.
Readers write of its 'cosseting embrace' and 'efficient staff'. The
17th-century Grade II listed mansion has been restored to its original
splendour by Historic House Hotels Ltd (see also *The Cadogan*,
London, *Hartwell House*, Aylesbury, and *Middlethorpe Hall*, York).
Its 'lovely grounds' include a 17th-century knot garden, a rockery
with a cascade, and an 18th-century walled rose garden. The spa, in a
converted farmhouse, has an 18-metre swimming pool, a gymnasium
and three beauty salons. The interior is impressive; panelled rooms,
ancestral portraits, splendid fireplaces and stone mullioned windows.
David Thompson's cooking is traditional, eg, artichoke soup with
home-smoked chicken; loin of venison with red cabbage; Bara Brith
and butter pudding with calvados ice cream. When booking dinner,
you should ask about table position: best ones have a garden view, and
you might not want to sit too near the weekend pianist. Most bedrooms
are large and elegant. The cottage suites, close to the spa, are good for
a family (provided the children are over eight). Local attractions
include Bodnant Garden, and the castles of Conwy, Caernarfon and
Beaumaris. More reports welcome.

Open All year.
Rooms 16 cottage suites, 19 double, 3 single. Some on ground floor.
Facilities Hall, drawing room, library, bar, dining room (pianist Fri, Sat); con-
ference centre. 220-acre parkland: gardens, tennis, croquet; spa: swimming
pool, gym, sauna, beauty treatment, club room (light meals and drinks).
Riding, shooting, fishing, sandy beaches nearby.
Location Follow A55 towards Llandudno. Take A470 exit; hotel 2 miles on
right. Train: Llandudno.
Restrictions No smoking: dining room, 3 bedrooms. No children under 8.
Dogs in cottages/parkland only (not in gardens).
Credit cards MasterCard, Visa.
Terms Room: single £114–£255, double £150–£255, cottage £175–£265.
Breakfast £14.50. Set lunch £19.50, dinner £34.90. Special breaks. Christmas
package.

St Tudno Hotel   *Tel* 01492-874411
The Promenade   *Fax* 01492-860407
Llandudno LL30 2LP   *Email* sttudnohotel@btinternet.com
                                            Website www.st-tudno.co.uk

♥ *César award in 1987*

Since 1972, Martin and Janette Bland have owned and run this fairly
luxurious hotel, in a Grade II listed house facing the ornate Victorian

pier: lounges have 'lovely views of the sea and the promenade'. Decor is also Victorian-style: lounges with much drapery, potted plants, and patterned wallpaper. The food was again this year found 'excellent', by a reader who says: 'Staff are obviously highly trained and service was charming. Add a delightful bedroom and superb location, and you have a top small hotel.' But some visitors thought the prices high, and the hotel 'self-satisfied', and one found the garden-style restaurant 'nice, but badly lit, so it was gloomy'. The owners are not always present. The bedrooms (the best are front ones) have lots of frills, pastel colours; some bathrooms have a spa bath. One suite is new this year. Another, good for a family, is named after Lewis Carroll's Alice Liddell, who holidayed here in 1861. Some rooms are 'small, but excellently appointed'. The chef, David Harding, serves modern British cooking, with 'classic sauces and intense flavours': eg, wild mushroom risotto with Parmesan and rocket; grilled cod with a parsley and garlic crust and red wine jus; Cointreau and orange cheesecake with a vanilla sauce. Mrs Bland's wine list has won awards. 'Breakfast was very good, with excellent coffee.' Children are welcomed, but in the evenings it is preferred that they eat with their parents in the coffee lounge, rather than the restaurant. There is a 'nice indoor swimming pool' and a 'secret garden', with flowers in baskets and tubs, at the rear. Parking can be difficult, but staff will help. Bodnant Garden, Conwy, Caernarfon and Penrhyn castles are nearby. So are three championship golf courses. (*Gordon Hands, and others*)

Open All year.
Rooms 2 suites, 16 double, 1 single. 1 on ground floor.
Facilities Lift. Sitting room, coffee lounge, lounge bar, garden room, restaurant; harpist Sat evening; small indoor swimming pool; front and rear patios, rear 'secret garden'. Sandy beach 60 yds.
Location Central, opposite pier. Secure car park, garaging.
Restrictions No smoking: restaurant, sitting room, some bedrooms. No very young children in restaurant at night. Dogs at proprietors' discretion; not in public rooms, unattended in bedrooms.
Credit cards All major cards accepted.
Terms B&B: single £60–£78, double £85–£190, suite £230–£280. Set lunch £17.50, dinner £36; full alc £39.50. Bar lunches. Midweek, weekend, off-season, Christmas, New Year breaks. 1-night bookings occasionally refused bank holiday Sat. *V*

LLANFACHRETH Gwynedd   **Map 3:B3**

Tŷ Isaf Farmhouse   BUDGET   *Tel/Fax* 01341-423261
Llanfachreth   *Email* raygear@tyisaf78.freeserve.co.uk
nr Dolgellau LL40 2EA   *Website* www.tyisaf78.freeserve.co.uk

'Is this the greenest place in your guide?' ask Ray and Lorna Gear, owners of this little guest house in a hamlet on a quiet road in the Snowdonia National Park. Found 'excellent, with a relaxed family atmosphere', it has an 'idyllic' setting opposite a church. In its garden are a stream where deer drink, two llamas, Math and Mathonwy (named after Celtic heroes), wild birds, and hens which supply free-range eggs. Wide views of fields and hills are on every side. Built in

1624, the longhouse has thick stone walls, oak rafters, an inglenook fireplace and a country decor. Mrs Gear's lavish no-choice dinners, found 'most imaginative' by a recent visitor, have a Welsh emphasis, eg, cawl cenin (herb roll); ragout of Welsh lamb; Snowdon pudding with fruit sauce; Welsh cheeses. Unlicensed; bring your own wine. The three bedrooms have pine furniture. There's a pretty study with an ancient butter churn, and 'books to inspire the heart'. The lounge has TV, video, games; the dining room has background music if wanted. Local outdoor activities include walking, climbing, fishing and sailing. Packed lunches are available. The Gears, who provide secure facilities for bicycles, say: 'The Coed y Brenin forest has one of the best cycling tracks in Europe.' More reports, please.

Open All year, except Christmas, New Year; advance notice required.
Rooms 3 double. No telephone/TV.
Facilities Lounge with TV (classical/Welsh music if requested), study, dining room. 3-acre grounds: garden, paddock, stream. Walking, cycling, climbing, riding, fishing, sailing, beaches, castles nearby. Unsuitable for &.
Location 3½ miles NE of Dolgellau. On A470 Dolgellau bypass, take 1st right after *Little Chef*, signposted Bala, 1st left, signposted Dolgellau, 1st right signposted Llanfachreth. Continue to village; *Tŷ Isaf* 1st house on right. Train: Machynlleth, 12 miles; then taxi.
Restrictions No smoking. No children under 13. Dogs by arrangement (only 1 at any time).
Credit cards None accepted.
Terms B&B £27. Set dinner £17.50. £10 single supplement sometimes levied. 3-night breaks. *V* (1 night only)

LLANGAMMARCH WELLS Powys   Map 3:D3

The Lake   *Tel* 01591-620202
Llangammarch Wells LD4 4BS   *Fax* 01591-620457
                                          Email info@lakecountryhouse.co.uk
                                          Website www.lakecountryhouse.co.uk

César award in 1992

'A lovely spot to stay, with good food and wonderful public rooms.' More praise (balanced by some caveats) came again this year for Jean-Pierre and Jan Mifsud's imposing turn-of-the-century hotel (Pride of Britain). It has 'a beautiful setting' amid unspoilt countryside, above lawns that slope down to the river Irfon. The 'warm welcome' is admired, also the swift and 'very pleasant' service by a 'friendly, helpful and happy' staff (though they weren't always available during the day). 'Mr Mifsud is constantly in evidence. Our suite was very comfortable.' Many bedrooms were recently refurbished; they vary in size; some suites are large, with a canopied or a four-poster bed; sherry and fruit are provided, and early morning tea is brought up. A generous afternoon tea is served in a huge lounge with deep sofas and armchairs, a log fire, family photographs on a grand piano, and magazines. The big dining room, with candlelit tables at night, serves modern English/French food, eg, warm scallop mousse with oyster and saffron sauce; loin of local venison; glazed orange tart with a lemon sorbet. Some ingredients are local and organically produced. The wines and

the cheeseboard are much admired. The 'very good' and vast breakfast includes Welsh laver bread, and is accompanied by practical
details about the weather and local sightseeing (excellent fishing rivers
are nearby). Dogs 'are welcomed, but not in the public rooms'. At dinner, men are expected to wear a jacket. The Mifsuds also own *Dinham
Hall*, Ludlow (*qv*). (*Sir John Hall, NM Mackintosh, Prof. David
Taylor, and others*)

Open All year.
Rooms 11 suites, 8 double. 2 on ground floor.
Facilities 2 lounges, bar, billiard room, restaurant. No background music. 50-
acre grounds: lake (fishing), river, tennis, croquet, 9-hole par 3 golf course,
clay-pigeon shooting, archery. Riding, pony-trekking, golf, rivers, fishing
(tuition available) nearby. Civil wedding licence.
Location 8 miles SW of Builth Wells. From A483 Builth–Llandovery follow
signs to Llangammarch Wells, then to hotel. Train: Swansea/Shrewsbury, then
scenic Heart of Wales line to Llangammarch Wells; guests will be met.
Restrictions No smoking: restaurant, bedrooms. No children under 7 in
dining room after 7 pm (high tea provided). No dogs in public rooms, except
guide dogs.
Credit cards All major cards accepted.
Terms B&B £70–£135; D,B&B (min. 2 nights) £85–£150. Set lunch £18.50,
dinner £32.50. Winter breaks. Christmas, New Year packages. 1-night bookings sometimes refused. *V*

LLANSANFFRAID GLAN CONWY Gwynedd   Map 3:A3

The Old Rectory Country House	*Tel* 01492-580611
Llanrwst Road	*Fax* 01492-584555
Llansanffraid Glan Conwy	*Email* info@oldrectorycountryhouse.co.uk
nr Conwy LL28 5LF	*Website* www.oldrectorycountryhouse.co.uk

🦆 *César award in 1994*

'Sheer joy.' Wendy Vaughan, chef and co-owner (with her husband
Michael) of this Georgian guest house, is the only woman in Wales to
win a *Michelin* star for cooking. Our readers, too, have found it 'excellent'. Menus offer no choice, but the food 'is interesting', eg, spiced
monkfish with vanilla risotto; Welsh lamb with spinach parcels; passion fruit tart with mango sorbet. Dinner is served at separate tables at
8 pm, after drinks and *amuse-gueules* in the 'most attractive' panelled
drawing room (a harpist sometimes plays). The eclectic wine list has
plenty of half bottles. Breakfasts include Welsh rarebit cooked in ale.
The house stands up a steep drive, with fine views over the Conwy
estuary towards Snowdonia. In front, descending in terraces to the
road, are gardens partly formal, partly wilder. Recent praise:
'Comfortable, and good value.' 'They provide many of the elegances
of a grand country hotel.' The house is full of antiques, ornaments and
bric-a-brac; board games, books and a piano in the drawing room; soft
yellow walls and elegant table settings in the dining room. The bedrooms (some are small) are 'lavishly decorated, with lots of cushions,
easy chairs or a sofa, and masses of goodies: fresh fruit, etc'.
Bathrooms are mostly large (one was described as 'way over the top').
Front rooms have double-glazed windows. The Vaughans (he is 'an

indefatigable host') are knowledgeable about Welsh history and culture. Bodnant Garden is just down the road; Conwy, Caernarfon and Beaumaris castles are within 25 miles; so is the Snowdon Mountain Railway. The Conwy Estuary Bird Sanctuary and three championship golf courses are close by. (*Brian Wicks*)

Open 1 Feb–1 Dec. Dining room closed for lunch, occasionally for dinner (guests warned when booking).
Rooms 6 double. 2 on ground floor in coach house.
Facilities Lounge (harpist twice-weekly pre-dinner), restaurant. 2½-acre grounds. Sea, safe bathing 3 miles; fishing, golf, riding, sailing, dry ski-slope nearby.
Location On A470, ½ mile S of junction with A55. Train: Conwy, 2 miles.
Restrictions No children under 5, except babies under 9 months. Smoking/dogs in coach house only.
Credit cards MasterCard, Visa.
Terms B&B: single £99–£129, double £109–£199. Set dinner £34.90. 2-day breaks: D,B&B: single £129–£159, double £169–£229. 1-night bookings refused high season weekends, bank holidays. *V* (Nov, Feb, Mar)

LLANWRTYD WELLS Powys   **Map 3:D3**

Carlton House   *Tel* 01591-610248
Dol-y-Coed Road   *Fax* 01591-610242
Llanwrtyd Wells LD5 4RA   *Email* info@carltonrestaurant.co.uk
                                                Website www.carltonrestaurant.co.uk

❦ *César award in 1998*

'The sybaritic delights' provided by Alan and Mary Ann Gilchrist were enjoyed again this year, at their 'mildly eccentric' small restaurant-with-rooms, in an Edwardian villa painted bright red. 'We took a house party of 12, and found it a perfect place for our group, their wives and dogs. The gourmet option of five courses with appropriate wines was worth every (modest) penny.' Others have praised the 'warm, attentive hosts, cheerful staff, superb food'. The Gilchrists write: 'We try to provide a relaxed atmosphere – no formal dress code. We do *not* provide trouser presses, "free" sherry, sweeping views of extensive grounds – so you are not asked to pay for them.' The restaurant is in the bright front room, the lounge is a cosy, darker room at the back. *Michelin* awards a *Bib Gourmand* (one of only eight in Wales) for Mrs Gilchrist's modern British cooking, based on fresh, free-range and organic ingredients. Both the *à la carte* and the fixed-price menu change daily. They include, eg, chicken and cep boudin blanc; supreme of Gressingham duck served with punchnep and a citrus and honey sauce; apple soufflé. Special dietary needs are 'sympathetically catered for'. The wine list is varied and fairly priced. Breakfast is enjoyed too: 'They really know how to scramble eggs'; these come with a rasher of thick bacon, fresh orange juice, and 'good and plentiful coffee'. The Gilchrists' daughter, Emma, and their basset hound, Cecily, are in attendance. One reader had a 'beautiful large corner bedroom', but some rooms can suffer traffic noise; and stairs to upper floors are steep. Llanwrtyd Wells is a small spa town below the Cambrian mountains, in Wales's red kite country; they can be seen feeding at Gigrin or at the RSPB's Dinas Reserve. (*Christine and Stephen Wright; also Sir Timothy Harford*)

Open All year, except 10–28 Dec.
Rooms 1 suite, 5 double, 1 single. No telephone.
Facilities Lounge, restaurant. No background music. Tiny garden. Fishing on Canmarch and Irfon rivers. Unsuitable for &.
Location Town centre. No private parking. Llanwrtyd Wells is on the scenic Heart of Wales railway line (Shrewsbury–Swansea).
Restrictions No smoking in restaurant. No dogs in public rooms.
Credit cards MasterCard, Visa.
Terms B&B: single £30, double £60, suite £75. Set dinner £24; full alc £32. Short breaks.

LLYSWEN Powys   **Map 3:D4**

Llangoed Hall	*Tel* 01874-754525
Llyswen	*Fax* 01874-754545
Brecon LD3 0YP	*Email* office@llangoedhall.com
	Website www.llangoedhall.com

 César award in 1991

'Perfection. Every detail is just right.' A new manager, Graham Steed, has taken over and 'spends a great deal of time working directly with guests', perhaps addressing last year's complaints of '*froideur*' in a peaceful and interesting hotel. It is a 17th-century mansion, redesigned by Sir Clough Williams-Ellis, which stands back from a main road, in 'beautifully kept' gardens with a maze, and 'wonderful views' across the river Wye to the Black Mountains. Its owner, Sir Bernard Ashley, aims to create 'the atmosphere of an Edwardian house party' (eg, no reception desk). His superb collection of pictures is distributed throughout. The public rooms are impressive: great hall with deep sofas and stone fireplace, morning room with piano, library with snooker table. Oriental rugs and 'fascinating antiques' abound. Bedrooms have Laura Ashley chintzes, period furniture (some four-posters); but bathroom showers are hand held. 'Our rooms were wonderful, huge, spacious and quiet, with beautiful views,' one visitor wrote. The 'very pretty' yellow-walled restaurant has a *Michelin* star (one of only two in Wales) for Daniel James's cooking – dishes like ragout of lobster and red mullet with poached oyster; breast of duck with plum tarte Tatin. 'I admired the pomp and ceremony,' a 2001 visitor wrote, 'but it came with formal service by French waiters, rather than Welsh warmth.' During the Hay-on-Wye book festival, 'the place becomes a hothouse of literati-glitterati – you crash into Martin Amis on the stairs, nod casually to Gerald Scarfe in the library, ogle Norman Mailer, and are in danger of greeting Gore Vidal like a long-lost friend on the way to dinner'. The conference facilities have been expanded. There is fishing on the Wye, walking nearby in the Black Mountains and the Brecon Beacons, and many other country pursuits are available (see below). Chepstow and Raglan castles are within easy reach. (*Barbara A Kreuter, Sam Lewis, SH*)

Open All year.
Rooms 3 suites, 19 double, 1 single.

Facilities Hall, 3 lounges, restaurant, billiard room; private dining room, function rooms. Background music at functions only. 17-acre grounds: tennis, croquet, maze, river Wye (200 yds), fishing (ghillie). Riding, golf, gliding, clay-pigeon shooting, canoeing nearby. Only ground floor suitable for &. Civil wedding licence.
Location 11 miles N of Brecon, on A470, 1 mile N of Llyswen. Train: Cardiff or Newport; regular bus service or hotel will meet.
Restrictions No smoking in restaurant. No children under 8. No dogs in house (heated kennels in grounds).
Credit cards All major cards accepted.
Terms [2001] B&B: single £110–£130, double £145–£270, suite £295–£315. Set lunch £16.50 (Sun £23.50), dinner £37.50. 2-day breaks. Christmas, New Year house parties. *V*

MUMBLES Swansea   **Map 3:E3**

Hillcrest House   NEW   *Tel* 01792-363700
1 Higher Lane, Langland   *Fax* 01792-363768
Mumbles SA3 4NS   *Email* stay@hillcresthousehotel.com
                            Website www.hillcresthousehotel.com

Dave and Liz Bowen are the new owners of this tiny, unusual hotel just outside Swansea. It is restored to the *Guide* by an inspector this year: 'It stands imposingly on a rise above Swansea Bay.' A daunting wall, called 'the Berlin Wall' by the Bowens, shields it from the car park. 'Liz Bowen is very friendly and chatty,' says our inspector. 'Each bedroom is themed on a country: Scotland, South Africa, etc. Ours (England), with mainly pink and apple-green decor, was not kitschy, though the straw hats hung with cheerful ribbons on one wall brought it to the verge of twee. It had good lighting, a bathroom with fairly fluffy towels. The public rooms on the ground floor, all open plan, have a somewhat 1920s feel, created in part by the bright jazz music: you half expect flappers with boyish haircuts to come in to dinner. The menu had a bright, fresh flavour too (starters such as salmon rösti with mozzarella). We enjoyed beetroot and bacon salad; excellent rack of pink lamb; spotted dick with custard – but my mousse with orange liqueur sauce was poor. Wines are fairly priced. A waitress turned down the music when we asked. Breakfast was adequate, with hot dishes and good coffee.' French windows lead to a terrace, where you can dine outdoors in warm weather. The Gower beaches are close by.

Open All year.
Rooms 5 double, 1 single.
Facilities Lounge, bar area, restaurant ('easy listening' background music at night). Terrace. Unsuitable for &.
Location 4 miles SW of Swansea centre. At Mumbles, right at main roundabout, 4th left at church; down Langland Road.
Restrictions No smoking: restaurant, 4 bedrooms. No dogs.
Credit cards Amex, MasterCard, Visa.
Terms [2001] B&B: single £50, double £70–£90. Full alc £25. *V*

Please never tell a hotel you intend to send a report to the *Guide*. Anonymity is essential for objectivity.

Norton House [NEW]

Norton Road, Mumbles
Swansea SA3 5TQ

Tel 01792-404891
Fax 01792-403210
Email nortonhouse@btconnect.com
Website www.nortonhousehotel.co.uk

'What a wonderful find, and so peaceful – it reminded us of a small family-run French hotel.' So write the nominators in 2001 of Jan and John Power's handsome little white-fronted Georgian manor, a former master mariner's house. It stands near the shore of Swansea Bay in a village three miles from the city centre. Others liked the four-poster beds in some rooms, and the smart restaurant with its chandeliers, circular mahogany tables, and lively Welsh atmosphere. Here the 'excellent chef', Mark Comisini, provides modern British cooking on a menu written in English and Welsh. Bara Lawr (laver bread with cockles and bacon) and Bwydlys Gwydd (salad of smoked goose breast) have been enjoyed; or you could try Cig Carw Gyda Reis a Madarch (venison steak on wild rice), or indeed Caws Pob (Welsh

rarebit). Breakfast is 'fabulous' (with muesli, porridge, thick toast). Heather, the assistant manager, is 'always helpful and smiling'. The best bedrooms have period furnishings and patterned rugs; flowery fabrics abound. The lovely Gower peninsula is nearby. (*Margaret Rogers and Elizabeth Oakley*)

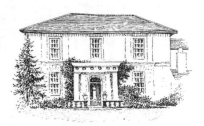

Open All year, except Christmas.
Rooms 15 double. 8 in annexe.
Facilities Bar, restaurant; background CDs. 1-acre garden. Sea, sandy and rock beach 100 yds. Unsuitable for &.
Location 3 miles SW of Swansea. Coast road to Mumbles; right into Norton Rd exactly 1 mile after 'Welcome to Mumbles' sign. Hotel 60 yds on left.
Restrictions No smoking: restaurant, some bedrooms. No children under 10. Guide dogs only.
Credit cards All major cards accepted.
Terms B&B: single £62.50–£72.50, double £72.50–£87.50. Set dinner £25.50.

NANTGWYNANT Gwynedd

Map 3:A3

Pen-y-Gwryd Hotel [BUDGET]

Nantgwynant
Llanberis LL55 4NT

Tel 01286-870211
Website www.pyg.co.uk

❧ *César award in 1995*

Rich in eccentricity, this 'unique old inn' is adored by readers for its 'wonderful atmosphere', and its low prices, but is *not* for those who want luxury. The owners, Brian and Jane Pullee, are 'great characters', 'the nicest possible hosts', and most of their guests are mountaineers. The inn (also a mountain rescue post) stands on a busy tourist road near the foot of the Llanberis Pass, in the Snowdonia National Park. In 1953, Hunt, Hillary and most of the Everest team used it as a training base before flying to Nepal; their signatures are scrawled on a ceiling. Climbing memorabilia – well-worn boots, ice picks, etc – fill the slate-floored bar. 'Not posh or sophisticated; run on house-party lines, with a great social mix of guests,' writes one devotee. A reader this year, who came with her two dogs, was bemused by the contrasts: 'A stream of one-nighters. Dark bedrooms, with old-fashioned furniture, no telephone or TV, but wonderful white fluffy monogrammed towels, masses of warm bedding. The food was fantastic: five courses, delicious home-made soups, loads of well-cooked vegetables, super puddings with local cream, very good coffee, served in the bar from a silver pot. Pleasant young Danish staff, vases with scented lilies. The original public toilets at the front have been converted into a chapel, which is super.' Mr Pullee writes: 'We are swimming against the tide, being somewhat old-fashioned. We insist on proper behaviour: no baseball caps indoors, no drinking straight from a bottle, no vests or bare feet, no uncontrolled children running around. I would also ban vegetarians and similar faddish eaters.' Welsh lamb with provençale sauce; steak and mushrooms braised in port with garlic; hot fudge surprise pudding, are among the 'tasty, plentiful' dishes of chef Lena Jensen, from Jutland. The 'substantial packed lunches' are also enjoyed. Breakfast (with porridge, kippers) at 8.50 am, and dinner at 7.30, are announced by a gong; everyone eats at the same time. The bedrooms are simple (no extras); five have facilities *en suite* (Rooms 15 and 17 are said to be the best). There are five public bathrooms, some with a massive old bath. The annexe room was completely refurbished this year. The panelled lounge, simply furnished, has a blazing log fire. The large games room has bar billiards, etc. Outside, there is a natural spring-fed pool fringed with ferns, and a sauna. (*Janice Carrera, Mrs Andrew Stainton, Amanda Barrow; also* Good Pub Guide)

Open Mar–end Oct, New Year, weekends Jan/Feb.
Rooms 15 double, 1 single. 3 with bath, 1 with shower. No telephone, TV. 1 on ground floor, across courtyard.
Facilities Lounge, bar, smoking room, games room, dining room; chapel. No background music. 2-acre grounds: natural swimming pool, sauna. Fishing nearby.
Location A498 Beddgelert–Capel Curig, at junction with A4086. Train: Bangor/Betws-y-Coed; local bus (frequent in summer).
Restriction No smoking: dining room, bedrooms.
Credit cards None accepted.
Terms B&B: single £24, double £48–£60. Bar lunch £5–£6, set dinner £17. 1-night bookings sometimes refused weekends.

NEWPORT Pembrokeshire   **Map 3:D1**

Cnapan   *Tel* 01239-820575
East Street, Newport   *Email* cnapan@online-holidays.net
nr Fishguard SA42 0SY   *Website* www.online-holidays.net/cnapan

'We were delighted. If every small hotel was like *Cnapan*, one could travel blissfully round the UK,' says a fellow *Guide* hotelier of this small restaurant-with-rooms. It is a family affair, run by John and Eluned Lloyd and their daughter and son-in-law, Judith and Michael Cooper (mother and daughter are the chefs). Other visitors wrote of 'a wonderful lunch, exceptionally friendly owners, fantastic value for money'; 'every meal was delicious'; 'we loved the bread'. In the middle of a pleasant old seaside town, this listed building is painted bright pink. Inside, it has 'comfortable rooms, superb food and an air of rural France, so welcoming, generous and cheerful'. A traditional Welsh dresser, crowded with family treasures, stands in the hall; a wood-burning stove warms the guests' sitting room; books, current magazines and local information are everywhere. The dining room is large and cheerful, with flowers and candles on lace-covered tables, plates, pictures and pieces of armour on walls, a large stone fireplace. For a set price, residents choose items from the *carte*, which might include spicy fish chowder with hot savoury bread; breast of duck with a plum and ginger sauce; gooey chocolate roll with raspberries and cream. There is always a vegetarian main course. The small bedrooms are 'ingeniously designed, if rather cluttered', with pine furniture, bright colours, knick-knacks and a tiny shower (there is also a massive bath along the corridor). Families can use a two-roomed suite. Huge breakfasts include home-made marmalade, warm croissants, free-range eggs (but not fresh orange juice). In summer, drinks and tea are served in the sheltered garden. Nearby are the Pembrokeshire Coast Path and lovely beaches. (*Robin Oaten, Russell England*)

Note: There is a larger Newport in Gwent, but you won't find *Cnapan* there.

Open Mar–Dec, except Christmas. Restaurant closed Tue.
Rooms 5 double. No telephone.
Facilities Lounge, bar, restaurant; occasional jazz/classical background music. Small garden. 10 mins' walk to sea; fishing, birdwatching, pony-trekking, golf, boating nearby. Unsuitable for &.
Location Centre of small town (quiet at night; windows double-glazed). Parking. Train: Fishguard; bus to Newport.
Restrictions No smoking: restaurant, bedrooms. Guide dogs only.
Credit cards MasterCard, Visa.
Terms B&B £31–£38; D,B&B £51–£58. Set lunch £12, dinner £20. 1-night bookings occasionally refused in season.

PENALLY Pembrokeshire   **Map 3:E2**

Penally Abbey NEW   *Tel* 01834-843033
Penally, nr Tenby   *Fax* 01834-844714
SA70 7PY   *Email* penally.abbey@btinternet.com
                                       Website penally-abbey.com

'A friendly hotel, in a spectacular setting above Carmarthen Bay.' It is on the green of a tiny village, across a golf course from the broad beach. 'Mysterious ruins are in the garden,' write reporters in 2001. 'Parts of the main building are centuries old, but its high, wide windows, large, airy rooms, give an Edwardian feel: we half expected to see Peter Pan and the Darling children fly out of a window.' Once owned by the Jameson Irish whiskey family, the house was bought in

1985 and converted into a hotel by Steve and Eileen Warren, 'a cheerful couple from Berkshire'. Other guests liked the 'ambience of a well-loved family home, enhanced by antiques, teddy bears, photos of the children in the lounge'. Mrs Warren's 82-year-old father tends the terraced gardens. The best bedrooms are in the main house, overlooking the bay. 'We had one of the finest, with a prince-sized bed, excellent lighting, free sweet sherry, large bathroom, towelling bath robes. The roomy lounge had a grand piano. Dinner was marred by slightly overloud music. The menu was over-long and helpings too large, but the food was good – devilled crab, baked ham, succulent venison, delicious roast potatoes and fresh vegetables, apple crumble. The young waitress was efficient.' Another reader found Eileen Warren's cooking 'imaginative and delicious', in the elegant candlelit dining room facing the sea. 'Our room in the coach house had a four-poster. There's a tiny indoor swimming pool, and informal gardens.' Off the coast is Caldey Island, home of a religious community for nearly 1,500 years, now owned by Cistercians and open to visitors. Tenby's 'lovely beaches', and the 180-mile Pembrokeshire Coast Path, are nearby. (*Sarah and Tony Thomas, Jean Marsh*)

Open All year.
Rooms 1 suite, 10 double, 1 single. 4 in coach house (100 yds). 2 on ground floor.
Facilities Lounge, bar, conservatory, restaurant; 'classic/romantic' background music. Small indoor swimming pool. 6-acre grounds. Beach 10 mins' walk. Civil wedding licence.
Location On green in Penally village, 2 miles SW of Tenby, off A4139 to Pembroke.
Restrictions No smoking: restaurant, some bedrooms. No children under 7 at dinner. No pets.
Credit cards Amex, MasterCard, Visa.
Terms B&B: single £98, double £112, suite £134; D,B&B £84–£126 per person. Set lunch £18, dinner £28.50; full alc £34. 25% discount 1 Nov–30 Mar. Child under 14 in parents' room: B&B £10. Christmas package.

PENMAENPOOL Gwynedd   **Map 3:B3**

Penmaenuchaf Hall	*Tel* 01341-422129
Penmaenpool	*Fax* 01341-422787
Gwynedd LL40 1YB	*Email* relax@penhall.co.uk
	Website www.penhall.co.uk

'Pleasant and unobtrusive' staff, and a 'gracious host' in Lorraine Fielding are to be found at this grey manor house. Built by a Bolton cotton magnate as his summer home, it stands inside the Snowdonia National Park, near Penmaenpool. It has large and lovely grounds with gardens and woodlands, and 'great views' over the Mawddach estuary. Beware, however, of the steep potholed drive ('an off-road experience'). The public rooms, elegant and spacious, have parquet floors, oriental rugs, log fires, fresh flowers. There is a Victorian billiard room and a pretty conservatory. The 'beautifully decorated' bedrooms vary in size; many have splendid views. 'We had the Leigh Taylor room, which is large, with windows on two sides; the bathroom, spacious too, had a wonderful array of towels.' In the 'lovely dining room', the food is modern British (eg, warm salad of mackerel with wild asparagus tips; tian of roast aubergine with Pant-Ysgawn goat's cheese; spiced duckling with sweet onion confit. Another new chef arrived in early 2001. Breakfasts are 'good and varied', but the orange juice is not freshly squeezed. There is a booking system, with time slots, for both breakfast and dinner. The house has a large bat roost. Good walking all around, also fishing, golf, birdwatching, castles. (*Dr Norman Waterman, Michelle Brown, JRCW*)

Open All year.
Rooms 14 double.
Facilities Ramps. Hall, morning room, library, snooker room, bar, restaurant (classical background music). 21-acre grounds: croquet, woodland walks. Free trout and salmon fishing on Mawddach estuary; golf, riding, white-water rafting, sailing, pony-trekking nearby. Only public rooms suitable for &. Civil wedding licence.
Location From Dolgellau bypass (A470), take A493 towards Tywyn and Fairbourne. Entrance drive to hotel ½ mile on left. Train: Morfa Mawddach; taxi.
Restrictions No smoking: restaurant, morning room, library, 5 bedrooms. No children under 6, except babies. Dogs by arrangement.
Credit cards All major cards accepted.
Terms B&B: single from £70, double £100–£170; D,B&B: single from £97.50, double £165–£225. Set lunch £14.25–£15.75, dinner £27.50; full alc £38. Weekend, midweek, special breaks. Christmas package. *V*

PORTHKERRY Vale of Glamorgan   Map 3:E3

Egerton Grey   *Tel* 01446-711666
Porthkerry, nr Cardiff CF62 3BZ   *Fax* 01446-711690
Email info@egertongrey.co.uk
Website www.egertongrey.co.uk

A former 19th-century rectory, now a small, luxurious hotel. It stands in broad gardens near the Bristol Channel, facing the Somerset coast over Porthkerry Park. Reporters this year recommend: 'It is worth paying the extra ten pounds for a room with a view down the valley that leads to the sea.' Earlier visitors wrote: 'Excellent, with good food, lovely atmosphere.' The house is 'full of country charm', with ornate mouldings, panelling, antiques, porcelain, paintings, a collection of old clocks. But one visitor disliked the background music: 'Loud jazz or Chopin in the restaurant; Classic FM in the hall all day.' The spacious bedrooms, in Victorian or Edwardian style, have bold colour schemes, antiques, thick carpets, and carefully restored bathrooms (some have an enormous tub). Guests' names are placed on their door, house-party style. Dinner, by candlelight, is in the former billiard room. On the 'country-house menu' of chef Nigel Roberts, you can take two or three courses: maybe chicken and asparagus terrine; salmon with dill and saffron beurre blanc; steamed coffee and walnut pudding ('but the menu did not change in two days,' said one guest). Good wine list. Lots of interesting choices for breakfast. Small children are 'warmly welcomed' (special meals, etc). The owner, Anthony Pitkin, has a new manager again this year, Richard

Morgan-Price. Local attractions: the Welsh Folk Museum at St Fagans, Caerphilly and Cardiff castles. The airport is quite close (some noise is possible) (*Christine and Stephen Wright, RC*)

Open All year.
Rooms 2 suites, 7 double, 1 single.
Facilities Drawing room, library, restaurant (background music); conservatory; private dining room, function facilities. 3½-acre garden: croquet. Beach 200 yds; golf nearby. Only restaurant suitable for &. Civil wedding licence.
Location 10 miles SW of Cardiff. From M4 exit 33 follow signs to airport, bypassing Barry. Left at small roundabout by airport, signposted Porthkerry; after 500 yds left again, down lane between thatched cottages. Train: Barry, 4 miles; bus from Cardiff.
Restrictions No smoking in restaurant. No dogs in public rooms.
Credit cards All major cards accepted.
Terms B&B: single £70–£89.50, double £95–£105, suite £110–£130; D,B&B £55–£95 per person. Set lunch/dinner £13.50; full alc £25. Special break: D,B&B £60–£75 per person. Christmas package. *V*

PORTMEIRION Gwynedd   **Map 3:B3**

Portmeirion Hotel   *Tel* 01766-770000
Portmeirion LL48 6ET   *Fax* 01766-771331
                                 Email hotel@portmeirion-village.com
                                      Website www.portmeirion.com

César award in 1990

The late Sir Clough Williams-Ellis's famous Italianate fantasy resort, on the steep hillside of a wooded peninsula above a wide estuary, has been extended this year. On its edge, *Castell Deudraeth*, a grey turreted 1850s folly in its original Victorian garden, was opened as a small luxury hotel with 'cutting edge design'. The *Portmeirion Hotel* itself continues to be enjoyed. Its guests are well protected from the tourists who throng in the village by day (it stands in Mediterranean-style gardens with peacocks and a swimming pool). Behind its early Victorian exterior is an exuberant decor: bright fabrics, carved panels, furniture and ornaments from Rajasthan. But the atmosphere is very Welsh: the 'delightful staff' are bilingual; so are the menus; there is a Welsh harpist and a resident bard. The bedrooms in the main house are thought 'stunning': the Peacock Room has 'a magnificent four-poster bed, and a lovely sitting room facing the estuary'. Bedrooms in the village, and the self-catering cottages, are simpler, 'but all are unusual'. In the handsome, curved dining room, Billy Taylor's cooking is modern Welsh, eg, local lamb with lyonnaise potatoes and black pudding; Brecon venison with a casserole of baby apples, apricots and walnuts; Bara Brith and butter pudding. 'The food is the best and most innovative I have tasted outside London,' said one reader. Another found much of it overcooked, but he liked the wines. Breakfast includes fresh fruit salad, plenty of cooked dishes. Videos of episodes of *The Prisoner*, which was filmed in the village, are shown each evening on a TV channel. Miles of paths lead along the headland and through woods to secret sandy beaches. Sir Clough's other life-work, the garden at nearby Plas Brondanw, is open every day; Snowdonia, and the castles of Caernarfon, Harlech, Criccieth and Dolwyddelan, are nearby. (*AG, and others*)

Open 6 Jan–1 Feb. Restaurant closed Mon midday.
Rooms 18 suites (11 in castle), 33 double (26 in village). Also self-catering cottages.
Facilities Lift in castle. Hall, 3 lounges, 2 bars, restaurants, grill, children's supper room; function room; beauty salon. No background music. 70-acre grounds: garden, swimming pool (heated May–Sept); spa, tennis, lakes, sandy beach. Free golf nearby. Unsuitable for &. Civil wedding licence.
Location Off A487 at Minffordd, between Penrhyndeudraeth and Porthmadoc. Street parking.
Restriction No dogs.
Credit cards All major cards accepted.
Terms Room: £115–£180, suite £145–£230. Breakfast £11. Set lunch £12, dinner £35. D,B&B double (min. 2 nights) £207–£322. 3 days for the price of 2, 31 Oct–13 Apr. Christmas, New Year packages.

PWLLHELI Gwynedd   **Map 3:B2**

Plas Bodegroes   *Tel* 01758-612363
Nefyn Road   *Fax* 01758-701247
Pwllheli LL53 5TH   *Email* gunna@bodegroes.co.uk
                                           Website www.bodegroes.co.uk

꩜ *César award in 1992*

'Marvellous. The house is elegantly Georgian, the food is superb' (*Michelin Bib Gourmand*). 'Spacious rooms, lovely house and grounds.' 'What a comfy, cosy place. We sat in the garden with coffee, watching family parties having fun with croquet.' Renewed praise this year for Chris and Gunna Chown's restaurant-with-rooms, its 'pleasant atmosphere and personal service'. It is a small, pretty, white house up an avenue of ancient beeches in wooded grounds. The 'attractively understated' Scandinavian interior has been designed by the elegant Mrs Chown, who is Faroese. The restaurant, with 'inspired decor' in shades of green, is hung with contemporary paintings by Welsh artists, such as Kyffyn Williams and Gwilym Pritchard. Chris Chown's 'modern Welsh' cooking is much enjoyed, though one reader felt that the menu does not change often enough. But it has lots of choice. Dishes include seafood cawl with onions and coriander; roast pork with black pudding, bacon and garlic sauce; bara brith and butter pudding with apricot and ginger yogurt rice. The bedrooms vary in size and price: some, simple but comfortable, are in the attic; larger ones, 'sensitively appointed', have a four-poster and tall windows. Two are in a cottage at the rear, facing a courtyard garden. The lounge, quite small, can get crowded with non-resident diners, but the veranda, draped with wisteria and roses, is a pleasant place for sitting. Breakfast has been thought 'excellent, with delicious Greek yogurt and apricots', but one reader found the service 'haphazard'. Pwllheli is in a popular sailing area, near rocky shores, cliffs and beaches. (*Meryl Chetwood, Lynn Wildgoose, BG*)

Open 12 Feb–30 Nov. Closed Mon, except bank holidays.
Rooms 10 double (2 in cottage), 1 single. Some on ground floor.

Facilities Lounge, bar, breakfast room, restaurant (occasional jazz/classical background music). 5-acre grounds. Safe, sandy beach 1 mile. Golf, sailing nearby. Unsuitable for &.
Location 1 mile W of Pwllheli, on A497 to Nefyn. Train: Pwllheli; taxi.
Restrictions No smoking: restaurant, bedrooms. Children 'not encouraged'. No dogs in public rooms.
Credit cards MasterCard, Visa.
Terms B&B £40–£80; D,B&B £60–£110. Set Sun lunch £14.50, dinner £29.50. 1-night bookings refused bank holidays. *V*

REYNOLDSTON Swansea   **Map 3:E2**

Fairyhill   *Tel* 01792-390139
Reynoldston, nr Swansea SA3 1BS   *Fax* 01792-391358
                                                 Email postbox@fairyhill.net
                                                 Website www.fairyhill.net

Paul Davies and Andrew Hetherington ('an excellent front-of-house') own and run this creeper-covered 18th-century mansion, where prices are high but recent visitors have mostly been happy. 'The owners and staff were unfailingly charming and cheerful.' 'We had a lovely big room facing the spacious grounds.' These include woodlands, a trout stream and a lake with wild ducks: but huge trees round the edge of the house make it sunless, which some find depressing. The bedrooms, recently redecorated (some are 'cramped'), have a good bathroom and a CD-player; there's a huge library of discs downstairs. In the green-and-yellow restaurant, Paul Davies and Adrian Coulthard's enterprising 'modern Welsh' food includes dishes such as laver bread tart; seared fillets of brill with noodles and saffron mussel sauce; fillet of Welsh black beef with sun-dried tomato polenta. The kitchen team makes its own jam, biscuits and bread, and herbs and fruit are from the garden. The wine list is 'excellent but expensive'. 'The cooking was very good, almost as good as the owners seemed to think it was,' said one critic who found service 'patronising' on the first night, but after that 'very warm'. The beautiful Gower coast is nearby. (*PD, SW, and others*)

Open 18 Jan–24 Dec, New Year.
Rooms 8 double.
Facilities Lounge, bar, 2 dining rooms; piped jazz/classical music. 24-acre grounds: croquet, woodland, stream, lake. Beaches, water sports nearby. Unsuitable for &.
Location 11 miles W of Swansea. M4 exit 47 to Gowerton, B4295 for 9 miles.
Restrictions No smoking in restaurant. No children under 8. No dogs.
Credit cards Amex, MasterCard, Visa.
Terms B&B: single £110–£210, double £125–£225. Set dinner £27.50–£35. Alc lunch £32. 2-day breaks. 1-night bookings sometimes refused Sat.

Many people are upset when they cancel a booking and discover that they have lost a deposit or been charged the full rate of the room. Do remember that when making a booking you are entering into a contract with the hotel. Always make sure you know what the hotel's policy about cancellations is.

RHYDGALED Ceredigion   **Map 3:C3**

Conrah Country House   *Tel* 01970-617941
Rhydgaled, Chancery   *Fax* 01970-624546
nr Aberystwyth SY23 4DF   *Email* enquiries@conrah.co.uk
                                          Website www.conrah.co.uk

More praise, but some of it modified, came again this year for 'this
lovely old hotel', a white-walled mansion set in landscaped grounds,
'with the largest ha-ha wall in Wales', just south of Aberystwyth. It is
full of flowers and antiques, and its owners, John and Pat Heading,
with son Paul and daughter-in-law Sarah, are 'excellent hosts'. Staff,
'caring and cheerful', are mainly Welsh, helped sometimes by young
French trainees in the dining room. In this 'beautiful room with wonderful views over the countryside', chef Stephen West provides 'international cooking', making imaginative use of local ingredients –
Welsh lamb and beef, Carmarthen ham, and Pencarreg cheese. Try the
smoked duck breast with chutney; fried fritters of laver bread, cockles
and capsicum; omelette of wild mushrooms, asparagus and smoked
cheese. But some readers have felt that the menu changes too rarely,
or that portions are too large. Breakfasts are mostly admired, save for
the coffee and sausages. Visitors have found bedrooms 'lovely'; one
has 'comfy armchairs, a bathroom tiled in blue and yellow'. But one
guest found pillows uncomfortable. The old 'courtyard motel' has
been converted into *Magnolia Court*, with three luxury bedrooms.
There is a heated swimming pool in a separate building, but it lacks
changing facilities. Paths through the estate lead to footpaths down to
the coast – a strenuous but bracing walk. (*Phyllida Flint, GK Clarke,
Richard Creed; also David Lodge, and others*)

Open All year, except Christmas.
Rooms 15 double, 2 single. 3 in cottage, 3 in *Magnolia Court*. 3 on ground
floor.
Facilities Ramp. 3 lounges, bar, restaurant. No background music. 20-acre
grounds: indoor swimming pool, sauna; croquet, table tennis; vegetable gar-
den, woodland walks. River ½ mile, sea 3 miles; golf, fishing, riding nearby.
Unsuitable for &. Civil wedding licence.
Location 3½ miles S of Aberystwyth on A487 coast road. Train:
Aberystwyth.
Restrictions No smoking: restaurant, some bedrooms. No children under 5.
No dogs.
Credit cards All major cards accepted.
Terms B&B: single £70–£80, double £100–£135; D,B&B (min. 2 nights):
single £97, double £140–£170. Full alc lunch £24; set dinner £27.

ST DAVID'S Pembrokeshire *See SHORTLIST*   **Map 3:D1**

SWANSEA *See SHORTLIST*   **Map 3:E3**

When you nominate a hotel, please, if possible, send us its
brochure.

TALSARNAU Gwynedd   Map 3:B3

Maes-y-Neuadd   *Tel* 01766-780200
Talsarnau LL47 6YA   *Fax* 01766-780211
                                           Email maes@neuadd.com
                                           Website www.neuadd.com

Two couples, the Slatters and the Jacksons, own and run this small
hotel in a grey granite-and-slate mansion (Pride of Britain), judged 'as
good as ever' this year by a returning devotee, and 'cheerful, even in
midwinter'. It stands amid lawns, orchards and paddocks, on a wooded
hillside with views across to the Snowdonia National Park. The
approach is by a narrow lane up a steep hill. Inside are oak beams, good
antique and modern furniture, photographs and watercolours, and a bar
with an inglenook fireplace. The bedrooms vary in style and size; some
are in the main house, four are in a converted coach house. They have
flowers, fresh fruit, good lighting and a smart bathroom. Some rooms
have pine furniture, others antiques; three have a spa bath. Informal
lunches (eg, salads; braised pork chop with pasta; seafood omelette),
and afternoon teas are served in the bar. In the panelled dining room
guests may choose three, four or five courses – dishes like warm mussel salad with melon; venison with braised shallots and bitter chocolate
sauce; always a vegetarian main course. The meal ends with
'Diweddglo Mawreddog' (the grand finale): Welsh cheeses followed
by three desserts (you can have the lot). The cooking, by Peter Jackson
and John Owen Jones, has been found 'imaginative and delicious', and

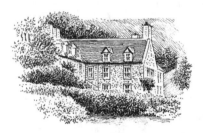

much produce is from the
superb kitchen garden. The
Royal St David's golf course,
Harlech and Caernarfon
castles and Portmeirion are
nearby. June Slatter runs
'Steam and Cuisine', a weekly
dining service on the narrow-
gauge Rheilffordd Ffestiniog
steam railway. (*Gordon
Hands*)

Open All year.
Rooms 2 suites, 13 double, 1 single. 4 in coach house, 10 yds. 3 on ground
floor.
Facilities Lift, ramps. Lounge, bar, conservatory, restaurant, business facili-
ties; terrace. No background music. 8-acre grounds: croquet, orchard, pad-
dock. Sea, golf, riding, sailing, fishing, climbing, clay-pigeon shooting nearby.
Civil wedding licence.
Location 3 miles NE of Harlech, signposted off B4573. ½ mile up steep lane.
Train: Harlech/Blaenau Ffestiniog; hotel will meet.
Restrictions No smoking in restaurant and lounge. No children under 7 in
dining room at night. Dogs by arrangement; not in public rooms.
Credit cards All major cards accepted.
Terms [2001] B&B: single £69, double £141–£177, suite £155–£169;
D,B&B: single £73–£94, double £158–£233, suite £168–£225. Bar lunches.
Set Sun lunch £14.95, dinner from £27. 2-night breaks all year; 3-day breaks
Nov–Mar. Christmas, New Year packages. *V*

THREE COCKS Powys   Map 3:D4

Three Cocks Hotel   *Tel* 01497-847215
Three Cocks, nr Brecon LD3 0SL   *Fax* 01497-847339
                                    Website www.threecockshotel.com

The high Brecon Beacons (good walking country) and the renowned second-hand book centre of Hay-on-Wye are both fairly close to this 15th-century ivy-clad inn, a restaurant-with-rooms in a village by the river Wye. 'It is very professionally run, everything is clean, tidy and punctual,' runs a new plaudit this year. It has big oak beams, a cobbled forecourt, a small flowery garden – and a Belgian accent, for its owners, Michael Winstone (chef) and his Belgian wife Marie-Jeanne (front-of-house), used to run a restaurant in Belgium; their son, who has worked at *Gidleigh Park*, Chagford, England (*qv*), has joined the kitchen team. The food also has some Belgian touches, eg, wild mussel soup, smoked Ardennes ham. 'An outstanding dinner, notably the scallops, duck and foie gras'; 'food is imaginative, generous, of high quality', were comments this year. But also: 'Lovely soups, lovely lamb, but boring veg, no dishes for vegetarians, and background music too noisy.' The spacious dining room has a massive French *armoire*, and tapestries on its stone walls. The 'excellent breakfasts' are cooked to order, the bread is freshly baked, and there's a good choice of Belgian beers. The sitting room has oak panelling, an open fire, fresh flowers, and new sofas. Bedrooms and bathrooms are small but comfortable, but plumbing can be noisy and bedside lighting poor. In this old house, floors can slope all ways. 'We had the "Drunkards' Room", with the floor at an interesting angle, but a very comfortable bed.' 'Children are made to feel very welcome, though there are no facilities for them.' (*Michael Forrest, Richard Green, Gill and Dave Crawshaw, SP, and others*)

Open Feb–end Nov. Restaurant closed Tues night, all day Sun.
Rooms 7 double. No telephone/TV (available on request).
Facilities 2 lounges, TV lounge, breakfast room, restaurant (piped classical music at night). ½-acre grounds. Golf, canoeing, riding, fishing nearby. Unsuitable for &.
Location 5 miles SW of Hay-on-Wye on A438 Hereford–Brecon. Rear rooms quietest. Large car park. Local buses.
Restriction No dogs.
Credit cards MasterCard, Visa.
Terms B&B: single £40–£67, double £67; D,B&B: single £68, double £123. Set lunch/dinner £29; full alc £37.50. 1-night bookings refused bank holiday weekends. *V*

TINTERN Monmouthshire   Map 3:E4

Parva Farmhouse   NEW/BUDGET   *Tel* 01291-689411
Tintern   *Fax* 01291-689557
nr Chepstow NP16 6SQ   *Email* parva_hoteltintern@hotmail.com
                                    Website www.hoteltintern.co.uk

Tintern's ruined abbey is a mile away from this 'very pretty' 17th-century farmhouse above the river Wye. Derek Stubbs is its 'cheerful owner/chef', and his wife, Vickie, is 'a friendly, chatty soul', say visitors in 2001, returning it to the *Guide*: 'We loved it. After negotiating a lethally sharp corner from the main road into the driveway, we found the garden merry with daffodils and primulas. Mrs Stubbs offered to carry our cases up two flights of stairs to our quiet room at the back, looking on to the Wye. Its furniture was repro Jane Austen, its bed was firm, with floral covers. The towels were agreeably fluffy. The lounge downstairs was large and comfortable, with an honesty bar, wooden beams, a friendly fire, and soft piped music by Handel and Mozart. Mrs Stubbs served us a very good meal: Sicilian prawns; cheese parcel; succulent lamb with rosemary and honey; lively scampi provençale; beautifully light lemon cheesecake. From the impressive wine list, we chose a Chilean Merlot. Breakfast, too, was excellent. And Mrs Stubbs, as we do, loves dogs: her King Charles spaniel patrols the garden.' Others too admired the service, the food and the 'stunning' location. Bedrooms vary in size, and have river or garden views. Some are good for a family. Children are welcomed: there are books, toys, cots, high teas, etc. Nearby are miles of footpaths (including Offa's Dyke): wardens conduct guided walks most weekends. Six golf courses, and Chepstow's racecourse, are close by. (*Sarah and Tony Thomas, Diana Hall Hall*)

Open All year, except annual holiday.
Rooms 9 double.
Facilities Lounge with honesty bar, restaurant; classical background music evenings. Small garden by river. Fishing, golf, riding nearby. Unsuitable for &.
Location 5 miles N of Chepstow, on A466 to Monmouth. At N end of village, opposite Offa's Dyke path (quietest rooms face river).
Restrictions No smoking in restaurant. No dogs in public rooms.
Credit cards Amex, MasterCard, Visa.
Terms B&B: single £48–£50, double £60–£74; D,B&B £44–£69 per person. Set dinner £19.50. 2-day breaks. Child under 12 in parents' room charged for meals only. 1-night bookings sometimes refused weekends. ***V***

WHITEBROOK Monmouthshire   Map 3:D4

The Crown at Whitebrook   **NEW**   *Tel* 01600-860254
Whitebrook, nr Monmouth NP25 4TX   *Fax* 01600-860607
                                   Email crown@whitebrook.demon.co.uk

Now with new resident owners, sisters Angela and Elizabeth Barbara, this 17th-century inn south of Monmouth, in a steep wooded valley near the river Wye, makes a welcome return to the *Guide*. An inspector writes: 'Reached via a narrow winding road, it is in a lovely position straight out of storybook rural Wales. It calls itself a restaurant-with-rooms – and while the food is splendid, the rooms are serviceable but slightly spartan. The Barbaras have created a warm and welcoming atmosphere, while the Roux-trained chef, Mark Turton, who has stayed on from the old regime, succeeds in his aim of "combining the best Welsh ingredients with the best traditions of French cuisine". We had fish terrine; mallard and dorade; pancakes flambéed at the table; vanilla soufflé – all excellent. Breakfast, with

ppers, was good, too. There is a very comfortable sitting area. In our
edroom, freshly made Welsh cakes awaited us. The room was compact, with good beds but a temperamental TV; the bathroom was a bit
too compact, but the towels were fluffy.' Another visitor this year also
liked the food and the 'friendly welcome', but thought the inn 'difficult to find'. Tintern Abbey, the Wye Valley and Offa's Dyke are
nearby. So are Raglan and Chepstow castles. (*RR, and others*)

Open All year, except Christmas, New Year.
Rooms 8 double (1 with spa bath), 2 single.
Facilities Lounge/bar, restaurant. No background music. 2-acre garden.
Location 6 miles S of Monmouth, just W of A466 to Chepstow. Turn off at
Bigsweir Bridge, go 2 miles W down narrow lane.
Restrictions No smoking: restaurant, bedrooms. No children under 12. No
dogs in public rooms.
Credit cards All major cards accepted.
Terms B&B £42.50–£52.50; D,B&B £68–£78. Set lunch £15.95, dinner
£29.95; full alc £21.50. Discount for 2–3-night stay. *V*

****

Traveller's tale Hotel in Lincolnshire. In this hotel we had a
lovely bedroom. The dining room was attractive, the waiter
charming, the food terrible. Starters were dull; meat dishes were
tough, prawns and fish tasteless though allegedly fresh. A dear
little chef came out each night to ask if everything was satisfactory and we did not have the heart to tell him what we really
thought, as he was so sweet. We noticed with amusement that
the Italian proprietor and his wife, who ate in the restaurant, had
nothing but pasta each night, so perhaps they had their own
view of their chef.

****

Traveller's tale Hotel in Scotland. We entered the newly
painted bedroom. It had an unloved feel. The proprietor said she
had put the heat on low, as she didn't know how we would feel.
Cold was a word that sprang to mind. A howling draught came
in through the windows, which would not shut thanks to the
recent decoration. We asked for extra pillows; this elicited a
sharp intake of breath. There was a nasty smell in the room; and
I had to sleep pressed up against a wardrobe.

****

Traveller's tale Hotel in Scotland. This was the worst hotel we
have found in the UK: expensive and pretentious. The marble
floor in the entrance hall was cold and uninviting; the rugs on it
old and tatty. We were shown to a suite in converted stables. In
the bathroom, flies were hatching – dozens of them. We complained and were moved to a cottage. This was cold, dark and
damp. We went to dinner expecting to be cheered up, but it was
an unmitigated disaster. The service was slow, the room cheer-
less and the food almost inedible. We returned to the cottage
and sat up most of the night. Next day we left. The staff were
uninterested.

****

Channel Islands

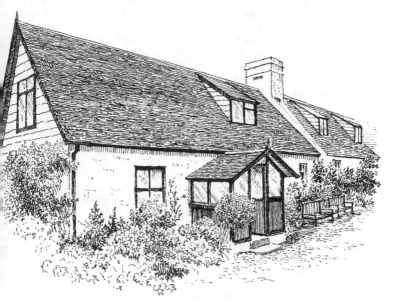

La Sablonnerie, Sark

Many of our entries for the Channel Islands are in out-of-the-way spots, well away from the holiday throng. One is on the tiny island of Herm; another, stylish and idiosyncratic, is a converted farmhouse on Sark. On Jersey, the much-admired *Château La Chaire* is tucked away in an unpopulated area. On the other hand, our two choices for St Brelade's, also on Jersey, are relatively large and opulent. So close to Normandy, these *Isles Anglo-Normandes*, as the French call them, have something of a French flavour – and that applies notably to the cooking, at least of the main meals. Breakfasts tend to be boldly British.

CASTEL Guernsey

Map 1:D:

La Grande Mare NEW
Vazon Bay, Castel
GY5 7LL

Tel 01481-256576
Fax 01481-256532
Email hotellagrandemare@gtonline.net
Website www.lgm.guernsey.net

Owned by Westward Investments, this solid modern 'hotel, golf and country club' stands alone beside a sandy bay on the rocky west coast of Guernsey, in its own huge grounds. On its 18-hole golf course, three resident professionals provide tuition. Its nominators this year were pleased: 'The view is spectacular. From our four-poster in our large, airy bedroom, we could watch the waves pounding over the sea wall, up to 30 feet high, across the coast road. The staff were very friendly and efficient, the nicest ever. Towels were thick, but pillows were hard and thin, and the ridge down the middle of the bed was not conducive to romance. The restaurant's awards are well deserved.' Fergus MacKay's cooking is traditional, using local vegetables, fish and shellfish; vegetarians are catered for. To end, you could choose 'The Ultimate Dessert' (crêpes Suzette). The polyglot staff include a Spanish restaurant manager. Functions are extensively catered for. Coarse fishing lakes are nearby. (*Valerie Phillips*)

Open All year.
Rooms 12 suites, 12 double. 10 self-catering units.
Facilities Lift, ramps. Lounge, conservatory, restaurant (classical background music). 110-acre grounds: tennis, indoor and outdoor swimming pools, gym, spa, sauna, steam room; sandy beach.
Location On W coast, 4 miles W of St Peter Port, 3 miles NW of airport.
Restriction No dogs.
Credit cards All major cards accepted.
Terms [2001] B&B £59–£104. Set lunch £12.95, dinner £19.95; full alc £30. 3-night breaks. Christmas package.

HERM

Map 1:D6

White House
Herm, via Guernsey GY1 3HR

Tel 01481-722159
Fax 01481-710066
Email hotel@herm-island.com
Website www.herm-island.com

César award in 1987

'An ideal location for a wonderful family holiday,' says one visitor to Herm, a tiny island two kilometres long. Others have written of 'perfect peace, no cars or TV'. It also has pristine beaches, high cliffs, a little harbour, pastel-painted cottages, three shops, an inn, a campsite, a 10th-century chapel – and just 97 inhabitants. Some of them work at this 'wonderful, friendly hotel', created from an old house in 1949. The lease to the island is owned by Pennie Heyworth, who runs the hotel with her husband, Adrian, and manager Sue Hester. Recent praise: 'A delightful staff, delicious food' (the Saturday night gala dinner is particularly enjoyed). 'A charming rustic experience. Great views of the rolling hills, the sea and Guernsey.' An enchanting island,

or children to explore. The hotel cleverly creates an atmosphere
mony, and is well geared for a family holiday: staff are helpful,
ger children can have separate meals. Catering is excellent, prices
incredibly reasonable: house wines only £6–£7 a bottle.'
mfortable lounges have plenty of board games; the 'delightful gar-
n' has a swimming pool by the sea. No telephones in the bedrooms,
t there is baby-listening. A conference room has just been added –
ut it's a small one. The hotel has its own oyster bed, and the island is
erfect for birdwatching, shell gathering, bathing, snorkelling and
ishing. Guernsey and Sark are a short boat-trip away, and visits to
Jersey and France can be arranged. In summer Herm is much visited
by day-trippers, but they are gone by the late afternoon. The hotel will
help with travel arrangements. (*JD, ES*)

Open Early Apr–early Oct.
Rooms 1 suite, 36 double, 2 single. 21 in 3 cottage annexes (some on ground floor). No telephone/TV. Also 18 self-catering cottages.
Facilities 3 lounges, 2 bars, carvery, restaurant; conference room. No background music. 1-acre garden: tennis, croquet, swimming pool; beach 100 yds. Boating, fishing, snorkelling.
Location By harbour. Air or sea to Guernsey; ferry to Herm. Travel arrangements ABC Travel, *tel* 01481-235551.
Restrictions No smoking: restaurant, 2 lounges. Guide dogs only.
Credit cards Amex, MasterCard, Visa.
Terms [2001] D,B&B £59–£85. Set lunch £13–£18, dinner £20. 2-night breaks: bluebells in bloom, wine tasting, etc.

ROZEL BAY Jersey   **Map 1:E6**

Château La Chaire	*Tel* 01534-863354
Rozel Bay	*Fax* 01534-865137
St Martin JE3 6AJ	*Email* res@chateau-la-chaire.co.uk
	Website www.chateau-la-chaire.com

Secluded above the Rozel valley in north-east Jersey, with beautiful
cliff walks, this small and stylish hotel is owned by the Hiscox family
and managed by Seán Copp. A devotee returning this year found it
better than ever: 'We had a huge, wonderful room on the first floor,
with a big bow window on one side, an enormous balcony on the
other, with access to the garden. The soft furnishings, though not new,
were very pretty in pink and blue. The food was wonderful, as ever;
the new cutlery shone; the staff are hard to beat.' Others have found
the hotel 'lovely and restful'. Its steep terraced gardens, home to red
squirrels and barn owls, overlook a pretty fishing harbour. The interior
is smart: panelled public rooms, mouldings with cherubs, chandeliers:
'The drawing room is a triumph of plasterwork.' Some bedrooms are
large and luxurious, with a spa bath. The attic rooms are much smaller,
'but sweet', and some bathrooms may have a low ceiling. The bar is
'old-fashioned, well mannered'. The 'inspired chef', Simon Walker,
serves modern British cooking, with an emphasis on seafood, eg, mussels steamed with coconut and coriander; roast black bream with
garlic and parsley noodles. 'The vegetarian alternatives are delicious,
for example wild mushroom risotto.' One visitor this year thought

presentation too fussy: 'Starters are laid out like a child's pa...
numbers picture. But desserts are good.' Tea is served on a terrac...
a fountain. No entertainments for children, so there tend to be f...
them. Cliff walks and safe beaches are close by, and various activ...
can be arranged, such as yachting and flying lessons. Jersey's cap...
St Helier, is nearby. (*Linda Brook, H and FE Dryden, and others*)

Open All year.
Rooms 1 suite, 13 double.
Facilities Drawing room, bar, 3 dining rooms; classical background music i...
public areas all day. 6-acre garden. Sandy beach, safe bathing nearby. Golf,
fishing, yachting, flying available. Only restaurant suitable for ♿.
Location 5 miles NE of St Helier. Follow signs for St Martin's church, then
Rozel. 1st left in village; hotel car park 200 yds on left.
Restrictions No smoking in conservatory restaurant. No children under 7. No
dogs.
Credit cards All major cards accepted.
Terms [2001] B&B: single £90–£115, double £120–£200, suite £210–£240;
D,B&B £75–£135 per person. Set lunch £17.50, dinner £28.50. Winter breaks.
Christmas package.

ST BRELADE Jersey   **Map 1:E6**

Atlantic Hotel   *Tel* 01534-744101
Le Mont de la Pulente   *Fax* 01534-744102
St Brelade JE3 8HE   *Email* info@theatlantichotel.com
                                          Website www.theatlantichotel.com

'Very enjoyable. The refurbished rooms and bathrooms are excellent
– even good light for reading in the bath,' says a visitor this year to this
member of the Small Luxury Hotels of the World group. It adjoins the
La Moye championship golf course, and overlooks the superb five-
mile beach of St Ouen's Bay. A large, modern, white building, it was
opened in 1970 by the father of the present owner, Patrick Burke. 'His
manager, Simon Dufty, is first rate, and room balconies have great
views,' runs a recent report. Staff are 'excellent', 'friendly'. The interior contains antique terracotta flagstones, a wrought iron staircase,
rich carpeting, urns, fountains, antiques and specially designed
modern furniture. The Palm Club leisure centre, free for guests, has an
indoor swimming pool, mini-gym, etc. In summer the hotel is popular
with families. In 2000, almost all bedrooms were enlarged and
upgraded, but a few rooms are on the small side, 'and the ones by the
lift are to be avoided'. Many rooms face the golf course, or look over
the swimming pool to pine trees and the sea beyond. The suites in a
ground-floor annexe are spacious, but have no view. The food is
mostly admired: 'It was quite good, but variable: interesting cheeses,
but some oversweet sauces,' said a visitor this year. Ken Healy's
enterprising menus include, eg, scallops in pancetta, black pudding
and quail egg salad; roast brill with leeks and wild mushrooms; hot
passion fruit soufflé with Jersey honey. The restaurant is now non-
smoking. Light lunches are served by the pool in fine weather.
'Excellent breakfasts.' 'The breaks are superb value.' The airport is
ten minutes' drive away. (*FE Dryden, and others*)

pen 8 Feb–31 Dec.
Rooms 2 suites, 48 double.
Facilities Lounges, cocktail bar, restaurant, 3 children's rooms; fitness centre: swimming pool, sauna; background CDs all day. 3-acre grounds: tennis, swimming pool. Golf club, beach ½ mile. Unsuitable for &.
Location 5 miles W of St Helier; taxi/bus.
Restrictions No smoking in restaurant. No dogs.
Credit cards All major cards accepted.
Terms [2001] B&B: double £175–£255, suite £250–£400. Set lunch £17.50, dinner £30; full alc £45. Special breaks. Christmas package.

St Brelade's Bay Hotel   *Tel* 01534-746141
St Brelade JE3 8EF   *Fax* 01534-747278
                                    Email info@stbreladesbayhotel.com
                                    Website www.stbreladesbayhotel.com

'The wonderful beach, just across the road' was much enjoyed this year at the Colleys' 'all-round-excellent family hotel, luxurious throughout'. It is a long white modern building, facing the sea on Jersey's loveliest bay. Earlier praise: 'Wonderful. It caters for children of all ages, without being like a holiday camp. For our three-year-old and twin babies, we were given cots, high chairs, a good range of baby food, etc (children have tea at 5 pm, and must not be in the dining room after 7 pm – heaven for parents!). There's a children's playroom, pool, playground, etc. Wonderful gardens with tennis courts, *boules*, etc. The staff are all friendly, and the food is a delight, with a superb English breakfast, choice of formal lunch or barbecue, fantastic six-course dinner' (dishes might include smoked salmon roulade with warm potato rösti; sautéed guineafowl with mixed pulses and thyme). Men are required to wear jacket and tie at night. The barbecue lunches, served in a pergola, are 'excellent and substantial'. Bedrooms are large and airy; front ones have a balcony and views over the bay; second-floor ones above the kitchen can be noisy. Moulded ceilings, chandeliers, lots of fresh flowers and large grounds complete the picture. The poolside areas, and the cocktail bar, gym, sauna and sun terrace have just been renovated, and the gardens have won the 'Best Garden in Jersey' award. (*Philippa Parker, EKE*)

Open End Apr–mid-Oct.
Rooms 1 suite, 75 double, 4 single.
Facilities Lift. Lounge, reception, TV room, cocktail bar (entertainment 4 nights a week), restaurant; 2 children's playrooms, sun veranda. No background music. 7-acre grounds: outdoor restaurant, swimming pool with bar, barbecue, sauna, exercise room; *boules*, children's play area. Beach across road. Golf nearby.
Location 5 miles W of St Helier. Bus from St Helier.
Restrictions No smoking in restaurant. No dogs.
Credit cards MasterCard, Visa.
Terms B&B: single £60–£98, double £120–£196, suite £170–£244; D,B&B £75–£137 per person. Set lunch £15, dinner £25; full alc £35.

There is no VAT in the Channel Islands.

ST PETER PORT Guernsey   Map 1:E

La Frégate   *Tel* 01481-724624
Les Côtils   *Fax* 01481-720443
St Peter Port GY1 1UT   *Email* lafregate@guernsey.net
                                        Website www.lafregate.guernsey.net

Much enjoyed by readers, the 'excellent' French cuisine here may
well be the best on Guernsey (eg, coquilles Saint Jacques au chou
piquant; paillard de filet de boeuf Strindberg). This 'outstanding hotel
in many ways' is an old converted manor house, set in terraced gardens on a hill above the harbour of the island's main town. There are
fine views from the restaurant, the front patio and from many bedrooms, notably those with a balcony (but a main road runs below, and
there can be noise at weekends from nightclub-goers). Rooms are
'fairly basic' but comfortable, with a large bathroom. Breakfasts are
good, generally served in one's room. The bar and restaurant have just
been smartened up, with 'designer decor'. The dining-room staff,
some of them Portuguese, are 'enthusiastic', but in the past, meal service has sometimes been found slow. The general manager and restaurant manager are new this year, so we'd like more reports, please. The
house has many stairs, but no lift.

Open All year, but may close briefly in Nov.
Rooms 9 double, 4 single.
Facilities Lounge/bar, restaurant; private dining/function room. No back-
ground music. Patio (alfresco dining), ½-acre terraced garden. Unsuitable
for &.
Location 5 mins' walk from centre. Hard to find; brochure gives directions.
Car park.
Restrictions No children under 4. No dogs.
Credit cards All major cards accepted.
Terms [2001] B&B: single £65, double £80–£110. Set lunch £14.50, dinner
£20, full alc £30–£35. ***V***

ST SAVIOUR Jersey   Map 1:E6

Longueville Manor   *Tel* 01534-725501
Longueville Road   *Fax* 01534-731613
St Saviour JE2 7WF   *Email* longman@itl.net
                                        Website www.longuevillemanor.com

César award in 1986

Jersey's most sumptuous hotel (Relais & Châteaux) is a 13th-century
manor house with newer additions. It stands in large grounds at the
foot of a lovely wooded valley just inland from St Helier. It has the
island's best restaurant: the gifted Andrew Baird was only 23 when he
came as head chef in 1990. Four years later he won a *Michelin* star,
which he retains. He often goes diving in the sea for scallops. Readers
love his 'modern English' cooking, very expensive, complex and
nouvelle: eg, salad of roast quail with foie gras and glazed pears;
grilled beef with sautéed calf's sweetbreads, white asparagus and
truffle jus; clafouti of berries with vanilla ice cream. 'Wonderful

rian dishes', 'superb cheese trolley'. For a splash, try the
net menu' (£52.50). Meals are served in a large, light room fac-
ne garden, or in a darker panelled one. The hotel's owners,
:olm Lewis and his sister Sue Dufty, the third generation here,
always attentive'. The staff are 'hard-working, willing to please'.
:ry well run', the hotel is 'unstuffy': 'guests share the reception
oms with the house cats and dogs'. The decor is smart – swagged
irtains, colourful oriental rugs, original paintings, antiques, good
epro furniture. 'Breakfasts are excellent, with lots of choice – a festival of cholesterol.' The spacious, chintzy bedrooms have a comfortable sofa, fresh flowers. 'No tea-making equipment; room service is
swift.' This year, 17 bedrooms have been refurbished, and a suite and
two small function rooms are new. There are colourful flowers in the
grounds, and a herb and vegetable garden. Lunches and teas by the
swimming pool (heated to a constant 80°F) are 'excellent'. Guests
may also dine at the nearby 'little sister' restaurant, *Suma's*. The Royal
Jersey Golf Club is not far. The winter package (with car hire) is good
value. Day-trips to France are arranged. More reports, please.

Open All year, except 3–17 Jan.
Rooms 2 suites (1 in cottage), 28 double.
Facilities Lift. 2 lounges, bar, restaurant; 2 function rooms; conference facilities. No background music. 16-acre grounds: gardens, woodland, croquet, tennis, swimming pool. Golf, bowls, squash nearby; beaches ¾ mile. Unsuitable
for &.
Location 1 mile E of St Helier by A3; hotel on left (double-glazed throughout).
Restriction No dogs in public rooms.
Credit cards All major cards accepted.
Terms B&B: single £165–£235, double £210–£350, suite £370–£410. Set
lunch £17.50, dinner £47.50; full alc £53. Winter weekend breaks. Christmas
package.

SARK **Map 1:E6**

La Sablonnerie *Tel* 01481-832061
Little Sark *Fax* 01481-832408
Sark, via Guernsey GY9 0SD

Long, low and white-walled, this converted 16th-century farmhouse is
now a stylish, idiosyncratic little hotel, much admired. Many guests
are returning visitors, which creates something of a club atmosphere,
'but a club that readily welcomes kindred spirits', says one visitor.
Another adds that the owner, Elizabeth Perrée, 'runs a well-organised,
comfortable, friendly hotel with outstanding food, in a rather remote
location (on Sark's southern peninsula). Everyone was warm and
friendly – rarely have I seen hotel staff so eager to please. All our
requests were met, including several tractor rides, courtesy of brother
Philip Perrée, for my three-year-old tractor-mad son, who also loved
the toy plane, which came stuck into his pizza as a surprise. We stayed
in a cottage next to the well-tended tea gardens with their sun parasols.
The grounds are lovely. Evening fare was elegant and inventive: venison with lavender sauce; lobster various ways.' And two 'sweaty

cyclists' found the hotel 'very welcoming, with some of the be.
we have had anywhere'. The 'young and enthusiastic' waiters c
in conversation (surely the sign of a happily managed hotel). The
erable Philip Perrée senior serves behind the bar. Beef, fruit
vegetables come from the hotel's farm; the menus often include c
ters, scallops, and lobster (you pay extra). Typical dishes: go£
cheese soufflé with roasted figs; tandoori spiced monkfish with gre
lentils. No TV or telephone in the 'quite small but elegant' bedroom
Guests are met at the port by the hotel's very stylish horse and cart, c
a tractor. They are advised to pack an old pair of rubber-soled shoes
for bathing from rocks or shingle, a torch for exploring caves, and a
dress or a tie for dinner. The coast nearby has beautiful cliffs, coves
and sandy beaches. More reports, please.

Open Easter–Oct.
Rooms 1 suite, 15 double, 6 single. Guests sometimes accommodated in
nearby cottages. No telephone/TV.
Facilities 3 lounges, 2 bars (background piano/ classical music), restaurant. 1-
acre garden: tea garden/bar, croquet. Bays, beaches, rock pools nearby. Sark
unsuitable for &.
Location Southern part of island. Boat from Guernsey; hotel will meet.
Restrictions No smoking in some bedrooms. Dogs at hotel's discretion; not in
public rooms.
Credit cards Amex, MasterCard, Visa.
Terms (*Excluding 10% service charge*) B&B £40–£77; D,B&B £51.50–
£89.50; full board £61.50–£94.50. Set lunch £22.80, dinner £28.50; full
alc £38.50.

****

Traveller's tale Hotel in Suffolk. In many ways this is quite
good: food excellent, staff pleasant. But we were surprised to
find a vase of dead carnations when we entered our bedroom.
The manager happened to be at Reception when I suggested the
flowers might have been removed. He thought it a great joke.
'Should have put live ones in, ho, ho!' Then we discovered that
beds were not being made properly – covers just pulled up.
Bathroom glasses were unwashed, dirty facecloths left on bath,
no vacuum-cleaning. When I moved my bed as I was remaking
it, I noticed a heap of papers underneath it, including a piece of
Christmas wrapping paper. All this in a 'superior' bedroom at
£95 a night each.

****

Traveller's tale Hotel in London. The restaurant was very
busy, and service was slow. But since we were staying the night,
we were relaxed and unhurried. After the main course, we
decided to wait a while before ordering a dessert. Eventually we
managed to catch the waiter's eye, and we ordered. He, looking
harassed, disappeared into the kitchen, only to return a few
minutes later to say: 'I'm sorry, you can't have dessert. The
chef's gone home.'

****

Ireland

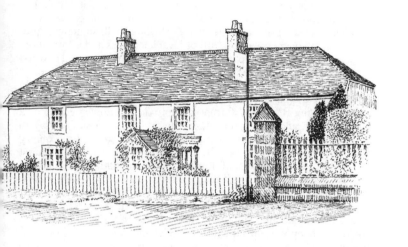

Buggys Glencairn Inn, Glencairn

This year, for the first time, we have put all of Ireland, North and South, into the same chapter. After all, in many ways this is one country: the two tourist boards now work closely together, and along many roads you can cross the border without realising that you have done so.

Of our several new Irish entries this year, most are in the west. One delightful hotel is at Caragh Lake, on the Ring of Kerry. Others are at Dingle and in Co. Galway. In the North, readers have enjoyed excellent hotels at Derry, and at Annalong and Portaferry in Co. Down. We have three entries for Belfast and its suburbs – an interesting city, now peaceful at last.

Our other Irish entries are in Dublin, where the giant new tourist boom has spawned some ambitious new hotels, or elsewhere in the Republic. There are a few small Irish chains, notably Fitzpatrick's and Jury's, but they do not feature in this chapter, and the big international chains are hardly represented in Ireland. Almost all Irish hotels are privately owned and run; indeed this country is a paradise of the kind of smallish, personal hotel of character that the Guide seeks and encourages.

Some of these are stately homes, still lived in by their ancestral owners, the Anglo-Irish gentry, who have turned them into private hotels or guest houses to defray the costs of keeping up a big estate. Or newer owners have acquired them, and run them in the same very personal way. Many belong to the Hidden Ireland association, which is affiliated to the Wolsey Lodge group in the UK. Guests may be surrounded by old family portraits and heirlooms, fine family antiques and furniture. It is all very civilised, though this kind of inspired amateurism in hotel-keeping can have its drawbacks. In many such places, the owners try to create a house party atmosphere, to give their paying clients the illusion that they are personal friends on a visit. Often they dine communally round one big table, at one sitting, and conversation is general, as at a private dinner party. The hosts will sometimes preside. Often they are great fun, full of local anecdotes and information, but the whole experience can sometimes be embarrassing, and at worst you may feel that you are paying your host to amuse him at dinner.

Most of the best of these stately home hotels are in this guide. In town and country alike, there are also guest houses of all kinds; private homes offering B&B, and farmhouses providing simple bedrooms, a big breakfast, and sometimes an evening meal too. You can stay in converted farm buildings or outhouses, get to know the country people, even share briefly in the life of the farm. The Irish Tourist Board, Bord Fáilte, grades all kinds of accommodation; the places it approves generally display at the gate its green shamrock sign.

Food in Irish hotels has improved greatly since the Guide's first edition. In some places today it is rather sophisticated; and out of national pride (as in Wales and Scotland), the chefs like to call it 'modern Irish cooking', though the specifically Irish element is not always evident. A few places win a Michelin star or bib gourmand for quality, and we identify these. But standards remain erratic, and attempts at sophistication do not always succeed. In the stately home hotels, you are more likely to find 'country house cooking' done by the hostess – simple, maybe too bland for some tastes, but generally reliable.

Ireland's economic boom has led to an influx of job-seekers from the rest of the EU, and in many hotels you may now find French, Italian or Spanish waiters. But service is still mostly by local people. It may sometimes lack polish, but it makes up for this by an almost universal Irish cheerfulness and readiness to oblige. And all Irish accommodation provides a cooked breakfast – ample, if sometimes a little monotonous. VAT is included in bills, but service is not: you should add about 10 per cent. The euro is becoming legal currency in Ireland in February 2002, as in many other EU countries. But in this section we still give the prices in Irish punts. For the exchange rate, please see page 549.

Some of the hotels in this section did not return their questionnaire, so the information given may be less accurate than we would wish.

RE Co. Limerick   **Map 6:D5**

raven Arms   *Tel* (+353) (0)61-396633
Fax (+353) (0)61-396541
Email reservations@dunravenhotel.com
Website www.dunravenhotel.com

big, traditional coaching inn, old, handsome and yellow-fronted, beside the river Maigue in a pretty village near Limerick. 'It is wonderfully stylish, a reliable old favourite,' runs one of two recent admiring reports. Bryan Murphy, the manager, and his son 'are much in evidence', and 'the large, highly professional staff make it all very civilised'. 'It is a rambling place, but the several newer wings match well with the older parts. The welcome was warm, the service excellent, and the tone in the dining room was of old-fashioned elegance.' The food is 'first class (superb seafood terrine, Irish rib of beef, full Irish breakfast with delicious bacon)'. Sandra Earl's cooking is traditional with a trolley roast each day. Bedrooms and public rooms are 'smart and comfortable', though one guest thought the decor in the bar 'too trendy'. Some bedrooms look on to gardens, but front ones face the busy main road. 'Our junior suite was spacious.' There are several small lounges with fires, 'for quiet reading', and a leisure centre with a gym, steam room and large swimming pool. Adorned with many paintings of local hunting scenes, the hotel is geared towards horse riding, and may not appeal to those who dislike blood sports; guests can hunt with the famous local packs. One gripe: 'The swimming pool is banned to under-16s after 5 pm.' Salmon and trout fishing, and an 18-hole championship golf course, are nearby. (*RP, LW*)

Open All year.
Rooms 20 suites, 54 double. Some on ground floor.
Facilities Lift. Lounge, writing room, library, residents' bar (pianist), public bar, restaurant, conservatory; conference/function facilities; leisure centre: swimming pool, steam room, gym. 3-acre gardens. River, fishing, golf, riding, fox-hunting nearby.
Location In village 10 miles SW of Limerick. Private parking.
Restrictions No smoking in restaurant. No dogs.
Credit cards All major cards accepted.
Terms Room: single IR£85–£110, double IR£105–£135, suite IR£160–£200. Breakfast IR£12. Set lunch IR£19.50, dinner IR£30. Christmas package.

AGLISH Co. Tipperary   **Map 6:C5**

Ballycormac House   `BUDGET`   *Tel* (+353) (0)67-21129
Aglish, nr Borrisokane   *Fax* (+353) (0)67-21200
Email ballyc@indigo.ie

An English couple, John and Cherylynn Lang, own and run this stylish little guest house, clad with flowers and well converted from a 350-year-old farmhouse. East of Lough Derg, it is not far from Birr with its fine castle. 'It was like staying with friends,' say recent visitors. 'The Langs made us very welcome and even took us to the pub one night.' Others wrote of 'superb hospitality'; they found the house and gardens 'charming', and their room 'very comfortable'. The 'delightfully

decorated suite' has a four-poster. Mrs Lang's 'very good cooki.
varied and eclectic, using the farm's organically grown fruit
vegetables, and other local produce. Thai-style prawn and sweet
soup; Irish lamb with a herb and oatmeal crust; crêpes Suzette m
be on the menu. The ambience is intimate: there are only six roor
Outdoor activities can be arranged (see below). The Langs, who 'a
keen horse people', have their own stable of hunters, and in seaso
they offer hunting holidays (several packs are nearby). They also offe

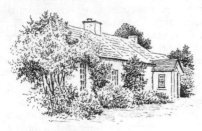

'weekend equestrian breaks'
with two experienced horse-
men, John, who has taken part
in eventing for years, and Jim,
an ex-national hunt jockey.
And they will put up visitors
to local hunt balls, arranging
transport 'so that everyone
can have a drink'. (*WR, and
others*)

Open All year.
Rooms 1 suite, 5 double, 1 single. 1 with TV. No telephone.
Facilities Sitting room, dining room; drying room. No background music. 2-
acre gardens, 20-acre pastures; horse riding, fox-hunting, shooting arranged.
Lough Derg (fishing, water sports) 5 miles; golf nearby. Unsuitable for &.
Location From Nenagh, N on N52 to Borrisokane, then N65. Right at signs to
hotel. Bus from Nenagh.
Restrictions No smoking. No dogs in house.
Credit cards MasterCard, Visa.
Terms B&B IR£28–£50; D,B&B IR£53–£75. Set lunch IR£15, dinner IR£25.
Child in parents' room: under 12, 40% reduction. Off-season, riding, hunting
breaks, etc. ***V***

ANNALONG Co. Down   Map 6:B6

Glassdrumman Lodge   *Tel* 028-4376 8451
85 Mill Road   *Fax* 028-4376 7041
Annalong BT34 4RH   *Email* glassdrumman@yahoo.com
                                 Website www.glassdrummanlodge.co.uk

Contrary to the popular song, the Mountains of Mourne sweep down
not quite to the sea: between them and the coast is a broad rural stretch
where this stylishly converted old farmhouse, long, low and white,
stands outside a village. 'The location is splendid; my dinner was
excellent,' says a report this year. Others wrote: 'The owner, Joan
Hall, is lovely, she treats you like a guest in her home.' 'All is a delight
inside, sophisticated yet intimate.' Most readers share this praise,
though one thought that, since reception is not always attended, 'a bell
would be a useful investment'. 'The lounge is graceful yet cosy – old
beamed ceiling, imposing open fireplace with a real log fire, velvety
sofas, nice lamps, lots of books.' Guests can watch, even take part in,
the life of the small home farm (pigs, poultry, horses and golden
retrievers are bred). It supplies many of the ingredients of the dinners
cooked by Mrs Hall's son, Jonathan (eg, Irish stew of Mourne lamb;

ıcking pig pie). Home-churned butter and free-range eggs are used; ısh and shellfish come from local ports. Dinner is served by candle-ıight with good silver, and guests usually dine together round one long pine table, though smaller ones are available. 'Our large bedroom was superb, with panoramic windows, big sofa, luxury bathroom, gas fire in chilly April' (other rooms vary in size, and some may be in need of maintenance). 'Good breakfasts' have 'lovely home-made breads'. Overnight shoe-polishing and car-washing are promised in the brochure. There's a well-kept garden with loungers. Many visitors are American golfers with Irish roots, come to play on the Royal County Down golf course close by; riding and pony-trekking can be arranged. (*FO, and others*)

Open All year. Lunch not served.
Rooms 2 suites (in garden), 8 double.
Facilities Drawing room/bar, library, dining room, restaurant (classical/Irish background music during dinner); meeting facilities. 7-acre grounds: fishing lake. Golf, sailing, fishing, riding nearby. Unsuitable for &.
Location 8 miles S of Newcastle, 1 mile inland from Annalong (turn off at *Halfway House* pub).
Restrictions No smoking: restaurant, bedrooms. No dogs in house (kennels available).
Credit cards Amex, MasterCard, Visa.
Terms B&B: single £50–£100, double £50–£110, suite £125–£135. Set dinner £32.50. Christmas package. *V*

ARTHURSTOWN Co. Wexford   Map 6:D6

Dunbrody Country House   NEW   *Tel* (+353) (0)51-389600
                                      Fax (+353) (0)51-389601
                                      Email dunbrody@indigo.ie
                                      Website www.dunbrodyhouse.com

'Quite superb,' says an inspector this year, bringing into the *Guide* this 'large grey Georgian pile', originally owned by Lord Donegal who still lives on the estate. It was bought five years ago by a young couple, Mark and Catherine Dundon – she is front-of-house, he won success as a chef in Canada, then was executive chef of the renowned *Shelbourne Hotel* in Dublin. 'Undoubtedly large sums of money have been spent on the conversion, with very good taste. Through the patrician gates we went up the long drive, and into the magnificent foyer with grand piano and splendid chandelier. A charming young lady escorted us to our rooms, reached by three fine staircases, all with expensive carpets and high-quality curtains. All the furniture in the house is either old, or good repro. Our room was more like a suite, with a huge bathroom, dressing gowns, apples and flowers. The bar downstairs is a fine room with an open fire; there was muzak, but soft. The large red dining room, with fresh flowers on each table, is impressive. On the set menu, our dishes included scallops, beef fillets, raspberry torte, apple Tatin – very good food, all served cheerfully and professionally. Coffee was taken in the lovely drawing room-cum-library. The good breakfast included scrambled eggs with smoked salmon. In the entrance hall, the original bell system to summon staff is still in place. From the large grounds, you can see the sea.' The house is beside the estuary of the Bannon river. The beaches of the lovely Wexford coast are not far away.

Open All year, except 23–26 Dec.
Rooms 6 suites, 13 double, 1 single. 1 with access for &.
Facilities Ramp. Sitting room, lounge, bar, restaurant; background jazz and light classical music 6–12 pm; terrace. 20-acre grounds: jogging track, croquet, clay-pigeon shooting. 14 beaches within 5–15 mins' drive.
Location 10 miles S of New Ross, by R733, on E side of Bannon estuary. From Wexford, by R733; hotel on left as you enter Arthurstown. Train: Waterford or Wexford; then taxi.
Restrictions No smoking in restaurant. No children under 12 in restaurant after 8 pm. No dogs in house.
Credit cards All major cards accepted.
Terms B&B IR£65–£85. Set lunch IR£16, dinner IR£35; full alc £40. Child under 12 in parents' room: 50% of adult rate. 2-night winter weekend rates. *V*

BALLINACURRA Co. Cork　　　　　　　　　　Map 6:D5

Rathcoursey House　NEW　　　　*Tel* (+353) (0)21-461 3418
Ballinacurra, nr Midleton　　　　　*Fax* (+353) (0)21-461 3393
　　　　　　　　　　　　　　　　Email beth@rathcoursey.com
　　　　　　　　　　　　　　　　Website www.rathcoursey.com

'We spent a rapturous week.' 'A lovely place.' There are two nominators this year (one from Spain) for this country guest house. 'Set in acres of woods and meadows, above a quiet inlet of Cork harbour, it is an enchanting Georgian house, exquisitely decorated, very comfortable, full of antiques, books, paintings and prints. Fresh flowers from the garden are in every room. Beth Hallinan is a delightful hostess, a superb professional cook and food writer; the grounds provide fruit, herbs and vegetables, eggs are from local farms. Breakfasts are delicious, the five-course dinners [by arrangement] are magnificent.' Cooking is 'Irish, traditional and modern'. The sea is visible from the grounds. Several golf courses are nearby, also the Midleton whiskey distillery, ancient castles like Blarney and Barryscourt. Good birdwatching, and walking. (*Angela Kirby, Charles A Da Costa*)

Open All year. Lunch not served.
Rooms 5 double. 1 on ground floor, suitable for &.
Facilities Drawing room, library, small TV room, dining room. No background music. 35-acre grounds: woods, meadow, pond. Horse riding, sailing, fishing, golf nearby.
Location 18 miles E of Cork city, 5 miles S of Midleton. At Midleton roundabout take Whitegate road. After *c.* 2½ miles turn right for East Ferry. Go through Rathcoursey; follow green arrows on left.
Restriction No dogs in house.
Credit cards MasterCard, Visa.
Terms B&B: single IR£65–£75, double IR£120–£130. Set dinner (by arrangement) IR£28. Christmas package negotiable.

Report forms (Freepost in UK) are at the end of the *Guide*.

LINDERRY Co. Tipperary   **Map 6:C5**

lenoe BUDGET   *Tel* (+353) (0)67-22015
llinderry, Nenagh   *Fax* (+353) (0)67-22275

irginia Moeran's 200-year-old stone house stands on a hilltop, with
ne views over Lough Derg and the country around – 'a lovely area'.
Another warm tribute came this year: 'All was first class. A charming
welcome from Mrs Moeran in her beautiful, restful home. We had a
comfortable bedroom with large bathroom, a superb dinner and breakfast. Dogs and horses made the whole thing perfect.' Others wrote
earlier: 'Excellent value.' 'Collapsing on a sofa by a huge log fire in
the lounge, we thought we'd arrived in heaven, and that Virginia
Moeran was an angel.' 'We felt we were staying with friends.' Guests
can roam in the huge grounds, with meadows, woods, apple orchards,
masses of wild flowers in spring, plenty of wildlife – foxes, deer,
badgers, red squirrels, wild birds, etc – and a small horse-breeding
farm. The informal atmosphere, the personal attention, and the cooking, 'in local and French style', are all enjoyed. Children are welcomed. The spacious bedrooms have fresh flowers and an electric
blanket. At breakfast 'everything is home-made including the gorgeous marmalade'; eggs are free-range. An evening meal, based on
local produce, is available by arrangement, eg, smoked salmon; roast
lamb. It is elegantly served at tables set with flowers and silver. Water
is from the estate's own spring. 'We are very quiet,' says Mrs Moeran,
'but buzzing night life and restaurants are ten minutes' drive away.'
Other local attractions: golf, fishing, sailing, 'beautiful walks', Birr
and Portumna castles. (*Penelope Spencer-Cooper, YB, and others*)

Open All year, except Christmas.
Rooms 3 double, 1 single. No telephone. TV in one room.
Facilities Stair lift. Drawing room (background music on request), dining
room. 150-acre estate with stud, woods, etc. Lake, fishing ½ mile. Golf nearby.
Unsuitable for ♿.
Location Between Ballinderry and Terryglass (signposted). 7 miles NW of
Borrisokane.
Credit cards MasterCard, Visa.
Terms [2001] B&B IR£30–£40. Set dinner IR£25–£30.

BALLYCOTTON Co. Cork   **Map 6:D5**

Bayview Hotel   *Tel* (+353) (0)21-464 6746
                                     Fax (+353) (0)21-464 6075
                                     Email bayhotel@iol.ie
                                     Website www.bayviewhotel.net

Set above a fishing village on the Atlantic coastline, this quite luxurious holiday hotel is owned by John O'Brien and managed by Stephen
Belton. Long, low and white, it has been much admired. The large
house looks Georgian/Victorian but was massively rebuilt in 1991. It
stands in its own grounds on the edge of the cliffs, with a pretty terraced garden and panoramic views of the bay. Steps lead down to the
sea. All bedrooms have sea views, and some take in the picturesque

harbour, full of boats. The bedrooms are spacious: many have length windows; housekeeping is good. 'The hotel is well furnis with lots of flowers and old paintings. We found it really peace Apart from a distant foghorn, the only sound is of the sea on the ro and seabirds at dawn.' One end of the large bar is furnished as a co library/lounge, with an open fire. The elegant dining room has wel spaced tables: 'On the short fixed menu, the food was good, cooke and served with style.' More reports welcome on Ciaran Scully's cooking, which might include roast quail with courgette risotto; brill with grilled asparagus. There are six golf courses in the area.

Open 6 Apr–28 Oct.
Rooms 2 suites, 33 double.
Facilities Lift. Bar, lounge, restaurant; 24-hour classical background music; 2 meeting rooms. 2-acre grounds. Access to public beach.
Location Near village centre and harbour, 20 miles SE of Cork city.
Restrictions No smoking in some bedrooms. No dogs.
Credit cards All major cards accepted.
Terms B&B: single IR£80–£95, double IR£120–£150, suite IR£170–£200. Set lunch IR£15, dinner IR£34.

BALLYLICKEY Co. Cork   **Map 6:D4**

Sea View House   *Tel* (+353) (0)27-50073 and 50462
Ballylickey, Bantry Bay   *Fax* (+353) (0)27-51555
                                    Email seaviewhousehotel@eircom.net
                                    Website www.cmvhotels.com

'As good as ever.' 'It's great.' Renewed praise this year for Kathleen O'Sullivan's large, white, many-windowed Victorian house near the waterfront, looking towards Bantry Bay. She grew up here, and now runs it as a guest house in cheery personal style, offering 'a warm welcome' and 'outstanding value'. 'It is a haven of peace. The gardens are magnificent.' The ambience and the decor (patterned carpets, flowery curtains) are not especially sophisticated, but 'everything is spotless, gleaming, run by Miss O'Sullivan with such charm and efficiency'. Her staff are 'friendly' and 'amusing'. 'She runs the restaurant as a benevolent despot,' says one reader this year. 'It is well known locally and is always full. The meals are well above average, and service is prompt and cheerful.' Others have enjoyed the 'good vegetables in sensible portions', the local fish and seafood, the 'mix of sauced and plain dishes': the latter tend to be the more successful. Breakfasts are 'outstanding', with fish, potato pancakes, omelettes and chunky marmalade. The best bedrooms are large, with some antiques: 'They are perhaps furnished in an old-fashioned way, but have every luxury.' Some have 'a wonderful view'. Some more have been added in a new wing this year, and the restaurant now has a conservatory extension. The large, comfortable public rooms include a well-stocked library. (*Ran Ogston*)

Open 15 Mar–15 Nov.
Rooms 4 suites, 19 double. 2 on ground floor adapted for &.
Facilities Lounge bar, library/TV room, restaurant/conservatory. No background music. 5-acre grounds on waterfront: fishing, boating; riding, golf nearby.

cation In village 3 miles N of Bantry towards Glengarff; 70 yds off main
ad. Bus from Cork, 48 miles.
estrictions No smoking: restaurant, some bedrooms. No dogs in public
ooms.
Credit cards All major cards accepted.
Terms B&B IR£45–£90. Set lunch IR£16, dinner IR£30. Special breaks on
request. *V*

BALLYMOTE Co. Sligo   **Map 6:B5**

Temple House   *Tel* (+353) (0)71-83329
Fax (+353) (0)71-83808
Email guests@templehouse.ie
Website www.templehouse.ie

Discerning Americans were 'mightily impressed' by this typical
stately home whose owners, Sandy and Deb Perceval, take paying
guests. Sandy Perceval's family has lived since 1665 in this
Georgian mansion of 'faded grandeur'. It stands in a large estate,
recently declared a European lichen conservation area, with terraced gardens, woods and farmland, a lake and a ruined 13th-cen-
tury Knights Templar castle. Inside are an imposing main hall and
stairway, antique furniture, turf and log fires, and canopied beds.
Some bedrooms are huge (one is nicknamed 'the half-acre'). The
house is well heated in winter, and it has been much redecorated this
year. 'Voltage has been increased,' the Percevals tell us in response
to earlier reports of dim lighting. They are friendly, and helpful with
advice about places to visit, and the style is informal. At dinner,
guests sit round one table to enjoy Deb's cooking ('Irish with
French connections'). No choice: a typical menu might be: leeks
and brie in a puff pastry tart; salmon with lime and coriander; ice-
cream gateau; Irish cheeseboard. Vegetarians are catered for if they
give advance notice. Much produce comes from the farm, which is
stocked with sheep and Kerry cattle; wildlife abounds. You can hire
a boat and fish in the lake (pike over 20 lb are not uncommon), and
shooting parties are held in winter. Children are welcomed (under-
sevens are given supper in the kitchen at 6.30). Because of
Mr Perceval's severe allergies, brought on by sheep dip, guests are
asked not to wear scented products. Yeats country is all around, and
traditional music and dancing sessions are held regularly in the
area. More reports, please.

Open 1 Apr–30 Nov.
Rooms 5 double, 1 single. No telephone/TV.
Facilities Sitting room, snooker room, dining room. No background music.
1,000-acre farm: 1½-acre terraced garden, croquet, woodlands, lake, coarse
fishing, boating. Golf, riding nearby. Unsuitable for &.
Location 12 miles S of Sligo by N17, then R293. Signposted beyond Esso
garage in Ballymote. Train: Ballymote, 4 miles; then taxi.
Restrictions No smoking in dining room. No children under 7 at dinner. Dogs
in cars only.
Credit cards Amex, MasterCard, Visa.
Terms B&B IR£51.19. Single supplement IR£15.81. Set dinner IR£23.63.
Reductions for long stays. 1-night bookings refused public holidays.

BALLYVAUGHAN Co. Clare   Map 6:C

Gregans Castle   *Tel* (+353) (0)65-707 700
                        Fax (+353) (0)65-707 711
                        Email res@gregans.ie
                        Website www.gregans.ie

The Burren is a curious region of rocky scenery, full of rare plants and flowers. On its edge, on a hill above Galway Bay, is Peter and Moira Haden's luxurious country house hotel (their son Simon is manager). 'It is an elegant and atmospheric haven,' runs recent praise. 'Our room had a cushioned window seat with views of the Burren, its own private garden and a huge double bath. The staff were helpful and warm. Turf fires and paintings of local Galway characters create an authentically Irish feel. Pictures of local flora hang in the drawing room, whose bay window looks over the lovely garden. The bedrooms (one has a four-poster) are admired for their 'sophisticated comfort'. The dining room offers views of the sun setting over the bay. Locally grown ingredients, organic when possible, are used, and locally caught fish and seafood. The cooking of the French chef, Régis Herviaux, is admired, eg, grilled monkfish with tapenade; Irish beef; Burren lamb; chocolate and orange mousse. Vegetarians are catered for too. The atmosphere is 'quite genteel'; a jacket and tie are expected of male guests at night. There is live classical harp or piano music during dinner, and a pianist plays Irish folk and jazz in the Corkscrew Bar, popular for pre-dinner drinks. The lounge is 'tranquil, full of books and board games'. The library has 'an interesting selection of books, including a history of the papacy in umpteen volumes'. The Burren is also a centre of Irish folk culture (you'll hear good Irish music in its pubs). Nearby are the 'awe-inspiring' cliffs of Moher, the golf courses of Lahinch – and Lisdoonvarna with its famous annual matchmaking festival. (*JE*)

Open 28 Mar–late Oct.
Rooms 6 suites, 18 double. Some on ground floor.
Facilities Hall, lounge, library, bar, dining room. No background music. 12-acre grounds: garden, ornamental lake, croquet. Safe sandy beach, swimming 4½ miles; golf, riding, hill-walking nearby.
Location At foot of Corkscrew Hill, 3½ miles SW of Ballyvaughan, on N67 to Lisdoonvarna.
Restrictions No smoking: restaurant, some bedrooms. No dogs.
Credit cards Amex, MasterCard, Visa.
Terms [2001] B&B: single IR£126–£178, double IR£146–£198, suite IR£230–£290. Set dinner IR£38; full alc IR£46. 3/4-day rates. Child in parents' room: under 5, IR£10; 5–10, IR£15.

BANTRY Co. Cork   Map 6:D4

Bantry House   *Tel* (+353) (0)27-50047
                        Fax (+353) (0)27-50795
                        Email bantry@hidden-ireland.com
                        Website www.hidden-ireland.com/bantry

A grand classical country house, enjoyed again this year. Set in wide wooded grounds, it has a 'stunning location' overlooking Bantry Bay

.d the Caha mountains on the Beara peninsula. It has belonged to the
⁄hite family since 1739: the present owner, Egerton Shelswell White,
⁚s a keen trombone player (as guests can hear) and he usually serves
⁚he wine at dinner. He is a scion of the Earl of Bantry, who received
the title for warning the British of the arrival of a French fleet in the
bay in 1796. Today the French still come: 'We liked the atmosphere,
the friendly owner and cook, and the snooker table,' said one Gallic
guest. The house is filled with furniture, paintings and *objets d'art* collected by the second earl on his travels in Europe in the 19th century.
He also laid out the formal gardens, with a fountain, parterres and a
'stairway to the sky'. The bedrooms are much admired: one is 'huge,
with breathtaking views of the bay, and modern furnishings chosen
with taste'. 'Very good' breakfasts, with fresh orange juice, fruit, kippers, etc, are served in a 'cosy, delightful room'. A 'simple and delicious' dinner is available, by arrangement, at 7.30 on weekdays.
Limited choice, eg, carrot and orange soup or melon; roast lamb or
baked sole. There is a short children's supper menu. The house is open
to visitors, and a tour is included in the room price. Guests have the
use of a separate sitting room, billiard room and television room, plus
free access to the main rooms of the house, notably the library, where
concerts are often held. (*N Kent*)

Open Mar -Oct inclusive, except 23 June–6 July. Dinner Mon–Fri by arrangement.
Rooms 1 suite, 7 double. No TV.
Facilities Hall, sitting room, TV room, library (2 or 3 concerts a month), bil-
liard room, bar dining room; craft shop, tea room. No background music. 100-
acre estate: formal gardens, woodland. Sea, sandy beach ½ mile; tennis,
sailing, fishing, golf, horse riding nearby. Unsuitable for &.
Location ½ mile NE of centre; signposted at Inner Harbour. Bus from Cork
(2½ hrs).
Restrictions No smoking: dining room, bedrooms. Dogs in grounds only.
Credit cards Amex, MasterCard, Visa.
Terms B&B 1R£85–95. Light lunch IR£5. Set lunch IR£10–£15, dinner
IR£25.

BEAUFORT Co. Kerry   **Map 6:D4**

Beaufort House   *Tel/Fax* (+353) (0)64-44764
                                   Email info@beaufortireland.com
                                   Website www.beaufortireland.com

The river Laune, with fishing for salmon and trout, flows through the
large wooded grounds of this big white Georgian house near
Killarney, owned and run by Donald and Rachel Cameron. 'They,
with their two children and two dogs, were extremely hospitable and
helpful,' say recent visitors. 'This was the jewel in the crown of our
Irish visit.' Others have enjoyed the 'warmth, food, and efficient, as
well as friendly, care'. The bedrooms have been lavishly decorated
with coordinated curtains and carpets: 'Our superb front room had a
bed wide enough for four.' The upper rooms offer a good view of
Macgillicuddy's Reeks, the range with Ireland's highest peak. 'There
are two excellent restaurants in the village, within walking distance,'

write the Camerons this year, 'so from 2002 we shall be providing dinner only for groups of six or more, by arrangement.' This served at 8 pm: a no-choice four-course menu ('modern country house cooking') might include ceviche of scallops and brill with home-made focaccia bread; monkfish fillets roasted in bacon; elderflower sorbet. The wine list is admired, as are the Irish cheeses. The Camerons join their guests over coffee. Breakfast is generous Irish, with freshly squeezed orange juice, a vast assortment of jams and spreads, as well as eggs cooked any way. The drawing room has 'a roaring log fire and plenty of magazines'. The four new self-catering cottages have well-equipped kitchens, terraces with mountain views, and lounges with open fires. Nearby are the Ring of Kerry, the lakes of Killarney and Tomies Wood, a huge natural oak forest; three 18-hole golf courses are within five minutes' drive. More reports welcome.

Open Easter–30 Sept; groups out of season by arrangement. Dinner (for groups) served Mon–Thurs, with 24 hours' notice.
Rooms 4 double. 4 self-catering cottages (open all year). No telephone/TV.
Facilities Drawing room, library, dining room. No background music. 42-acre grounds: river, trout/salmon fishing. Golf nearby. Unsuitable for &.
Location 6 miles W of Killarney on N72. Left over stone bridge opposite petrol station. House immediately on left.
Restrictions No smoking in library. No dogs.
Credit cards MasterCard, Visa.
Terms B&B: single IR£75–£80, double IR£140–£150. Set dinner (by arrangement, min. 6 guests) IR£27.50.

BELFAST   Map 6:B6

Ash-Rowan	*Tel* 028-9066 1983
12 Windsor Avenue	*Fax* 028-9066 3227
Belfast BT9 6EE	*Email* ashrowan@hotmail.com

One delight of Evelyn and Sam Hazlett's much-admired guest house is the enterprising cooked breakfasts (ordered the night before). They include 'Ulster Fry (not for the faint-hearted)', 'Irish Scramble', and the house speciality, mushrooms flambéed with sherry and cream. Plus fresh orange juice, home-baked bread, 'gorgeous' home-made jams, fresh fruit salad. An early breakfast, if needed, is 'cheerfully given'. Set in a tree-lined street not far from Queen's University, the spacious Victorian house has pots of flowers and hanging baskets by the front door, and is full of old furniture, lace, curios and plants. The owners, 'genuinely kind and welcoming' (and supported by a black Labrador), have done much redecoration. The well-equipped bedrooms, all with a shower, are 'cosy, with lovely linen', and pine and cane furniture. There's a lounge for residents, with daily papers, and a large conservatory. An evening meal is available by arrangement, with main courses like fillet steak flambéed in whiskey, and other restaurants are nearby (*Cayanne* in Shaftesbury Square is recommended). Thomas Andrews, designer of the *Titanic* (built in Belfast), lived in *Ash-Rowan*, and from here, with his wife, he set out on its maiden voyage, never to return. More reports, please.

pen All year, except 24 Dec–2 Jan, 11–17 July.
Rooms 3 double, 2 single.
Facilities Lounge, dining room, conservatory. No background music. ½-acre garden. Unsuitable for &.
Location Just off Lisburn Rd, 1½ miles SW of centre. Car park. Bus from centre.
Restrictions No smoking: breakfast room, bedrooms. No children under 12. No dogs.
Credit cards MasterCard, Visa.
Terms B&B: single £48–£69, double £77. Evening meal by arrangement.

McCausland Hotel	*Tel* 028-9022 0200
34–38 Victoria Street	*Fax* 028-9022 0220
Belfast BT1 3GH	*Email* info@mccauslandhotel.com
	Website www.mccauslandhotel.com

In the city's commercial heart, near the river Lagan, two adjacent 1850s red brick industrial warehouses have been stylishly converted into a fairly luxurious hotel of modern design. Opened in 1998, it is a welcome venture for Belfast, and is 'most attractive, with lots of exposed brick and girders in the rooms', says a recent visitor. 'Reception was friendly and professional, my bathroom was luxurious, and I had reasonable food in the café/bar/bistro.' The bedrooms have 'environmentally aware services', says the hotel. Some are designed for female travellers, and three are suitable for disabled guests. In the main restaurant, Sandy Plum is the new chef, offering such dishes as lamb samosa on wilted rocket; confit of duck on warm crispy noodles, bock choi and black beans; sticky toffee steam pudding. We'd be glad of reports on this 'contemporary Irish cooking', as he describes it. Under the same ownership as *The Hibernian*, Dublin (*qv*), and the *Woodstock* at Ennis, near Shannon. (*PD*)

Open All year, except 24–27 Dec.
Rooms 9 suites, 51 double. 3 adapted for &.
Facilities Lift. 2 bars, café, restaurant; business centre; classical/'easy listening' background music in public areas. Free use of local leisure centre.
Location Central, just W of river Lagan, between Anne St and the Albert clock tower. Private parking.
Restrictions No smoking in 33 bedrooms. Guide dogs only.
Credit cards All major cards accepted.
Terms [2001] Room: single £120–£150, double £120–£170, suite £170–£190. Breakfast £12. Set lunch £11.95, dinner £18.95. *V*

See also SHORTLIST

BIRR Co. Offaly	**Map 6:C5**

Spinners Town House NEW/BUDGET	*Tel/Fax* (+353) (0)509-21673
& Bistro	*Email* spinners@indigo.ie
Castle Street	

In the thinly populated Irish Midlands, Birr is a pleasant small town whose imposing 17th-century castle has large, attractive gardens. Just

opposite, and next to a ruined church, *Spinners* is a small hotel c
character, converted from a terrace of Georgian houses. Its nominators
write: 'Furnished in minimalist Scandinavian style, it has been decorated by someone with a good eye for colour. Restaurant food was
good but not exceptional; the breakfast was the best we had in Ireland
[it can include kippers, smoked mackerel or Irish cheese plate as well
as scrambled eggs]. All excellent value – and lots of trouble taken by
hosts, eg, electric blanket in bed, tea brought to us in lounge where
there was a great fire.' Bedrooms face the castle walls; three are
'medieval' in style. The courtyard garden is sometimes used as an outdoor theatre. In the bistro, lit with lanterns and candles, and hung with
contemporary prints and oil paintings, soft music plays. A 'postmod-
ern dining experience' is promised . . . the kitchen's policy is 'buy
local, think global'. Its short menu includes seafood chowder, prawns
in garlic and chilli, summer fruit cup Greek-style. Herbs are from the
garden, bacon is organic. (*Richard and Helen Firth*)

Open All year. Bistro closed Mon.
Rooms 1 family, 10 double, 2 single.
Facilities Lounge, breakfast room, bistro (background music); conference
room; garden.
Location Central. Birr is 87 miles W of Dublin.
Restriction No dogs in house.
Credit cards All major cards accepted.
Terms B&B: single IR£20, double IR£50–£70. Full alc IR£12–£25. Child in
parents' room: under 2, free; under 12, 50% discount.

BUSHMILLS Co. Antrim *See SHORTLIST*   **Map 6:A6**

CAHERLISTRANE Co. Galway   **Map 6:C5**

Lisdonagh House NEW	*Tel* (+353) (0)93-31163
Caherlistrane, nr Headford	*Fax* (+353) (0)93-31528

Email cooke@lisdonagh.com
Website www.lisdonagh.com

'Tucked away in the countryside', north of Galway city, this big
Georgian house (1720s), on a large estate with ancient trees, has a
colourful history. One former owner, Walda Palmer, loved hunting
and shooting, and would sometimes fire shotguns at intruders. No such
welcome faced our inspectors in 2001: 'We were greeted by a charming young lady, immaculately dressed. The house was bought in 1996,
in a run-down state, by John and Finola Cooke from London, who
have renovated it lovingly, using materials of the highest quality. The
magnificent spiral staircase, and the frescoes in the fine oval hallway,
painted by John Ryan in 1790, have been restored. The drawing room
is superb, yellow walled, impeccably furnished by Mrs Cooke – a
delightful place in which to sit. In the basement, the library/bar offers
drinks on an honesty basis. In the compact blue-walled dining room,
the original dado rail has been kept; and fortunately the muzak was
soft. We were well looked after by three girls in smart monogrammed
outfits, led by the receptionist, doubling as head waiter. She and the

chef, Liebe van Deventer, are from South Africa, as are many of wines, such as our fine Sauvignon Blanc (IR£19). The set dinner, n little choice, was enjoyable: red pepper soup; crispy duck breast; sational, if fattening, date and nut pudding. Breakfast was also well ne, with good fresh products: porridge with honey and cream; moked salmon and scrambled egg; an Irish fry; leaf tea. The five first-loor bedrooms all look towards Lough Hackett; others are on the lower ground floor. Mrs Cooke, most friendly, told us that they plan to reclaim the kitchen garden. Maybe they should re-landscape the grounds in front of the house. The car park, 50 yards away, is awkward.'

Open Mid-Mar–end Oct. Lunch not served. Non-residents must book dinner.
Rooms 2 suites, 9 double. 2 in gate lodge.
Facilities Lounge, library/bar, dining room (piped music). 250-acre estate on lake (fishing); walled garden, kitchen garden; horses.
Location 26 miles N of Galway city, off R333 Headford–Tuam. In Caherlistane, take Shule road for 1½ miles, turn left (house signposted).
Restrictions Smoking in lounge only. No children under 11. No dogs in house.
Credit cards Amex, MasterCard, Visa.
Terms [2001] B&B IR£50–£100. Set dinner IR£30.

CARAGH LAKE Co. Kerry   **Map 6:D4**

Caragh Lodge	*Tel* (+353) (0)66-976 9115
Caragh Lake	*Fax* (+353) (0)66-976 9316
Killorglin	*Email* caraghl@iol.ie
	Website www.caraghlodge.com

'We fell in love with this hotel. It was like staying in the country house of delightful friends' – more admiration this year for the ever-present Mary Gaunt's Victorian fishing lodge. Set in seven acres of 'incredibly beautiful' gardens, with rare trees and shrubs, it stands by the shore of Caragh Lake, and has views of the high Macgillicuddy's Reeks. 'Our spacious bedroom was finely furnished, with a marvellous view and a large bathroom. The dining room, with a lovely view of the garden, offers good food with a menu changing daily. The home-made cake served with afternoon tea was superb. We loved the roaring fires in the two finely furnished drawing rooms. The staff were helpful, full of friendly smiles, and our fellow guests were charming and discerning.' Others wrote of 'a warm welcome, and an outstanding dinner'. The bedrooms in the main building have splendid views; those in the new wing are 'superbly decorated'. In the restaurant, facing the lake, the food is modern Irish, eg, tuna tartar with chilli and ginger; rack of Kerry lamb with spicy chickpeas; plum and peach crumble with cream. Breads are home-baked, and the wine list is large. Breakfasts include smoked salmon and scrambled eggs. The hotel has two boats for the use of guests. There is unpolluted swimming in the lake, and free trout fishing. The Ring of Kerry and the sandy beaches of Dingle Bay are a short drive away, and there are ten golf courses nearby. (*P de B Hart, DC*)

Open Mid-Apr–mid-Oct.
Rooms 1 suite, 13 double, 1 single. 3 in garden annexe. Some on ground floor. No TV.

Facilities 2 lounges, restaurant (varied background music during din
meeting room. 7-acre grounds: garden, tennis, sauna, lake, swimming, fish
boating. Sea 4 miles. Unsuitable for &.
Location 22 miles W of Killarney, off N70. From Killorglin towa
Glenbeigh, take road signposted *Caragh Lodge* 1 mile. Left at lake, lodge
right.
Restrictions No smoking in restaurant. No children under 12. No dogs.
Credit cards All major cards accepted.
Terms [2001] B&B: single IR£85, double IR£125–£160, suite IR£220. Set
dinner IR£33.

Carrig House NEW	*Tel* (+353) (0)66-976 9100
Caragh Lake	*Fax* (+353) (0)66-976 9166
Killorglin	*Email* info@carrighouse.com
	Website www.carrighouse.com

A splendid newcomer. Very near *Caragh Lodge* (above), and 'with a
much better view of the lake', *Carrig House* is owned and run by Mary
and Frank Slattery. 'He is a large jovial man, full of *bonhomie*, and we
rapidly got on first-name terms,' says our inspector, whose visit was
just before the opening of an extension that brings the number of
rooms from six to 16. We trust this will not affect the 'homeliness' and
very personal ambience. 'Approached down a narrow twisty lane, the
bright yellow house stands right by the lake, a superb location.
Entering a small porch littered with wet-weather footwear, you
squeeze through narrow doors into a cramped foyer with a loud carpet. Our very cosy ground-floor room had a spacious bathroom, but
my reverie there was disturbed by the central heating boiler close by.
There are open fires in the comfortable drawing room and in the
"snug". The dinner menu is adventurous, and the French chef's cooking is very accomplished: we enjoyed an unusual warm salmon salad,
shallot tarte Tatin, and large helpings of duck. The wine list is extensive and, for Eire, reasonably priced. Frank explains the dishes in
advance to the guests, and a group of four French visitors regarded
him in awe as he detailed the intricacies of "black-and-white seafood
pudding" (many guests are from the Continent). Breakfast, with a
stunning view of the lake, was good Irish country house fare: delicious
wheaten bread, but canned orange juice.' The new extension, says
Mr Slattery, has Victorian furnishings, in keeping with the main house
which is 1850s. He adds: 'By policy, we do not have TV in the bedrooms, as we want our guests to meet each other, and not hide.' He is
proud of the 950 species of trees, rare flowers and shrubs in his large
and lovely gardens: there are marked walks, a stream and waterfalls.

Open Mar–Nov. Lunch not served.
Rooms 2 suites, 14 double. No TV.
Facilities 2 lounges, snug, library, TV room, dining room; sauna (opening
summer 2002). 4-acre garden on lake: private jetty, boat, fishing; walks, cro-
quet. 10 golf courses locally.
Location 22 miles W of Killarney. From Killorglin: N70 to Glenbeigh, left to
Caragh Lake after 2½ miles; after 1½ miles sharp right at Caragh Lake school
and shop; entrance ½ mile on left. From Glenbeigh: N70 to Killorglin
2½ miles, turning right over bridge. Right on to Caragh Lake road before *Red
Fox* inn. House on right after 1½ miles.

Restrictions No smoking in some bedrooms. No children under 10. No dogs in house.
Credit cards Diners, MasterCard, Visa.
Terms [2001] B&B IR£60–£100. Full alc dinner IR£40.

CARRIGBYRNE Co. Wexford   Map 6:D6

Cedar Lodge   *Tel* (+353) (0)51-428386
Carrigbyrne, Newbawn   *Fax* (+353) (0)51-428222
                                Email cedarlodge@eircom.net
                                Website www.prideofeirehotels.com

Not a converted old house, but a low, white, modern building, *Cedar Lodge* stands beneath wooded slopes, west of Wexford. 'A very good overnight stop,' said a devotee returning recently. 'The owner Tom Martin chats away; his wife, Ailish, is up at crack of dawn carrying breakfast trays for people leaving on the Rosslare ferry.' Recent improvements and additions include a new wing with spacious bedrooms, refurbishment of older rooms, and a facelift for the motel-like facade. Rooms on the main road now have triple glazing, 'to remove traffic noise', says Mr Martin, 'a talented hotelier', 'very attentive'. 'His staff were welcoming, the rooms are large and well furnished in executive style,' reports one visitor. But the bar lunch was thought 'overpriced' this year. 'At dinner, in a pleasant conservatory, the chairs were comfortable and the food was excellent, notably crab, scallops, steak.' Mrs Martin's other dishes include smoked ostrich; fillets of turbot with vermouth. Logs burn in the big brass-canopied fireplace in the middle of the dining room. Ask for Mrs Martin's Irish brown bread at breakfast. There is a garden, and good walking locally (a guide is provided). Nearby are the John F Kennedy Arboretum, which has trees and shrubs from all over the world, and the lovely Wexford coast. (*CB, RW, and others*)

Open 1 Feb–1 Dec.
Rooms 28 double. Some on ground floor.
Facilities Ramp. Lounge, lounge bar, breakfast room, restaurant; varied background music. 1½-acre garden. Golf nearby, sandy beaches 12 miles.
Location On N25, 14 miles W of Wexford.
Restrictions No smoking in restaurant. Dogs by arrangement.
Credit cards All major cards accepted.
Terms B&B: single IR£55–£80, double IR£80–£130. Set lunch IR£17.50, dinner IR£27.50.

CASHEL BAY Co. Galway   Map 6:C4

Zetland Country House   *Tel* (+353) (0)95-31111
                                          Fax (+353) (0)95-31117
                                Email zetland@iol.ie
                                Website www.zetland.com

Set in wide grounds on the edge of Cashel Bay, amid wild Connemara scenery, this handsome white 1850s hunting lodge was built for the Earl of Zetland. Its owners today, John and Mona Prendergast and their son, Ruaidhri, offer 'genuine Irish hospitality'. Recent guests thought it 'an excellent place, with tasteful decor, beautifully cooked food' (this is served by 'a variety of nationalities'). The lounges are large, with peat fires, antiques, soft colour schemes, fresh flowers, books, porcelain, varied paintings. The dining room is 'exquisitely decorated, with dreamy views over the sea and mountains in the setting sun'. The 'progressive Irish' cooking of local salmon, lobster and lamb, by chef Jason Le Gear, is generally admired. Other dishes might include salad of aubergine and feta cheese; fried sea bass in fennel sauce; bread-and-butter pudding. Many vegetables are from the garden. Afternoon tea comes with home baking. Most bedrooms are spacious, with views of the bay. Fishing can be arranged, in local lakes and rivers. Two championship golf courses are nearby, also good beaches with safe swimming, and other sporting activities (see below). Shooting parties sometimes fill the place. (*WR*)

Open Apr–Oct.
Rooms 17 double, 2 single. 1 on ground floor.
Facilities Drawing room, lounge, bar, restaurant. No background music. 10-acre grounds: tennis; rocky shore 200 yds. Golf, water sports, river/lake fishing, sea angling, cycling, shooting, pony-trekking available.
Location 40 miles NW of Galway. Take N59 towards Clifden; turn left after Recess, follow hotel signs. Bus from Galway.
Restrictions No smoking: restaurant, bedrooms. No dogs in public rooms.
Credit cards All major cards accepted.
Terms (*Excluding 12½% service charge*) B&B: single IR£79–£89, double IR£110–£130. Set lunch IR£15, dinner IR£33.50. Child in parents' room: 50% of adult rate. 3-night D,B&B rates.

CASTLEBALDWIN Co. Sligo   Map 6:B5

Cromleach Lodge   *Tel* (+353) (0)71-65155
Castlebaldwin, via Boyle   *Fax* (+353) (0)71-65455
                                     Email info@cromleach.com
                                     Website www.cromleach.com

🦢 *César award in 1999*

'It is really lovely, its *César* is well deserved,' runs one plaudit in 2001. Another: 'We enjoyed Christy and Moira Tighe's warmth of welcome, the quality of the food, the ambience of the lounge, the stunning situation.' One of the *Guide*'s most admired rural entries, this small, sophisticated hotel is a striking modern building, grey-gabled and glass-fronted, set on a hillside above Lough Arrow; all bedrooms have good views across the lake to the mountains. Mrs Tighe's modern Irish cooking, 'with an emphasis on lightness', does not come cheaply, but is much admired: 'This is serious and not pretentious food.' The six-course gourmet menu for residents might include warm smoked salmon with champagne sauce; duck wrapped in pastry with orange and ginger glaze; iced almond and apricot nougat. Vegetarians are catered for. 'The desserts are a work of art, and the staff are well trained.' But wine-list mark-ups are thought too high. Guests rotate to different tables each night, so that all get a turn for the best views. Families with young children can use a separate dining room. As for the 'large, warm, sunlit' bedrooms:

rs was delightful, with luxurious bathroom and tempting exotica he fruit bowl.' The design in the public rooms is thought 'a bit er-the-top' by some guests, but 'lovely' by others. The large black abrador, Rocky, will accompany guests on walks. There is good shing and golf in the area, also archaeological tours. (*PD, Simon nd Pearl Willbourn*)

Open 1 Feb–1 Nov. Lunch not served.
Rooms 10 double. Some on ground floor.
Facilities 2 lounges, bar, 2 dining rooms, conservatory. No background music. 30-acre grounds: forest walks; private access to Lough Arrow: fishing, boating, surfing; walking, hill climbing.
Location 9 miles NW of Boyle, off N4 Dublin–Sligo. Turn E at Castlebaldwin. Train: Boyle; taxi.
Restrictions No smoking: restaurant, 1 lounge, bedrooms. No dogs in public rooms.
Credit cards All major cards accepted.
Terms B&B IR£85–£139; D,B&B IR£125–£179. Set dinner IR£40. 2- to 5-day rates.

CLARECASTLE Co. Clare   Map 6:C5

Carnelly House   *Tel* (+353) (0)65-682 8442
                                            Fax (+353) (0)65-682 9222
                                            Email rgleeson@iol.ie
                                            Website www.carnelly-house.com

Ten miles N of Shannon, between airport and Ennis, on 100-acre estate with farm, woodlands and wildlife: creeper-covered Georgian house 'most impressive'. Friendly owners, Rosemarie and Dermot Gleeson; house-party atmosphere. Elegant period furnishings, beautiful drawing room, tall windows, open fires, wide staircase, spacious bedrooms, 'splendid' bathrooms. Good home cooking (no choice), eg, wild Irish salmon; pheasant in port; communally served in red and white dining room. Generous breakfasts. Classical background music. Fishing, fox-hunting, beaches, surfing, golf nearby. Unsuitable for ♿. Dogs in grounds only. Amex, MasterCard, Visa accepted. 5 bedrooms. B&B IR£70–£90. Set lunch IR£25, dinner IR£35 [2001]. More reports, please.

CLIFDEN Co. Galway   Map 6:C4

The Quay House   *Tel* (+353) (0)95-21369
Beach Road   *Fax* (+353) (0)95-21608
                                            Email thequay@iol.ie
                                            Website www.thequayhouse.com

'A lovely hotel, wonderful breakfast, gorgeous new rooms,' runs praise this year for Paddy and Julia Foyle's small B&B enterprise. Trim, white and Georgian, it is Clifden's oldest building, once the harbourmaster's house, then a convent and Franciscan friary; and it stands in a garden with tropical plants, beside the harbour with its fishing and pleasure boats. 'The amusingly eccentric decor' is an eclectic mix of serious Irish antiques and paintings, and 'the kitschy-cute'. The pictures are 'fascinating but hardly jolly – Joan of Arc at prayer death of General Wolfe'. 'In the hallway is a cabin trunk full of [and a couple of battered toppers hanging from antlers on the wall.' Foyles 'couldn't be more hospitable' and the 'friendly informality enjoyed. Bedrooms in the main house have garden or bay views, sor have a working fireplace; most are spacious, though some at the to are small. The rooms are as full of character as the rest: one is 'superb with marble wall scrolls, a fabulous bed, and French doors leading on to a tiny flower-filled balcony facing the harbour'. Another has a huge baroque mirror as a bedhead. 'The bath was vast, and the water ran peaty and soft.' A new section has studios, each with a kitchenette. Breakfasts have 'generous servings of fresh orange juice, good yogurt, and scrambled eggs and smoked salmon'. The Foyles formerly ran *Destry's* restaurant, nearby, but they have closed it.

Open Mid-Mar–end Oct.
Rooms 14 double. 2 on ground floor. 7 self-catering studios in annexe.
Facilities Ramps. 2 sitting rooms, breakfast room, conservatory. No background music. ½-acre garden. Fishing, sailing, golf, riding nearby.
Location Harbour; 3 mins' walk from centre. Courtyard parking.
Restrictions No smoking: breakfast room, bedrooms. No dogs.
Credit cards MasterCard, Visa.
Terms B&B: single IR£60–£70, double IR£95–£110. Child under 12 free in parents' room.

Rock Glen
Tel (+353) (0)95-21035
Fax (+353) (0)95-21737
Email rockglen@iol.ie
Website www.connemara.net/rockglen-hotel

Large open turf fires are among the pleasures of this converted 1815 hunting lodge, a low white building. It stands in large grounds by Ardbear Bay, with the wild Connemara Twelve Pins mountains behind, and is 'beautifully quiet'. John and Evangeline Roche, the owners, and their daughter Siobhán (she is manager), are all 'most welcoming', while their friendly and efficient young staff include 'locals, a Breton head waiter, a Dane and some French trainees'; Gee Nazri is head chef. The clientele is equally cosmopolitan. 'Great comfort, very good dinner,' ran recent praise. There are chandeliers and large sofas, chess and Scrabble in the drawing room; a resident pianist plays at weekends in the cocktail bar; there is a full-size snooker table, and the candlelit restaurant 'is a fine setting for the imaginative, strongly flavoured food'. You can take the five-course dinner for IR£35, or pay per course. Local seafood and shellfish are cooked in a modern style 'with a French/Asian influence'. A menu might include: crabmeat ravioli; roast Connemara lamb; pistachio crème brûlée. The best bedrooms, in front, are 'light and attractive; we enjoyed splendid views of hills, water and boats as we lay in bed'. Most rooms are now redecorated; some bathrooms are small. The generous breakfast includes scrambled eggs with smoked salmon, and they will cook fish caught by the guests. Children are welcomed. A floodlit tennis court is in the grounds. Plenty of outdoor activities are available locally (see below); sandy beaches are nearby. Painting courses are sometimes held by an artist member of the family, Tom Roche. (*MB, and others*)

Open Mid-Feb–mid-Nov, New Year.
Rooms 1 suite, 24 double, 1 single. 15 on ground floor.
Facilities Drawing room, cocktail bar/conservatory (pianist weekends), snooker room, TV room, restaurant. No background music. 50-acre grounds: tennis, croquet, putting. Riding, pony-trekking, river/deep-sea fishing, mountaineering nearby.
Location 1½ miles S of Clifden on Ballyconneely road. Bus from Galway.
Restriction No smoking in restaurant. No dogs in public rooms; in bedrooms by arrangement.
Credit cards Amex, MasterCard, Visa.
Terms [2001] B&B: single IR£92–£109, double IR£116–£140, suite IR£174–£210; D,B&B: single IR£122–£134, double IR£178–£267. Set dinner IR£35; full alc IR£50. 1-night bookings refused bank holiday weekends.

CLONES Co. Monaghan   **Map 6:B6**

| **Hilton Park** | *Tel* (+353) (0)47-56007 |
| Scothouse, Clones | *Fax* (+353) (0)47-56033 |

Email jm@hiltonpark.ie
Website www.hiltonpark.ie

🦢 *César award in 1994*

Enjoyed by inspectors in 2001, this imposing Italianate mansion is run in house-party style by 'genial hosts' Lucy and Johnny Madden (it has been his family's home since 1734). It stands near the border with Fermanagh, in a wooded park, with fields of sheep, three lakes, a golf course, and pleasure gardens laid out in the 1870s. 'Here we were bathed in birdsong at dusk: bliss. In the beautiful house, the halls and passages are much lived in, but spick and span. Interesting books of eclectic taste and vintage abound. Our bedroom was very comfortable, its bathroom had a splendidly authentic claw-foot bath, with lots of hot water during published hours of availability. The dining and drawing rooms, on the first floor, have stunning views. One has a welcoming log fire and Johnny offering you glasses of what-you-will while informing you of Lucy's impending culinary masterpieces. Her dinner started with "cosseting by cheese", a dish in between quiche and soufflé, stunning and unique. A rich dark green soup was delicious. Duck breasts were tender and beautifully presented, but bland. The lemon-balm jelly for pud had a subtle and delicious flavour. Breakfast was in the vaulted basement, a bit like a cheerful and brightly decorated cloister, with reassuring kitchen noises; a buffet of delicious fruits and cereals, plus cooked dishes with the bonus of potato cake (Lucy has published a book on 365 ways of cooking potatoes).' She makes her own bread and preserves, and her cooking draws on the estate's produce, including organically grown vegetables. In the baronial dining room, meals are served round one big table (but there are separate ones, too). The high-windowed public rooms are elegantly furnished, and full of memorabilia. The bedrooms, some with a four-poster bed, are huge; all have fine views. At Clones, the lace museum is worth a visit.

Open 1 Apr–end Sept; to pre-booked groups all year. Closed 2 days a week, generally Sun/Mon. Dining room closed midday, and to non-residents.
Rooms 1 suite, 5 double. No telephone/TV.
Facilities Drawing room, sitting room, TV room, games room, smoking room, dining room, breakfast room. No background music. 500-acre grounds: 20-acre gardens, golf, 3 lakes, swimming, boating, fishing. Unsuitable for ♿.
Location 4 miles S of Clones, on L46 to Ballyhaise. Bus: Clones; then taxi.
Restrictions No smoking. No children under 8. Dogs in cars.
Credit cards MasterCard, Visa.
Terms [2001] B&B IR£64–£75. Single supplement £20. Set dinner IR£27.50. Reductions for children 8–16 in parents' room. 1-night bookings refused for Sat if too far in advance.

CONG Co. Mayo Map 6:C4

Ballywarren House NEW   *Tel/Fax* (+353) (0)92-46989
Cross   *Email* ballywarrenhouse@eircom.net

Between Lough Corrib and Lough Mask, set in idyllic solitude amid pastures where sheep and cows graze, is this country house with just three guest bedrooms, owned and run by David and Diane Skelton. 'It is a really lovely country home,' say its German nominators this year. 'Very comfortable and welcoming, it has luxurious bedrooms and excellent food, all home-made. The breads and marmalade are delicious. David and Diane were most kind.' Peat and log open fires are in the public rooms; bedrooms are large, with a king-size bed; one has an oak four-poster, another a hand-carved pine bed. Small wonder that *Michelin* bestows its coveted red print. Diane Skelton's cooking, 'traditional French and Irish', might embrace dressed Connemara crab in Irish malt whiskey; rack of lamb with port and redcurrant; lemon cake with mascarpone. Served at about 8 pm, at separate tables, the four-course set meals offer no choice, but a vegetarian alternative is available. With a dairy farm next door, all meat and fish is local, and eggs are free-range. The surrounding grounds are being planted with trees, and a croquet lawn is planned. You can take a cruise on huge Lough Corrib, or roam in the wide grounds of mighty Ashford Castle, now a large luxury hotel: among its guests, President Reagan stayed here while seeking out his forebears. Parts of *The Quiet Man* were filmed at Corrib village. (*Holger and Brigitte Wulf*)

Open All year.
Rooms 3 double.
Facilities Reception hall, sitting room, dining room. No background music. 7-acre grounds: 1-acre garden. Lake, fishing nearby. Unsuitable for ♿.
Location 2 miles E of Cong. From Galway city, take N84 to Headford, R334 to Cross. House on right ¾ mile further, towards Cong.
Restrictions No smoking: dining room, bedrooms. No children under 12. Dogs by arrangement, not in public rooms.
Credit cards Amex, MasterCard, Visa.
Terms B&B: single IR£60–£75, double IR£75–£98. Set dinner IR£25. 1-night bookings sometimes refused.

The *Guide* takes no free hospitality and no advertisements.

STELLO Co. Galway   **Map 6:C4**

rmoyle Lodge   *Tel* (+353) (0)91-786111
Fax (+353) (0)91-786154
Email fermoylelodge@eircom.net
Website fermoylelodge.com

Secluded in a lovely setting amid trees and heather, beside Fermoyle Lake on the south side of Connemara, this small hotel was built in the late 19th century as a sporting lodge. Found 'wonderful' by recent visitors, it has 'engaging young owners', Nicola Stronach and her husband Jean-Pierre Maire (he is chef). They 'provide intimate hospitality, yet space and privacy'. Bedrooms are 'well laid out yet simple' (they have antiques and original paintings). 'I revelled in the luxury of the thick duvets, and the views.' 'Our room faced the garden, river and lough: the distant Twelve Pins completed the wild and tumbling view.' The dining room has huge windows overlooking spectacular scenery. The lakeside setting can bring midges in the late summer. The three-course set dinner (24 hours' notice is required) is served at 7.30. A typical menu this year: fresh local langoustine in Pernod vinaigrette; fillet of Irish beef with wild mushrooms; orange and lemon tart. After dinner, coffee and drinks are taken by a wood fire in a sitting room, where guests are joined by their hosts, 'who clearly enjoy their work'. 'They cater for the serious fisherman, while also offering all the creature comforts a non-fisherperson could want.' Good lough and sea fishing is nearby. Five golf courses are within 90 minutes' drive, and trips can be made to the Aran Islands. (*FG*)

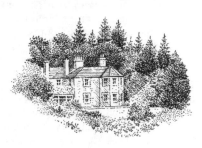

Open Apr–Oct.
Rooms 6 double. No telephone/TV. 2 ground-floor rooms in adjoining mews.
Facilities 2 sitting rooms, dining room. No background music. 11-acre garden leading to lough. Sea, sandy beaches, fishing, golf nearby.
Location From Galway, take N59 towards Clifden. Left before bridge in Oughterard, follow signs for Costello for 11 miles; lodge on right. Bus: Costello or Oughterard; taxi.
Restrictions No smoking: dining room, bedrooms. Unsuitable for young children. No dogs.
Credit cards MasterCard, Visa.
Terms B&B IR£45–£75. Set dinner IR£25.

****

Traveller's tale Hotel in Cardiff. I noticed a mouse scurrying across the car park. It disappeared through an open door of the kitchen. The area around the kitchen was distinctly unhygienic. Discarded food littered the ground round the dustbins.

****

CROSSMOLINA Co. Mayo   **Map 6**

Enniscoe House	*Tel* (+353) (0)96-311
Castlehill	*Fax* (+353) (0)96-317

Email mail@enniscoe.co
Website www.enniscoe.cor

'It was wonderful, full of family history,' said one enthusiastic report
on this handsome Georgian country house which the Kelletts have
owned for centuries. It stands in large grounds beside Lough Conn, not
far from Ballina, where former president Mary Robinson grew up and
her family still lives. Today, Susan Kellett runs it as a private hotel;
she has much redecorated it this year. A party of 28, including
14 children under ten, spent three nights here over the New Year: 'We
all found Mrs Kellett, her son and staff, to be helpful, efficient and
friendly. The food was excellent, particularly the leisurely breakfasts.'
The setting is peaceful, and there are nice views over the lake. 'We
enjoyed sitting in front of the peat fire after a long walk, with a drink,
anticipating a great dinner.' The menu, with limited choice, is Irish
country house cooking, eg, kidneys in mustard sauce; casserole of
spring lamb; sticky toffee pudding. Behind the house's plain facade
are elegant 18th-century plasterwork, a sweeping staircase, and two
large sitting rooms with their original furniture, family portraits and
bookcases; family memorabilia are everywhere, and polished wood
floors with rugs. Some bedrooms, with a comfortable four-poster, are
huge; only three overlook the lough. There's a working farm on the
estate, an organic vegetable garden which supplies the kitchen, a
walled garden with a tea room, and a resident fishing manager – brown
trout can be caught in the lough; other fishing is nearby. Mrs Kellett
also runs a heritage centre, helping returning emigrants to trace their
Irish roots; it includes a museum of old farm machinery. Nearby are
the great cliffs of north Mayo, and three golf courses. (*MH*)

Open 1 Apr–14 Oct. Dining room closed midday. Groups only for New Year.
Rooms 2 suites, 4 double. 1 on ground floor. No TV. Self-catering units
behind house.
Facilities 2 sitting rooms, dining room. No background music. 150-acre
estate: garden, tea room, farm, heritage centre, lake frontage, fishing (tuition,
ghillie). Golf, riding, cycling, shooting nearby. Unsuitable for &.
Location 2 miles S of Crossmolina on R315 to Pontoon and Castlebar.
Train/bus: Ballina, 10 miles; then taxi.
Restrictions No smoking: restaurant, 2 bedrooms. Dogs by arrangement.
Credit cards Amex, MasterCard, Visa.
Terms B&B IR£56–£78; D,B&B IR£84–£106. Set dinner IR£28. 10% dis-
count for 3 or more nights. Child in parents' room: under 2, free; 2–12, 50% of
adult rate.

****

> **Traveller's tale** Hotel in Cornwall. The hotel bore no resem-
> blance to *Fawlty Towers*, but there was more than a hint of Basil
> and Sybil about the proprietors. Accusatory comments, *sotto
> voce*, could be heard from behind the bar. The garden was
> watered copiously, regardless of relaxing visitors. Best of all
> was an audible mutter: 'Bloody guests.'

****

ERRY Co. Londonderry   Map 6:B6

Beech Hill House   Tel 028-7134 9279
32 Ardmore Road   Fax 028-7134 5366
Derry BT47 3QP   Email info@beech-hill.com
                                Website www.beech-hill.com

One of the most admired hotels in the North, with 'warm and always friendly service', *Beech Hill* was built in 1729 as the private home of a sea captain. It is now owned by local people, Mr Donnelly and Mrs O'Kane, and is managed by Crawford McIlwaine, all of them 'full of kindness'. The handsome pale pink house stands outside the interesting and attractive town of Derry, in a large park with ponds, waterfalls, birds and wildlife and beech trees. Celebrities often visit (Senator Edward Kennedy came recently) and locals use the big bar as a kind of pub. 'The bedrooms were comfortable, warm and tastefully furnished, partly with antiques,' says a recent guest. They are bright and spacious, and many have lovely views. The *Ardmore Restaurant* (with bare floor and pine-clad ceiling), open all day, looks over the landscaped gardens. Here Adrian Catterall's cooking, much enjoyed, is 'classical French with a modern Irish influence', and is based on fresh local beef, poultry and game, and home-grown vegetables. There is a short vegetarian menu. Light lunches are served, and a hefty Ulster Fry at breakfast, for those who wish it. Breads at all meals 'are superb'. The private chapel, on the first floor, can be used for christenings, wedding blessings and mass. The lovely scenery of Donegal is just across the border, and this is a good base for exploring the Antrim coast. (*SWH*)

Open All year, except 24/25 Dec.
Rooms 4 suites, 22 double, 1 single. 1 with access for ♿.
Facilities Lift. Lounge, morning room, bar, restaurant; conference facilities; fitness club; chapel. Classical background music all day in public areas. 32-acre grounds: tennis, ponds, waterfall. Fishing, golf, sailing, flying nearby.
Location 2 miles SE of Derry, off Belfast road (signposted to right). Car park.
Restriction No dogs.
Credit cards Amex, MasterCard, Visa.
Terms B&B: single £80, double £100–£120, suite £150. Set lunch £18.95, dinner £28.95; full alc £40. 2- and 3-day breaks. Christmas package.

DINGLE Co. Kerry   Map 6:D4

Benners   BUDGET   Tel (+353) (0)66-915 1638
Main Street   Fax (+353) (0)66-915 1412
                               Email benners@eircom.net
                               Website www.bennershotel.com

On the main street of the old fishing port, Thomas Garvey's 'typical small-town hotel' (Best Western), managed by Pat Galvin, is 'unpretentious, convenient, quiet and comfortable', says an inspector in 2001. Behind the 250-year-old facade, it has been renovated and modernised – crystal chandeliers were added this year – but old photographs and repro country furniture maintain a traditional feel. 'All is fresh, and the atmosphere is easy-going. Our quiet bedrooms looked

up the green hill at the back, and were attractive in cream and rush
Our main course at dinner was good, though the waiter was inflexible
House wines came in small screw-top bottles.' The traditional cooking includes local seafood. At breakfast, orange juice was commercial,
but tea, toast and cooked dishes were fine. Our day was made when we
asked for natural yogurt. The waitress replied confidentially: "I am
sorry, but the chefs have used it for their sunburn."' The 'sociable bar'
opens on to Dingle's main street.

Open All year, except 25 Dec.
Rooms 52 double. 2 suitable for &.
Facilities 2 lounges (1 no-smoking), bar, restaurant. Irish/classical back-
ground music in public areas all day. Access to leisure centre at sister hotel;
special rates at championship golf course nearby.
Location Central. Street parking.
Restrictions No smoking: 1 lounge, 1 floor of bedrooms. Guide dogs only.
Credit cards All major cards accepted.
Terms B&B IR£45–£95. Set lunch (Sun) IR£13.50, dinner IR£19.50. Full alc
from IR£22. Child in parents' room: from 50% of adult rate. *V*

Greenmount House   NEW   *Tel* (+353) (0)66-915 1414
John Street   *Fax* (+353) (0)66-915 1974
                                     Email mary@greenmounthouse.com
                                     Website www.greenmounthouse.com

This little fishing-port-cum-resort, 'squeezed between sea and mountains', is a good centre for exploring the lovely Dingle peninsula,
where David Lean filmed *Ryan's Daughter*. Here, John and Mary
Curran's beguiling B&B makes its *Guide* debut: 'It is an extended
bungalow, plus an architect-designed block of luxury bedrooms – all
very neat and pristine outside, with a faintly disconcerting suburban
air. But our room, with oodles of space, gave an excellent impression:
its bottled water and fresh fruit were replenished daily. And the breakfasts were superb: home-made breads and jams, muesli, black-and-
white pudding, smoked salmon, fish, even fried banana. One day,
when we went out early and came back at 10 am, we found bowls of
fruit and cereal in our fridge. Such acts of thoughtfulness, and
Mr Curran's Jeeves-like efficiency, made our stay a real pleasure. For
dinner, there are two seriously good restaurants within walking distance' (*The Chart House* has a *Michelin Bib Gourmand*). The local
crafts are interesting, and the offshore Blasket islands are worth
exploring. (*Tom Mann*)

Open All year, except 10–27 Dec.
Rooms 7 junior suites, 5 double.
Facilities 2 lounges (1 with TV), reading room, breakfast room. No back-
ground music. 1 acre-garden. Unsuitable for &.
Location Central (on quiet cul-de-sac). 2nd right turn after entering Dingle;
house on left.
Restrictions No smoking: breakfast room, bedrooms. No children under 8. No
dogs.
Credit cards MasterCard, Visa.
Terms B&B: single IR£30–£60, double IR£60–£100. 1-night bookings
refused July/Aug.

Anglesea Town House	*Tel* (+353) (0)1-668 3877
63 Anglesea Road	*Fax* (+353) (0)1-668 3461
Ballsbridge, Dublin 4	

South-east of the city centre, on a busy road in select Ballsbridge, is this handsome Edwardian house where Helen Kirrane runs a 'luxurious B&B'. Her 'warm welcome, with tea and apple tart' has recently been admired. 'Our bedroom was large and attractive; the bathroom was modern.' Another visitor wrote of a 'huge, comfy bed and a beautiful vase of roses'. Lavish breakfasts are served in a room with family portraits, an oak table set with fine china and silver: they include fruit compote, baked cereal, porridge, freshly baked breads, kedgeree, sole and salmon. Only drawback: front rooms get traffic noise. The DART station and buses nearby provide transport to the centre. More reports, please.

Open All year.
Rooms 6 double, 1 single.
Facilities Drawing room, breakfast room. No background music. Small garden. Unsuitable for &.
Location 2 miles SE of centre, reached by buses and DART railway. Limited parking.
Restrictions No smoking. No dogs.
Credit cards Amex, MasterCard, Visa.
Terms B&B: single IR£50–£60, double IR£90–£120.

Ashbrook House **NEW**	*Tel/Fax* (+353) (0)1-838 5660
River Road	
Ashtown, Dublin 15	

Five miles NW of centre, near ring road to airport, but quiet: Eve and Stan Mitchell's 'beautiful' Georgian house in big garden, now comfortable and stylish B&B. 'Excellent breakfasts.' TV room. No smoking. Large walled garden, grass tennis court. Closed 20 Dec–1 Jan. MasterCard, Visa accepted. 6 rooms. B&B: single IR£45, double IR£70 [2001].

Belcamp Hutchinson	*Tel* (+353) (0)1-846 0843
Carrs Lane, Malahide Road	*Fax* (+353) (0)1-848 5703
Balgriffin, Dublin 17	

More eulogies came this year for this 'wonderfully hospitable' guest house, a creeper-covered Georgian manor, in a garden with a pond, on the north-east fringe of Dublin. Former home of Francis Hely-Hutchinson, Earl of Donoughmore, it is now very well run by the 'charming' Doreen Gleeson, who co-owns it with Karl Waldburg. 'She introduces all her guests to each other by name, even when they are one-nighters.' 'Warm and spacious rooms with candles and chocolates by the bed, lovely views of well-kept grounds. Doreen, warmly welcoming, even served us breakfast at 5.30 am so we could catch our flight.' 'Very peaceful, with large and comfortable bedrooms', the house has high ceilings, smart furnishings and moulded fireplaces. Breakfasts are 'prodigious, across the Irish and continental range'. Nearby are good bathing beaches and the lovely old village of Malahide. Dublin airport is 15 minutes' drive away. (*Prof. David C Taylor, Miss D Tressider*)

Open All year, except Christmas, 1 week Nov.
Rooms 8 double.
Facilities Drawing room with TV, breakfast room. No background music. 4½-acre garden. Golf, riding, horse racing nearby. Unsuitable for &.
Location 20 mins' drive NE from centre. Take Malahide road, turn left at Balgriffin. Parking. Buses from city.
Restrictions Not suitable for children. No dogs in breakfast room.
Credit cards MasterCard, Visa.
Terms [2001] B&B IR£44.

The Hibernian
Eastmoreland Place
Ballsbridge, Dublin 4

Tel (+353) (0)1-668 7666
Fax (+353) (0)1-660 2655
Email info@hibernianhotel.com
Website www.hibernianhotel.com

'Very enjoyable, with a warm welcome, excellent food and service.' 'Fantastic food, comfort and a friendly atmosphere' – two more thumbs-up (but also one gripe) in 2001 for this peaceful city hotel, managed by David Butt. It inhabits a red brick late Victorian building down a side street in Ballsbridge, about a mile from the centre. Once a nurses' home, it is furnished with bright colours and floral displays. The 'intimate public rooms' are well designed in country house style. Bedrooms are mostly admired, though this year one reader found his much too small, with poor upkeep. He also complained of a 'tasteless' meal. But since then another change of chef has brought Norbert Neylon to the kitchen of the hotel's *Patrick Kavanagh* restaurant (named after the poet). We'd be glad of reports on his 'contemporary Irish' cooking – ambitious dishes such as roast stuffed quail with wild mushrooms in a red wine sauce; fillet of lamb stuffed with foie gras with a courgette clafoutis; passion fruit soufflé. Light meals are served in the lounge. Women on their own are treated well, but tour parties 'can lead to overcrowding at times'. One reader this year felt that the influx of European staff, typical of today's Dublin, was diluting the hotel's 'Irish' atmosphere. Under the same management are the *McCausland Hotel* in Belfast (*qv*) and the *Woodstock Hotel* in Co. Clare. (*ER Lynas, Val Hennessy, WR, and others*)

Open All year, except 24–27 Dec.
Rooms 10 suites, 30 double. 2 adapted for &.
Facilities Lift, ramp. Drawing room, library, sun lounge, conservatory, restaurant; 'easy listening'/classical background music round the clock. Small garden.
Location Off Baggot St Upper, ⅔ mile SE of St Stephen's Green. Private parking. Bus 10 from centre.
Restrictions No smoking: drawing room, 14 bedrooms. Guide dogs only.
Credit cards All major cards accepted.
Terms [2001] (*Excluding 12½% service charge on meals*) Room: single IR£150, double IR£150–£170, suite IR£190. Breakfast IR£12. Set lunch IR£17.95, full alc dinner IR£47. Child in parents' room: under 2, free; 2 and over, 50% of adult rate. *V*

Number 31 `NEW`
31 Leeson Close
Dublin 2

Tel (+353) (0)1-676 5011
Fax (+353) (0)1-676 2929
Email number31@iol.ie
Website www.number31.ei

Noel and Deirdre Comer are the new owners of this unusual B&B hotel, renominated by two readers this year. Set in the heart of Georgian Dublin, it consists of a converted coach house and a Georgian mansion across the garden. The former was once the home of the controversial architect Sam Stephenson, who gutted its centre to create a huge drawing room. This year's reports: 'Noel Comer is hyperactive with the gabbest gift ever, and very welcoming. He addresses you by name from the moment of arrival. We stayed in one of the great Georgian rooms, which had to be spoilt to accommodate a bathroom, but was comfortable.' 'Our luxury room was big enough to play hockey in. Noel is up on what's playing in the local theatres.' Mrs Comer 'cooks a great breakfast': served in the rooftop conservatory, it is an informal affair, taken at 'large, common room-style tables'. Bedrooms vary: some are small, some have thin walls, but those on the street are soundproofed. Some in the new building, where there is no lift, are up several flights of stairs. The 'beautiful yellow Labrador', Homer, is in evidence. (*John Crisp, Jim and Lucy Bowers*)

Open All year.
Rooms 4 suites, 14 double. Some on ground floor.
Facilities Lounge, bar, rooftop conservatory/breakfast room. No background music. Patio garden.
Location Central, off St Stephen's Green. Garage.
Restrictions No smoking: breakfast room, bedrooms. No children under 10.
Credit cards Amex, MasterCard, Visa.
Terms [2001] B&B: single IR£85, double IR£120–£180.

Simmonstown House
Sydenham Road
Ballsbridge, Dublin 4

Tel (+353) (0)1-660 7260
Fax (+353) (0)1-660 7341
Email info@simmonstownhouse.com
Website www.simmonstownhouse.com

'Not cheap, but by far the best place we stayed at on our Irish trip,' say recent admirers of this 'superb B&B', in a quiet cul-de-sac near the sea, a mile or so south-east of the centre. The setting of the terraced house in a side road may be unappealing, 'but James and Finola Curry have smothered it outside with flowers, and added a pretty courtyard garden at the rear'. Inside, 'they have contrived an extremely elegant decor, using bold colours'. The antique-furnished lounge and dining room are painted dark blue, the bedrooms have some Laura Ashley fabrics. 'Our room had twin beds, lots of freshness, all comforts, plus a bathroom with a luxuriously powerful shower. Breakfast was served with exquisite china and silver: a platter of fresh berries with hot croissants and four types of home-made jams, and for my husband the full Irish, with black pudding.' Others wrote of the 'endlessly helpful' hostess, and admired the 'good, mainly modern, paintings'. 'You feel like honoured private guests.' (*PF, and others*)

Open Mid-Jan–mid-Dec.
Rooms 4 double.
Facilities Drawing room, breakfast room. No background music. Patio garden.
½ mile from seafront. Unsuitable for &.
Location 1½ miles SE of centre, in cul-de-sac off Merrion Rd opposite Royal
Dublin Society. Many buses, and DART rail services close by.
Restrictions No smoking. No dogs.
Credit cards Amex, MasterCard, Visa.
Terms B&B IR£45–£65. Child in parents' room: under 2, free; 2–12, 50% of
adult rate. 1-night bookings occasionally refused weekends.

See also SHORTLIST

ENNISCORTHY Co. Wexford   **Map 6:D6**

Salville House   *Tel/Fax* (+353) (0)54-35252
Salville   *Email* info@salvillehouse.com
                                          Website www.salvillehouse.com

'It continues to be my favourite place in Ireland,' says a connoisseur
this year, revisiting Jane and Gordon Parker's small, neat guest
house, 'wonderfully quiet'. A light, bright mid-Victorian building
with large windows and 'beautifully simple' decor, it stands on a hilltop outside the town, with views over the river Slaney and the
Blackstairs Mountains. Rosslare ferry is 30 minutes' drive away. The
Parkers are 'carefully preserving the ambience: no television, no
radio'. The four-course dinner (no choice), served at 8 pm at one long
table by an open fire, is by arrangement. 'Gordon Parker's cooking is
exquisite. His forte is fish, very fresh, and the taste of the food sings
through his wonderful recipes.' Others enjoyed the king prawn tem-
pura, and marinaded squid with peppers, of this 'outstanding culinary
enthusiast', and found his wife 'an all-round friendly person with a
nice Dalmatian, Jack'. No wine licence, no corkage charge.
Bedrooms are 'impeccable', spacious and elegant, even if 'ours was
home-from-home and most unhotel-like: creaky floorboards, eccentric shower, but a "we don't want to get out of it" bed, and stunning
views over the valley. Breakfast was special, with fruit compote
which had fallen straight off the bush.' There are cooked dishes too
(scrambled eggs and smoked salmon, etc), and newspapers.
Enniscorthy has a fine cathedral and 13th-century castle; bird sanctu-
aries, beaches and golf courses are nearby; Wexford is not far.
(*Catherine Fraher, and others*)

Open All year. At Christmas by arrangement only.
Rooms 3 double in house. 2-bedroom apartment (can be self-catering) at rear.
No telephone/TV.
Facilities Drawing room, dining room. No background music. 5-acre grounds:
tennis, badminton. Golf nearby; beach, bird sanctuary 10 miles. Unsuitable
for &.
Location 2 miles S of town. Take N11 to Wexford. 1st left after hospital;
uphill, bear left. Entrance sign on left. Train/bus to Enniscorthy; taxi.
Restrictions No smoking in bedrooms. Dogs by arrangement; not in house.
Credit cards None accepted.

erms [2001] B&B IR£27.50–£35. Set dinner IR£22.50. Child in parents' oom: under 1, free; 1–12, half price.

FERRYCARRIG Co. Wexford   **Map 6:D6**

Slaney Manor   BUDGET   *Tel* (+353) (0)53-20051
                                       Fax (+353) (0)53-20510
                                       Email slaneymanor@eircom.net
                                       Website www.new-zealands.com/slaney

A mud-walled cabin with guest bedroom and bathroom, and a murdered British minister in the founding family, make this an intriguing entry. It is a stone manor house deep in the country near Wexford, built in the 1820s by the Anglo-Irish Perceval family (Spencer Perceval was killed by a madman in the House of Commons in 1812). Our reporter found the place 'delightful and peaceful', well restored by its owners, Esther and James Caulfield. 'They are charming and attentive, and their prices are very reasonable, even at Wexford festival time,' runs an endorsement this year. Some bedrooms have a four-poster; many have 'wonderful views' over the Slaney estuary; some are in a converted building on a courtyard. 'The owners take real pride in their home', which they call 'a pre-Famine time capsule' – being tradition-minded, they have installed in the large grounds an 18th-century mud-walled cabin, 'a typical residence of the native Irish' in former days. Mrs Caulfield's simple no-choice meals use local produce (eg, wild mushroom and garlic soup; roast beef with red wine jus): we'd be glad of reports. The cooked breakfasts and coffee are 'very good', though marmalade and butter 'are packaged'. Wine is available until 11 pm in the large 'common room'. A conservatory is new. Nearby are an Irish National Heritage Park, a museum of the John F Kennedy family, good walks amid plenty of wildlife, and plenty of pubs. (*Richard Parish, KH*)

Open All year, except Christmas. Dining room closed midday, and to non-residents.
Rooms 2 suites, 36 double. 26 in courtyard, 1 in mud cabin. Some on ground floor (some have facilities for &). Telephone in manor house bedrooms only.
Facilities Lift. Sitting room, dining room, conservatory, courtyard. No background music. 150-acre grounds: woodland walks. River: fishing, boating nearby.
Location 3 miles W of Wexford, on N25, near junction with N11.
Restrictions No smoking. No dogs.
Credit cards All major cards accepted.
Terms B&B: single IR£35–£75, double IR£50–£110, suite IR£110–£140. Set dinner (5 courses) IR£25–£30. 10% reduction for extended stays. Reduced rates for children.

GALWAY   **Map 6:C5**

Norman Villa   *Tel* (+353) (0)91-521131 and 521380
86 Lower Salthill   *Fax* (+353) (0)91-521131
                              Email normanvilla@oceanfree.net

Galway is the liveliest Irish town outside Dublin. A focus for the young and the artistic, it has many fringe theatres, musical pubs, folksy bistros, and a big summer arts festival. A mile from the centr⌐ this restored Victorian coach house is run as a B&B by Mark and De⌐ Keogh. 'The finest inn we found in Ireland,' one couple thought it. 'The beautiful breakfast is garnished with edible flowers from the dazzling garden.' Others said: 'We loved this place.' Not luxurious, it is run 'with the emphasis on quality and personal attention'. It is 'like an art gallery', with contemporary paintings (lots of nudes) and sculpture in the public rooms and bedrooms, along with old pine furniture and unusual decorative rustic items. 'Good crisp linen on antique brass beds' (but some rooms, baths and wardrobes are small). The copious breakfast includes home-made muesli and 'superb porridge'. The Keoghs will help you plan day trips to Connemara, the Burren and the spectacular cliffs of Moher. Limited parking space in the courtyard. (*KC and SW*)

Open 1 Feb–30 Nov.
Rooms 6 double. No telephone/TV.
Facilities Drawing room, breakfast room (jazz/classical background music). ¼-acre garden. Sandy beach, river, fishing nearby. Unsuitable for &.
Location 1 mile W of centre. Follow signs for Salthill, then Lower Salthill. Limited courtyard parking.
Restrictions No smoking: breakfast room, bedrooms. No children under 6. No dogs.
Credit cards MasterCard, Visa.
Terms B&B: IR£37.50–£50. Child in parents' room: under 12, 25% discount.

GLASLOUGH Co. Monaghan   Map 6:B6

Castle Leslie	*Tel* (+353) (0)47-88109
Glaslough	*Fax* (+353) (0)47-88256
	Email ultan@castle-leslie.ie
	Website www.castle-leslie.ie

A famously eccentric hotel. 'Outrageous but amusing', it has been called; 'so extraordinary it is almost shocking'. A hefty Victorian castle in a vast estate near the Border, it was built in 1878 by the titled Leslie family, who claim descent from Attila the Hun and have lived on the site since 1661. Crammed with Victoriana and hand-me-downs from the Churchill family (relatives by marriage), it has changed little, save for the addition of modern comforts, and is run in high Victorian style, with a great sense of fun. Sir John, the fourth baronet, now 83, presides, but the place is run by his 'charismatic' niece Samantha (Sammy) (the last of the line) and her husband, Ultan Bannon. Meals are served in the candlelit banqueting hall by waitresses in Victorian dress. The new young chef, Noel McMeel, has worked in Paris and the USA, and this year his 'modern Irish' cooking was enjoyed – roast quail, followed by red snapper with a spiced couscous, sun-dried tomato and tarragon dressing. Or you could try wild mushroom and goat's cheese tart; white chocolate soup with a blueberry cookie. 'An off-beat Oz wine, a Tarrango, was good value. A pseudo-theatrical troupe, the Plurabelles, entertained us with Joyce and Beckett during and after dinner.' The huge public rooms have fine old tapestries, suits of armour, and other heirlooms – a painted Della Robbia fireplace from a chapel in Florence, a harp given by Wordsworth, an emerald bracelet from the Empress of China. As for bedrooms, one reader's was 'mind-blowing in its uniqueness, with deep green walls, teddy bears, painted furniture'. One room has a big four-poster with heavy velvet drapes, and a wooden 'thunderbox' loo. Some rooms are intentionally comic, some 'truly beautiful'; in the former nursery, a vast doll's house facade conceals the bathroom. Lighting can be poor. Business seminars are held; also tourist banquets, at the end of which Sammy, in hooded cloak, tells ghost stories of the house. The dogs will take you for a walk in the grounds. So will the 'dryly amusing' Sir John. He acts in the film, recently made at the Castle, of Spike Milligan's classic novel *Puckoon*. Ten more bedrooms are being added this year. (*Simon and Pearl Willbourn, RW*)

Open All year.
Rooms 4 suites, 9 double, 1 single. 10 more by 2002. No telephone/TV, etc.
Facilities Drawing room, dining room, gallery; conference/function facilities. No background music. 1,000-acre grounds: 14-acre pleasure gardens, tennis, wildlife, lakes, boating, fishing. Unsuitable for &.
Location On N edge of Glaslough village, 6 miles NE of Monaghan town.
Restrictions Smoking in drawing room only. No children under 18. No dogs in house (kennels available).
Credit cards MasterCard, Visa.
Terms [2001] D,B&B: double IR£135–£240. Single room supplement IR£20. Gourmet lunch IR£55. Set dinner IR£31.50; full alc IR£39. Christmas/New Year packages. 1-night bookings refused weekends.

GLENCAIRN Co. Waterford   **Map 6:D5**

Buggys Glencairn Inn   *Tel/Fax* (+353) (0)58-56232
Glencairn, Tallow   *Email* buggysglencairninn@eircom.net
                                                    Website lismore.com

César award: Irish inn of the year

'It is delightful in every way,' runs an inspector's glowing report in 2001 on this small pink house (1720) in a hamlet below the Knockmealdown Mountains. Run as a B&B, inn and restaurant by its owners, Ken and Kathleen Buggy ('interesting talkers'), it has always enchanted readers. 'It is comfortable, friendly and quaint; sparklingly clean, with good service, excellent food. It is beside the road, but very peaceful. The door is unlocked, there is no bell, you just push. The dog (or two) may receive you. The host or hostess will carry your bags up the steep stairs. The decor includes a vast amount of memorabilia/Victoriana which was earlier displayed in the Buggys' former guesthouse, *The Old Presbytery* at Kinsale. The host's drawings, cartoons and paintings are everywhere. No sitting or lounge area. In the dining room/bar are red-and-white gingham cloths, and beams hung with all imaginable pieces of brass. Copper vessels gleam in the firelight. Mirrors abound. All food was fresh, and guests are met by the appetising smell of dinner. Ken Buggy's dishes included very good marinated herring pâté, various seafood in puff pastry, exquisite brill, quail in jus, plum crumble with almonds. Fish is delivered straight from Helvick harbour. Breakfast includes fresh fruit salad, excellent porridge, smoked salmon, perfect scrambled egg, outstanding home-made breads. Bedrooms are somewhat small, but well heated; beds blissfully comfortable. My room was fascinating; pictures every-where. The style of the place includes some eccentricities which one might expect, like crooked walls, creaky boards in sloping floors. Probably the most relaxed place I have ever stayed in – amid quiet country where walks can lead to fields full of rabbits and flowers, with birdsong everywhere.' 'We are a quiet inn, not a noisy pub,' write the Buggys. In the low-ceilinged rooms, the brass beds have patchwork quilts. The Blackwater river and the old fortified port of Youghal are not far off.

Open All year, except Christmas.
Rooms 5 double. No telephone.
Facilities Bar, 2 dining rooms (background jazz/classical music at night – switched off on request). ½-acre grounds. Fishing nearby. Unsuitable for ♿.
Location By crossroads in Glencairn hamlet, off R627, between Lismore and Tallow (both 3 miles).
Restrictions No smoking in bedrooms. No children under 8. No dogs in restaurant.
Credit cards MasterCard, Visa.
Terms (*Excluding 10% service charge*) B&B IR£33–£48; D,B&B IR£60–£75. Full alc IR£34. ***V***

GLIN Co. Limerick   **Map 6:D4**

Glin Castle   *Tel* (+353) (0)68-34173
                                   Fax (+353) (0)68-34364
                                   Email knight@iol.ie
                                   Website www.glincastle.com

'We could not have been better looked after. The staff were extremely friendly and professional. Our room had views across the river; we walked in the wonderful gardens. Everything was done to make us feel at home.' Set by the banks of the Shannon estuary, in a large wooded estate with formal gardens and a dairy farm, this magnificent Georgian Gothic castle stands on the site of a former medieval one. It is the country seat of Desmond and Olda FitzGerald. His family has owned the land for 800 years, and he is the 29th Knight of Glin (nicknamed 'Knightie'). Bob Duff is his manager. The interiors are impressive, with original plasterwork, family antiques, secret doorways, Corinthian pillars, and an unusual flying staircase. The drawing room has an Adam ceiling and huge windows facing the garden. Dinner is served in the formal dining room with baronial oak furniture and family portraits. The guest bedrooms are lavishly done, with *chaises longues*, blue-and-white porcelain plates on walls, and views of the river or the garden. Despite the grandeur, the castle 'has a welcoming feel'. 'You are looked after on a very personal basis.' The cooking is 'superb': 'imaginative dishes use the best of ingredients'. The set menu offers two choices for each course, dishes like spinach and mushroom strudel; grilled monkfish with a lime, honey and chilli glaze. Many ingredients are grown on the estate. Breakfasts are excel-lent too, with 'wonderful summer berry compote'. Once a week there is live Irish music in the main hall. Glin village, with its very pretty pub, is at the gate. (*John Vigar*)

Open 16 Mar–9 Nov.
Rooms 2 suites, 13 double. 3 in castle wing.
Facilities Drawing room (classical background music evenings), sitting room, library, dining room. 500-acre estate: 5-acre garden, parkland, dairy farm, tennis, croquet, shooting, tea/craft shop, clay-pigeon shooting. On Shannon estuary: boating, fishing; golf nearby. Unsuitable for &.
Location On edge of village 32 miles W of Limerick. Bus: Foynes, 7 miles.
Restrictions No smoking in public rooms, except sitting room. No children under 10. No dogs in house (kennels available).
Credit cards All major cards accepted.
Terms B&B double IR£190–£300. Set lunch IR£23, dinner IR£35. Weekend midweek rates in low season. Can be taken over by house party (max. 20 people).

GOREY Co. Wexford   **Map 6:D6**

| Marlfield House | *Tel* (+353) (0)55-21124 |
| Courtown Road | *Fax* (+353) (0)55-21572 |

Email info@marlfieldhouse.ie
Website www.marlfieldhouse.com

❦ *César award in 1996*

'Much enjoyed' again this year, Mary and Ray Bowe's sophisticated country house hotel (Relais & Châteaux) stands in 14 hectares of woodlands and beautiful gardens, two miles from a sandy beach. Once the main Irish residence of the Earls of Courtown, it is a fine Regency building, with white easy chairs on its neat lawns, also a herb garden, a wildfowl reserve, and a lake with ducks, geese and black swans. The entrance is impressive, with goldfish ponds and a peacock, Kane, by the front door; inside are smart antique furniture, spectacular flower displays. The luxurious best bedrooms have antiques, dramatic wallpapers and curtains, hand-embroidered sheets, real lace pillows, a splendid marble bathroom; but some rooms are small, and not all have a good view. The dining room, with its large domed conservatory extension, frescoes and silver, is 'a glorious place to eat'. Service can be slow, but chef Henry Stone's cooking is always admired. His elaborate dishes might embrace terrine of foie gras and confit rabbit leg; fried fillet of beef with sautéed oyster mushrooms; chocolate marquise with a brunoise of mango. Herbs, vegetables and fruit are grown in the gardens. Light lunches are served in the library, and 'excellent breakfasts' include a generous buffet. Despite *Marlfield*'s grandeur, children and dogs are welcomed. 'Mrs Mary Bowe, entertaining and welcoming to the manner born, makes every effort to have personal contact with her guests', and her junior staff are 'delightful and extremely helpful'. (*Prof. TM and Dr Eirlys Hayes*)

Open All year, except mid-Dec–31 Jan.
Rooms 6 state rooms, 12 double, 2 single. Some on ground floor.
Facilities Reception hall, drawing room, library/bar, restaurant with conservatory. No background music. 36-acre grounds: gardens, tennis, croquet, wildfowl reserve, lake. Sea, sandy beaches, safe bathing 2 miles. Fishing, golf, horse riding nearby.

Location 1 mile from Gorey on Courtown road, R742. Train: Gorey, from Dublin/Waterford.
Restrictions No smoking: restaurant, bedrooms. Dogs by arrangement, with own basket in bedrooms; not in public rooms.
Credit cards All major cards accepted.
Terms B&B: single IR£90–£100, double IR£170–£190, state room IR£325–£550. Set lunch IR£26, dinner IR£41. 1-night bookings sometimes refused Sat.

HOLYWOOD Co. Down   Map 6:B6

Rayanne Country House   *Tel/Fax* 028-9042 5859
60 Demesne Road
Holywood BT18 9EX

In affluent coastal suburb, 5 miles E of Belfast (bus or train to centre): Anne McClelland's small upmarket hotel (her son Mark is chef), set back from road in ³/₄-acre garden. Lavish Victorian decor, 2 lounges, large bedrooms, friendly staff – 'atmosphere of welcome and culture'. Good dinners (24 hours' notice needed). Award-winning breakfasts with unusual dishes, eg, raspberry porridge, prune soufflé. No smoking: breakfast room, 1 lounge, bedrooms. No background music. MasterCard, Visa accepted. 7 bedrooms (1 family). B&B £35–£55. More reports, please.

INISTIOGE Co. Kilkenny   Map 6:D5

Cullintra House   `BUDGET`   *Tel* (+353) (0)51-423614
The Rower   *Email* cullhse@indigo.ie
                                         Website http://indigo.ie/~cullhse

🐾 *César award in 2001*

'Unusual, eccentric, quixotic. Hospitable, and that's not just the lovely log fire, and the offer of cream tea on arrival. Even the six cats, one with only three legs and a minute tail, do their best to welcome you by curling up on your lap. We were invited out to the yard to see Sally, the fox, having her grub. A great experience, and such wonderful value.' Last year's *César* was for 'utterly enjoyable mild eccentricity' – well deserved, according to the many admirers of the exuberant Patricia Cantlon. Her family has owned this handsome 18th-century farmhouse, 'where honest, affordable accommodation teams up with pure theatre', for 100 years. It stands quietly at the end of a long drive amid farmland, at the foot of Mount Brandon. Ms Cantlon is hostess, chef, entertainer and artist (her paintings fill the house, and are for sale). 'Some adjustment of one's internal clock' may be necessary, as the leisurely candlelit dinners (good French-influenced home cooking, communally served) are scheduled for 9 pm, but may take place much later: 'It was nearly 1 am before pudding was brought, followed by Patricia's Irish homilies and a sing-song.' Breakfast is served till midday ('preferably not before 10.30 if you want bacon and eggs'). Children are given an early supper 'and then to bed'. The bedrooms are 'delightfully pretty and individual', in plush-rustic style, with period furnishings, but the *en suite* showers are simple, and the only bathroom is communal. There is a conservatory studio with a piano, where guests can have fun. The hostess will accept guests' dogs only if she is certain that they will behave. No licence; bring your own wine. Inistioge has a tree-lined square beside a fine stone bridge. The grounds of the local estate, Woodstock, are open to the public. Nearby Kilkenny is a picturesque town, with a splendid historic castle. (*James Kavanagh*)

Open All year.
Rooms 6 double. 3 with bath, 1 with shower. 2 in barn. No telephone/TV.
Facilities Drawing room, dining room, studio conservatory. No background music. 230-acre grounds: 1-acre garden, woodland, private path to Brandon Hill with 4,000-year-old cairn. River bathing, fishing nearby. Unsuitable for &.
Location 6 miles NW of New Ross, off New Ross–Kilkenny road. Take turning E (signposted); hotel 1 mile. Bus to main road (1 mile) once a day.
Restrictions No smoking: dining room, gallery. Dogs by arrangement.
Credit cards MasterCard, Visa (3% extra).
Terms B&B: single IR£33–£43, double IR£46–£60. Set dinner IR£18–£20. 10% reduction for children. Christmas package. 1-night bookings refused weekends.

KANTURK Co. Cork   **Map 6:D4**

Assolas Country House   *Tel* (+353) (0)29-50015
Kanturk   *Fax* (+353) (0)29-50795
                                   Email assolas@eircom.net
                                   Website www.assolas.com

❧ *César award in 1995*

'The house-party atmosphere, over a pre-dinner drink in the lounge' has been especially enjoyed at this handsome creeper-covered 17th-century manor house, set in lovely grounds, with a grass tennis court, a lake and a weir. It has been the Bourke family's home for over 70 years, and since the 1970s they have welcomed guests ('we are not a hotel,' they point out). Joe Bourke and his widowed father are front-of-house, his wife Hazel is the chef. Also admired: 'Joe's warm sense of humour, the fabulous breakfasts, the swans, five cats and a dog or two.' 'The food, oh, the food – notably the tomato tarte Tatin.' 'The house and grounds are lovely, the housekeeping is impeccable, and our room in the courtyard was pleasant.' The bedrooms are large and quite plainly furnished, but very comfortable. Some bathrooms are 'magnificent, with a whirlpool bath'. 'Everything is presented so elegantly. One feels utterly pampered.' Afternoon tea, with lemon or chocolate cake, is served in the garden or by a log fire. There is sparkling glass in the dining room, and damask napkins. The 'progressive Irish' cooking

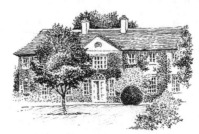

puts its accent on fish, shellfish and local meat, eg, baked brill with olive oil and herbs; roast duck with apricot and pineapple stuffing; rhubarb and strawberry crumble. The soups and sauces are much admired; and the wine list is well chosen. Many herbs and vegetables come from the house's organic garden. Good hill-walking and forest walks are nearby, also Millstreet Country Park and Annesgrove Gardens at Castletownroche. (*AD*)

Open Mid-Mar–1 Nov. Whole house booking only, New Year. Dining room closed midday.
Rooms 9 double. 3 in courtyard annexe, 20 yds. No TV.
Facilities Hall, drawing room, dining room; private dining room. No background music. 15-acre grounds: gardens, tennis, croquet, river, boating, trout fishing. Salmon fishing, golf nearby. Unsuitable for &.
Location 3½ miles NE of Kanturk; turn off N72 Mallow–Killarney towards Buttevant.
Restrictions No children under 8 at dinner. No dogs in house (accommodation in stables).
Credit cards MasterCard, Visa.
Terms [2001] B&B: single IR£70–£75, double IR£120–£170. Set dinner IR£30. Child in parents' room: 25% of adult rate. 1-night bookings sometimes refused. *V* (low season)

## KENMARE Co. Kerry					Map 6:D4

Hawthorn House		BUDGET			*Tel* (+353) (0)64-41035
Shelbourne Street					*Fax* (+353) (0)64-41932
						Email hawthorn@eircom.net

Noel and Mary O'Brien (she has 'a bubbly sense of humour') are the friendly owners of this sympathetic B&B, much admired for its 'excellent' bedrooms and good value. It stands inside this small resort town at the east end of the Ring of Kerry, and makes a contrast with our two other Kenmare entries, grand and pricey. Tea and cake are served in the drawing room to arriving guests; bedrooms, of different shapes and sizes, are all 'cheerful, welcoming and pretty', nicely furnished in pine, with fresh fruit and flowers. Most have a shower rather than a bath. Breakfast, in a room decorated in pink, is good, with freshly made porridge and Irish fries. Plenty of restaurants are nearby. And you can take a long scenic walk along the Kerry Way. More reports welcome.

Open All year, except Christmas.
Rooms 7 double, 1 single. No telephone.
Facilities TV lounge, breakfast room (mixed background music). Sea ¼ mile; walking, cycling, golf, water sports, fishing nearby. Unsuitable for &.
Location On S edge of village, close to centre. Private parking.
Restrictions No smoking: restaurant, bedrooms. No dogs.
Credit cards MasterCard, Visa.
Terms B&B IR£22–£28.

> The Irish punt and the pound sterling do not have the same value. Be sure to check the exchange rate. And remember that from the beginning of 2002 Ireland will be using the euro.

Park Hotel Kenmare   *Tel* (+353) (0)64-41200
                                          Fax (+353) (0)64-41402
                                          Email info@parkkenmare.com
                                          Website www.parkkenmare.com

More plaudits this year for the *Park*, one of two very grand country
hotels, both Relais & Châteaux, both with four red gables in *Michelin,*
that stand on the edge of this attractive but touristy village, amid fine
mountain scenery on the Ring of Kerry. The *Park*, owned and run by
the Brennan family, has a peaceful parkland setting, with lovely views
of the Kenmare estuary and the west Cork mountains. Outwardly, the
long grey building (built in the 19th century by the Great Southern and
Western Railway Company as an overnight stop for the gentry) is no
beauty, but inside are elegant public rooms with open fires, sculptures,
'dazzling paintings' and flowers. 'No conference centre or other dis-
tractions, to detract from the well-being of guests,' say the Brennans.
And most visitors enjoy it greatly. 'I had two excellent dinners and a
splendid room. Room service was very prompt. Even at 6.30 am, the
breakfast tray was embellished with a vase of flowers.' The restaurant
and lounges look over the sea. A terrace for tea has just been added, and
verandas for 15 rooms. The 'gorgeous' bedrooms have smart antiques
and fine china; some bathrooms are 'splendid', but others can be poorly
lit. The staff are 'delightful', 'truly professional'. The chef, Joe Ryan,
provides 'modern Irish cooking with French influences' (eg, honey-
roasted quail on potato pancake with French bean salad; caramelised
breast of duck on a noodle salad with pickled ginger jus). 'The food is
terrific', the bar is 'most pleasing'. The lounge is enlivened at night by
the 'charming in-house pianist'. In the large grounds there are tennis,
croquet and garden walks; Kenmare golf course is adjacent, and fishing with a ghillie can be arranged. 'At meals, no one said, every time
they brought a course, "You're welcome", or "No problem", or
"Enjoy!" – our bugbears.' (*Esler Crawford, Jean and George Dundas*)

Open 13 Apr–29 Oct; 23 Dec–2 Jan.
Rooms 9 suites, 36 double, 4 single.
Facilities Lift, ramps. Lounge (classical background music all day; pianist at
night), bar, restaurant; terrace; fitness suite. 12-acre grounds: tennis, croquet;
18-hole golf course adjacent. Rock beach, safe bathing, water sports 5 mins'
walk; fishing, horse riding arranged. Civil wedding facilities.
Location 60 miles W of Cork, adjacent to village. Signposted. Train:
Killarney/bus: Kenmare; then taxi.
Restriction No smoking: restaurant, bedrooms. No dogs in building (kennels
in grounds).
Credit cards All major cards accepted.
Terms [2001] B&B IR£132–£262. Set lunch IR£10–£20, dinner IR£44; full
alc IR£47. Christmas, New Year packages.

Sheen Falls Lodge   *Tel* (+353) (0)64-41600
                                          Fax (+353) (0)64-41386
                                          Email info@sheenfallslodge.ie
                                          Website www.sheenfallslodge.ie

A large Cromwellian manor house, much extended, is now a luxurious
resort hotel (Relais & Châteaux), again this year judged 'superb'. It

stands in wide grounds of woods and fields beside the Sheen Falls, with glorious views of Kenmare Bay. With a Danish owner, and under Adriaan Bartels's management, it has a cosmopolitan ambience: yet 'the welcome and impeccable service are wonderfully Irish, and the atmosphere is family-like'. A guest found the staff 'incredibly kind and helpful' and the food 'excellent', notably the breakfast buffet with fresh fruit, porridge, cold meats, etc. In the *Cascade* restaurant (with live piano music), Chris Farrell's ambitious 'modern Irish' dishes could include hot foie gras with braised apple and wild mushrooms; Irish beef on grilled polenta with truffle-scented cream; pistachio soufflé with rum and raisin ice cream. A bar/bistro, overlooking the falls, is named for Oscar, the heron resident on the river. It is open from 6 am to 10 pm, and serves children's suppers. The public rooms are 'cosy and delightful'. The 'wonderful library' has up-to-date magazines such as the *New Yorker*, and books in many languages. The bedrooms are huge, with crisp linen sheets and duvets, a CD-player, and a large marble bathroom. Outdoor pursuits include golf, waterskiing and riding. There is a health spa with beauty treatments, and a thalassotherapy centre; also a discreet conference centre. Guided hill-walks are arranged, and guests are sometimes taken sightseeing in the hotel's 1936 Buick convertible. Or they are shown the wine cellars, with over 950 different varieties. More reports, please.

Open 2 Feb–2 Jan.
Rooms 9 suites, 52 double. 1 adapted for &. Self-catering cottage in grounds.
Facilities Lift, ramps. 2 lounges, billiard room, study, library, bar/bistro, restaurant; health and fitness centre: swimming pool, spa bath, sauna, gym, beauty treatments; extensive business facilities. Background music in public areas all day; piano nightly. 300-acre grounds: river, fishing, riding, croquet, tennis, clay-pigeon shooting; hill-walking with local guide. Golf, lake/river fishing, windsurfing, boating nearby; sea 6 miles.
Location 1½ miles SE of Kenmare, just off N71 to Glengariff. Bus from Kenmare.
Restrictions No smoking bar/bistro, 10 bedrooms. No dogs in house.
Credit cards All major cards accepted.
Terms [2001] Room: single/double IR£180–£295, suite IR£310–£450. Breakfast IR£12–£17. Set dinner £42. Spring rates. Christmas package.

Shelburne Lodge   NEW   *Tel* (+353) (0)64-41013
Cork Road   *Fax* (+353) (0)64-42135
                              Email shelburne@kenmare.com

'Heartily recommended' this year, Maura and Tom O'Connell-Foley's stylish B&B is a 1740s house, on the eastern edge of Kenmare. 'Set back from the road, with spacious grounds, it is quiet. The interior is elegant: polished wooden floors, rugs, real fires. Spotlessly clean. Tea and cakes offered on arrival. Amazing breakfasts, with fish, and different choice of fresh fruit each day, eg, melon with strawberries. The owners' restaurant in town, *Packies* (about five minutes' walk), is excellent, with friendly staff. Need to book, as it's very popular.' (*Mr and Mrs MC Bradshaw*)

Open Mar–Nov. *Packies* (dinner only) closed Sun, Mon.
Rooms 1 family, 8 double.

Facilities Lounge, breakfast room, restaurant. Garden: tennis.
Location On R569 to Cork, ½ mile E of town centre.
Restrictions No smoking in bedrooms. No dogs.
Credit cards MasterCard, Visa.
Terms [2001] B&B IR£30–£50. *Packies*: full alc IR£26–£36.

KILLEAGH Co. Cork   **Map 6:D5**

Ballymakeigh House   *Tel* (+353) (0)24-95184
Killeagh, nr Youghal   *Fax* (+353) (0)24-95370
                                    Email ballymakeigh@eircom.net
                                Website www. ballymakeighhouse.com

Enjoyed by American visitors in 2001 ('very special: we could not
have been better looked after'), Margaret Browne's old but well-mod-
ernised farmhouse, now a stylish guest house, stands amid the green
fields of prosperous east Cork. 'She, husband Michael and daughter
Kate were much in evidence.' Over the years she has won plenty of
awards: Landlady of the Year, Housewife of the Year, Farm Guest
House of the Year, and she has published a best-selling cookbook. She
serves lunches in the farmhouse, and dinners in her restaurant,
Browne's, two miles away, beside her equestrian centre. Here, she
offers 'modern Irish' dishes, effusively described on the menu: eg,
Clonality black pudding with lakeshore mustard sauce; fried fillet
steak topped with Café de Paris butter, with a lively cracked pepper
sauce. Desserts include 'love bytes: special homemade ice cream
kissed with hot blackberry sauce'. Visitors this year found *Browne's*
'truly delightful and different, with the best seafood chowder ever'.
The 'wonderful home-baking' is always admired, so is the 'swift,
friendly and personal' service. Breakfasts are thought 'excellent'.
There is a spacious, flowery conservatory, facing south. The bedrooms
are mostly liked, though one was found 'dismal'. 'Done with style and
taste, and without TV, they have views of lush farmlands.' Your wake-
up call is provided by the cows brought in for milking. Being on a
working dairy farm, this is a good place for children. The equestrian
centre offers riding courses and treks to local sandy beaches.
Mrs Browne is 'full of local knowledge'. The old port of Youghal is
nearby. (*Amanda Molloy, and others*)

Open Mar–Nov.
Rooms 6 double, 1 single. No telephone/TV.
Facilities TV room, conservatory, restaurant (harpist Sat night); 200-acre
farm: 2-acre garden, tennis, children's play area, equestrian centre. Blue Flag
beaches nearby. Unsuitable for &.
Location 6 miles W of Youghal, 1 mile NE of Killeagh. Buses from Cork.
Restrictions No smoking in bedrooms. No dogs in house.
Credit cards MasterCard, Visa.
Terms B&B IR£35–£50. Set lunch IR£15, dinner IR£25; full alc IR£30. Child
in parents' room: 50% of adult rate.

Some of the hotels in this section did not return their questionnaire, so the information given may be less accurate than we
would wish.

KILMALLOCK Co. Limerick   Map 6:D5

Flemingstown House   BUDGET   *Tel* (+353) (0)63-98093
Kilmallock   *Fax* (+353) (0)63-98546
                                   Email flemingstown@keltec.ie
                                   Website www.ils.ie/flemingstown

'She is a treasure' – much liked for her friendly informality, and her
'scrumptious food'. Imelda Sheedy-King owns and runs a dairy farm
with a large 18th-century farmhouse, just outside Kilmallock, amid
pleasant open country by a river. Recent praise: 'The warmth of her
welcome, the superb quality of her cooking, and the comfort, all made
our stay a treat.' The 'plentiful menus' include, eg, home-made soups,
avocado and blue cheese puffs; roast leg of lamb, carved at the table;
chocolate soufflé with raspberry coulis. 'Imelda even wrote out
recipes for some of her dishes. Our small daughter was made very welcome.' 'She always has time for a chat and advice on places to visit.'
The bedrooms have just been enlarged, and given new king-size beds.
Visitors can be shown round the farm. Kilmallock, south of Limerick,
is an interesting medieval town with a fine Dominican friary. For traditional music (three times a week), visit the local pub. More reports
welcome.

Open 1 Feb–1 Dec.
Rooms 1 suite, 4 double. No telephone.
Facilities Lounge, dining room ('tranquil' background music during dinner).
2-acre garden. Golf, riding, fishing, cycling nearby. Unsuitable for &.
Location 2 miles SE of Kilmallock on R512 to Fermoy. Bus from Kilmallock.
Restriction No smoking. No dogs.
Credit cards MasterCard, Visa.
Terms B&B: single IR£35–£40, double IR£50–£60. Set dinner
IR£20–£22.50.

KINSALE Co. Cork   Map 6:D5

The Old Presbytery   BUDGET   *Tel* (+353) (0)21-477 2027
Cork Street   *Fax* (+353) (0)21-477 2166
                                   Email info@oldpres.com
                                   Website www.oldpres.com

Much enjoyed again this year, notably for its lavish breakfasts, Noreen
and Philip McEvoy's stylish B&B lies down a quiet street in the town
centre. It is in a Georgian house with a red door, once the home of
priests at the nearby church of St John the Baptist. 'An amazing warren of a house, lovely bedlinen on high brass beds, gentle and pretty
colour schemes.' 'Perfect mattress under canopied bed. The better-
than-excellent breakfast made lunch a superfluous word' (it can
include mango, home-made muesli, pancakes stuffed with apples and
maple syrup, fresh fish). The McEvoys are 'chatty and friendly', 'very
helpful'. One bedroom had 'a balcony with superb views, old pine furniture and Victorian light fittings – but modern plumbing'. Four bathrooms have a claw-foot Victorian bath. And spa baths have been
added to three rooms this year. The public rooms have coal fires; the
sitting room is 'Victorian in every detail, down to the music on the

upright piano'. Kinsale is an attractive old fishing port, today rather fashionable, with an annual gourmet festival and several good fish restaurants: *Jim Edwards* is recommended. (*Ray and Angela Evans, Mr and Mrs MC Bradshaw, N Kent, SW*)

Open 14 Feb–30 Nov.
Rooms 5 double, 1 single. 3 with spa bath. Some on ground floor. 3 2-bed-room self-catering suites.
Facilities Lounge with TV, conservatory, breakfast room (classical background music). Sea/river fishing, water sports, golf nearby. Unsuitable for &.
Location 2 mins' walk from centre, near parish church. Car park. Bus from Cork city.
Restrictions No smoking. No dogs.
Credit cards Amex, MasterCard, Visa.
Terms B&B: single IR£30–£40, double IR£60–£90. *V*

LEENANE Co. Galway   **Map 6:C4**

Delphi Lodge   *Tel* (+353) (0)95-42222
Leenane, Connemara   *Fax* (+353) (0)95-42296
                                               Email delfish@iol.ie
                                          Website www.delphilodge.ie

The former sporting lodge of the Marquis of Sligo, now Peter Mantle's very personal little enterprise, stands amid dramatic mountain country just north of Connemara. It is 'a charming old house', set by a lake in a large estate – 'most civilised and relaxing'. A notice at the gate says 'Private House', and it 'does not consider itself a hotel' (there is no room service – 'if your day has to start with a cuppa, you totter along to the deserted kitchen in your dressing-gown'). But the welcome is 'the warmest'. Mr Mantle 'has the knack of getting on with people', and the evenings are usually convivial. The 'excellent cooking', by Cliodhna Prendergast, is 'traditional Irish country house', eg, roast beef with olive champ and béarnaise sauce; roast wild duck with a blackberry jus; spiced ginger cake. The 'serious wine list' is praised. The menu is no-choice, and guests eat together around one big table. The captor of the day's biggest salmon presides. Mr Mantle is a keen fly-fisherman, and his Delphi fishery is famous for its salmon and sea-trout fishing on three lakes and on the pretty Delphi river; fishing courses are held, and ghillies are available; advance booking is essential. Non-fishermen enjoy the peaceful atmosphere, the open fires and old pine furniture, and the walks amid wild scenery. Most of the bed-rooms are large, and some have a four-poster with 'the softest cotton linen'; towels are huge and fluffy. Empty sandy beaches lie within easy reach, and the wildlife is exceptional: badgers, peregrines, pine martens, otters, etc, and masses of wild flowers. The house can be taken for small conferences and 'executive brainstorming sessions'. 'Due to the remote location and the house-party style, there is little point in making a one-night booking, and even less point in not having dinner,' writes Mr Mantle. (*JG*)

Open 15 Jan–15 Dec.
Rooms 12 double. 2 on ground floor. No TV. Also 5 self-catering cottages.
Facilities Drawing room, library, billiard room, dining room; function/

business facilities. No background music. 600-acre estate: 15-acre gardens, lake, fishing (pre-booking essential), bathing. Golf, riding, beaches nearby.
Location 9 miles N of Leenane on Louisburgh road. 20 miles SW of Westport.
Restrictions Young children discouraged. No dogs.
Credit cards MasterCard, Visa.
Terms B&B IR£47–£106; D,B&B from IR£57. Set lunch IR£10, dinner IR£31. 3-night rates. Fly-fishing tuition weekends.

LOUGH ESKE Co. Donegal　　　　　　　　　　　Map 6:B5

Ardnamona House　　　　　　　　　*Tel* (+353) (0)73-22650
Lough Eske　　　　　　　　　　　　　*Fax* (+353) (0)73-22819
　　　　　　　　　　　　　　　　　　Email info@ardnamona.com
　　　　　　　　　　　　　　　　　　Website www.ardnamona.com

Run in house-party style by Kieran Clarke, a Donegal man, and his English wife, Amabel, this pink 1830s shooting lodge stands amid wild scenery below the Blue Stack Mountains. It has a 'staggeringly beautiful' position on the shores of Lough Eske, plus a superb and unusual National Heritage garden, created in the 1880s in Himalayan style, with plants from the palace gardens in Kathmandu and the Imperial Gardens in Peking. The ancient rhododendrons (some are 60 and 70 feet high) are at their best in March and April. All around is a primeval oak forest of ecological and botanical importance. Recent praise: 'The quiet pleasantness of the hosts and their staff greatly enhance the setting.' 'Wonderful views across the lough.' 'A relaxed and friendly place. An excellent dinner, by a warming fire, and civilised conversation with other guests. Breakfasts were equally good.' Mr Clarke is 'a great talker'. His wife's menus, based on organic vegetables and salads, might include fennel and Parmesan gratin; duck legs with cabbage and red onions; chocolate truffle cream with spiced plums. When dinner is not available, you could try *Harvey's Point*, 'a rather expensive but good Swiss-run restaurant', two miles away. The bedrooms, south-facing, are brightly decorated; all but one have a bathroom *en suite*. 'The ambience and the dawn and dusk chorus are beyond price.' The house rambles round a courtyard. It has a sunroom and sitting room, and lots of books, especially on music. Mr Clarke is a musician who restores pianos; he will let guests try his Steinway grand, which was once used by Paderewski. Children are welcomed. The Clarkes' two horses will come to join you, if you leave their paddock gate open. Plenty of beaches within a half-hour drive. More reports, please.

Open All year. Dining room closed Sun night.
Rooms 6 double, 5 with facilities *en suite*. No telephone/TV.
Facilities Sitting room, snug, sunroom, dining room, music room. No background music. 100-acre grounds: garden, lake, fishing, swimming, boating. Unsuitable for &.
Location 7 miles NE of Donegal town. Turn left off N15 3 miles N of Donegal, towards Harvey's Point.
Restrictions No smoking in bedrooms. No dogs in house.
Credit cards Amex, MasterCard, Visa.
Terms B&B IR£45–£55. Single supplement £10. Set dinner IR£25. Special breaks negotiable. *V*

MAYNOOTH Co. Kildare   Map 6:C6

Moyglare Manor   *Tel* (+353) (0)1-628 6351
Maynooth   *Fax* (+353) (0)1-628 5405
                                     Email moyglare@iol.ie
                              Website www.iol.ie/moyglaremanor

'Magical, hedonistic,' says a recent visitor to Nora Devlin's sturdy
Georgian country manor house. It stands imposingly in large grounds,
up a long tree-lined avenue. Chairs and tables and statuary stand on the
wide lawn. The large and small public rooms are 'sumptuously furnished, with a clutter of ornaments, antiques, oriental rugs and old
paintings'. The manager, Shay Curran, 'has a very Irish mixture of
sound advice and good-humoured chuckling blarney'. 'Our bedroom,
with a four-poster and flowery fabrics, was large and beautiful. Dinner
was excellent, pianist serenading.' Chef Jim Cullinane's menus,
served by candlelight in the deep pink chandeliered dining room,
might include crab claws in garlic butter; roast breast of duckling with
cranberry and orange sauce. Fruit and vegetables are grown on the
estate. Log fires, patterned wallpaper, tasselled lampshades, opulent
flower displays, and the scent of roses from the garden, all create an
aura of 'fabulous decadence', quite at odds with the 'dour reputation'
of Maynooth, two miles away. This small town west of Dublin houses
Ireland's principal Catholic college, the leading venue of the meetings
of the Irish bishops. Its moral influence on the nation has been huge:
'This ye may do, but that ye may nooth', goes an old quip, while Seán
O'Casey called the high spire of its church 'a dagger through the heart
of Ireland'. The Curragh horse country is quite close. (*JM*)

Open All year, except 24–26 Dec.
Rooms 1 suite (for 3), 15 double. 2 on ground floor.
Facilities Ramps. 2 lounges, 2 bars (pianist sometimes), TV room, 3 dining
rooms; conference facilities. No background music. 17-acre grounds. Golf,
shooting, hunting, horse riding, tennis nearby.
Location 2 miles N of Maynooth. Bus/train from Dublin; taxi.
Restrictions No smoking in some bedrooms. No children under 12. No dogs.
Credit cards All major cards accepted.
Terms (*Excluding 12½% service charge*) B&B: single IR£110, double
IR£180, suite IR£290. Set lunch IR£25, dinner IR£35; full alc IR£40.

MIDLETON Co. Cork   Map 6:D5

Glenview House   *Tel* (+353) (0)21-463 1680
Ballinaclasha   *Fax* (+353) (0)21-463 4680
                                Email glenviewhouse@esatclear.ie
                         Website www.dragnet-systems.ie/dira/glenview

Midleton is a historic whiskey-producing village: here you can visit
the Jameson Whiskey Centre. Nearby, amid quiet wooded country, is
this small white Georgian manor house, 'the model of a quality rural
guest house'. The long-time owners, Ken Sherrard, a local gentleman
farmer, and his Scottish wife, Beth, who run it on very personal lines,
write: 'We take a warm approach to our guests. We sit with them
round the fire and talk, or we take them to a local pub.' 'You feel like

a cherished guest,' one visitor wrote. A report this year adds: 'The
dining room is beautiful; breakfast is good; dinner was well cooked
and plentiful. We spent a day on the beautifully maintained grass tennis court, chasing the hens away from the action.' The house is 'well
restored and elegant', with fine antique pieces. Persian carpets have
been added this year. Each bedroom is large, lovely and well
equipped, with a king-size bed and superior bathroom, and views over
the landscaped flower garden and the fields beyond, where horses
graze. Two ground-floor rooms have facilities for wheelchair guests.
Families can stay in the two self-catering units. The residents' lounge
has a log fire on chilly days. Good silver gleams in the dining room,
where 'excellent meals', cooked by Beth Sherrard, are served by candlelight round one big table. No choice of the first two courses, but
preferences are discussed: lavish servings of, eg, fresh seafood cocktail; beef casserole with Guinness; bramble fool. Guests can help
themselves to seconds. Breakfast, 'imaginative and elegantly laid out',
has fresh orange juice, home-made marmalade and soda bread. Fifty
hens provide free-range eggs. Three German shepherd dogs (one is
said to be 'very excitable'), and Burmese and Siamese cats, add to the
family feel. All types of fishing can be arranged. There are 16 golf
courses in the area. The place is often taken over by a house party.
(*E and P Thompson*)

Open All year.
Rooms 3 suites (with TV, can be self-catering) in coach house; 4 double.
2 equipped for &. No telephone.
Facilities Ramp. Lounge, wine bar, dining room. No background music. 20-
acre grounds: patio, garden, tennis, croquet, woodland walks. River/lake fish-
ing, golf nearby; sea, safe sandy beaches ½ hour's drive.
Location 13 miles E of Cork, 3 miles N of Midleton. From Midleton take L35
towards Fermoy; turn left after 2½ miles (signposted).
Restrictions No smoking: dining room, bedrooms. Guide dogs only.
Credit cards Amex, MasterCard, Visa.
Terms B&B IR£50–£62; D,B&B IR£75–£87. Set lunch IR£8, dinner IR£25.
Child in parents' room: under 4, 25% of adult rate; 4–12, 75% of adult rate.

MOATE Co. Meath   **Map 6:C5**

Temple Country House   *Tel* (+353) (0)506-35118
Horseleap   *Fax* (+353) (0)506-35008
                                      Email info@templespa.ie
                                      Website www.templespa.ie

&) *César award in 2001*

Down the end of a winding lane is this 'paradise', an 18th-century
farmhouse which Declan and Bernadette Fagan, 'young and quiet',
with three children, have turned into a small, superior guest house,
with a health spa in buildings in the grounds. Here you can take beauty
treatments, hydrotherapy, reflexology, aromatherapy, and enjoy a
steam bath or sauna. 'All the therapists were professional, pleasant,
well dressed,' one admirer said. 'I strongly recommend the massage
and yoga.' Around is a large farm with pastures, and a garden where
hens strut on the croquet lawn. Other guests wrote: 'Declan is a

generous host with a nifty palate, so his wine list is fairly priced and interesting. His wife is a very proficient cook. Both are completely unpretentious.' 'Flights of birds in the evening, and a spectacular red sunrise.' The bedrooms have a simple decor, matching fabrics, good lights. Rooms above the spa are 'small but tastefully done, with views to sheep and cows'. In the main house they are bigger and grander: 'They catch the morning sun, and are the epitome of the perfect country bedroom: high ceilings, a fireplace and rugs, no TV.' 'No one bothers to lock the doors.' Dinner is served by candlelight at 8 pm. 'The communal dining table provided agreeable ambience and company. Food was first class'; eg, red peppers stuffed with pine nuts and mushrooms; roast pork with caramelised plums; tiramisu, chocolate bavarois. Vegetables are often home-grown. Vegetarians are catered for. The 'restful sitting room' has a log fire, books and board games. Breakfast includes local yogurt, good breads, porridge, home-made jams, a fry-up if wanted. Cycles are available to borrow, 'and guided walks will exercise the outer man' – wellies are provided. Nearby are golf courses, and the peat bogs and lakes of West Meath. The main Dublin to Galway road is only half a mile away. (*SW*, *ES*)

Open All year, except 6 Dec–28 Jan. Dining room closed Sun/Mon.
Rooms 7 double, 1 single. 5 in adjacent building.
Facilities 2 lounges, dining room; health spa: sauna, steam room, spa bath, aromatherapy, etc. No background music. 100-acre farm: 1-acre garden. Walking, cycling, riding, golf, dinghy sailing nearby. Unsuitable for ♿.
Location Just N of N6, 1 mile W of Horseleap, 4 miles E of Moate.
Restrictions No smoking in restaurant. No children, except in July/Aug school holidays. No dogs in house.
Credit cards Amex, MasterCard, Visa.
Terms B&B: single IR£60–£80, double IR£100–£120. Set dinner (Tues–Sat) IR£22. Spa packages. 1-night bookings refused weekends.

MOUNTRATH Co. Laois — Map 6:C5

Roundwood House

Tel (+353) (0)502-32120
Fax (+353) (0)502-32711
Email roundwood@eircom.net
Website www.hidden-ireland.com/roundwood

César award in 1990

A 'wonderful Georgian mansion', set in 20 acres of gardens, pastures and woodlands, at the foot of the Slieve Bloom mountains in the largely empty Irish Midlands. The 'cheerful, delightful' owners, Frank and Rosemarie Kennan, 'joined us after dinner for talk and gossip over much whiskey and coffee: most enjoyable', say visitors this year. Mr Kennan is 'always ready with an amusing anecdote'. The house, full of books and pictures, has creaking floorboards, 'a staircase to die for', and a 'slightly shabby Irish charm'. Bedrooms are 'a bit sparse', but large and well appointed. Dinner (no choice) is communal, though you can have a separate table if you prefer. Mrs Kennan's 'very adventurous' cooking is 'based on what is in the market – nothing frozen except the ice creams'. Much enjoyed by readers, it features such dishes as smoked salmon trout roulade; lamb with rosemary and olive sauce; lemon soufflé pudding. There's a choice of desserts (you can try them all). Portions are large, and the wine list is especially good. Breakfast is 'highly enjoyable'. The house has been partly refurbished, with bathrooms upgraded (some now have a shower as well as a tub). Children are welcomed (there is a 'wet day' nursery), and are encouraged to feed the animals, which include donkeys, ducks, horses and a Labrador. A coach house, forge and cottage have been restored as self-catering units this year. (*John Crisp, RW*)

Open All year, except Christmas, Jan.
Rooms 10 double. 4 in annexe. No telephone/TV.
Facilities Drawing room, study, dining room; nursery. No background music. 20-acre grounds: croquet, *boules*, swings, stables. Golf, walking, river fishing nearby. Unsuitable for &.
Location N7 Dublin–Limerick. Right at T-junction in Mountrath, then left to Kinnitty. *Roundwood* 3 miles exactly. Train: Portlaoise; they will meet.
Restrictions No smoking: restaurant, some bedrooms. No dogs in house.
Credit cards All major cards accepted.
Terms [2001] B&B IR£47.25. Single room supplement IR£11.81. Evening meal IR£27.56. Child in parents' room: 50% of adult rate. 3-night breaks. ***V***

MULRANNY Co. Mayo   **Map 6:B4**

Rosturk Woods   `BUDGET`   *Tel/Fax* (+353) (0)98-36264
Mulranny   *Email* stoney@iol.ie

❦ *César award in 2000*

Louisa and Alan Stoney (he grew up in the castle next door) 'make a handsome couple, and provide the friendliest of welcomes', say visitors in 2001 to their civilised guest house, 'lovely and peaceful'. It is a trim white building set alone amid trees by a sandy shore, outside a village on Clew Bay (at low tide, you can walk among the tiny offshore islands). 'We liked the views over the sound towards that iconic mountain Croagh Patrick.' Though quite modern, the house has an old, cottagey atmosphere, 'an artistic quality and a family feel', with some antique furnishings, interesting books and pictures. The bedrooms 'have every comfort, no fussiness' – stripped pine doors, soft colours, bay views. Sherry is served by a log fire, before the home-cooked dinner, discussed in advance and based on local ingredients, eg, wild salmon, turbot and lamb; starters such as organic spinach soup; puddings like apple and rhubarb pie; chocolate mousse. 'Louisa is a sound cook, not over-ambitious, using the freshest of produce.' Wines come from a 'limited but well-chosen list'. There are 'glorious views from the dining room as the sun sets'. When dinner is not available, the Stoneys help guests book at local restaurants (eg, *Newport House*, Newport, *qv*). Breakfast, 'in a gorgeous room, with a fire', includes organic muesli, yogurt, scrambled eggs. With its toys, swings, tennis court ('in excellent repair'), beach close by, owners' children and small dogs, the place is good for families, and is very popular. There are also self-catering cottages, whose residents may dine in the main house. This is real *Playboy of the Western World* country – the remote west coast of Mayo, between the neat, historic town of Westport and the cliffs of Achill Island. (*Simon Willbourn*)

Open Feb–Dec. Closed Christmas/New Year. Self-catering accommodation open all year.
Rooms 3 double. 1 on ground floor. No telephone.
Facilities Ramp. Sitting room with TV, games room, dining room. No background music. 5-acre wooded grounds: garden, tennis, seashore, bathing, sea angling. Riding, golf, lake/river fishing, sailing nearby.
Location 7½ miles W of Newport, between main road and sea.
Restrictions No smoking: dining room, bedrooms. No dogs in public rooms.
Credit cards None accepted.
Terms B&B double IR£60–£70. Set dinner IR£25.

NEWPORT Co. Mayo   **Map 6:B4**

Newport House   *Tel* (+353) (0)98-41222
Fax (+353) (0)98-41613
Email kjtl@anu.ie

'The public rooms are splendid, and the food was very good,' runs a 2001 endorsement of this creeper-covered Georgian mansion, former home of a branch of the O'Donnells. Facing towards Achill Island, it stands near the sea in a much-visited little town on lovely Clew Bay, with superb scenery all round. Owned and run by Thelma and Kieran Thompson, who offer 'great hospitality', it is a Relais & Châteaux member, but has an 'unstuffy atmosphere' and friendly service. The public rooms have fine plasterwork, chandeliers, 'cheerful fires burning', and there is a grand staircase with a lantern and dome. The wine list is 'astonishing' and the gourmet menu was thought 'outstanding value' at IR£34, notably the tomato and pepper soup; scallops in leeks and vermouth; home-made blackcurrant ice cream. Chef John Gavin's ambitious dishes might also include poached turbot with garlic spinach; roast duck with rillettes in pastry and orange and blackcurrant sauce. Earlier visitors called the hotel 'marvellous, with wonderful staff'; and wrote of 'gloriously old-fashioned bedrooms' (some have a four-poster; some are suitable for a family). You can have eggs Benedict for breakfast, but there is no buffet, and service might be slow. The house has its own fishery on the Newport river. (*SW*)

Open 19 Mar–5 Oct.
Rooms 16 double, 2 single. 5 in courtyard. 2 on ground floor. No TV.
Facilities Drawing room, sitting room, bar, restaurant, billiard room, table-tennis room. No background music.15-acre grounds: walled garden. Private fishing on Newport river, 8 miles; golf, riding, walking, shooting, hang-gliding nearby. Unsuitable for ♿.
Location In village, 7 miles N of Westport. Bus 25 from Westport 3 times daily.
Restrictions No smoking in restaurant. No dogs.
Credit cards All major cards accepted.
Terms [2001] B&B: single IR£75–£99, double IR£150–£198; D,B&B: single IR£111–£135, double IR£222–£270. Set dinner (6 courses) IR£34; full alc IR£32. Child in parents' room: under 2, free; in own room: 2–10, 70% of adult rate.

NEWRY Co. Down *See SHORTLIST*   **Map 6:B6**

OUGHTERARD Co. Galway   **Map 6:C4**

Currarevagh House   *Tel* (+353) (0)91-552312
Oughterard   *Fax* (+353) (0)91-552731
                                     Email currarevagh@ireland.com

Ⓒ *César award in 1992*

'A wonderful refuge, absurdly good value,' says a devotee returning
this year to a mid-Victorian country house that has featured in every
edition of the *Guide*. It stands in large grounds beside Lough Corrib,
on the edge of Connemara. The Hodgson family have owned it for five
generations; Harry and June Hodgson have been resident hosts since
1970, helped now by their 'charming daughter'. 'A warm welcome;
cheerful personal attention from the local staff, gleaming glass and
cutlery in the elegant dining room, excellent food and wines – a good
Irish breakfast, and a well-balanced traditional five-course dinner (but
they tend to over-cook the meat). As a single guest, I was made to feel
entirely at ease. My room was in the (semi-derelict) coach house. The
ethos would not appeal to all (no TV). But the relative shabbiness of
some surroundings is exactly right, and complemented by huge
towels.' Indeed the house is not smart, but 'rather shambolically comfortable', with a 'hotchpotch of furniture', hot-water bottles in huge
beds. 'It has high standards and original style, reflecting the warm personalities of the owners.' 'The views over the lough are lovely.'
Afternoon teas are 'exceptional'. Guests are expected to be punctual
for the four-course, no-choice dinner, prepared by Mrs Hodgson.
Second helpings are offered. One visitor had 'the best roast duck ever'
and adored the breakfast, 'served in the country house manner of the
last century' – an old-style buffet, with a range of hot dishes (local
trout, kedgeree, blood pudding, etc) on the sideboard. There is good
fishing, swimming and boating in the lough. (*Richard Parish, RF*)

Open Apr–20 Oct. Only parties of 10 or more in winter (not Christmas/New
Year). Lunch by arrangement (residents only).
Rooms 13 double, 2 single. 2 on ground floor, in mews. No telephone/TV.
Facilities Drawing room, sitting room, library/bar, dining room. No back-
ground music. 150-acre grounds: lake, fishing (ghillies available), boating,
swimming, tennis, croquet. Golf, riding nearby. Unsuitable for &.
Location 4 miles NW of Oughterard. Take N59 (Galway–Clifden) to
Oughterard. Right in village square; follow Glann lakeshore road for 4 miles.
Restrictions No smoking in dining room. Children under 12 by arrangement.
Dogs by arrangement; not in restaurant.
Credit cards MasterCard, Visa.
Terms B&B: single IR£55–£80, double IR£115–£130; D,B&B: single
IR£80–£105, double IR£165–£180. Set dinner IR£25. 3-day, weekly rates.
Winter house parties. 1-night bookings sometimes refused if too far ahead.

The Irish punt and the pound sterling do not have the same
value. Be sure to check the exchange rate. And remember that
from the beginning of 2002 Ireland will be using the euro.

Ross Lake House   *Tel* (+353) (0)91-550109
Rosscahill   *Fax* (+353) (0)91-550184
                             Email rosslake@iol.ie
                             Website www.rosslakehotel.com

S of Oughterard and 14 miles NW of Galway city, in lovely wild
Connemara: fine Georgian estate house in 5-acre wooded grounds
with hard tennis court. Once the home of landed gentry, now owned
and run by Henry and Elaine Reid as a relaxed and intimate country
house – 'a gem'. Warm period furnishings. Irish cooking using local
produce; vegetarians well catered for. Ramp. Large drawing room,
bar; light classical background music. Golf and good fishing nearby.
Closed 2 Nov–13 Mar. No smoking in dining room. No dogs in public
rooms. All major credit cards accepted. 3 suites, 10 double rooms,
some on ground floor. B&B IR£50–£90. Set dinner IR£29 [2001]. New
chef this year. More reports welcome. *V*

PORTAFERRY Co. Down   **Map 6:B6**

The Narrows   *Tel* 028-4272 8148
8 Shore Road   *Fax* 028-4272 8105
Portaferry BT22 1JY   *Email* info@narrows.co.uk
                             Website www.narrows.co.uk

Portaferry is a delightful village at the mouth of the huge Strangford
Lough, a marine nature reserve. By the waterside, with fine views
across the lough, stands Will and James Brown's 'engaging and stylish', yet unpretentious, little hotel. Formerly their father's home and
its neighbour, it is built round an 18th-century courtyard. Its restaurant
is considered to be one of Ireland's finest. The chef, Danny Millar,
serves 'excellent contemporary cooking' in the light, airy restaurant,
looking across the water. Seafood is a speciality, eg, mussels with
bacon and garlic; roast hake with cannellini beans, fennel and shellfish
broth. The 'stupendous breakfasts' are admired, and so are the staff –
'both friendly and professional'. The pleasant bedrooms have a
modern decor: simple colours, pale wooden floors, white bedlinen. All
look over the lough. Some rooms are interconnecting and good for a
family. The house is wheelchair accessible throughout. 'We serve
any combination of sausages, chicken nuggets, chips and baked
beans (£3.95),' say the Browns, 'but we also encourage children to
experiment with our *à la carte* menu.' Vegetarians are well catered
for, too. (*AN*)

Open All year.
Rooms 12 double, 1 single. Some on ground floor. Some suitable for &.
Facilities Lift. 2 lounges, restaurant (classical/'easy listening' background
music); conference facilities. Courtyard, large walled garden.
Location On shorefront. Bus from Belfast.
Restrictions No smoking: restaurant, bedrooms. Dogs allowed in 1 bedroom
only.
Credit cards Amex, MasterCard, Visa.
Terms [2001] B&B: single £57.50, double £85; D,B&B: single £74, double
£118. Full alc £27. Christmas package.

Portaferry Hotel   *Tel* 028-4272 8231
10 The Strand   *Fax* 028-4272 8999
Portaferry BT22 1PE   *Email* info@portaferryhotel.com
                                 Website www.portaferryhotel.com

'A lovely place,' say visitors this year. Set peacefully by the ferry
landing in a pleasant village (see above), it is a traditional quayside
pub, owned and run by John and Marie Herlihy. Quite plain outside
but nicely modernised within, it is 'very sympathetic', with 'a warm,
unpretentious' atmosphere. Mr Herlihy, 'charming, urbane and
breezy', is often around, chatting with guests. The staff are 'friendly,
smartly dressed and courteous'. The public rooms overlook the broad
entrance to Strangford Lough. There is a pleasant residents' lounge,
with Irish paintings, fresh garden flowers and *objets d'art*. The lively
bar has 'an informal ambience, good food and youthful service'. In the
restaurant, 'said to be one of the best for miles around', Ann
Truesdale's 'modern British' cooking embraces such dishes as
Portavogie prawn soup; sautéed monkfish with capers; pork fillet in
smoked bacon; prune and Armagnac tart. The bedrooms are well furnished, but some beds are small. With a busy tourist trade in season,
this enterprising hotel offers painting, opera, sailing and riding
courses; there are fine walks and cycle trails all round and eight golf
courses within reach. The lough is a marine nature reserve and bird
sanctuary, also a yachting centre. (*Oliver and Rosanna James*)

Open All year, except 23–25 Dec.
Rooms 12 double, 2 single.
Facilities 2 lounges, residents' lounge, bar, restaurant; light instrumental
background music. Golf, riding, sailing, cycling, birdwatching nearby. Only
public areas suitable for &.
Location Village seafront. Parking. Bus from Belfast.
Restrictions No smoking in some bedrooms. No dogs.
Credit cards All major cards accepted.
Terms B&B £45–£65. Full alc £35. *V*

RATHMULLAN Co. Donegal   **Map 6:B5**

Rathmullan House   *Tel* (+353) (0)74-58188
Rathmullan, Letterkenny   *Fax* (+353) (0)74-58200
                              Email info@rathmullanhouse.com
                              Website www.rathmullanhouse.com

'Superbly comfortable, professionally run, with very good food and a
famous breakfast. Like home from home in its understated way.' A
regular visitor again this year enjoyed the Wheeler family's enterprising country hotel, a longtime *Guide* favourite. Mark and William
Wheeler are managers. Set on Lough Swilly (not a lake, but an inlet of
the sea), it is a handsome white 1800s mansion outside a sleepy village. 'Spacious well-furnished' public rooms have high ceilings,
chandeliers, antiques, marble fireplaces, log fires, oil paintings. 'A
bonus is the large indoor swimming pool.' There are also tennis courts
and a steam room. The courteous, long-serving staff are supported by
'well-coached students'. 'For 15 years, I have been looked after by the

same two waitresses.' The striking conservatory-style dining room, with a tented ceiling, serves an ambitious mix of modern and classical cooking by chef Seamus Douglas, eg, brandade of cod; fillet of beef with red onion marmalade; roast monkfish wrapped in Parma ham. The menu format has changed this year, and is now more comprehensive, if less changing. But rather than the five-course dinner, you could eat a simpler meal in the cellar bar/bistro; it serves lunches on a terrace in fine weather. The bedrooms vary: 'superior' ones have a sitting area; some have a balcony; lough-view rooms cost extra. The simpler rooms, good for a family, were recently renovated. One guest had 'a hard single bed and ancient wardrobe with creaking door'. 'Enjoyable breakfasts' offer a wide choice. A 'holistic week', with yoga and beauty treatments, is offered in early November. Outside the gates are some ugly holiday bungalows. But inside is a well-tended garden with access to a 'glorious beach', and you can go for pleasant walks up the Fanad peninsula, with fine views. Four championship golf courses are nearby. (*Esler Crawford, AD and JL*)

Open All year, except Jan–mid-Feb, Christmas.
Rooms 11 superior, 9 double, 4 single. 2 on ground floor.
Facilities Ramps. 4 lounges, TV room, cellar bar/bistro, restaurant; indoor swimming pool, steam room. No background music. 10-acre grounds: tennis; direct access to sandy beach, safe bathing. Golf, boating, riding, hill-walking nearby.
Location ½ mile N of village. From Letterkenny, take road to Ramelton (Rathmelton); at bridge in Ramelton turn right to Rathmullen; go through village and head N. Hotel's large gates are just past chapel, on right. Bus: Letterkenny; hotel will meet.
Restrictions No smoking in restaurant. Dogs by arrangement; not in public rooms.
Credit cards All major cards accepted.
Terms (*Excluding 10% service charge*) B&B IR£60–£80; D,B&B IR£97–£118. Set dinner IR£32.50. Holistic weeks May, Nov. Garden tours. 1-night bookings refused weekends, bank holidays. *V*

RATHNEW Co. Wicklow   **Map 6:C6**

Hunter's Hotel   *Tel* (+353) (0)404-40106
Newrath Bridge   *Fax* (+353) (0)404-40338
                Email reception@hunters.ie
                Website www.hunters.ie

Run 'with old-style charm' by Maureen Gelletlie and her son, Richard (he is manager), this 'supremely welcoming' old coaching inn has been owned by the family since 1825. It stands by the river Vartry, north-west of Wicklow. 'One of my favourite hotels, exceptionally good value. I had a newly refurbished room with a lovely view over the garden,' says a returning visitor this year, echoing last year's praise: 'It was super, very comfortable, with friendly staff, and very Irish in the nicest way. Our spacious room had a large bed, antique furniture. It was pleasant to sit and drink in the flowery garden. Fires were lit in the public rooms. The hotel was very busy, with residents and locals: it seemed a real part of the community.' Renovation has been 'carefully done': some of the decor is traditional, with antiques, polished brass and open fires, but the house also 'gleams with fresh paint and polished wood'. The bedrooms are 'comfortable in a homely style, with plenty of space, a large, pristine bathroom'. Even the singles are sizeable. The extensive dinner menu provides 'hearty fare, if not *haute cuisine*', cooked by Martin Barry, eg, mussel and tomato gratin; roast Wicklow lamb with herb stuffing; glazed orange tart. This year, the 'vast selection' of home-grown vegetables was enjoyed, and the varied wine list. But service can be slow. The 'very good' breakfast is 'full Irish', with freshly squeezed juice. Whiskey and tea are on offer throughout the day: tea is served on the lawn in summer. There are 15 golf courses within an hour's drive. Nearby sights include Mount Usher and Powerscourt gardens, Russborough and Avondale houses. (*Thomas Ender, LW*)

Open All year, except 3 days over Christmas.
Rooms 13 double, 3 single. 1 on ground floor.
Facilities Residents' lounge, bar lounge, dining room; conference room. No background music. 7-acre grounds: 2-acre garden, river, fishing. Golf, tennis, riding, sea, sandy beach, fishing nearby.
Location 28 miles S of Dublin. Take N11; left at bridge in Ashford, hotel 1½ miles. From S, take N11; right on leaving Rathnew, hotel ½ mile. Car park. Bus from Ashford/Wicklow.
Restrictions No smoking in dining room. No dogs.
Credit cards Amex, MasterCard, Visa.
Terms B&B IR£65–£75; D,B&B IR£98–£108. Set lunch IR£16.50, dinner IR£33. 1-night bookings refused holiday weekends.

Tinakilly House
Tel (+353) (0)404-69274
Fax (+353) (0)404-67806
Email reservations@tinakilly.ie
Website www.tinakilly.ie

'Very comfortable, with superb views and well-appointed rooms; the staff were particularly friendly,' says a visitor in 2001 to this superior country hotel. 'Very popular, and often booked up weeks ahead', it stands in large wooded grounds above the Irish Sea (no direct access). The original grey stone mansion was built in the 1870s as a retirement home, by the great navigator Captain Robert Halpin, who laid the first successful transatlantic telephone cable in 1866. It has been much enlarged; most bedrooms are in a new block at the back; they are spacious, and individually furnished in period style. Most have a view to the coast – 'a magical mixture of the bucolic and the marine, with cows grazing and the sea beyond'. The public rooms have gilt chandeliers and sconces, polished dark wood, rococo fireplaces, softly upholstered formal sofas and chairs, bright red carpets, potted plants, assorted glittering bric-a-brac, and good reproduction pictures. Bee and William Power, who ran the hotel for many years, have handed over to their son, Raymond, and his wife, Josephine. The food was thought good this year, 'though the newly built, modern restaurant seemed out of character with the elegance of the rest of the building'. Chef Chris Daly's modern Irish dishes include starters such as caramelised scallops on a parsley and potato cake, or chargrilled asparagus tips with roast aubergine; main courses like loin of Wicklow lamb with fondant potato and pistachio cream, or wild mushroom risotto with scallions, Parmesan crisps and truffle oil. Small business functions are held midweek, and Irish entertainments and theatrical evenings can be arranged. Local sightseeing includes Powerscourt, 'the last of the great formal gardens of Europe' (laid out in the 1740s), and the bird sanctuary of Broadlough lagoon; Glendalough monastery and the Wicklow mountains are not far off. Convenient for the ferry from England (30 minutes' drive down the coast). (*John Vigar, ES*)

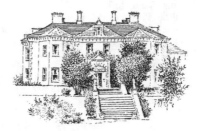

Open All year.
Rooms 29 suites, 22 double. Some on ground floor.
Facilities Lift. Great Hall (pianist Fri/Sat nights), drawing room, bar lounge, 3 dining rooms; small meeting facilities. Classical background music in public areas 'when appropriate'. 7-acre grounds: marked walks, tennis, putting. Golf, sailing, hill-walking, bird sanctuary, riding, hunting, shooting nearby.
Location Off N11 Dublin–Wicklow. Take R750 through Rathnew. Entrance on left after ¼ mile. Train: Wicklow, 2 miles.
Restriction No dogs.
Credit cards All major cards accepted.
Terms [2001] B&B IR£74–£130; D,B&B IR£113–£169. Bar lunches. Set dinner IR£39. Short breaks. Dickensian Christmas, New Year packages. 1-night bookings sometimes refused Sat.

RECESS Co. Galway   **Map 6:C4**

Ballynahinch Castle   **NEW**   *Tel* (+353) (0)95-31006
                                   Fax (+353) (0)95-31085
                           Email bhinch@iol.ie
            Website www.commerce.ie/ballynahinch

'The location is superb, in the wild heart of Connemara,' says an inspector in 2001, restoring to the *Guide* this bulky building, 'sort of baronial, no great beauty, but with presence', in a large wooded estate. 'We were warmly welcomed, given a second-floor room with views towards the mountains. Those at the back look over the scenic Ballynahinch river (good for salmon). The room, with a four-poster, was drab but restful, with a good bathroom. The drawing room downstairs is magnificent, the conservatory is very light, the bar is atmospheric, the chess room is dignified and quiet, a log fire burns in reception. Everywhere are polished wood floors, good rugs, lots of pictures, a feeling of cosiness, despite the size. In the spacious dining room, the headwaiter had a good sense of humour. On the fairly extensive menu, we enjoyed seafood soup, and seasonal salad; wild salmon with turnip purée; fillet of beef. Main dishes arrived with a flourish, under domes. Good vegetables, adequate wine list. Over-casual dress is not encouraged, but this did not deter some guests: one was in combat trousers and a T-shirt. Breakfast, with fresh flowers on the tables, was very good' (the menu includes fish, lamb's liver, potato cakes).

This is the ancestral home of the Martin family: 'Humanity Dick' Martin founded the RSPCA; it was also owned by an Indian cricketer, Maharajah Ranjitsinji.

Open All year except Christmas, Feb.
Rooms 18 double.
Facilities Lounge, dining room, conservatory, bar, chess room. 350-acre grounds: river, fishing, shooting. Golf, tennis nearby. Unsuitable for &.
Location 36 miles NW of Galway. Turn left towards Roundstone off N59 to Clifden; entrance 2 miles.
Restriction No dogs in house.
Credit cards All major cards accepted.
Terms [2001] B&B: single IR£72–£120, double IR£104–£200. Set lunch IR£20, dinner IR£30.

RIVERSTOWN Co. Sligo   **Map 6:B5**

Coopershill   *Tel* (+353) (0)71-65108
                                                  Fax (+353) (0)71-65466
                                                  Email ohara@coopershill.com
                                                  Website www.coopershill.com

  César award in 1987

'Splendid; efficiently but informally run; perfect for a relaxing break.' More adulation for this Palladian mansion 'filled with real antiques', and with a 'comfortable, lived-in feeling: amiable dogs help, and a grey parrot potters around the ground floor'. Set in a large estate, near the knobbly hills that Yeats loved (his grave is nearby), it has been the home of the O'Hara family since they built it in 1774. Mrs O'Hara senior, who turned it into a hotel many years ago, is still around, 'bright-eyed and jolly', aged 89. Her son, Brian, and his wife, Lindy, are 'caring hosts', 'so comfortable in their role that guests feel at home too'. 'Staff are wonderful. Meticulous thought has gone into every detail.' Dinner, cooked by Lindy O'Hara and served by candlelight, starts at 8.30 or so and can be leisurely – all guests are served each course at the same time – but diners talk to each other. The five-course meal is mostly thought 'superlatively good', 'very rich', eg, roasted red peppers; loin of lamb with a creamy pesto. But one visitor found it 'a bit bland'. The long wine list is 'a gem, very fairly priced'. Breakfasts include 'fresh fruit juices, superior porridge', but cooked dishes may be 'nothing special'. 'Afternoon tea, with home-baked scones and cakes, is most civilised.' There are plenty of books and guides on the area. Children are genuinely welcomed. The bedrooms are 'large, and luxuriously homely'; most have a four-poster or a canopied bed. A visitor this year had a 'vast, magnificent bathroom, with a huge Victorian bath', and admired the housekeeping, but found a confusion over booking. Other pleasures: 'Walks through the woods; peacocks; the gathering of guests in the drawing room (with an open fire) before and after dinner. Wonderful fudge and chocolate with coffee.' The interior is something of a time warp: spears, hunting trophies, stags' heads and ancestors decorate the walls. 'Brian bustles about, and runs a sizeable farm as well': much of the estate is given over to deer farming (lots of high fences), 'but there is no shortage of Arcadian vistas, with sheep grazing.' (*Andrew Wardrop, and others*)

Open 1 Apr–31 Oct. Out-of-season house parties by arrangement.
Rooms 8 double. No TV.
Facilities 2 halls, drawing room, TV room, dining room; snooker room. No background music. 500-acre estate: garden, tennis, croquet, woods, farmland, river (trout fishing). Sandy beach nearby; championship golf course 18 miles. Unsuitable for &.
Location 11 miles SE of Sligo. Turn off N4 towards Riverstown at Drumfin; follow *Coopershill* signs. Train: Ballymote. Air: Sligo/Knock.
Restrictions No smoking: dining room, bedrooms. No dogs in house.
Credit cards All major cards accepted.
Terms [2001] B&B IR£52–£73; D,B&B IR£81–£105. Light/picnic lunch IR£7; set dinner IR£31. Discounts for 3 or more nights.

ROSSLARE Co. Wexford   **Map 6:D6**

Churchtown House   *Tel* (+353) (0)53-32555
Tagoat   *Fax* (+353) (0)53-32577
                    Email churchtown.rosslare@indigo.ie
                    Website www.churchtown-rosslare.com

Patricia and Austin Cody's handsome white Georgian house stands in large grounds with lawns and old trees, in a hamlet ('just a pub, a shop and a church', they say) west of Rosslare. It has been called 'charming', 'excellent value', with a 'good ambience', and the Codys are 'superb hosts, very professional' – 'the welcome was good, even at nearly 11 pm'. 'Everywhere is warm; a nice fire in the drawing room.' Bedrooms are 'sparkling clean', with a 'sink-into bed'. Guests meet in the Garden Room for a sherry before dinner, which is based on 'traditional Irish country cooking', and may include local seafood, Wexford lamb, and vegetables from the garden. The food may be 'unexciting', but the wine list is 'reasonably priced, with some reassuring eclecticism'. Breakfast is 'superb'; it can be served early to guests catching a crack-of-dawn ferry to Fishguard. The medieval walled town of Wexford is also near, and many guests come here for its opera festival in October (early suppers are served). (*John Crisp, Simon Willbourn*)

Open Mar–Oct.
Rooms 1 suite, 10 double, 1 single. 5 on ground floor.
Facilities 2 lounges, dining room, private dining room. No background music. 8-acre grounds. Golf, fishing, riding, beaches nearby.
Location ½ mile N of Tagoat, on R736; 2½ miles W of Rosslare.
Restrictions Smoking in 1 lounge only. No children under 12. No dogs.
Credit cards Amex, MasterCard, Visa.
Terms [2001] B&B IR£45–£70. Single room supplement £IR20. Set dinner IR£27.50.

SCHULL Co. Cork   **Map 6:D4**

Rock Cottage   `BUDGET`   *Tel/Fax* (+353) (0)28-35538
Barnatonicane   *Email* rockcottage@eircom.net
                    Website www.mizen.net/rockcottage

'An oasis of tranquillity and good taste,' says a returning guest to this trim Georgian hunting lodge, which stands peacefully near Dunmanus

Bay, north-west of the lively holiday village. The 'beautiful old house' overlooks a tree-filled paddock. 'Good housekeeping; quiet good taste with wonderful art on the walls.' In the large wooded grounds are a garden, a walled courtyard, old farm buildings, a large rock which gives the cottage its name. 'Excellent breakfasts' are continental, traditional, healthy, or fish (smoked salmon, mackerel or kipper with scrambled eggs). Barbara Klötzer is owner/chef. Reports praise her 'upmarket home cooking, German, French, Italian': dishes like warm lamb's liver salad; duck breast with orange and ginger; lobster and seafood platter by arrangement. You can walk into the hills for fine views over the bay, or drive to nearby sandy beaches; the lovely south Cork coast is worth exploring. (*Catherine Fraher*)

Open All year.
Rooms 2 family, 1 double. Also 1 self-catering cottage.
Facilities Lounge (mixed background music 'when guests like it', dining room. 17-acre grounds. Sea, sandy beaches nearby. Unsuitable for &.
Location 8 miles NW of Schull. Go W towards Goleen. At Toormore, turn right on to R591 to Durrus. B&B signpost on left, after 1½ miles. Bus: Schull; then taxi.
Restrictions No smoking: restaurant, bedrooms. Guide dogs only.
Credit cards MasterCard, Visa.
Terms (*Not VAT-rated*) B&B IR£25–£45. Set dinner IR£25.

SHANAGARRY Co. Cork   **Map 6:D5**

Ballymaloe House   *Tel* (+353) (0)21-465 2531
                                              Fax (+353) (0)21-465 2021
                                              Email res@ballymaloe.ie
                                              Website www.ballymaloe.com

✤ *César award in 1984*

Headed by the veteran Myrtle Allen, this famous and 'marvellous' hotel in a handsome ivy-covered Georgian house has had an entry in every edition of the *Guide*. It is a true family enterprise: one daughter-in-law, Hazel, is manageress; head chef is Rory O'Connell, brother of another daughter-in-law, Darina, who runs the Ballymaloe Cookery School and is a well-known cookery writer. Recent plaudits: 'We enjoyed it immensely.' 'To stay is a great pleasure, with some of the best food in the British Isles. The atmosphere is relaxed and warm; service is efficient.' The house still has its Norman keep (which includes some bedrooms); graceful and rambling, it stands amid a large home farm, which provides much of what you eat – 'Irish country house cooking' at its best. The restaurant, with five rooms and a conservatory, draws a civilised clientele from many lands. Its atmosphere is 'friendly, with everyone talking and laughing'. It serves 'the freshest ingredients of the day'. The daily-changing menu might include: wild garlic soup; warm salad of quail with grapes; sauté of lamb's kidney and liver flamed in whiskey. Plenty of choice for vegetarians. 'Breakfasts are outstanding, with a range of mueslis.' The comfortable lounges have log fires in winter; walls are hung with modern Irish paintings. 'After dinner, by the wood fire, we unwound to Rory's Irish singing, and guests were encouraged to join in.' 'Our huge pretty room, with fresh lilies, opened on to lawns, lake and pea-cocks.' Bedrooms vary in size; those in the main house tend to be larger than annexe ones. Some bathrooms may be cramped. Children are warmly welcomed: they can enjoy a slide or sandpit, explore the farm, and are given high tea at 5.30 pm. (*Mr and Mrs ER Birch, DC, and others*)

Open All year, except 22–26 Dec.
Rooms 30 double, 3 single. 10 in adjacent building. 3 on ground floor. TV on request.
Facilities Drawing room, 2 small sitting rooms, conservatory, 5 dining rooms; conference facilities. No background music. Irish entertainment weekly in summer. 40-acre grounds: farm: gardens, tennis, swimming pool (heated in summer), 6-hole golf course, croquet, children's play area; craft shop. Cookery school nearby. Sea 2 miles: sand and rock beaches; fishing, riding by arrangement.
Location On L35 Ballycotton road, 2 miles E of Cloyne, 20 miles E of Cork. Train: Cork; taxi.
Restrictions No smoking in some dining rooms. No dogs.
Credit cards All major cards accepted.
Terms B&B: single IR£85–£115, double IR£140–£200; D,B&B: single IR£123–£153, double IR£216–£276. Set lunch IR£24, dinner IR£38. Child in parents' room: 50% of adult rates. Winter, conference rates.

THOMASTOWN Co. Kilkenny   **Map 6:D5**

Mount Juliet   *Tel* (+353) (0)56-73000
                Fax (+353) (0)56-73019
             Email info@mountjuliet.ie
          Website www.mountjuliet.com

'The first sight is breathtaking' – one of Ireland's stateliest houses, this large creeper-covered mansion was built in the 1750s by the first Earl of Carrick and named for his wife Julianna ('Juliet'). It stands in a huge estate of well-kept parkland, where the river Nore offers fishing for salmon and trout. It has an 18-hole championship golf course designed by Jack Niklaus, tennis, cycling, archery and an equestrian centre. Now a superior hotel, often catering for the conference trade, it keeps 'a warm personal feel', with family portraits, log fires – and it has been thought 'superb'. There are Adam fireplaces, hand-carved marble, and stucco work on the walls and ceilings of the public rooms. The smart dining room serves modern Irish cooking: you might find ham and foie gras terrine; velouté of white beans with chorizo oil; roast chump of lamb; Irish whiskey bread-and-butter pudding on the *table d'hôte* menu. 'The food is uniformly excellent,' says a reader this year, adding: 'This is a family run hotel. The indoor heated pool and health spa are a godsend for parents on a rainy day. My five-year-old started a major passion for riding. We could find no fault.' But one 2001 visitor, while praising the 'beautiful surroundings and accomo-dation', found the meals disappointing. The bedrooms have a country house decor: period furniture, chandeliers, luxurious fabrics. there are large suites, ech with a kitchen, in *Rose Garden Lodges*. Simpler bed-rooms are around a courtyard, in the *Hunter's Yard*, which has its own less formal restaurant, *Kendals*. A conference facility is new this year;

also five new treatment rooms (including flotation rooms) in the spa. Kilkenny town with its superb old castle is ten miles away. (*Michael Kavanagh, and others*)

Open All year.
Rooms 4 suites, 52 double, 3 single. 16 in *Hunter's Yard*, 11 in *Rose Garden Lodges*. Some on ground floor. 1 equipped for &.
Facilities 2 lounges, TV room, 4 bars, 2 restaurants; mixed background music in public areas; conference facilities. 1,500-acre estate: garden, tennis, 18-hole golf course, 18-hole putting course, golf academy, equestrian centre, archery, clay-target shooting, fishing, hunting, leisure centre: indoor swimming pool, sauna, steam room, gym, beauty treatment; bicycles available, helipad.
Location 4 miles NW of Thomastown, 9 miles S of Kilkenny. Train/bus from Kilkenny or Waterford.
Restrictions No smoking: 1 restaurant, 3 bedrooms. No dogs.
Credit cards All major cards accepted.
Terms [2001] Room: single IR£150–£200, double IR£180–£310, suite IR£240–£400. Breakfast IR£12.50. Set dinner IR£40; full alc IR£55. 2-day breaks off-season. Christmas package. 1-night bookings refused peak weekends.

THURLES Co. Tipperary   Map 6:C5

Inch House   *Tel* (+353) (0)504-51348 and 51261
Inch, Thurles   *Fax* (+353) (0)504-51754
                                        Email inchhse@iol.ie
                                        Website www.tipp.ie/inch-house

Reached up a long drive on the land of a large working farm, this elegant mansion was owned for nearly 300 years by the Ryan family (their chapel still stands). The 'lovely owners' since 1985, John and Nora Egan, have sensitively restored the old building, and this year have redecorated all five bedrooms. 'The abode is truly glorious and its entrance is awe-inspiring,' say recent American visitors, who 'met some lovely local people'. Others have enjoyed the 'old-style living', and the 'magnificent dining and drawing rooms': these are decorated in Adam style, with period furniture. The dining room, elegant in red and green, has a log fire; the drawing room has a huge stained-glass window. The split staircase 'is a sight to behold', and the bedrooms are 'huge and lovely'. 'Ours had wonderful views of the crops being harvested as the sun set. Breakfasts, with fruit, yogurt, home-made jams and soda bread, were excellent.' The chef, Kieran O'Dwyer, is back in the job he held three years ago, and offers 'modern Irish dishes with a French influence' – eg, crêpes filled with smoked chicken in a white wine and mushroom cream sauce; grilled steak with a cognac and pepper cream sauce; roast duckling with orange and ginger sauce. Vegetables and herbs are home-grown; meat often comes from the estate. Some of the 'interesting wines' are available by the glass. The restored Holy Cross Abbey, four miles away, by the river Suir, is worth a visit. (*CS, and others*)

Open All year, except Christmas. Dining room closed Sun, Mon.
Rooms 5 double.
Facilities Drawing room, bar, dining room (soft Irish background music at dinner); chapel; conference/function facilities. 4-acre garden in 250-acre farm. Golf, riding, fishing nearby.

Location 4 miles W of Thurles on Nenagh road.
Restrictions No smoking in dining room. No dogs.
Credit cards MasterCard, Visa.
Terms B&B IR£40–£45. Set dinner IR£29. Child in parents' room: 20% of adult rate.

WATERFORD Co. Waterford *See SHORTLIST*   **Map 6:D5**

WEXFORD Co. Wexford   **Map 6:D5**

McMenamin's Townhouse **BUDGET** *Tel/Fax* (+353) (0)53-46442
3 Auburn Terrace   *Email* mcmem@indigo.ie
Redmond Road   *Website* www.wexford-bedandbreakfast.com

Called 'amazing value for money', Seamus and Kay McMenamin's B&B is a dark red brick bay-windowed late Victorian house in the town centre. Standards are said to drop when the owners are away, but when they are around, say devotees, it is 'as good as ever'. 'The usual incredible array of goodies at breakfast, with about ten different home-made breads' (also scrambled eggs with smoked salmon; lamb's kidneys in sherry; porridge cooked slowly all night, then crusted with brown sugar, and with rum added). 'Our hosts, true professionals, exuded charm and honesty.' High ceilings, interesting Victorian objects, and a decor of dark red, pink and green, go with framed early 20th-century opera posters reflecting Wexford's annual music festival. There is a pleasant lounge and a 'cosily pretty' breakfast area. One bedroom has 'a spectacular carved canopied bed'. Loungers and tables stand in the garden. Nearby are fine beaches, the Wexford wildfowl reserve and the Irish National Heritage Park. (*A and RE*)

Open All year, except 20–30 Dec.
Rooms 6 double, 1 single. No telephone.
Facilities Lounge, breakfast room. No background music. Small garden. Unsuitable for &.
Location Central, opposite rail/bus station. Parking.
Restrictions No smoking: breakfast room, bedrooms. No dogs.
Credit cards MasterCard, Visa.
Terms B&B IR£27.50–£40. Child in parents' room: under 12, half price.

****

Traveller's tale Hotel in the home counties. You can tell a lot about a hotel by the way your initial telephone enquiry is handled. The young lady I spoke to had been trained at the Hitler charm school, and was very abrupt. We were advised that we could not have our room until 4 pm, and we were expected to leave by 11 am next day. During our stay, we met only the young French staff and the receptionist, who was as lacking warmth in the flesh as she had been on the telephone. Breakfast was supervised by this same hatchet-faced lady. When we left, nobody asked whether we had enjoyed ourselves, and the chef was sound asleep on a settle.

****

Shortlist

The following hotels, guest houses and B&Bs are listed, in order to plug gaps in our maps. Many are in, or within commuting distance of, major cities and towns that do not at present have a *Guide* entry, or that are inadequately represented. We have given the weekday rates for 2001. Many of the city hotels offer remarkably good weekend reductions.

We must emphasise that, while some Shortlist hotels are potential full entries – it includes new businesses, recommendations that arrived too late for us to check this year, and places on which we lack recent reports – many, particularly those in cities, are not typical *Guide* entries. The information is taken from various sources, including reports from readers and inspectors. A few of the hotels are large, and some belong to a chain, but we have tried, as usual, to seek out small, owner-managed establishments. Some lack the character of a true *Guide* entry. Some may be altogether too flamboyant. A number of them are designer hotels, a vast improvement on the impersonal blocks which were once the only choice for the city visitor. We recognise that this selection is somewhat haphazard, and the standards may be inconsistent. We'd like reports and nominations, please.

Those places which do not also have a full entry in the *Guide* are indicated on the maps with a triangle.

Note It is vital that, when discussing tariffs, you check whether or not VAT is included. Many hotels, particularly in London, quote tariffs without VAT.

LONDON   **Map 2:D4**

Abbey House, 11 Vicarage Gate W8 4AG. *Tel* 020-7727 2594. Family-run B&B in Victorian house (attractive entrance hall and staircase), in quiet road off Kensington Church St. Small lounge; basement breakfast room. 19 simple rooms, none *en suite*. B&B £37–£45. (Underground: Kensington High St)
Academy, 21 Gower Street WC1E 6HG. *Tel* 020-7631 4115, *fax* 020-7636 3442, *email* res_academy@etontownhouse.com, *website* www.etontownhouse.com. Extensively refurbished by new owners: boutique hotel in 5 Georgian town houses near British Museum. Bar, restaurant; limited conference facilities. 49 bedrooms. B&B: single £130, double £152–£225. (Underground: Goodge St)
Blooms, 7 Montague Street WC1B 5BP. *Tel* 020-7323 1717, *fax* 020-7636 6498, *email* blooms@mermaid.co.uk, *website* www. bloomshotel.com. 18th-century town house near British Museum. Breakfast room, bar/lounge, restaurant, library, small meeting room;

courtyard garden. 27 bedrooms (some small; largest/quietest at rear): single £130–£175, double £200–£205. (Underground: Russell Sq)

Charlotte Street Hotel, 15 Charlotte Street W1P 1HB. *Tel* 020-7806 2000, *fax* 020-7806 2002, *email* charlotte@firmdale.com, *website* www.charlottestreethotel.com. Victorian town house in 'Fitzrovia', opened June 2000. Modern decor. Lounge, library, juice bar, brasserie; gym; entertainment centre; 2 meeting rooms. 52 bedrooms: single from £175, double from £195. (Underground: Goodge St, Tottenham Court Rd)

County Hall Travel Inn Capital, Belvedere Road SE1 7PB. *Tel* 020-7902 1600, *fax* 020-7902 1619, *website* www.travelinn.co.uk. Large hotel in old County Hall building, S of Thames between Westminster and Waterloo bridges. 'Good value; spotless.' Bar, restaurant. 300 uniform bedrooms: single/double/family £74.95. Breakfast £4.50–£6.50. (Underground: Waterloo)

Covent Garden Hotel, 10 Monmouth Street WC2H 9HB. *Tel* 020-7806 1000, *fax* 020-7806 1100, *email* covent@firmdale.com, *website* www.firmdale.com. Former French hospital, now smart hotel with colourful decor. Classy foyer; wrought iron staircase leads to large lounge. Lift; brasserie; gym. Public car park nearby. 58 bedrooms (with cellular phone, CD-player, etc): single from £190, double from £220. (Underground: Leicester Sq, Covent Gdn)

Cranley Gardens Hotel, 8 Cranley Gardens SW7 3DB. *Tel* 020-7373 3232, *fax* 020-7373 7944, *email* cranleygarden@aol.com. Conversion of 4 Georgian terrace houses in South Kensington across quite busy road from garden square. Simple decor, friendly staff. Basement breakfast room; bar snacks served. 85 bedrooms. B&B £57.50–£95. (Underground: Gloucester Rd, South Kensington)

Dorset Square Hotel, 39–40 Dorset Square NW1 6QN. *Tel* 020-7723 7874, *fax* 020-7724 3328, *email* dorset@firmdale.com, *website* www.firmdale.com. Lavish conversion of Regency town houses on garden square near Marylebone Rd, Regent's Park. *Potting Shed* restaurant/bar open all day (live jazz week nights). Public car park nearby. 38 bedrooms: single from £98, double from £140. (Underground: Baker St)

Five Sumner Place, 5 Sumner Place SW7 3EE. *Tel* 020-7584 7586, *fax* 020-7823 9962, *email* reservations@sumnerplace.com, *website* www.sumnerplace.com. B&B in Victorian terrace. Buffet breakfast in conservatory. Small garden. 13 bedrooms, most *en suite*. B&B £65–£85. (Underground: South Kensington)

41 Buckingham Palace Road, 41 Buckingham Palace Road SW1W 0PS. *Tel* 020-7300 0041, *fax* 020-7300 0141, *email* reservations@41club.redcarnationhotels.com, *website* www. redcarnationhotels.com. Overlooking palace, 'all-inclusive luxury hotel' aimed at business market. Rates include 24-hour dining/snacks, drinks, minibar, national phone calls, business centre, butler service. 20 bedrooms: double £295–£325, suite £400–£525. (Underground: Victoria)

La Gaffe, 107–111 Heath Street NW3 6SS. *Tel* 020-7435 8965, *fax* 020-7794 7592, *email* la-gaffe@msn.com, *website* www.lagaffe.co.uk. Italian restaurant-with-rooms in Hampstead village, near heath, underground. Friendly proprietor (for 39 years) Bernardo Stella. Roof garden for tea; breakfast in coffee bar. 16 small, no-smoking bedrooms, most with shower; quietest (rear) ones overlook garden square. B&B £45 £80. (Underground: Hampstead)

The Gate, 6 Portobello Road, W11 3DG. *Tel* 020-7221 0707, *fax* 020-7221 9128, *email* gatehotel@thegate.globalnet.co.uk, *website* www.gatehotel.com. Near Portobello Rd market: Brian Watkins's Georgian terrace house: cottage-like exterior. 6 small bedrooms, with fridge (continental breakfast delivered at bedtime). B&B £42.50–£70. (Underground: Notting Hill Gate)

The Gore, 189 Queen's Gate SW7 5EX. *Tel* 020-7584 6601, *fax* 020-7589 8127, *email* reservations@gorehotel.co.uk, *website* www.gorehotel.com. Peter McKay's idiosyncratic hotel, with laid-back style: 2 large Victorian houses in tree-lined terrace near Albert Hall. Attractive decor: antiques, oriental rugs, open fires, potted palms, 5,000+ paintings and prints. 54 bedrooms, varying greatly; best with sitting room; some no-smoking; some get noise (traffic, TV, etc). Bar, *Bistrot 190*; *Fish Restaurant at One Ninety*. Public car park nearby. Room: single £120–£140, double £155–£285. Breakfast £8–£11. (Underground: Gloucester Rd)

The Milestone, 1 Kensington Court W8 5DL. *Tel* 020-7917 1000, *fax* 020-7917 1010, *email* guestservices@milestone.redcarnationhotels.com, *website* www.redcarnationhotels.com. Opposite Kensington Palace, 2 late 19th-century townhouses sumptuously refurbished: original architectural features; antiques. Lounge, bar, restaurant, conservatory; health club; function/conference facilities. 57 bedrooms (some with terrace or balcony): double from £250, suite from £530. (Underground: High St Kensington)

Montcalm, Great Cumberland Place W1A 2LF. *Tel* 020-7402 4288, *fax* 020-7724-9180, *email* reservations@montcalm.co.uk, *website* www.montcalm.co.uk. Owned by Japanese Nikko chain, managed by Jonathan Orr-Ewing, on elegant crescent by Marble Arch. Air-conditioned throughout. 'Delightful staff; pretty restaurant; good-value meals.' 120 bedrooms: single £230, double from £250. (Underground: Marble Arch)

La Reserve, 422–428 Fulham Road SW6 1DU. *Tel* 020-7385 8561, *fax* 020-7385 7662, *email* reservation@la-reservehotel.co.uk, *website* www.lareservehotel.co.uk. On Chelsea/Fulham border, by Chelsea Football Club. Purpose-built hotel: contemporary decor; all-day restaurant. 43 smallish bedrooms. Car park. B&B £67.50–£115. (Underground: Fulham Broadway)

Rookery, Peter's Lane, Cowcross Street EC1M 6DS. *Tel* 020-7336 0931, *fax* 020-7336 0932, *email* reservations@rookery.co.uk, *website* www.rookeryhotel.com. Near St Paul's Cathedral/City, owned by Peter McKay. Smart decor: panelling, antiques, Victorian bathroom fittings. Library, conservatory, tiny garden. Some noise from nearby nightclub. 33 bedrooms: single £175–£190, double £205, suite from £265. Breakfast £7.25. (Underground: Barbican, Farringdon)

Royal George House, 30 Bristol Gardens W9 2JQ. *Tel* 020-7289 6146, *fax* 020-7266 3143. Privately owned hotel in Little

Venice residential area. Panelled breakfast/bar area. Snacks available all day; evening meal by arrangement. 14 bedrooms (some *en suite*). B&B £35–£95. (Underground: Warwick Ave)

Searcy's Knightsbridge Roof Garden, 30 Pavilion Road SW1X 0HJ. *Tel* 020-7584 4921, *fax* 020-7823 8694, *email* rgr@searcys.co.uk, *website* www.searcys.co.uk. In small street off Sloane St. No public rooms, no extras. 13 good-sized, well-equipped bedrooms; access to fully equipped kitchen. B&B £65–£120. (Underground: Knightsbridge, Sloane Sq)

Sloane Hotel, 29 Draycott Place SW3 2SH. *Tel* 020-7581 5757, *fax* 020-7584 1348, *email* sloanehotel@btinternet.com. Victorian house in Chelsea. Exotic decor: lavish drapes, antiques, *objets d'art* (many for sale). Rooftop breakfast room/lounge, terrace. Snacks available. Business facilities. 12 bedrooms: double from £150, suite from £240. Breakfast £9–£12. (Underground Sloane Sq)

The Stafford, 16–18 St James's Place SW1A 1NJ. *Tel* 020-7493 0111, *fax* 020-7493 7121, *email* info@thestaffordhotel.co.uk, *website* www.thestaffordhotel.co.uk. In quiet backwater off St James's St: sedate hotel. Traditional restaurant; trophy-filled American bar. Access to nearby health club. 81 bedrooms. B&B: single £220, double £290, suite £360. (Underground: Green Pk)

Ten Manchester Street, 10 Manchester Street W1M 5PG. *Tel* 020-7486 6669, *fax* 020-7224 0348, *email* stay@10manchesterstreet.co.uk, *website* www.10manchesterstreet.com. Near Marylebone High St: red brick B&B hotel. 'Pleasant staff; no-frills service; user-friendly lounge.' Breakfast room. 46 bedrooms (largest overlook Manchester Sq; quietest ones at rear). B&B: single/double £120–£150, suite £195. (Underground Baker St, Bond St)

Thanet Hotel, 8 Bedford Place WC1B 5JA. *Tel* 020-7636 2869, *fax* 020-7323 6676, *email* thanetlon@aol.com, *website* www.freepages.co.uk/thanet hotel. Bloomsbury B&B, near British Museum: Richard and Lynwen Orchard's Grade II listed Georgian terrace house. Plain decor. 16 bedrooms (rear ones quietest), with shower/WC. B&B £44–£67. (Underground: Holborn, Russell Sq)

Twenty Nevern Square, 20 Nevern Square SW5 9PD. *Tel* 020-7565 9555, *fax* 020-7565 9444, *website* www.small-hotel.com/nevern. Victorian town house in Earl's Court. Newly restored (silks, velvets, plush carpets, hand-carved furniture). Drawing room, restaurant, conservatory. Parking. 20 bedrooms. B&B £87.50–£135.

Westbourne Hotel, 165 Westbourne Grove W11 2RD. *Tel* 020-7243 6008, *fax* 020-7229 7201, *email* wh@zoohotels.com, *website* www.zoohotels.com. Near Notting Hill: Giles Baker, Benjamin Fry and Orlando Campbell's '21st-century home-from-home'. Contemporary interior (modern art, design and technology). Lounge, bar/restaurant. B&B double £175–£277. (Underground: Notting Hill Gate)

Many people are upset when they cancel a booking and discover that they have lost a deposit or been charged the full rate of the room. Do remember that when making a booking you are entering into a contract with the hotel. Always make sure you know what the hotel's policy about cancellations is.

ENGLAND

ALFRISTON East Sussex   **Map 2:E4**
White Lodge, Sloe Lane BN26 5UR. *Tel* 01323-870265, *fax* 01323-870284, *email* sales@whitelodge-hotel.com, *website* www. whitelodge-hotel.com. Extended Edwardian house in 5-acre garden overlooking Cuckmere valley. Traditional decor, log fires. 'Good value; excellent service and food.' 19 bedrooms (some with 4-poster, balcony). B&B £45–£75.

ASHFORD Kent   **Map 2:D5**
Eastwell Manor, Eastwell Park, Boughton Lees TN25 4HR. *Tel* 01233-213000, *fax* 01233-635530, *email* eastwell@btinternet.com, *website* www.eastwellmanor.co.uk. Grand Tudor-style 1920s house in 3,000-acre estate, near Channel Tunnel: moulded ceilings, huge fireplaces. Restaurant, brasserie, bars, lounges; spa; indoor/outdoor swimming pools, gym, tennis; extensive function facilities. 61 bedrooms ('marvellously equipped') – family apartments in stable block (children welcomed). B&B £80–£175.

BIRMINGHAM West Midlands   **Map 2:B2**
Jonathans', 16 Wolverhampton Road, Oldbury B68 0LH. *Tel* 0121-429 3757, *fax* 0121-434 3107, *email* bookings@jonathans.co.uk, *website* www.jonathans.co.uk. Two Jonathans (Bedford and Baker) have re-created Victorian era (patterned wallpapers, heavy fabrics, bric-a-brac) behind 1930s facade on busy road, 4 miles W of centre. Bar, bistro, restaurant. Small conference facilities. Parking. 31 bedrooms. B&B £55–£155.

Further afield:
Grafton Manor, Grafton Lane, Bromsgrove, Worcestershire B61 7HA. *Tel* 01527-579007, *fax* 01527-575221, *email* grafton@ bestloved.com, *website* www.graftonmanorhotel.co.uk. 17 miles from Birmingham, overlooking motorway: Norman house in 26-acre grounds: herb garden, lake, 16th-century fish stew, chapel. 'Work needed in some areas but wonderful place to stay.' Indian cuisine a speciality. 9 bedrooms. B&B £52.50–£95.

BLACKBURN Lancashire   **Map 4:D3**
Millstone, Church Street, Mellor BB2 7JR. *Tel* 01254-813333, *fax* 01254-812628, *email* millstone@shireinns.co.uk. Former coaching inn. 2 bars, restaurant; conference facilities. Parking. 24 bedrooms (1 suitable for &). B&B £34–£98.

BLACKPOOL Lancashire   **Map 4:D2**
River House, Skippool Creek, Thornton-le-Fylde FY5 5LF. *Tel* 01253-883497, *fax* 01253-892083, *email* enquiries@theriverhouse.org.uk, *website* www.theriverhouse.org.uk. Bill and Linda Scott's restaurant-with-rooms in 1830s house, 4 miles NE of Blackpool. Log fires, antiques; Victorian conservatory. Hearty breakfasts. 4 bedrooms. B&B £45–£70.

BOURNEMOUTH Dorset   **Map 2:E2**
Langtry Manor, Derby Road, East Cliff BH1 3QB. *Tel* 01202-553887, *fax* 01202-290115, *email* lillie@langtrymanor.com, *website* www.langtrymanor.com. Mock-Tudor house near sea, built by Prince of Wales (later Edward VII) for his mistress, Lillie Langtry. Ornate restaurant (high ceiling, minstrels' gallery, tapestries, stained glass) sometimes serves an Edwardian feast. Lounge, conservatory; function room. Garden. 28 bedrooms. B&B £54.75–£104.75.

BRADFORD West Yorkshire   **Map 4:D3**
Quality Victoria, Bridge Street BD1 1JX. *Tel* 01274-728706, *fax* 01274-736358, *email* admin@gb646.u-net.com, *website* www.hotelnet.co.uk/friendly/home. Opposite coach and rail stations, imposing 19th-century purpose-built hotel, chain-owned. Pub, restaurant; leisure centre. 60 bedrooms (with CD-player, etc.): single £75–£83, double £90–£108. Breakfast £7.95–£9.95.

BRIGHTON East Sussex   **Map 2:E4**
Adelaide, 51 Regency Square BN1 2FF. *Tel* 01273-205286, *fax* 01273-220904, *email* adelaide@pavilion.co.uk. Grade II listed Regency house on seafront square. NCP car park opposite. 12 bedrooms. B&B £34–£46.
Ainsley House 28 New Steine, Marine Parade BN2 1PD. *Tel* 01273-605310, *fax* 01273-688604, *email* ahhotel@fastnet.co.uk, *website* www.searchl.co.uk/ainsleyhouse. Laurence and Christine King's B&B on E side of square near seafront. 11 bedrooms, most *en suite*. 'Considerate hosts. Good value. Faultless breakfast' (vegetarian, continental, English). B&B £22–£36.
Granville, 124 Kings Road BN1 2FA. *Tel* 01273-326302, *fax* 01273-728294, *email* granville@brighton.co.uk, *website* www.granvillehotel.co.uk. Pet-friendly Regency seafront hotel, 'furnished with flair' by owners, Sue and Mick Paskins. Organic restaurant, café/bar. 24 no-smoking bedrooms. B&B £50–£77.50.
Pelirocco, 10 Regency Square BN1 2FG. *Tel* 01273-327055, *fax* 01273-733845, *email* info@hotelpelirocco.co.uk, *website* www.hotelpelirocco.co.uk. Jane Slater and Mick Robinson's B&B, 'a shrine to youth culture', opposite West Pier. 18 themed bedrooms by sundry trendsetters (but attic room found 'dark and cramped'). Bar/lounge. Conference centre. B&B £32.50–£55.

BRISTOL   **Map 1:B6**
Berkeley Square Hotel, Berkeley Square, Clifton BS8 1HB. *Tel* 0117-925 4000, *fax* 0117-925 2970, *email* berkley@cliftonhotels.com, *website* www.cliftonhotels.com/berkeley. Conversion of 2 houses on Georgian square ½ mile from centre, near university. Pleasant decor; helpful staff; good breakfast. No residents' lounge. Basement bar. Modern cooking in *Nightingales* restaurant. Secure parking. 43 bedrooms (25 single). B&B from £53.50.

BROXTED Essex   **Map 2:C4**
Whitehall, Church End CM6 2BZ. *Tel* 01279-850603, *fax*

01279-850385, *email* sales@whitehallhotel.co.uk, *website* www.
whitehallhotel.co.uk. Elizabethan manor house, 10 mins' drive from
Stansted airport; easy access M11. 15th-century timbered dining hall;
function/conference facilities. Walled garden. 26 bedrooms: single
£95–£195, double £120–£220. Breakfast £6–£10.

CAMBRIDGE Cambridgeshire   Map 2:B4
Arundel House, 53 Chesterton Road CB4 3AN. *Tel* 01223-367701,
fax 01223-367721, *email* info@arundelhousehotels.co.uk, *website*
www.arundelhousehotels.co.uk. Near Cam and Jesus Green, privately owned hotel (converted Victorian town houses). Families
welcomed. Some conference trade. 105 unfussy bedrooms, most
en suite, all no-smoking. Small garden. Private parking. B&B
£36.25–£49.50.

Further afield:
Church Farm, Gransden Road, Caxton CB3 8PL. *Tel* 01954-
719543, *fax* 01954-718999, *email* churchfarm@aol.com, *website*
www.wolsey-lodges.co.uk. Peter and Maggie Scott's 17th-century
farmhouse, 8 miles SW of Cambridge. Communal breakfast; dinner
by arrangement. 3-acre garden: tennis. No smoking. 6 bedrooms.
B&B £35–£45.
Melbourn Bury, Melbourn, nr Royston SG8 6DE. *Tel* 01763-
261151, *fax* 01763-262375, *email* mazecare@aol.com. Anthony and
Sylvia Hopkinson's Tudor manor house: antiques, fine paintings, log
fires; garden (lake, wildfowl). 3 no-smoking bedrooms. Bus/train
from nearby Royston to Cambridge (10 miles N). B&B £47.50–£65.
Evening meal by arrangement.

CANTERBURY Kent   Map 2:D5
Ebury, 65–67 New Dover Road CT1 3DX. *Tel* 01227-768433,
fax 01227-459187, *email* info@ebury-hotel.co.uk, *website* www.
ebury-hotel.co.uk. 1 mile SE of centre, set back from main road in 2-
acre garden: 2 adjoining Victorian houses owned by Mason family.
Period decor (collection of 'bulls eye' clocks). English cooking in
no-smoking restaurant. Indoor swimming pool. 15 bedrooms. B&B
£32.50–£50.
Greyfriars House, 6 Stour Street CT1 2NR. *Tel* 01227-456255, *fax*
01227-455233, *email* christine@greyfriars-house.co.uk, *website*
www.greyfriars-house.co.uk. Keith and Christine Chapman's guest
house in quiet cul-de-sac. Children welcomed. Secure parking.
9 bedrooms (some 'tiny'). B&B £22.50–£30.
Magnolia House, 36 St Dunstan's Terrace CT2 8AX. *Tel/fax* 01227-
765121, *email* magnolia house canterbury@yahoo.com, *website*
www.freespace.virgin.net/magnolia.canterbury. Ann and John
Davies's late Georgian house on residential street. 'Friendly; excellent breakfasts.' Walled garden. No smoking. 7 bedrooms. B&B
£39–£55. Evening meal in winter by arrangement.

CARLISLE Cumbria   Map 4:B2
Crosby Lodge, High Crosby, Crosby-on-Eden CA6 4QZ. *Tel*

01228-573618, *fax* 01228-573428, *website* www.crosbylodge.co.uk. 5 miles NE of city: Sedgwick family's turreted mansion in parkland overlooking river Eden. Lounge, bar, restaurant. 11 bedrooms. B&B £57.50–£95.

CHELTENHAM Gloucestershire   **Map 3:D5**
Cleeve Hill Hotel, Cleeve Hill GL52 3PR. *Tel* 01242-672052, *fax* 01242-679969. Bob and Georgie Tracey's no-smoking B&B in area of outstanding natural beauty, 4 miles NE of town. Lounge, bar, breakfast room. ½-acre garden. 9 bedrooms. B&B £35–£60.

CHESTER Cheshire   **Map 3:A4**
Chester Bells, 21 Grosvenor Street CH1 2DD. *Tel* 01244-324022. Central: beamed building run by Ian and Jane Turner. 'Friendly, good decor, excellent value.' Parking. 6 bedrooms. B&B: single £20 (shared bathroom), double £50 (*en suite*).
Green Bough, 60 Hoole Road CH2 3NL. *Tel* 01244-326241, *fax* 01244-326265, *email* greenboughhotel@cwcom.net, *website* www. smoothound.co.uk/hotels/greenbo. Janice and Philip Martin's late Victorian house in leafy avenue. 'Civilised, friendly, with first-class restaurant.' Parking. 16 bedrooms (3 suitable for &). B&B from £42.50.
Redland Hotel, 64 Hough Green CH4 8JY. *Tel* 01244-671024, *fax* 01244-681309. B&B in red brick house 1 mile E of centre; ample parking. Victorian ambience. Lounge, bar, solarium, sauna. 12 bedrooms. B&B £32.50–£45.
Crabwall Manor, Parkgate Road, Mollington CH1 6NE. *Tel* 01244-851666, *fax* 01244-851400, *email* crabwallmanor@marstonhotels.com, *website* www.marstonhotels.com. Large turreted building, part 16th-century, in own park, 2¼ miles from centre. Spacious public rooms. Extensive leisure facilities; 18-metre indoor swimming pool, big gym; beauty treatments. 48 bedrooms: single £116–£140, double £140–£175, suite £185–£270.

CHICHESTER West Sussex   **Map 2:E3**
Crouchers Bottom, Birdham Road PO20 7EH. *Tel* 01243-784995, *fax* 01243-539797, *email* crouchers-bottom@btinternet.com, *website* www.crouchersbottom.com. Owned by Wilson family: group of old buildings and modern extensions on A286 to the Witterings, 2 miles S of centre. Lounge, restaurant. ½-acre garden. Parking. 17 bedrooms (quietest ones on courtyard; 2 with & access). B&B £42.50–£59.
Suffolk House, 3 East Row PO19 1PD. *Tel* 01243-778899, *fax* 01243-787282, *email* reservations@suffolkhshotel.demon.co.uk. Near cathedral and theatre: 18th-century house. 'Excellent service, comfortable room'; simple decor. Lounge, restaurant (no smoking); alfresco breakfast in summer. 11 bedrooms. B&B £44.50–£84.

COLCHESTER Essex   **Map 2:C5**
Rose and Crown, East Street CO1 2TZ. *Tel* 01206-866677, *fax* 01206-866616, *email* info@rose-and-crown.com, *website* www. rose-and-crown.com. Timber-framed former posting house (Best

Western) at road junction on edge of town. Exposed brick and beams. *Tudor Bar* (meals available); conference/function facilities; beauty treatments. Parking. 30 bedrooms (5 no-smoking): single £74, double £79–£99. Breakfast £5.95–£8.95.

CORNHILL-ON-TWEED Northumberland   **Map 4:A3**
Tillmouth Park TD12 4UU. *Tel* 01890-882255, *fax* 01890-882540, *email* reception@tillmouthpark.f9.co.uk, *website* www.tillmouthpark.co.uk. Victorian mansion in 15-acre woodlands (with ruined castle) on banks of river Till. Period decor ('slight Scottish feel'). Families welcomed. Galleried lounge, restaurant, bistro. 14 bedrooms. B&B £65–£115.

COVENTRY West Midlands   **Map 2:B2**
Coombe Abbey, Brinklow Road, Binley CV3 2AB. *Tel* 024-7645 0450, *fax* 024-7663 5101, *website* www.coombeabbey.com. 3½ miles E of centre. Atmospheric 12th-century Cistercian abbey (with moat, portcullis) in 500-acre park (lake, formal gardens by Capability Brown). Medieval evenings, banquets in baronial hall; weddings. 63 'bedchambers' (some with 4-poster, throne loo): single from £125, double from £135. Breakfast £10–£12.
Haigs, 273 Kenilworth Road, Balsall Common CV7 7EL. *Tel* 01676-533004, *fax* 01676-535132, *website* www.haigshotel.co.uk. Hester and Alan Harris's hotel on A452, 4 miles from Coventry, 5 miles from Birmingham airport/NEC. 'Real family feel; superb food.' Lounge bar, restaurant; function room. 23 bedrooms. B&B £45–£77.
Nailcote Hall, Nailcote Lane, Berkswell CV7 7DE. *Tel* 024-7646 6174, *fax* 024-7647 0720, *email* info@nailcotehall.co.uk, *website* www.nailcotehall.co.uk. 6½ miles SW of centre on B4101 to Knowle,10 mins from airport/NEC. Rick Cressman's Tudor-style manor house with subterranean extensions. French cooking in *Oak Room* restaurant; Mediterranean-style café/bar. Extensive leisure facilities. 15-acre grounds. 38 bedrooms. B&B £75–£140.

DARLINGTON Co. Durham   **Map 4:C4**
Clow-Beck House, Monk End Farm, Croft on Tees DL2 2SW. *Tel* 01325-721075, *fax* 01325-720419, *email* heather@clowbeckhouse.co.uk, *website* www.clowbeckhouse.co.uk. David and Heather Armstrong's 'informal, friendly' farmhouse, 2 miles SW of centre. 2 acre gardens, 90 acres farmland (fishing on river Tees). Flamboyant decor. 14 themed bedrooms (Camelot is 'dazzling'). Good breakfast; traditional evening meal. B&B £37.50–£47.
Headlam Hall, Headlam, nr Gainford DL2 3HA. *Tel* 01325-730238, *fax* 01325-730790, *email* admin@headlamhall.co.uk, *website* www.headlamhall.co.uk. In lower Teesdale hamlet, amid 200-acre farmland: Robinson family's rambling building, half Jacobean, half 18th-century. Lounges, small bar, restaurant. Indoor swimming pool, sauna, billiard room; conference/function facilities. Garden: lake, tennis, golf, croquet. 34 bedrooms. B&B £42–£99.

DOVER Kent   **Map 2:D5**
Loddington House, 14 East Cliff, Sea Front, Marine Parade
CT16 1LX. *Tel/fax* 01304-201947. Kathy and Mike Cupper's
Grade II listed guest house in seafront Regency terrace, near termi-
nals/Hoverport. Lounge, dining room – evening meal sometimes
served. 6 bedrooms (4 *en suite*; quietest ones at rear). B&B
£27.30–£45.
Old Vicarage, Chilverton Elms, Hougham CT15 7AS. *Tel* 01304-
210668, *fax* 01304-225118. Judy and Bryan Evison's large Victorian
house, 2 miles from port. Children welcomed. Evening meal by
arrangement. Secure parking. 3 bedrooms. B&B: double £65–£70.

DURHAM Co. Durham   **Map 4:B4**
Georgian Town House, 10–11 Crossgate DH1 4PS. *Tel/fax* 0191-
386 8070, *email* enquiries@georgian-townhouse.fsnet.co.uk. 'Good
value, excellent service' in Mr and Mrs Weil's 300-year-old Grade II
listed terrace house. 'Sat night can be noisy (pub opposite).' 7 bedrooms. B&B £30–£50.
Lumley Castle, Chester-le-Street DH3 4NX. *Tel* 0191-389 1111, *fax*
0191-387 1437, *email* lumcastl@netcomuk.co.uk, *website* www.
lumleycastle.com. 14th-century moated castle, remodelled by
Vanbrugh, above river Wear, 5 miles N of city. Thick walls, dimly
lit corridors, spiral staircases; vaulted restaurant; *Baron's Hall*
(Elizabethan banquets); extensive function/conference facilities;
whimsical style. 60 bedrooms (some no-smoking): single £95–£135,
double £135–£275. Breakfast £9–£12.50.

FLITWICK Bedfordshire   **Map 2:C3**
Flitwick Manor, Church Road MK45 1AE. *Tel* 01525-712242,
fax 01525-718753, *email* info@menzies-hotels.co.uk, *website* www.
menzies-hotels.co.uk. Georgian manor house, now chain-owned
hotel. 3 miles from M1 exit 12. 50-acre grounds: lake, deer park,
12th-century church. Traditional decor/food. 17 bedrooms: single
£120, double £145–£175, suite £195–£275.

GATWICK West Sussex   **Map 2:D4**
Alexander House, Ten Place, East Street, Turners Hill RH10 4QD.
Tel 01342-714914, *fax* 01342-717328, *email* info@
alexanderhouse.co.uk. Part 17th-century house in 135-acre grounds.
Elaborate decor (chandeliers, ruched curtains, murals). Drawing
room, library, bar, restaurant; conference facilities. 15 bedrooms.
B&B £79–£142.50.
Copperwood Guest House, Massetts Road, Horley RH6 7DJ.
Tel 01293-783388, *fax* 01293-420156, *email* copperwood@
blueyonder.co.uk, *website* www.copperwood.co.uk. Paul and
Caroline Hooks's no-smoking B&B. Near airport, off busy road.
Parking (£14 per week). B&B £25–£35.
Vulcan Lodge, 27 Massetts Road, Horley RH6 7DQ. *Tel* 01293-
771522, *fax* 01293-786206, *email* reservations@vulcan-lodge.com,
website www.vulcan-lodge.com. Half mile from Gatwick airport,
late 17th-century house: Colin and Karen Moon's B&B. Lounge,

breakfast room. Parking for guests making short trips abroad. 6 bedrooms (2 family). B&B £27.50–£38.50.

Wayside Manor Farm, Norwood Hill, Charlwood, Surrey RH6 0ET. *Tel* 01293-862692, *fax* 01293-863417, *email* plumbs@waysidemf.freeserve.co.uk, *website* www.waysidemf.freeserve.co.uk. Viv and Phil Plumb's Edwardian house, 8 mins' drive from airport (transport arranged). 'Personable owners; good breakfasts.' Pub opposite. 3 bedrooms, some *en suite*. B&B £27.50–£50.

GUILDFORD Surrey   Map 2:D3

The Angel, 91 High Street GU1 3DP. *Tel* 01483-564555, *fax* 01483-533770. Historic black-and-white inn on cobbled high street (pedestrianised 11 am–4 pm). Galleried lounge; panelled dining room; restaurant in crypt; conference facilities. 21 bedrooms: double £135–£140, suite £150–£200. Breakfast £8.50–£12.50.

HARROGATE North Yorkshire   Map 4:D4

Crescent Lodge, 20 Swan Road HG1 2SA. *Tel* 01423-503688. Julia Humphris's B&B in Grade II listed early Victorian house in quiet terrace near centre. Drawing room with books, ceramics. Garden. Limited parking. 4 bedrooms (2 *en suite*). B&B £26–£36.

Rudding Park, Follifoot HG3 1JH. *Tel* 01423-871350, *fax* 01423-872286, *email* sales@rudding-park.co.uk, *website* www.rudding-park.co.uk. On 2,000-acre estate (with 18-hole golf course, holiday park), 3 miles S of city centre: business/function-oriented hotel. 'Motivated, friendly staff. Excellent bedrooms.' Lounge, bar, restaurant, dining terrace. 50 bedrooms. B&B £72.50.

HASTINGS East Sussex   Map 2:E4

Beauport Park, Battle Road TN38 8EA. *Tel* 01424-851222, *fax* 01424-852465, *email* reservations@beauportprkhotel.demon.co.uk, *website* www.beauportprkhotel.demon.co.uk. Georgian country house (Best Western), 3 miles N of centre. Traditional decor; no-smoking restaurant; brasserie/conservatory. 37-acre grounds: woodland, gardens, swimming pool, tennis; golf adjacent. 25 bedrooms: single £85, double from £110.

HENLEY-ON-THAMES Oxfordshire   Map 2:D3

Thamesmead House, Remenham Lane RG9 2LR. *Tel* 01491-574745, *fax* 01491-579944, *email* thamesmead@supanet.com, *website* www.thamesmeadhousehotel.co.uk. B&B hotel overlooking cricket green, 3 mins' walk from centre. 'Friendly welcome. Bright Scandinavian-style decor. Immaculate rooms. Good breakfast.' No smoking. Drinks/sandwiches available. Small conference facilities. 6 bedrooms. B&B £62.50–£110.

HUDDERSFIELD West Yorkshire   Map 4:E3

The Lodge, 48 Birkby Lodge Road, Birkby HD2 2BG. *Tel* 01484-431001, *fax* 01484-421590. Garry and Kevin Birley's stone-built house in garden in prosperous suburb, 1½ miles from centre. Sitting room with Art Nouveau panelled walls, plaster ceiling. Good modern cooking in popular restaurant. Meeting rooms. Children welcomed. 11 no-smoking bedrooms. B&B £35–£60.

HULL East Yorkshire   Map 4:D5
Willerby Manor, Well Lane, Willerby HU10 6ER. *Tel* 01482-652616, *fax* 01482-653901. Edwardian mansion (Best Western), 10 mins from centre. Restaurant, brasserie; health club; business facilities. 3-acre mature gardens. 51 bedrooms: single £74.50, double £85–£99. Breakfast £6.20–£9.50.

LEAMINGTON SPA Warwickshire   Map 2:B2
Lansdowne, 87 Clarendon Street CV32 4PF. *Tel* 01926-450505, *fax* 01926-421313, *website* www.thelandsdowne.cwc.net. Now with Swiss-trained resident directors: small town house at road junction near centre (double glazing). Lounge, bar, restaurant. 14 small bedrooms. B&B £34–£59.95.
Leamington Hotel & Bistro, 64 Upper Holly Walk CV32 4JL. *Tel* 01926-883777, *fax* 01926-330467. Frank Nixey and Hilary Ashover's hotel/bistro (Best Western). Lounge, function/conference facilities. Children welcomed. 30 bedrooms, 'spacious, simply furnished'. B&B £40–£80.

LEDBURY Herefordshire   Map 3:D5
Feathers, High Street HR8 1DS. *Tel* 01531-635266, *fax* 01531-638955, *email* mary@feathers-ledbury.co.uk, *website* www. feathers-ledbury.co.uk. 16th-century half-timbered inn 'in best tradition of small town hotels'. Brasserie ('outstanding dinner'); spa; function/conference facilities. Parking. 19 bedrooms. B&B £44.75–£77.50.

LIVERPOOL Merseyside   Map 4:E2
Bowler Hat, 2 Talbot Road, Prenton, nr Birkenhead CH43 2HH. *Tel* 0151-652 4931, *fax* 0151-653 8127, *website* www.corushotels.com. 3 miles SW of centre, on Wirral peninsula. Late Victorian house. Restaurant; club bar; garden. 32 bedrooms. B&B £35–£60.
Thornton Hall, Neston Road, Thornton Hough, Wirral CH63 1JF. *Tel* 0151-336 3938, *fax* 0151-336 7864. In central Wirral village: hotel/health club in 18th-century house (Best Western). 2 bars, 2 restaurants; conference centre. 7-acre grounds. 63 bedrooms. B&B £50–£90.
Woolton Redbourne, Acrefield Road, Woolton L25 5JN. *Tel* 0151-421 1500, *fax* 0151-421 1501, *email* wooltonredbourne@cwcom.net, *website* www.merseyworld.com/woolton-redbourne. 'Very special': Grade II listed Victorian mansion in residential area, 25 mins' drive from centre. Period decor. Lounge, bar, restaurant (residents only). Garden. 21 bedrooms (rear ones quietest). B&B from £45.50.

LYME REGIS Dorset   Map 1:C6
Alexandra Hotel, Pound Street DT7 3HZ. *Tel* 01297-442010, *fax* 01297-443229, *email* alexandra@lymeregis.co.uk, *website*

www.hotelalexandra.co.uk. In superb position above The Cobb: Mr and Mrs Haskins's traditional hotel. Families and dogs welcomed. Lounge, conservatory; restaurant; garden. Parking. Beach 300 yds. 27 bedrooms. B&B £43–£110.

MANCHESTER and area   Map 4:E3

Crescent Gate, Park Crescent, Victoria Park, Rusholme M14 5RE. *Tel* 0161-224 0672, *fax* 0161-257 2822. Run for many years by Terry Hughes: guest house in quiet crescent off Wilmslow Rd, 2 miles S of centre. Car park. 25 bedrooms, most *en suite*. B&B £26–£38.50. Evening meal available.

Malmaison, Piccadilly M1 3AQ. *Tel* 0161-278 1000, *fax* 0161-278 1002, *email* manchester@malmaison.com, *website* www.malmaison.com. City-centre designer hotel, recently much extended, on busy street by Piccadilly station. Bar, brasserie; leisure centre. Valet parking. 167 bedrooms (many no-smoking): single/double £115, suite £175. Breakfast £9.95–£11.95.

Le Meridien Victoria & Albert, Water Street M3 4JQ. *Tel* 0870-4008585, *fax* 0161-834 2484, *email* gm1452@forte.hotels.com, *website* www.lemeridien-hotels.com. Two converted warehouses on river Irwell: decor themed to productions by Granada TV studios adjacent. Pub, café, restaurant; conference/function facilities; health club. 156 rooms (wing for lone female guests): single/double from £165, suite from £225.

Alderley Edge Hotel, Macclesfield Road, Alderley Edge, Cheshire SK9 7BJ. *Tel* 01625-583033, *fax* 01625-586343, *email* sales@ alderley-edge-hotel.co.uk, *website* www.alderley-edge-hotel.co.uk. By famous beauty spot, 14 miles S of centre, 7 miles from airport: red sandstone mansion, much extended. Smart restaurant. 46 bedrooms: single £109–£125, double £130–£140, suite from £145. Breakfast £8.50–£10.50.

Etrop Grange, Thorley Lane, Manchester Airport M90 4EG. *Tel* 0161-499 0500, *fax* 0161-499 0790, *email* etropgrange@ corushotels.com, *website* www.corushotels.com/etropgrange. Georgian Grade II listed house, much extended, by airport. Edwardian decor; antique/repro furniture; function facilities. Light meals all day; restaurant specialising in fish. 40 bedrooms. B&B £71–£155.

Hazeldean, 467 Bury New Road, Kersal, Salford M7 3NE. *Tel* 0161-792 6667, *fax* 0161-792 6668. Graham Chadwick's Victorian house in residential area of Salford, 2 miles N of Manchester centre. Lounge, bar, dining room (evening meals weekdays). Garden; car park. 21 bedrooms. B&B £26.50–£47.

Springfield, 99 Station Road, Marple, Cheshire SK6 6PA. *Tel* 0161-449 0721, *fax* 0161-449 0766. In dormitory town 11 miles SE of Manchester centre: Mrs Giannecchini's Victorian house, 5 mins' walk from station, 15 mins' drive from Stockport. Lounge, bar, breakfast room. Car park. 7 bedrooms. B&B £25–£40.

Stanneylands, Stanneylands Road, Wilmslow, Cheshire SK9 4EY. *Tel* 01625-525225, *fax* 01625-537282, *website* www.stanneylands. co.uk. Beech family's Edwardian house. Central Manchester

10 miles, airport 3 miles. Country-house decor; sophisticated Franco-British cooking. Conference/function facilities. Beautiful gardens. 32 bedrooms: single £94, double £108–£118.

Woodland Park, Wellington Road, Timperley, Cheshire WA15 7RG. *Tel* 0161-928 8631, *fax* 0161-941 2821, *email* info@woodlandpark. co.uk, *website* www.woodlandpark.co.uk. Brian and Shirley Walker's hotel in residential area, 4 miles from airport, 8 miles from centre (Metrolink 300 yds). Elaborate decor. Lounge, restaurant, conservatory; conference/function facilities. Parking. 45 bedrooms. B&B £50–£90.

MILTON KEYNES Buckinghamshire   Map 2:C3
Different Drummer, 92 High Street, Stony Stratford MK11 1AH. *Tel* 01908-564733, *fax* 01908-260646, *email* sales@ thedifferentdrummer.co.uk, *website* www.thedifferentdrummer. co.uk. NW of centre: old coaching inn, quirkily restored. Good Italian cooking in *Al Tamborista* restaurant. 14 bedrooms. B&B £32.50–£120.

NANTWICH Cheshire   Map 3:B5
Rookery Hall, Worleston CW5 6DQ. *Tel* 01270-610016, *fax* 01270-626027, *email* rookery@arcadianhotels.co.uk, *website* www. arcadianhotels.co.uk. Georgian mansion in 38-acre grounds on river Weaver (lake, fountain, tennis, croquet, fishing). Sumptuous decor. 'Excellent, good-humoured staff; lovely lounge.' Modern cooking. Conference suite. 45 bedrooms. B&B £55–£110.

NEWBURY Berkshire   Map 2:D2
Newbury Manor, London Road RG14 2BY. *Tel* 01635-528838, *fax* 01635-523406, *email* enquiries@newbury-manor-hotel.co.uk, *website* www.newbury-manor-hotel.co.uk. Georgian house in 9-acre wooded grounds (with rivers Kennet and Lambourn), 5 mins' drive W of Newbury. Traditional decor; specially commissioned paintings. Lounge, riverside bar (meal service), 'excellent restaurant'; conference/function facilities. 33 bedrooms. B&B £77.50–£250.

NORWICH Norfolk   Map 2:B5
Norfolk Mead, Church Lane, Coltishall NR12 7DN *Tel* 01603-737531, *fax* 01603-737521, *email* info@norfolkmead.co.uk, *website* www.norfolkmead.co.uk. Don and Jill Fleming's Georgian manor house, ½ mile from conservation village, 7 miles N of Norwich. 12-acre grounds on river Bure (garden, swimming pool, pasture, fishing, mooring). Lounge, bar, restaurant (no-smoking; modern British cooking); spa. 9 no-smoking bedrooms. B&B £39–£90.

NOTTINGHAM Nottinghamshire   Map 2:A3
Hotel des Clos, Old Lenton Lane NG7 2SA. *Tel* 0115-986 6566, *fax* 0115-986 0343, *website* www.hoteldesclos.com. Ralley family's Victorian farmhouse on banks of river Trent, reopened April 2001 following extensive refurbishment. 'Small, efficient, well decorated', but setting less than bucolic, by dual carriageway, industrial estate

and electricity pylons. Restaurant; function/conference facilities. Free parking. 8 bedrooms: single/double £85, suite £100–£125.

OXFORD Oxfordshire   Map 2:C2

Galaxie, 180 Banbury Road OX2 7BT. *Tel* 01865-515688, *fax* 01865-556824, *website* www.oxlink.co.uk/oxford/hotels/galaxie. Gwyn and Mair Harries-Jones's ivy-clad red brick B&B hotel, 'bright and cheerful', in Summertown (residential area). Breakfast conservatory. Garden. Parking. 30 bedrooms. B&B from £40.

Marlborough House, 321 Woodstock Road, OX2 7NY. *Tel* 01865-311321, *fax* 01865-515329, *email* enquiries@marlbhouse. win-uk.net, *website* www.oxfordcity.co.uk/hotels/marlborough. Purpose-built hotel in N Oxford, 1½ miles from centre; 10 mins' walk to restaurants. Street parking. Lounge. 16 bedrooms with kitchenette: breakfast tray brought to room previous evening. B&B £39.50–£68.

Further afield:

The Feathers, Market Street, Woodstock OX20 1SX. *Tel* 01993-812291, *fax* 01993-813158, *email* enquiries@feathers.co.uk, *website* www.feathers.co.uk. 8 miles NW of Oxford: 17th-century coaching inn near Blenheim Palace. Rambling interior, lots of steps. Drawing room, study, bar, restaurant (*Michelin* star, but new chef in 2001); function facilities; courtyard. 21 bedrooms. B&B £67.50–£115.

Studley Priory, Horton-cum-Studley OX33 1AZ. *Tel* 01865-351203, *fax* 01865-351613, *email* res@studley-priory.co.uk, *website* www.studley-priory.co.uk. Parke family's large Elizabethan house in 13-acre wooded grounds (tennis, croquet) in village 7 miles NE of Oxford. Drawing room, bar, restaurant. 17 bedrooms. B&B £75–£175.

PLYMOUTH Devon   Map 1:D4

Bowling Green Hotel, 9–10 Osborne Place, Lockyer Street, The Hoe PL1 2PU. *Tel* 01752-209090, *fax* 01752-209092, *email* info@bowlinggreenhotel.co.uk, *website* www.bowlinggreenhotel. co.uk. David and Paddy Dawkins's no-frills B&B, opposite The Hoe. 'High standards.' Small garden. 12 bedrooms. B&B £25–£38.

Invicta, 11–12 Osborne Place, Lockyer Street, The Hoe PL1 2PU. *Tel* 01752-664997, *fax* 01752-664994. Family-run guest house opposite The Hoe. Plain decor. 'Friendly welcome and service.' Mediterranean-style cooking. Car park. 23 bedrooms (3 family). B&B £31–£52.

Oliver's, 33 Sutherland Road PL4 6BN. *Tel* 01752-663923. Joy and Mike Purser's hotel/restaurant in residential area. 'Perfectly cooked food,' says nominator. Lounge/library, bar. Car park. 6 bedrooms. B&B £20–£30.

Kitley House, Kitley Estate, Yealmpton PL8 2NW. *Tel* 01752-881555, *fax* 01752-881667, *email* sales@kitleyhousehotel.com, *website* www.kitleyhousehotel.com. Large grey stone house in 300-acre estate, 7 miles E of centre. Lounge, bar, restaurant; health/beauty salon; function facilities. 20 bedrooms. B&B £49.50–£69.50.

POOLE Dorset **Map 2:E1**
Salterns, 38 Salterns Way, Lilliput BH14 8JR. *Tel* 01202-707321, *fax* 01202-707488, *website* www.salterns.co.uk. Looking across Poole Harbour; Best Western member in 14-acre grounds with marina. Unimpressive exterior hides 'warm interior'. 'Staff exceptionally helpful. Good meals.' Bar snacks; seafood bistro, restaurant; waterside patio. Conference facilities. 20 bedrooms: single from £76, double from £106. Breakfast £8–£10.

PORTSMOUTH Hampshire **Map 2:E3**
Beaufort, 71 Festing Road, Southsea PO4 0NQ. *Tel* 023-9282 3707, *fax* 023-9287 0270, *email* enq@beauforthotel.co.uk. Penny and Tony Freemantle's hotel in residential area, near sea. Lounge, bar, restaurant ('good home-cooked fare'). Garden; car park. 20 bedrooms (8 no-smoking). B&B £29–£48.
Sally Port Inn, High Street, Old Portsmouth PO1 2LU. *Tel* 023-9282 1860, *fax* 023-9282 1293. Built 1947 using timbers salvaged from 16th/17th-century building/19th-century ships, Georgian cantilever staircase and ship's top-spar. Pub meals; restaurant ('good fresh fish'). 14 bedrooms (exposed beams, period furniture, some *en suite*). B&B £27.50–£45.
Upper Mount House, The Vale, off Clarendon Road, Southsea PO5 2EQ. *Tel/fax* 023-9282 0456, *email* rlmoth@uppermount. fsbusiness.co.uk. 19th-century listed building in residential area, 5 mins' drive from ferry terminal. Lounge, bar, dining room (evening meal by arrangement). Garden. Parking. 12 bedrooms. B&B £24–£30.

REIGATE Surrey **Map 2:D4**
Cranleigh, 41 West Street RH2 9BL. *Tel* 01737-223417, *fax* 01737-223734. Carol and Pino Bussandri's hotel at end of high street, in garden (swimming pool, tennis). Italian restaurant (weekday dinners only); conservatory for functions. 10 bedrooms. B&B £45–£76.

RYE East Sussex **Map 2:E5**
Mermaid Inn, Mermaid Street TN31 7EY. *Tel* 01797-223065, *fax* 01797-225069, *email* mermaidinrye@btclick.com. *website* www. mermaidinn.com. 15th-century inn (old timbers, panelling, log fires). Lounges, bar, restaurant. 31 bedrooms. B&B: double from £70.

ST ALBANS Hertfordshire **Map 2:C3**
St Michael's Manor, Fishpool Street, St Michael's Village AL3 4RY. *Tel* 01727-864444, *fax* 01727-848909, *email* smmanor@ globalnet.co.uk, *website* www.stmichaelsmanor.com. 10 mins' walk from abbey and Roman city: 16th-century house run by Newling Ward family for 3 generations. Restaurant/conservatory, terrace; function facilities. 5-acre lakeside gardens. 23 bedrooms. B&B £77.50–£240.

SALISBURY Wiltshire **Map 2:D2**
Leena's, 50 Castle Road SP1 3RL. *Tel/fax* 01722-335419. Leena and Malcolm Street's Edwardian house on busy Amesbury road

(windows double-glazed). 15 mins' riverside walk to centre. Lounge; good breakfasts. Garden; parking. 6 bedrooms, most no-smoking. B&B £24–£38.

Red Lion, Milford Street SP1 2AN. *Tel* 01722-323334, *fax* 01722-325756, *email* reception@the-redlion.co.uk, *website* www. the-redlion.co.uk. Historic coaching inn (Best Western) in centre: creepered courtyard, clock collection, popular restaurant: 'Well-cooked meals; good breakfasts.' Limited parking. 54 bedrooms: single £84–£99, double £104–£122. Breakfast £5.50–£9.50.

Rose and Crown, Harnham Road, Harnham SP2 8JQ. *Tel* 01722-399955, *fax* 01722-339816. 13th-century inn on river Avon, short walk from centre. No-frills cooking in riverside restaurant. 28 bedrooms: single £110, double from £140. Breakfast £10.50.

Further afield:
Little Langford Farmhouse, Little Langford SP3 4NP. *Tel* 01722-790205, *fax* 01722-790086, *email* bandb@littlangford.co.uk, *website* www.dmac.co.uk.llf. Patricia Helyer's B&B in Victorian house in Wylye valley, on large working farm, 8 miles N of Salisbury. Relaxed atmosphere; children welcomed. Lounge, billiard room. 3 simple bedrooms. B&B £25–£26.

SCARBOROUGH North Yorkshire   Map 4:C5
Tall Storeys, 131 Longwestgate, Old Town YO11 1RQ. *Tel/fax* 01723-373696. Colin Milne's Grade II listed Regency house, over-looking castle, harbour. Slightly eccentric decor – lots of clocks. Lounge, bar, dining room, conservatory; snacks available; evening meal by arrangement. 7 no-smoking bedrooms. B&B £28–£32.

SHEFFIELD South Yorkshire   Map 4:E4
Hotel Bristol, Blonk Street S1 2AU. *Tel* 0114-220 4000, *fax* 0114-220 3900, *email* sheffield@bhg.co.uk. 'Inexpensive, unpretentious', near station: unprepossessing exterior; cheerful, modern interior; humorous style. Bar, *Picasso* restaurant ('food cooked with care'). Free parking (NCP adjacent). 112 bedrooms: £49.50–£64.50. Breakfast £5.95–£7.95.

Whitley Hall, Elliott Lane, Grenoside S35 8NR. *Tel* 0114-245 4444, *fax* 0114-245 5414, *website* www.whitleyhall.com. 4½ miles N of centre. Fearn family's part Elizabethan house: mullioned windows, flagstone floors, gallery, panelling. English cooking in large restau-rant. 30-acre grounds: 2 lakes, croquet, putting, peacocks. 19 bedrooms. B&B £47.50–£85.

SHREWSBURY Shropshire   Map 3:B4
Albright Hussey, Ellesmere Road SY4 3AF. *Tel* 01939-290571, *fax* 01939-291143, *email* abhhotel@aol.com, *website* www. albrighthussey.co.uk. Subbiani family's hotel/restaurant: Tudor house, much extended, 2½ miles N of Shrewsbury. Antiques, pan-elling, open fireplaces, beams. 4-acre garden with moat. 14 bedrooms. B&B £55–£93.50.

SIDMOUTH Devon   **Map 1:C5**
Hotel Riviera, The Esplanade EX10 8AY. *Tel* 01395-515201,
fax 01395-577775, *email* enquiries@hotelriviera.co.uk, *website*
www.hotelriviera.co.uk. 'Old-fashioned', white, bow-windowed
Regency hotel, 'very well run' by Wharton family owners. Large
lounge, piano bar, smart restaurant; function facilities; terrace overlooking seafront road. 27 bedrooms. B&B £69–£107.
Victoria, The Esplanade EX10 8RY. *Tel* 01395-512651, *fax*
01395-579154, *email* info@victoriahotel.co.uk, *website* www.
victoriahotel.co.uk. Brend family's holiday hotel on seafront.
Traditional decor. 'Good value, warm welcome, good comfort;
excellent food; affordable wine list.' Many sporting/health facilities.
40 bedrooms. D,B&B £75–£133.

SOUTHAMPTON Hampshire   **Map 2:E2**
Highfield House, Highfield Lane, Portswood SO17 1AQ. *Tel* 023-
8035 9955, *fax* 023-8058 3910, *email* highfield@zoffanyhotels.
co.uk, *website* www.zoffanyhotels.co.uk. Purpose-built hotel on out-
skirts, near Ocean Village. Restaurant, conference rooms. Parking.
66 bedrooms. B&B £52.25–£96.50.

STAMFORD Lincolnshire   **Map 2:B3**
Garden House, St Martin's PE9 2LP. *Tel* 01780-763359, *fax* 01780-
763339, *email* gardenhousehotel@stamford60.freeserve.co.uk,
website www.gardenhousehotel.com. Chris and Irene Quinn's 18th-
century house near centre. Bar, conservatory, dining room with
tapestries. Function/wedding facilities. Garden. 20 bedrooms. B&B
£44–£75.

STOKE-ON-TRENT Staffordshire   **Map 3:B5**
Haydon House, Haydon Street, Basford ST4 6JD. *Tel* 01782-
711311, *fax* 01782-717470. Red brick Victorian mansion, run by
Machin family for over 40 years. In quiet residential street near
centre, overlooking countryside. Conference/function/wedding facilities; 'adequate, unfussy' cooking. 30 bedrooms: single £55–£70,
double £65–£80. Breakfast £6.

TORQUAY Devon   **Map 1:D5**
Mulberry House, 1 Scarborough Road TQ2 5UJ. *Tel* 01803-
213639. 5 mins' walk from seafront, Lesley Cooper's no-smoking
guest house: listed Victorian white stucco villa in quiet street.
Restaurant ('excellent dinners'). 3 'calm, beautifully furnished' bedrooms. B&B from £25.
Orestone Manor, Rockhouse Lane, Maidencombe TQ1 4SX. *Tel*
01803-328098, *fax* 01803-328336, *email* enquiries@orestone.co.uk,
website www.orestone.co.uk. Hotel/restaurant on wooded hillside
overlooking Maidencombe beach. Reopened May 2000 following
extensive renovation. Drawing room, seafood restaurant, conservatory. Garden: swimming pool. 12 bedrooms. B&B £50–£80.

TRESCO Isles of Scilly   **Map 1:C1**
New Inn, Isles of Scilly TR24 0QQ. *Tel* 01720-422844, *fax* 01720-423200, *email* newinn@tresco.co.uk. Run by Graham and Sue Shone: small, family-friendly inn. Bar (focal point for islanders), colourful restaurant. Swimming pool. 14 bedrooms. D,B&B £62–£94.

WELLS Somerset   **Map 1:B6**
Market Place Hotel, Market Place BA5 2RW. *Tel* 01749-672616, *fax* 01749-679670, *email* marketplace@bhere.co.uk, *website* www.bhere.co.uk. 16th-century former temperance inn (Best Western) by cathedral; family run. Contemporary decor/medieval features. Bar, restaurant; conference/function facilities; courtyard garden. Car park. 34 bedrooms. B&B £42.50–£79.50.

WHITBY North Yorkshire   **Map 4:C5**
Dunsley Hall, Dunsley YO21 3TL. *Tel* 01947-893437, *fax* 01947-893505, *email* reception@dunsleyhall.com, *website* www.dunsleyhall.com. Carol and Bill Ward's Victorian mansion in hamlet 3 miles NW of centre. 'Excellent.' 'Very quiet; delicious breakfasts.' Lounge, bistro/bar, no-smoking restaurant. Indoor swimming pool. 4-acre garden: putting, tennis. Sea 1 mile. 18 bedrooms. B&B £54.85–£94.85.
Saxonville, Ladysmith Avenue YO21 3HX. *Tel* 01947-602631, *fax* 01947-820523, *email* saxonville@onyxnet.co.uk, *website* www.yorkshirenet.co.uk/saxonville. On West Cliff, 400 yards back from seafront, near cliff lift: Newton family's conversion of red brick terrace houses. Efficient staff, friendly feel, good conventional food. Lounge, bar, restaurant. Parking. 22 bedrooms. B&B £40.

WINDSOR Berkshire   **Map 2:D3**
Castle Hotel, High Street, Windsor SL4 1LJ. *Tel* 0870-400 8300, *fax* 01753-830244, *email* heritagehotels_windsor.castle@forte-hotels.com, *website* www.heritage-hotels.com. White Georgian building in centre. 'Comfortable public rooms, good main meals and breakfast; friendly service.' Bar, café, 2 restaurants. Car park. 111 bedrooms (many in annexe). B&B £60–£90.

WOLVERHAMPTON West Midlands   **Map 3:C5**
Ely House, 53 Tettenhall Road WV3 9NB. *Tel* 01902-311311, *fax* 01902-421098. June and Catherine Sanders's 18th-century former private school. On A41, just off ring road, near shopping centre. 18 bedrooms. B&B £29.50–£59.

WORCESTER Worcestershire   **Map 3:C5**
Diglis House, Severn Street WR1 2NF. *Tel* 01905-353518, *fax* 01905-767772, *website* www.jks.org/diglis. Georgian house by river Severn, near cathedral. Lounge, conservatory restaurant. Garden. Parking. 26 bedrooms. B&B £45–£105.

YORK North Yorkshire   **Map 4:D4**
Dean Court, Duncombe Place YO1 2EF. *Tel* 01904-625082, *fax* 01904-620305, *email* deancourt@btconnect.com, *website* www.deancourt-york.co.uk. Traditional hotel (Best Western), opposite minster. Children welcomed. Restaurant, conservatory tea room. Free valet parking. 40 bedrooms (12 no-smoking). B&B £50–£85.
Holmwood House, 114 Holgate Road YO24 4BB. *Tel* 01904-626183, *fax* 01904-670899, *email* holmwood.house @dial.pipex.com, *website* www.holmwoodhousehotel.co.uk. Rosie Blanksby and Bill Pitts's no-smoking B&B, 10 mins' walk from Micklegate, on A59, backs on to pretty square. Parking. 14 bedrooms. B&B £32.50–£52.50.

SCOTLAND

ABERDEEN   **Map 5:C3**
Ardoe House, South Deeside Road, Blairs AB12 5YP. *Tel* 01224-860600, *fax* 01224-861283, *email* info@ardoe.macdonald-hotels.co.uk, *website* www.macdonaldhotels.co.uk. 4 miles E of centre: baronial granite mansion, much extended. Mature grounds, views of river Dee. 'First-rate staff.' *À la carte* restaurant; informal meals in *Soapies Lounge*; banqueting suites. Leisure club. 108 bedrooms (40 no-smoking). B&B £55–£102.50.
Atholl, 54 King's Gate AB15 4YN. *Tel* 01224-323505, *fax* 01224-321555, *email* info@atholl-aberdeen.co.uk, *website* www.atholl-aberdeen.com. In West End, 5 miles S of airport: granite house. Restaurant; function/conference facilities. Car park. 35 no-smoking bedrooms. B&B £41.50–£75.
Craiglynn, 36 Fonthill Road AB11 6UJ. *Tel* 01224-584050, *fax* 01224-212225, *email* info@craiglynn.co.uk, *website* www.craiglynn.co.uk. Chris and Hazel Mann's Victorian guest house in residential area. 9 bedrooms (some *en suite*). Evening meal. B&B £38–£62.50.
Marcliffe at Pitfodels, North Deeside Road, Pitfodels AB15 9YA. *Tel* 01224-861000, *fax* 01224-868860, *email* reservations@marcliffe.com, *website* www.marcliffe.com. In 8-acre landscaped grounds in West End: Stewart and Sheila Spence's large, white 'country house in the city'. Restaurant, conservatory restaurant; large function facilities. 42 bedrooms (1 adapted for &). B&B £60–£165.
Simpson's, 59 Queens Road AB15 4YP. *Tel* 01224-327777, *fax* 01224-327700, *email* address@simpsonshotel.com. Simpson family's hotel in West End. Exuberant decor: Mediterranean-style bedrooms; Moroccan columns, palm trees in split-level bar; brasserie reminiscent of Alhambra. Wheelchair access throughout. 37 bedrooms. B&B £62.50–£145.

ANNAN Dumfries and Galloway   **Map 5:E2**
Warmanbie, Annan DG12 5LL. *Tel/fax* 01461-204015, *email* info@warmanbie.co.uk, *website* www.warmanbie.co.uk. Duncan family's Georgian hotel/restaurant. River Annan flows through 45-acre wooded grounds; old roses in walled garden. Old-fashioned decor;

'friendly service; informal atmosphere; good meals'. 7 bedrooms. B&B £37–£46.

DUNDEE   **Map 5:D3**
Invercarse, 371 Perth Road DD2 1PG. *Tel* 01382-669231, *fax* 01382-644112. Near university: extended Victorian mansion (Best Western) in large grounds on hill, overlooking river Tay. Large function facilities. 35 bedrooms (17 no-smoking). B&B £45–£78.
Strathdon, 277 Perth Road DD2 1JS. *Tel/fax* 01382-665648, *email* strathdon.dundee@tinyworld.co.uk. John and Mo Melville's Edwardian terrace guest house, near university (unlimited parking). 8 bedrooms. B&B £21–£26.

EDINBURGH   **Map 5:D2**
Acer Lodge, 425 Queensferry Road EH4 7NB. *Tel* 0131-336 2554, *fax* 0131-336 1112, *email* ejohn81068@aol.com, *website* www. acerlodge.co.uk. No-smoking guest house 10 mins' bus ride from centre. Car park. 4 bedrooms. B&B £20–£35.
Channings, South Learmonth Gardens EH4 1EZ. *Tel* 0131-315 2226, *fax* 0131-332 9631, *email* reserve@channings.co.uk, *website* www.channings.co.uk. On cobbled street near centre, composed of 5 Edwardian town houses. Lounge, library, wine bar, conservatory, restaurant. 48 bedrooms. B&B £77.50–£117.50.
The Grange, 8 Whitehouse Terrace EH9 2EU. *Tel* 0131-667 5681, *fax* 0131-668 3300, *email* grange-hotel@talk21.com, *website* www.grange-hotel-edinburgh.co.uk. Baronial house with garden, squirrels, putting, 1½ miles S of centre. Country house decor. Hall, library, bar, conservatory/restaurant, small conference room. 15 bedrooms. B&B £62.50–£80.
Parliament House, 15 Calton Hill EH1 3BJ. *Tel* 0131-478 4000, *fax* 0131-478 4001, *email* phhadams@aol.com, *website* www. scotland-hotels.co.uk. Near castle/Princes Street. Georgian facade; smart interior. Lobby; *MP's Bistro*. 53 bedrooms: single £90, double £140. Breakfast £7.50–£10.50.
17 Abercromby Place, 17 Abercromby Place EH3 6LB. *Tel* 0131-557 8036, *fax* 0131-558 3453, *email* eirlys.lloyd@virgin.net, *website* www.abercrombyhouse.com. Eirlys Lloyd's Wolsey Lodge: New Town terrace house overlooking tree-filled square, 5 mins' walk from centre. Lounge/library, dining room. No smoking. 'Great breakfast.' Evening meal by arrangement. Ample parking. 9 bedrooms. B&B: double £90–£120.

ELGIN Moray   **Map 5:C2**
Mansion House, The Haugh IV30 1AW. *Tel* 01343-548811, *fax* 01343-547916, *email* reception@mhelgin.co.uk. 19th-century baronial mansion in mature woodland; river Lossie nearby. Period decor. Piano lounge, bar, snooker room, restaurant, bistro; function room; country club (indoor swimming pool, gym, etc). 22 bedrooms. B&B £55–£95.

Make sure the hotel has included VAT in the prices it quotes.

FORRES Moray   **Map 5:C2**
Knockomie, Grantown Road IV36 2SG. *Tel* 01309-673146, *fax* 01309-673290, *email* stay@knockomie.co.uk, *website* www. knockomie.co.uk. 1 mile S of centre, in 25-acre park (Highland cattle). Renovated Arts and Crafts house. Restaurant, bistro. 15 bedrooms. B&B £46.50–£118.

GLASGOW   **Map 5:D2**
ArtHouse, 129 Bath Street G2 2SY. *Tel* 0141-572 6000, *fax* 0141-221 6777, *email* info@arthousehotel.com, *website* www. arthousehotel.com. Opened 1999, central, near Sauchiehall Street. Theatrical modern decor in listed building. Restaurant, bar/grill; beauty salon; function facilities. 65 bedrooms: £90–£180.
Cathedral House, 28–32 Cathedral Square G4 0XA. *Tel* 0141-552 3519, *fax* 0141-552 2444. Just off M8, 19th-century Scottish baronial house. Restaurant, café/bar; regular live music; function facilities. 8 bedrooms. B&B £34.50–£49.

INVERNESS Highland   **Map 5:C2**
Moyness House, 6 Bruce Gardens IV3 5EN. *Tel/fax* 01463-233836, *email* info@moyness.co.uk, *website* www.moyness.co.uk. Jenny and Richard Jones's 'meticulously kept' guest house, built 1880, in large garden. 10 mins' walk to centre. Old-fashioned decor. Sitting room, breakfast room. 7 no-smoking bedrooms. B&B £29.50–£35.

MARYCULTER Aberdeenshire   **Map 5:C3**
Maryculter House, South Deeside Road AB12 5GB. *Tel* 01224-732124, *fax* 01224-733510, *email* info@maryculterhousehotel.co.uk, *website* www.maryculterhousehotel.co.uk. Former Templar priory in 5-acre grounds on river Dee, 8 miles W of Aberdeen. Ample public rooms; efficient management; business-oriented clientele. 23 bedrooms. Bar meals; French cuisine in restaurant. B&B from £35.

MELROSE Scottish Borders   **Map 5:E3**
Burts, Market Square TD6 9PN. *Tel* 01896-822285, *fax* 01896-822870, *email* burtshotel@aol.com, *website* www.burtshotel.co.uk. Henderson family's 18th-century house in centre. Residents' lounge. Bar meals; formal restaurant. Garden. 20 no-smoking bedrooms (some small). B&B £46–£52.

MOFFAT Dumfries and Galloway   **Map 5:E2**
Auchen Castle, Beattock DG10 9SH. *Tel* 01683-300407, *fax* 01683-300667, *email* reservations@auchen.castle.hotel.co.uk, *website* www.auchen.castle.hotel.co.uk. Keith Parr's imposing grey stone building (Best Western), in 30-acre grounds (loch, fountain), 1 mile E of town. 15 bedrooms in main house; 11 (simpler) in lodge. B&B £47.50–£75.

OBAN Argyll and Bute   **Map 5:D1**
The Manor House, Gallanch Road PA34 4LS. *Tel* 01631-562087, *fax* 01631-563053, *email* manorhouseoban@aol.com, *website*

www.manorhouseoban.com. New owners (2001) are redecorating/ upgrading this Georgian house on quiet road ½ mile from centre. 2 lounges, bar, restaurant (Scottish traditional). Garden. 11 bedrooms. D,B&B £52–£110.

OLDMELDRUM Aberdeenshire   Map 5:C3
Cromlet Hill, South Road AB51 0AB. *Tel* 01651-872315, *fax* 01651-872164. In old town 16 miles NW of Aberdeen, 15 mins from airport. John Page's listed neo-classical Georgian mansion in conservation area. Garden; fine views. 3 bedrooms. B&B £27.50–£32.50. Communal evening meal by arrangement.
Meldrum House AB51 0AE. *Tel* 01651-872294, *fax* 01651-872464, *email* dpmeldrum@aol.com, *website* www.meldrumhouse.com. 1½ miles from centre, on A947. Douglas and Eileen Pearson's part 13th-century baronial house in 15-acre grounds (garden, woods, golf course). Restaurant (traditional/international dishes); conference facilities. 9 bedrooms. B&B £55–£85.

PEEBLES Scottish Borders   Map 5:E2
Park Hotel, Innerleithen Road EH45 8BA. *Tel* 01721-720451, *fax* 01721-723510, *email* reserve@parkpeebles.co.uk. Just outside town: turreted, gabled white building with views over hills. Lounges, restaurant; access to sport/health facilities at large sister, *Peebles Hotel Hydro* (700 yds). 24 bedrooms. D,B&B £64–£80.50.

PITLOCHRY Perth and Kinross   Map 5:D2
Pine Trees, Strathview Terrace PH16 5QR. *Tel* 01796-472121, *fax* 01796-472460, *email* info@pinetrees-hotel.demon.co.uk, *website* www.pinetrees-hotel.demon.co.uk. Brian Waller's Victorian mansion in 10-acre gardens, 5 mins' walk NE of centre. Traditional decor; 'willing staff; adequate restaurant'. 19 bedrooms. B&B £29–£58.

ST ANDREWS Fife   Map 5:D3
Old Manor, Lundin Links KY8 6AJ. *Tel* 01333-320368, *fax* 01333-320911, *email* enquiries@oldmanorhotel.co.uk, *website* www. oldmanorhotelco.uk. Overlooking 2 championship golf courses and Largo Bay: country house in seaside village 12 miles S of centre. 'Friendly service; good food.' Traditional decor. Lounge/bar, terrace, restaurant, bistro; function facilities. Parking. 24 bedrooms. B&B £60–£80.
Rufflets, Strathkinness Low Road KY16 9TX. *Tel* 01334-472594, *fax* 01334-478703, *email* reservations@rufflets.co.uk, *website* www.rufflets.co.uk. In 10-acre grounds, Ann Russell's creeper-covered hotel, built 1924. 1½ miles from golf course. Paintings by Sir William Russell Flint. Library, dining room, brasserie, meeting room. 25 bedrooms (1 suitable for &). B&B £91–£96.

THURSO Highland   Map 5:B2
Pentland Hotel, Princes Street KW14 7AA. *Tel* 01847-893202, *fax* 01847-892761. Mr and Mrs Mancini's hotel in northerly-most town

on British mainland. Near sea, empty beaches, golf. Half modern, half old building; plain decor. 'Helpful staff; good bar meals; pleasant restaurant.' 25 bedrooms. B&B £30–£35.

WALES

ABERYSTWYTH Ceredigion   Map 3:C3
Belle Vue Royal, The Promenade SY23 2BA. *Tel* 01970-617558, *fax* 01970-612190, *email* reception@bellvueroyalhotel.fsnet.co.uk, *website* www.bellevueroyal.co.uk. Alan and Marilyn Davies's 2-storey seafront hotel, 'truly family run: high standard of service and food'. 3 bars, dining room, conference room. Car park. 37 bedrooms (34 *en suite*, some family). B&B £45–£60.

CAERNARFON, Gwynedd   Map 3:A1
Seiont Manor, Llanrug LL55 2AQ. *Tel* 01286-673366, *fax* 01286-672840. In 150-acre park (jogging track, fishing): Georgian farmstead now holiday/business hotel. Library, bar, restaurant, conservatory; leisure facilities (swimming pool, etc). 28 bedrooms. B&B £47.50–£78.

CARDIFF   Map 3:E4
The Big Sleep, Bute Terrace CF10 2FE. *Tel* 029-2063 6363, *fax* 029-2063 6364, *email* bookings@thebigsleephotel.com, *website* www.thebigsleephotel.com. Cosmo Fry's affordable designer B&B hotel (backers include actor John Malkovich), aimed at business market, in former British Gas office building. Formica, PVC, Ikea furniture create 'millennium retro' style. 'Helpful service; excellent breakfast.' Bar, breakfast room. Parking. 81 bedrooms (1 suitable for &). B&B double £45–£99.
Churchills, Cardiff Road, Llandaff CF5 2AD. *Tel* 029-2040 1300, *fax* 029-2056 8347, *email* reservations@churchillshotel.co.uk, *website* www.churchillshotel.co.uk. Large white stuccoed town house owned by Brains, the national brewer of Wales. 5 mins W of centre, near Llandaff cathedral. Lounge/bar (snacks served), restaurant; function facilities. Parking. 22 bedrooms, 13 mews suites. B&B £30–£52.50.
The Town House, 70 Cathedral Road, CF1 9LL. *Tel* 029-2023 9399, *fax* 029-2022 3214, *email* thetownhouse@msn.com, *website* www. thetownhousecardiff.co.uk. Iris and Bart Zuzik's B&B in Victorian Gothic town house in conservation area by castle. 'High standard of housekeeping; good communal breakfast.' Secure parking. 7 simple bedrooms. B&B £24.75–£39.50.

ST DAVID'S Pembrokeshire   Map 3:D1
Warpool Court, St David's SA62 6BN. *Tel* 01437-720300, *fax* 01437-720676, *email* warpool@enterprise.net. Peter Trier's grey stone hotel in magnificent setting above St Bride's Bay. Unique hand-painted tiles throughout. Lounge, restaurant. 7-acre grounds: covered swimming pool, gym, tennis, croquet. 25 bedrooms. B&B £61–£118.

SWANSEA   **Map 3:E3**
Windsor Lodge, Mount Pleasant SA1 6EG. *Tel* 01792-642158, *fax* 01792-648996. 'Extremely pleasant: agreeable staff, good restaurant.' Ron and Pam Rumble's blue Grade II listed 18th-century house with modern decor, central location, parking. 19 bedrooms. B&B £32.50–£55.

IRELAND

BELFAST   **Map 6:B6**
Oakdene Lodge, 16 Annadale Avenue BT7 3JH. *Tel* 028-9049 2626, *fax* 028-9049 2070, *email* peter@oakdenelodge.com, *website* www.oakdenelodge.com. Stephens family's budget B&B in leafy avenue 2 miles from centre. 'Quiet, friendly, comfortable; good breakfast. Minimal public rooms; excellent bedrooms.' Car park. 17 rooms (1 suitable for &), 8 apartments. B&B £27.50–£38.50.

Further afield:
Dunadry, 2 Islandreagh Drive, Dunadry, Co. Antrim BT41 2HA. *Tel* 028-9443 4343, *fax* 028-9443 3389, *email* mooneyhotelgroup@talk21.com. 15 miles NW of Belfast, 5 miles NE of airport. In quiet countryside, unusual modern white building, now large hotel, much used for functions. Impressive public rooms; restaurant, bistro. 10-acre grounds: health club. 67 bedrooms: single £65–£89, double £85–£108. Breakfast £8–£10.
Old Inn, 15 Main Street, Crawfordsburn, Co. Down BT19 1JH. *Tel* 028-9185 3255, *fax* 028-9185 2775, *email* info@theoldinn.com, *website* www.theoldinn.com. In village 10 miles E of centre, 1 mile from sea. Historic inn: panelling, chintz, pastels; canopied 4-posters; honeymoon cottage. Bistro; conservatory-style restaurant, specialising in seafood. Function facilities. 32 bedrooms. B&B: single/double £65–£90; cottage £150.

BUSHMILLS Co Antrim   **Map 6:A6**
Bushmills Inn, 9 Dunluce Road BT57 8QG. *Tel* 028-207 32339, *fax* 028-207 32048, *email* good@bushmillsinn.com, *website* www.bushmillsinn.com. Award-winning conversion of old coaching inn and mill house on river Bush ½ mile from spectacular Giant's Causeway coast. Bars, restaurant (new Irish cooking). 32 bedrooms (some family; 1 designed for &). B&B £44–£78.

DUBLIN   **Map 6:A6**
Aberdeen Lodge, 53 Park Avenue, off Ailesbury Road, Ballsbridge, Dublin 4. *Tel* (+353) (0)1-2838155, *fax* (+353) (0)1-2837877, *email* ireland@greenbook.ie, *website* www.greenbook.ie/aberdeen. Pat Halpin's B&B (Relais du Silence) in 3-storey house. Modern interior: lounge, breakfast room (snacks available); gym; conference facilities. Garden. Car park. DART to centre. 20 bedrooms. B&B IR£49.50–£112.
Albany House, 84 Harcourt Street, Dublin 2. *Tel* (+353) (0)1-4751092, *fax* (+353) (0)1-4751093, *email* albany@indigo.ie, *website*

www.byrne-hotels-ireland.com. Near St Stephen's Green: Richard Byrne's Georgian house. Traditional decor, 'generous, inventive breakfast', pleasant staff. Minor maintenance problems reported, but 'good value'. 33 bedrooms (some small; quietest ones at rear). B&B IR£45–£70.

Butlers Town House, 44 Lansdowne Road, Ballsbridge, Dublin 4. *Tel* (+353) (0)1-6674022, *fax* (+353) (0)1-6673960, *email* info@ butlers-hotel.com, *website* www.butlers-hotel.com. B&B in Victorian house: smart drawing room, breakfast conservatory; room-service meals. Walled garden. Car park. 20 bedrooms. B&B IR£75–£110.

Charles Stewart, 5–6 Parnell Square, Dublin 1. *Tel* (+353) (0)1-8780350, *fax* (+353) (0)1-8781387, *email* cstuart@iol.ie, *website* www.iol.ie/~cstuart. Budget accommodation in listed Georgian building. 'Central, clean, well maintained, friendly.' 44 bedrooms (many *en suite*). B&B IR£25–£45.

Harrington Hall, 70 Harcourt Street, Dublin 2. *Tel* (+353) (0)1-4753497, *fax* (+353) (0)1-4754544, *email* harringtonhall@eircom.net, *website* www.harringtonhall.com. B&B in 2 Georgian town houses, 'elegantly converted'; central; safe parking. 30 bedrooms (quietest ones at rear). B&B IR£55–£90.

Kilronan House, 70 Adelaide Road, Dublin 2. *Tel* (+353) (0)1-4755266, *fax* (+353) (0)1-4782841, *email* info@dublinn.com, *website* www.dublinn.com. Terry and Rosemary Masterson's B&B near St Stephen's Green. 'Spotless, quiet, friendly; great breakfast.' TV lounge, wine licence. 12 bedrooms. B&B IR£48–£55.

Longfield's, 10 Fitzwilliam Street Lower, Dublin 2. *Tel* (+353) (0)1-6761367, *fax* (+353) (0)1-6761542, *email* lfields@indigo.ie. In 2 Georgian houses. Elegant furnishings; attractive lounge; restaurant. 26 bedrooms. B&B IR£67.50–£105.

The Morgan, 10 Fleet Street, Temple Bar, Dublin 2. *Tel* (+353) (0)1-6793939, *fax* (+353) (0)1-6793946, *email* sales@themorgan.com, *website* www.themorgan.com. Modern hotel in lively central area: minimalist decor; contemporary Irish paintings. Restaurant/bar, café. 61 bedrooms (with CD-player, modern telecommunications): from IR£105. Breakfast IR£7.

Raglan Lodge, 10 Raglan Road (off Pembroke Road), Ballsbridge, Dublin 4. *Tel* (+353) (0)1-6606697, *fax* (+353) (0)1-6606781. In tree-lined residential street, 1 mile SE of centre, is Helen Moran's B&B: Victorian house; some antiques; award-winning breakfast. Small garden. Car park. 7 bedrooms. B&B IR£40–£60.

Trinity Lodge, 12 South Frederick Street, Dublin 2. *Tel* (+353) (0)1-6795044, *fax* (+353) (0)1-6795223, *email* trinitylodge@eircom.net. Georgian town house in quiet street by Trinity College. Bright colours, modern pictures. 13 bedrooms. B&B IR£52.50–£90.

Further afield:

Barberstown Castle, Straffan, Co. Kildare. *Tel* (+353) (0)1-6288157, *fax* (+353) (0)1-6277027, *email* castleir@iol.ie, *website* www.barberstowncastle.com. 13th-century castle plus Elizabethan and Victorian houses now traditional country hotel, 30 mins' drive from centre/airport. Bar, restaurant; conference facilities. 22 bedrooms. B&B IR£60–£175.

Leixlip House, Captain's Hill, Leixlip, Co. Kildare. *Tel* (+353) (0)1-6242268, *fax* (+353) (0)1-6244177, *email* manager@leixliphouse.com, *website* www.leixliphouse.com. Georgian house, 8 miles from centre. Country-house decor; 'modern Irish' restaurant; conference centre. Safe parking. 15 bedrooms. B&B IR£65–£125.

NEWRY Co. Down   **Map 6:B6**
Canal Court, Merchants Quay BT35 8HF. *Tel* 028-3025 1234, *fax* 028-3025 1177, *email* rooms@canalcourthotel.com, *website* www.canalcourthotel.com. 'Excellent' new hotel by Newry Canal. Traditional decor. Bar, restaurant, conservatory; conference/function facilities; leisure club. Parking. 51 bedrooms. B&B £50–£75.

WATERFORD Co. Waterford   **Map 6:D6**
Waterford Castle, The Island, Ballinakill. *Tel* (+353) (0)51-878203, *fax* (+353) (0)51-878342, *email* info@waterfordcastle.com, *website* www.waterfordcastle.com. Former home of Edward Fitzgerald: Norman castle on private 310-acre island reached by car ferry (3 miles from centre). Now a smart hotel/country club: championship golf course, indoor swimming pool, tennis; conference facilities. 19 bedrooms: single IR£120–£175, double IR£140–£315. Breakfast IR£12.50–£15.50.

****

Traveller's tale Hotel in Birmingham. We arrived on a Saturday afternoon. Reception was in chaos. No one greeted us as we walked through the door. A young lad and an older lady behind the desk seemed preoccupied. Standing on one side was a woman talking loudly to her husband. She was cursing 'the bloody hotel'. We were given the key to our room and made our way there. It stank of cigarette smoke. We opened the window to let in some air, and found two stubbed-out half cigarettes on the windowsill.

****

Traveller's tale Hotel in Leicestershire. In this hotel we had a really nice bedroom with a lovely view, but the food was awful. After unripe melon, I had stuffed chicken breast with tomato sauce. The chicken was all right, but the unpleasant sauce had probably come straight out of a tin, and the piece of bacon that adorned the chicken was so tough it would have defeated teeth younger than mine. The vegetables were so undercooked that it was difficult to bite into them. At the end of our main course, the waiter came to ask if all was well. I asked him if he would like an honest answer. He looked amazed, but said he would. I told him I had just had the worst chicken dish I had ever been served, picked up the piece of bacon and said he could return it to the chef with my compliments and tell him that if anyone could eat it, I'd be surprised.

****

Alphabetical list of hotels

(S) indicates a Shortlist entry

A

Abbey Penzance 225
Abbey House Abbotsbury 20
Abbey House London (S) 507
Abbey Inn Byland Abbey 75
Aberdeen Lodge Dublin (S) 531
Academy London (S) 507
Acer Lodge Edinburgh (S) 527
Adelaide Brighton (S) 512
Ainsley House Brighton (S) 512
Airds Port Appin 380
Albannach Lochinver 368
Albany House Dublin (S) 531
Albright Hussey Shrewsbury (S) 523
Alderley Edge Manchester (S) 519
Alexander House Gatwick (S) 516
Alexandra Lyme Regis (S) 518
Altnaharrie Inn Ullapool 394
Amberley Castle Amberley 21
Amerdale House Arncliffe 27
Angel Bury St Edmunds 72
Angel Guildford (S) 517
Anglesea Town House Dublin 471
Apple Lodge Lochranza 370
Apsley House Bath 38
Ardanaiseig Kilchrenan 364
Ardnamona House Lough Eske 488
Ardoe House Aberdeen (S) 526
Ardsheal House Kentallen 363
Ardvourlie Castle Ardvourlie 325
Argyll Iona 361
Arisaig Hotel Arisaig 326
Arisaig House Arisaig 326
Ark Erpingham 114
Arkleside Reeth 234
ArtHouse Glasgow (S) 528

Arundel House Cambridge (S) 513
Arundell Arms Lifton 184
Ascot House Harrogate 142
Ashbrook House Dublin 471
Ashburn House Fort William 352
Ashelford East Down 112
Ashfield House Grassington 133
Ash-Rowan Belfast 456
Ashwick House Dulverton 110
Assolas Country House Kanturk 481
At the Sign of the Angel Lacock 171
Atholl Aberdeen (S) 526
Atlantic St Brelade 440
Auchen Castle Moffat (S) 528
Auchendean Lodge Dulnain Bridge 342
Avondale Carlisle 79
Aynsome Manor Cartmel 80

B

Baile-na-Cille Timsgarry 392
Balcary Bay Auchencairn 327
Bales Mead West Porlock 302
Balgonie Country House Ballater 331
Ballycormac House Aglish 447
Ballymakeigh House Killeagh 485
Ballymaloe House Shanagarry 502
Ballynahinch Castle Recess 499
Ballywarren House Cong 466
Bank House Oakamoor 219
Bantry House Bantry 454
Barberstown Castle nr Dublin (S) 532
Barcelona Exeter 118
Bark House Bampton 32
Basil Street London 2

Champagne winners: Report of the Year competition

As usual we have awarded a dozen bottles of champagne for the best reports of the year. A bottle apiece, and a free copy of the *Guide*, will go to the following generous and eloquent readers for their contributions to this volume.

Felicity Chadwick-Histed of Teddington, Middlesex
Ann Evans of Oxford
Michael Kavanagh of Haywards Heath, Sussex
Nigel M Mackintosh of Pewsey, Wiltshire
Jonathan and Michelle Ray of Edwalton, Nottinghamshire
Robert Sandham of Darlington, Co. Durham
Kay and Martin Slingsby of Cottingham, East Yorkshire
Anthony Stern of London
H J Martin Tucker of Winchester, Hampshire
Benjamin Twist of Edinburgh
Andrew Wardrop of London
Deborah Zachary of Blandford, Dorset

A further dozen bottles will be awarded to readers who write to us about hotels on the Continent when the 2002 guide to Continental Europe is published, and another case will be on offer for reports to the 2003 edition of this volume. No special entry form is required; everything we receive in the course of the year will qualify. A winner may be someone who nominates a new hotel or comments on an existing one. We award champagne to those whose reports are consistently useful, as well as to individually brilliant examples of the art of hotel criticism.

Exchange rates

This guide is also published in the United States. For the benefit of the readers of that edition, here are some exchange rates at the time of publication. They may well have changed considerably since then, so it is vital that you check up-to-date rates when planning your visit.

Pound sterling

£1 = US $1.42

£1 = Canadian $2.14

Irish punt

IR£1 = US $1.08

IR£1 = Canadian $1.63

Euro (this will be legal currency in Ireland from February 2002)

€1 = US $0.85

€1 = Canadian $1.29

How it was

1994 was Robert Deville's 25th year at *Heddon's Gate Hotel,* Heddon's Mouth (see page 154). In an article he wrote for the *Guide* that year, he looked back at the changes in taste over a quarter of a century, and remembered nostalgically the ascetic conditions that prevailed in his parents' guest house in Jersey. Here we reprint the article, with a 21st-century footnote from Mr Deville.

'FOR SALE: Large country house with fine views, situated within Exmoor National Park. 15 bedrooms and suitable for use as hotel or guest house. £15,000 ono.'

So ran the estate agent's advertisement in 1967. After some haggling, I bought it for £12,500 and spent a winter trying to turn a run-down Victorian house into a pleasant but simple holiday hotel with 13 bedrooms. I opened for business the following Easter, never dreaming that I would still be here over a quarter of a century later.

Twenty-five years ago guests never came for less than a week unless they were touring, because it wasn't worth making the long journey for a short break. There were no motorways, and the West Country was reached by the A38 or the winding A39. This often meant leaving the night before in order to arrive in daylight and in time for dinner. Everyone had his or her own horror story of delays on the Exeter by-pass, at Scotch Corner or through Birmingham. Nowadays the journey from the Midlands or London takes three-and-a half to four hours.

Had you visited us in 1968, you would have found a warm reception and a jolly atmosphere, but few creature comforts. Our weekly tariff was 11 to 12 guineas (£11.55–£12.60 per person) for half board. A lunch of lamb chop and chips followed by ice-cream could be had for about three shillings and sixpence (18p) and morning tea cost one shilling per person (5p). Dinner, not the refined affair it is today, was served at 7 pm in a most spartan dining room with 'brick' wallpaper, bentwood chairs, and chipboard tables covered with a cheap tablecloth; not much of the crockery and cutlery matched. Tables were advertised as 'separate' but were about an inch apart. Guests dined on soup, a roast with one vegetable, generally peas, cabbage, carrots or runner beans (courgettes were unknown), and about a pound of potatoes each, followed by fruit pie with custard, and, because it was Devon, clotted cream. The floor was covered by thick rubber treated with Linopaint. If you lingered over your cheese you might find your chair firmly stuck to it. The room was heated by a small fan heater which I turned towards whoever complained most vociferously about the cold. In hot weather diners in the big bay window were quite likely to pass out from the heat.

None of us had much knowledge of wine. Our list had about a dozen wines, stored in an unused fireplace; the most popular were Sauternes, Mateus Rosé and Liebfraumilch. After dinner, guests crowded into the bar; there was a great consumption of spirits, accompanied by a hubbub of conversation and laughter. In these sophisticated days far fewer spirits are taken after dinner, and though things are still pleasant, the absolute conviviality has gone.

Upstairs, bedrooms were, at least, fully carpeted, and had a wash-basin and 'interior sprung mattresses', quite a special feature. Unlike other hotels, we never descended to nylon sheets. On the first floor, up to 20 guests had the use of one WC and one bathroom. We allotted times for use of the bathroom, usually unsuccessfully, because of our uncertain water supply; our solid fuel boiler either blew like a blast furnace or went out, sometimes of its own accord, sometimes because I was reluctant to refuel it sufficiently on account of the rattle of the coke in the early hours. From about 6 am bedroom doors opened and shut endlessly. The WC could be seen from most door-ways, and folk would peep out to see if it was occupied and if there was a competitor in the offing. The bathroom became, in the words of one loyal guest, 'the white knee, sponge-bag, 7 am shuffle'. No one would tolerate it now. Bedroom heating was non-existent, apart from 'hot-water bottles on request', but guests only came from Easter to mid-September. There was no business to be had for the rest of the year.

We had our first inspection by the Automobile Association in1968 and were given a star. The inspector, who was unmistakable, hid toffee papers in odd places to see if they had gone by morning. He 'disappeared' at dinner time and we had to find him and bring him in to dine. Such darling dodos, I wonder if they still do the same? Hotel inspectors of many sorts came here, but few ever sought the soul of the place. We had a lengthy correspondence with one of the tourist boards about fire-proof waste baskets in the bedrooms.

My earliest experience of catering for the public was in 1950 when I was 13. My parents bought a guest house in Jersey and my memo-ries of this are still crystal clear, probably because of the effect of the change from a very private to a public existence at that age. Before going to school I had to make up the Ideal boiler, riddling and re-coking it, and breaking up the crust of tea leaves placed on the fire to keep it going overnight. During school holidays I earned my pocket money by hand-peeling the potatoes and helping with the bedrooms. They had wood-stained polished floorboards, a small carpet square, marble-topped washstands and iron-framed beds, some with crank-ing handles to adjust the 'bounce'. No private facilities; I had to carry up yellow tapered enamelled jugs of hot water for washing and shav-ing. Large cups of strong, sugary tea were also delivered to each inmate. Later in the day I helped with removing the 'soils' – the slop-pail full of scummy water and the chamber pots, most of which had been used. We never looked into them; they were decently covered with a cloth and brought down three flights of stairs to the only WC in the house, washed, disinfected and returned. We had one bath-room, and guests could rent a plug for 6p.

We were licensed for 16 guests, but my mother would squeeze in more by boarding them out at neighbouring houses. It was a short but hectic season of about 16 weeks. My mother did the cooking and my father the washing up; they charged four guineas (£4.60) per person per week half board. The food was very basic by today's standards, but most things were still on ration – guests gave up their ration tokens for the time they spent with us. The gong was sounded at 6 pm sharp (this early time gave folks a chance to see a show later) and dinner started with a bowl of the ubiquitous Maggi soup, put on the table whether or not anyone was seated. It was followed by dishes such as shepherd's pie and peas, bought puff-pastry mince pies with cream and a minuscule cup of Camp coffee [coffee extract], only one per person. Friday's dinner was the highlight of the week: tomato soup, tinned salmon salad, and trifle topped with tinned peaches.

Saturday was 'change-over' day so on Friday evening we had a get-together in the lounge, often ending with a glorious session around the piano. A sign: 'Lounge closed at 11 pm for your rest and comfort' actually meant that we could go to bed, as during the season we had given up our rooms to guests and slept in the lounge on 'put-u-up beds'. I hated it, and one year made myself a bedroom out of a bicycle shed in the yard. To my horror, my mother let it the following year as a guest bedroom. One of my earliest resolutions was never again to have anything to do with catering. Forty-three years later I can't imagine doing anything else.

Heddon's Gate in 1993 is a very comfortable place. All bedrooms have *en suite* bathroom, telephone, TV, central heating and other luxuries. We also have a large overdraft. Improved standards have to be paid for, and we charge over twice as much in real terms as when we started.

Winter has always been spent trying to put right some of the worst defects and making general improvements. In 1969 we installed the first private bathroom. In 1982 the 18th and final one. Each year some major project has been tackled. The first part of the central heating system was installed in 1969; it was completed ten years later. We remade the quarter-mile-long drive in 1972, built the dining room wing in 1977, and between 1984 and 1998 converted the old annexe into three cottage-style suites. After all these years there is still much to be done. It's a 'painting the Forth Bridge job' which will never be finished. We still sound the gong at 8 pm. No longer intended to be a peremptory instrument, it's just a signal that the dining room is open. It gives me a lovely nostalgic feeling too, a reminder of gongs sounding in the guest houses lining that high street in Jersey.

Postscript in 2001

The above article was written during the despondent years of the 1992/93 recession, after which business did start to improve but never to the levels of the late 1980s. Since then we have had BSE, the petrol crisis and a foot-and-mouth epidemic! Couple all these things with the strong pound, 17½ per cent VAT, high business rates, and a complete lack of interest in rural tourism from successive governments, and it is not surprising that many of our country hotels, guest houses and even farms have been sold as private houses or converted into self-catering apartments.

In the last eight years, nothing much has changed here, and while we now have more creature comforts and more sophisticated menus than 50 years ago, my mother's nostrum of 'make your guests happy and they will want to come again' still says it all.

The magnificent seven

This is what we said in our first edition about the seven hotels that have had an entry in every edition of the *Guide*.

Rothay Manor, Ambleside
There are hotels which offer a particularly friendly ambience, others which are in an exhilarating location, and others again which concentrate on haute cuisine. Hotels which combine all three virtues are comparatively rare, but *Rothay Manor* belongs to this class. The Nixons, who run this handsome Georgian house close to the head of Lake Windermere and within a few minutes' walk of Ambleside, have managed to preserve the atmosphere of a private house. 'The cooking is imaginative (though a bit on the rich side if you are staying a long time) and the service excellent. Naturally it makes a good centre for exploring the Lake District; but because of the friendly relaxed atmosphere, it is also a good place for just doing nothing.' (*Dr PJ Glenny*)
   B&B (including early morning and afternoon tea and a newspaper) £11; 5-course dinner £6.25.

Lastingham Grange, Lastingham
'My husband and I have stayed here many times over the last 11 years, at first with our three children (the youngest aged six when we first went), and we have never failed to enjoy it. It is a true English country house hotel, dating back to the 17th century, run by a family, and situated in a charming village within yards of superb walking country – the road peters out at *The Grange* and becomes a bridle path stretching across the moors to Rosedale. It is very quiet – a blessing, we think – with a residential licence, but no bar and no TV. The menus are limited but usually excellent. Lunches and dinners are served at set times. Most of the double rooms are very pleasant. The single rooms can be rather hot in warm weather as they are over the kitchen quarters. Although the average age of the guests is middle to elderly, children are always welcome and great kindness was always shown to ours.' (*Margaret Fell*)
   B&B £7.50; half board (min. 3 days) £11.50.

The Connaught, London
At the top of the price scale, but with one of the great restaurants of London, intimate and welcoming public rooms and simply lovely bedrooms.
   Room (excluding service) from £19. Meals à la carte.

Chewton Glen, New Milton
'This charming and luxurious country house hotel of Georgian

origins stands at the southern fringe of the New Forest; the stream that now forms the boundary between Dorset and Hampshire runs through the thirty acres of grounds and parkland. *Chewton Glen* achieves a standard of excellence through the personal enthusiasm and vigilance of Martin Skan and his wife who, like all the best hoteliers, combine high management skills with an obvious pleasure in caring for their visitors' well-being. Big log fires burn when days or nights are chilly; the main rooms are spacious and almost outrageously comfortable; the restaurant, softly lit and intimate, with fine linen and silver, blesses its diners with the kind of high quality cooking and imaginative menus, combined with impeccable service, that mark it as outstanding. There is no lift, but there are most elegant staircases to the two upper floors; and there are also ground-floor rooms which open on to the garden terrace. Bedrooms have blissful country views and are delightully furnished with an impressive care for detail.' (*Diana Petry*)

B&B £15.25; lunch from £3.50, dinner from £5.

Sharrow Bay, Ullswater

A quiet road runs along the eastern shore of Ullswater from Pooley Bridge, eventually petering out on Martindale Common, and one of the small bays on its course is Sharrow Bay. But to many people, both in Britain and abroad, the name *Sharrow Bay* means not an indentation in the lake shore, but a splendid hotel with a remarkable view of this most romantic lake. Built originally as a desirable residence, the house has many of the characteristics of an Italian villa: flowery terrace with statuary, elegant furnishings, antiques, *objets d'art* and books, all in an incomparable setting above the lake in woodland gardens with lodge and cottages and waterside walks. 'Here you will be not only peaceful but pampered. The meals are a villainously stern test for those guests who hope to leave at least not heavier than when they arrived. It is hard not to dwell on the food, which is superb and for which Francis Coulson is internationally famous, but just as important is the skill with which he and his partner, Brian Sack, unobtrusively make you feel most welcome and at home through all the day. A highly civilised and most distinguished hotel.' (*Tom and Christine Seddon; also Roger Smithells*)

Half board from £19.50.

Currarevagh House, Oughterard

'The Hodgson family have been living in this mid-Victorian country house on the banks of Lough Corrib for five generations, and June and Harry Hodgson now run it as an unstuffy, personal hotel. It is set in 150 acres of its own grounds, and there is beautiful wild country around for walks and golf, and riding nearby, but it is particularly popular with fishermen. There's a book in the hall where you can enter the number of fish caught, and that is a characteristic of the "private house" approach of the owners. There are no keys to the bedrooms – not that one would be likely to take one's diamonds to this remote spot. The decor hasn't changed much since 1900: the beds are marvellously capacious, with heavy linen sheets; splendid bathroom fittings, lots of Edwardian furniture. There are huge baskets of turf and large open fires in the two reception rooms – and the public rooms and hall are so spacious that it is easy enough to be on one's own. The food is good plain home cooking, such as one would get if one were lucky as a weekend guest in the country. Excellent home-made brown bread for breakfast, for instance, and first-rate coffee, kept hot over individual spirit lamps. Trout from the lough for dinner, simply cooked with melted butter. This is not a place I would bring small children to – it is full of the hush of grown-ups relaxing – but I know the owner would be too polite to demur at the idea.' (*Mirabel Cecil*)

Full board (min. 3 days) £13; full board weekly £84.

Ballymaloe House, Shanagarry

'I first went to this hotel years ago, when we dropped in for lunch and found ourselves staying several days. I went there for my honeymoon, and whenever we feel we deserve a treat, we go there again. It's a beguiling place. The Allen family who run it are in evidence everywhere – Mrs Allen is in the kitchen, various children driving tractors on the Home Farm, helping in the office, etc, and grandchildren eating in the dining room. The service is efficient and relaxed. On our way here for our honeymoon, we were delayed by a meandering Irish cow on the road and rang the hotel, who sympathised and promised that they would have a cold meal waiting for us when we arrived late at night. There was a beautifully arranged cold supper with a half-bottle of Pommard waiting for us in our room. This summer we stayed in the *Gatehouse*, a pretty white cottage a mile away at the end of the drive, with two rooms, a little kitchen and a bathroom. There are also lofts above the converted stables in the courtyard where you can stay very cheaply in simple whitewashed bedrooms and still enjoy the marvellous food in the main house. The hotel is as popular with the Irish as with the tourists. I would thoroughly recommend it for children: there are so many jolly friendly families staying there in summer, that the kids have a wonderful time together. The sea is about three miles away . . . The house itself, which is 17th century (though with a 14th-century keep), is very pretty. The dining room is in splendid William Morris greens, and is called the Yeats room after its collection of Jack Yeats pictures. The decor may have got shabbier over the years, which rather becomes it, but isn't significant of any decline in the standard of cooking. The menus are very imaginative, and make full use of the fish caught in Ballycotton Bay nearby. The home-made bread is out of this world, and the mushrooms alone at breakfast are worth staying there for several days. Helpings are generous. There is an interesting cold buffet lunch, so it doesn't matter whether you are in on time or not. Dinner is slightly more of a dressed-up occasion, though not oppressively so.' (*Mirabel Cecil; also Len Deighton*)

B&B £6.25; lunch (residents only) £2, dinner £5.50.

Readers' bouquets

This is what some famous readers of the *Guide* have said about it:

David Lodge: 'The guides are invaluable.'

Susan Hill: 'Quite simply, it's indispensable. You don't need any other hotel guide. The *Good Hotel Guide* is the best.'

Jan Morris: 'Unique – I never travel without it.'

Timothy West: 'Good hotels are getting better, the bad ones are getting worse. The *Good Hotel Guide* is more important than ever.'

Simon Jenkins: 'It offers the certainty of a communality of taste which no other guide remotely approaches . . . I cannot imagine a visit to the Continent without your splendid guide in my pocket.'

Lord Jenkins of Hillhead: 'I regard the *Good Hotel Guide*, edited by the Raphaels, both in its Continental and Britannic isles editions as invaluable: accurately informative for practical use and with a penetrating edge of comment which makes it also a browsing pleasure.'

Claire Bloom: 'I consult the *Good Hotel Guide* on every trip I make. The guide is invaluable and has never given me wrong advice.'

Sue MacGregor: 'Not only highly useful – it's a very good read.'

Media reviews

A selection of comments from the media over the last decade is given below:

'An indispensable companion of our travel writers as well as of discerning travellers . . . a uniquely reliable reference work.' *Daily Telegraph*, November 1993

'Wickedly incisive characterisation and an overriding sense of place . . . Gripping stuff, faultlessly edited.' *Daily Telegraph* Books of the year, November 1998

'Ruthlessly honest . . . eclectic in the best sense of the word . . . A rattling good read.' Derek Cooper, *Saga Magazine*, December 1998

'Not a perfect guide, but all things considered, it is the best. Its great strength lies in its squeaky clean integrity ' no free hospitality accepted, no payment solicited from hotels and no advertisements allowed . . . conveys the spirit of a hotel better than any of its competitors.' *The Sunday Times*, January 1997

'Its fierce independence precludes free hospitality, payments or advertising.' *Legal Executive*, December 1997

'Authoritative and entertaining.' *The Evening Standard*, February 1998

'Unbiased, candid and comprehensive.' *Business Traveller*, April 1998

'A boon for self-directed travellers seeking a break from the monotony and boring sameness of the giant chain hotels.' *International Travel News*, September 1998

'A voice of sanity in a country in which hotel classification systems are notoriously confusing.' *The Times*, September 1998

'For all its middle class prissiness . . . remains the one source that offers any . . . sense of what a place is really like. Inspirational at its best, maddening at its worst.' *The Mail on Sunday*, September 1999

'An independent guide and an entertaining read to boot.' *Radio Times*, February 2000

'This is simply one of the best reference guides that you can buy. The focus is on smallish hotels with their own individual character. Basic information on each hotel includes their facilities, location, restrictions and booking terms. Entries tell it like it is and are not afraid to criticise if necessary. The compilers do not accept any advertising or hospitality.' *The Times*, August 2000

'Were I ever to open my own hotel, the accolade that I would relish above all others would be a glowing report in the *Good Hotel Guide*. Unlike many other publications, the entry would not cost me so much as a bean.' *The Sunday Times*, September 2000

'Such squeaky-clean integrity, coupled with descriptions that convey the spirit of the place rather than the number of trouser presses, explains why the *Guide* is held in such high regard.' *The Sunday Times*, September 2000

'Refreshingly honest.' *Daily Express*, January 2001

'Thoroughly entertaining and ruthlessly honest.' *In Britain*, January 2001

Hotel reports

The report forms on the following pages may be used to endorse or criticise an existing entry or to nominate a hotel that you feel deserves inclusion in the *Guide*. But it is not essential that you use our forms or restrict yourself to the space available.

All reports (*each on a separate piece of paper, please*) should include your name and address, the name and location of the hotel, and the date and length of your stay. Please nominate only places that you have visited in the past 12 months, unless you are sure from friends that standards have been maintained. And please be as specific as possible, and critical where appropriate, about the character of the building, the public rooms and the bedrooms, the meals, the service, the night-life, the grounds.

If you can give some impression of the location as well as of the hotel, particularly in less familiar regions, that is very helpful. Comments about worthwhile places to visit in the neighbourhood and, in the case of B&B hotels, recommendable restaurants, would also be much appreciated.

Do not feel embarrassed about writing at length. We want the *Guide* to convey the special flavour of its hotels, and any small details that you give will help to make a description come alive. Many nominations just don't tell us enough. We mind having to pass up a potentially attractive place because the report is too brief. You need not bother with prices and routine information about the number of rooms and facilities; we obtain such details direct from the hotels. We want readers to supply information that is not accessible elsewhere. And we should be extremely grateful, particularly in the case of new nominations and foreign hotels, if you would include brochures whenever possible.

Please never tell a hotel that you intend to file a report. Anonymity is essential to objectivity.

The 2003 edition of this volume will be written between mid-March and the end of May 2002, and published in early September 2002. Nominations should reach us not later than 25 May 2002. The latest date for comments on existing entries is 1 June 2002.

Please let us know if you would like us to send you more report forms. Our address for UK correspondents (no stamp needed) is: *The Good Hotel Guide*, Freepost PAM 2931, London W11 4BR.

Reports can also be faxed to us on 020-7602 4182, or sent by email to Goodhotel@aol.com. Reports posted outside the UK should be stamped normally and addressed to: *The Good Hotel Guide*, 50 Addison Avenue, London W11 4QP, England.

To: *The Good Hotel Guide*, Freepost PAM 2931, London W11 4BR

NOTE: No stamps needed in UK, but letters posted outside the UK should be addressed to 50 Addison Avenue, London W11 4QP and stamped normally. Unless asked not to, we shall assume that we may publish your name if you are recommending a new hotel or supporting an existing entry. If you would like more report forms please tick ☐

Name of Hotel _____

Address _____

_____

Date of most recent visit   Duration of visit
☐ New recommendation   ☐ Comment on existing entry
Report:

Please continue overleaf

I am not connected directly or indirectly with the management or proprietors

Signed _____

Name (CAPITALS PLEASE)_____

Address _____

_____

[2002]

To: *The Good Hotel Guide*, Freepost PAM 2931, London W11 4BR

NOTE. No stamps needed in UK, but letters posted outside the UK should be addressed to 50 Addison Avenue, London W11 4QP and stamped normally. Unless asked not to, we shall assume that we may publish your name if you are recommending a new hotel or supporting an existing entry. If you would like more report forms please tick ☐

Name of Hotel _____

Address _____

_____

Date of most recent visit   Duration of visit
☐ New recommendation   ☐ Comment on existing entry
Report:

Please continue overleaf

I am not connected directly or indirectly with the management or proprietors

Signed _____

Name (CAPITALS PLEASE)_____

Address _____

_____

[2002]

To: *The Good Hotel Guide*, Freepost PAM 2931, London W11 4BR

NOTE: No stamps needed in UK, but letters posted outside the UK should be addressed to 50 Addison Avenue, London W11 4QP and stamped normally. Unless asked not to, we shall assume that we may publish your name if you are recommending a new hotel or supporting an existing entry. If you would like more report forms please tick □

Name of Hotel _____

Address _____

_____

Date of most recent visit   Duration of visit
□ New recommendation   □ Comment on existing entry
Report:

Please continue overleaf

I am not connected directly or indirectly with the management or proprietors

Signed _____

Name (CAPITALS PLEASE)_____

Address _____

_____

[2002]

To: *The Good Hotel Guide*, Freepost PAM 2931, London W11 4BR

NOTE: No stamps needed in UK, but letters posted outside the UK should be addressed to 50 Addison Avenue, London W11 4QP and stamped normally. Unless asked not to, we shall assume that we may publish your name if you are recommending a new hotel or supporting an existing entry. If you would like more report forms please tick ☐

Name of Hotel _____

Address _____

_____

Date of most recent visit   Duration of visit
☐ New recommendation   ☐ Comment on existing entry
Report:

Please continue overleaf

I am not connected directly or indirectly with the management or proprietors

Signed _____

Name (CAPITALS PLEASE)_____

Address _____

_____

[2002]

To: *The Good Hotel Guide*, Freepost PAM 2931, London W11 4BR

NOTE: No stamps needed in UK, but letters posted outside the UK should be addressed to 50 Addison Avenue, London W11 4QP and stamped normally. Unless asked not to, we shall assume that we may publish your name if you are recommending a new hotel or supporting an existing entry. If you would like more report forms please tick ☐

Name of Hotel _____

Address _____

_____

Date of most recent visit   Duration of visit
☐ New recommendation   ☐ Comment on existing entry
Report:

Please continue overleaf

I am not connected directly or indirectly with the management or proprietors

Signed _____

Name (CAPITALS PLEASE)_____

Address _____

_____

[2002]

To: *The Good Hotel Guide*, Freepost PAM 2931, London W11 4BR

NOTE: No stamps needed in UK, but letters posted outside the UK should be addressed to 50 Addison Avenue, London W11 4QP and stamped normally. Unless asked not to, we shall assume that we may publish your name if you are recommending a new hotel or supporting an existing entry. If you would like more report forms please tick ☐

Name of Hotel _____

Address _____

_____

Date of most recent visit   Duration of visit
☐ New recommendation   ☐ Comment on existing entry
Report:

Please continue overleaf

I am not connected directly or indirectly with the management or proprietors

Signed _____

Name (CAPITALS PLEASE)_____

Address _____

_____

[2002]

To: *The Good Hotel Guide*, Freepost PAM 2931, London W11 4BR

NOTE: No stamps needed in UK, but letters posted outside the UK should be addressed to 50 Addison Avenue, London W11 4QP and stamped normally. Unless asked not to, we shall assume that we may publish your name if you are recommending a new hotel or supporting an existing entry. If you would like more report forms please tick ☐

Name of Hotel _____

Address _____

_____

Date of most recent visit   Duration of visit
☐ New recommendation   ☐ Comment on existing entry
Report:

Please continue overleaf

I am not connected directly or indirectly with the management or proprietors

Signed _____

Name (CAPITALS PLEASE)_____

Address _____

_____

[2002]

To: *The Good Hotel Guide*, Freepost PAM 2931, London W11 4BR

NOTE: No stamps needed in UK, but letters posted outside the UK should be addressed to 50 Addison Avenue, London W11 4QP and stamped normally. Unless asked not to, we shall assume that we may publish your name if you are recommending a new hotel or supporting an existing entry. If you would like more report forms please tick ☐

Name of Hotel _____

Address _____

_____

Date of most recent visit   Duration of visit
☐ New recommendation   ☐ Comment on existing entry
Report:

Please continue overleaf

I am not connected directly or indirectly with the management or proprietors

Signed _____

Name (CAPITALS PLEASE)_____

Address _____

_____

To: *The Good Hotel Guide*, Freepost PAM 2931, London W11 4BR

NOTE: No stamps needed in UK, but letters posted outside the UK should be addressed to 50 Addison Avenue, London W11 4QP and stamped normally. Unless asked not to, we shall assume that we may publish your name if you are recommending a new hotel or supporting an existing entry. If you would like more report forms please tick ☐

Name of Hotel _____

Address _____

_____

Date of most recent visit   Duration of visit
☐ New recommendation   ☐ Comment on existing entry
Report:

Please continue overleaf

I am not connected directly or indirectly with the management or proprietors

Signed _____

Name (CAPITALS PLEASE)_____

Address _____

_____

[2002]

To: *The Good Hotel Guide*, Freepost PAM 2931, London W11 4BR

NOTE: No stamps needed in UK, but letters posted outside the UK should be addressed to 50 Addison Avenue, London W11 4QP and stamped normally. Unless asked not to, we shall assume that we may publish your name if you are recommending a new hotel or supporting an existing entry. If you would like more report forms please tick □

Name of Hotel _____

Address _____

_____

Date of most recent visit   Duration of visit
□ New recommendation   □ Comment on existing entry
Report:

Please continue overleaf

I am not connected directly or indirectly with the management or proprietors

Signed _____

Name (CAPITALS PLEASE)_____

Address _____

_____

[2002]

To: *The Good Hotel Guide*, Freepost PAM 2931, London W11 4BR

NOTE: No stamps needed in UK, but letters posted outside the UK should be addressed to 50 Addison Avenue, London W11 4QP and stamped normally. Unless asked not to, we shall assume that we may publish your name if you are recommending a new hotel or supporting an existing entry. If you would like more report forms please tick ☐

Name of Hotel _____

Address _____

_____

Date of most recent visit
☐ New recommendation
Report:

Duration of visit
☐ Comment on existing entry

Please continue overleaf

I am not connected directly or indirectly with the management or proprietors

Signed _____

Name (CAPITALS PLEASE)_____

Address _____

_____

Maps

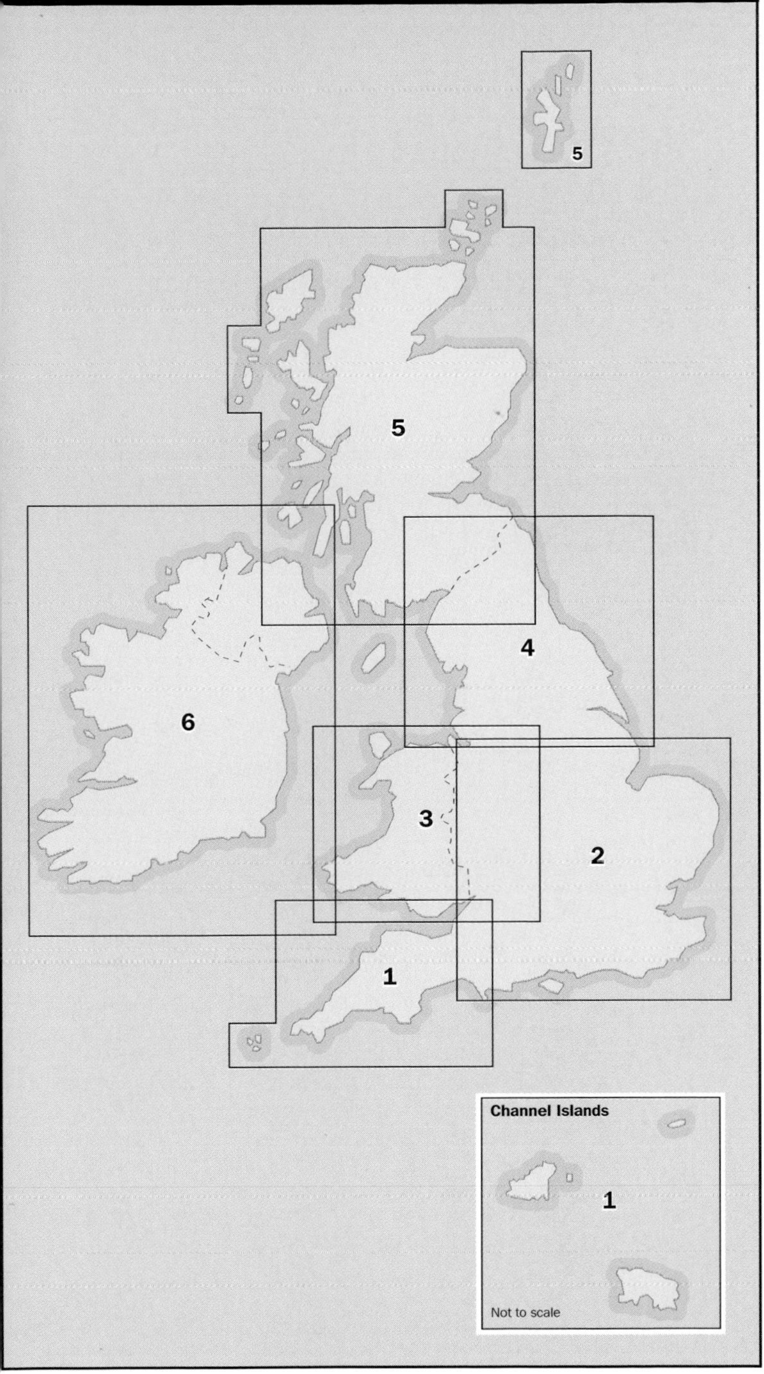

5

5

4

6

3

2

1

1

Channel Islands

1

Not to scale

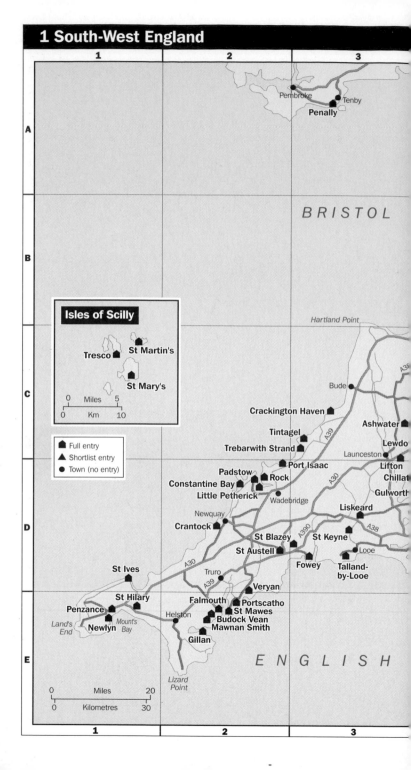

1 South-West England

Isles of Scilly

Tresco
St Martin's
St Mary's

0 Miles 5
0 Km 10

Full entry ■
Shortlist entry ▲
Town (no entry) ●

BRISTOL

Hartland Point

Bude ●

Crackington Haven ■

Ashwater ■

Tintagel ■
Trebarwith Strand ■
Port Isaac ■

Lewdo
Launceston ●
Lifton
Chillat

Padstow ■
Rock ■
Constantine Bay ■
Little Petherick ■

Wadebridge ●

Gulworth

Newquay ●

Crantock ■

Liskeard ■

St Blazey ■
St Keyne ■

St Austell ■

Looe ●

Fowey ■

Talland-
by-Looe ■

St Ives ■

Truro ●

Veryan ■

St Hilary ■
Penzance ●
Newlyn ■

Falmouth ■
Portscatho ■
St Mawes ■
Budock Vean ■
Mawnan Smith ■
Gillan ■

Helston ●

Land's End
Mount's Bay

Lizard Point

ENGLISH

0 Miles 20
0 Kilometres 30

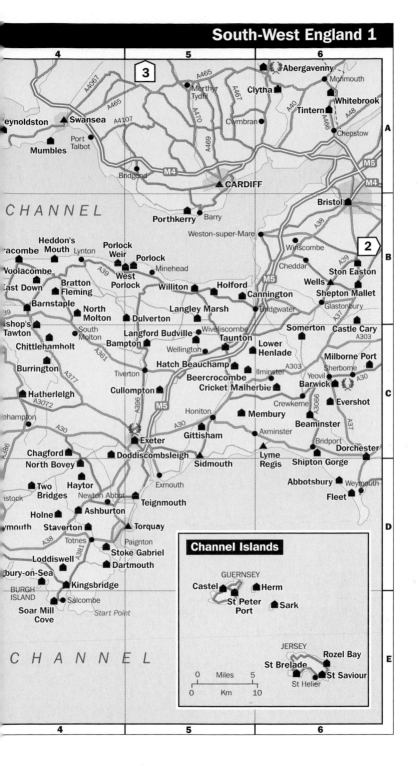

3

2

Abergavenny
Monmouth
Clytha
Whitebrook
Merthyr Tydfil
Cwmbran
Tintern
Chepstow
eynoldston
Swansea
Port Talbot
Mumbles
Bridgend

CHANNEL

CARDIFF

A

Bristol

Porthkerry
Barry
Weston-super-Mare

Heddon's Mouth
Lynton
Porlock Weir
Porlock
Minehead
Winscombe
Cheddar
Ston Easton
Wells
racombe
Voolacombe
West Porlock
Williton
Holford
Cannington
Shepton Mallet
:ast Down
Bratton Fleming
Bridgwater
Glastonbury
Barnstaple
North Molton
Dulverton
Langley Marsh
B

ishop's Tawton
South Molton
Langford Budville
Wiveliscombe
Taunton
Somerton
Castle Cary
Chittlehamholt
Bampton
Wellington
Lower Henlade
Milborne Port
A303
Burrington
Tiverton
Hatch Beauchamp
Ilminster
Sherborne
Yeovil
Hatherleigh
Cullompton
Beercrocombe
Cricket Malherbie
Barwick
ehampton
Honiton
Crewkerne
Evershot
Membury
Beaminster
C
Chagford
Exeter
Gittisham
Axminster
Bridport
Dorchester
North Bovey
Doddiscombsleigh
Lyme Regis
Shipton Gorge
Sidmouth
Two Bridges
Haytor
Exmouth
Abbotsbury
Weymouth
istock
Newton Abbot
Teignmouth
Fleet
Holne
Ashburton
D
ymouth
Staverton
Torquay
Totnes
Paignton
Loddiswell
Stoke Gabriel
Dartmouth
bury-on-Sea
Kingsbridge
Salcombe

Channel Islands

BURGH ISLAND
Soar Mill Cove
Start Point
GUERNSEY
Castel
Herm
St Peter Port
Sark

CHANNEL

JERSEY
Rozel Bay
St Brelade
St Saviour
St Helier

0   Miles   5
0   Km   10

E

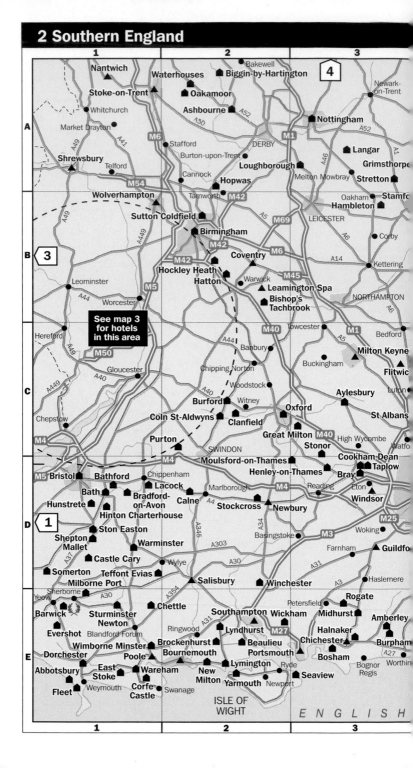

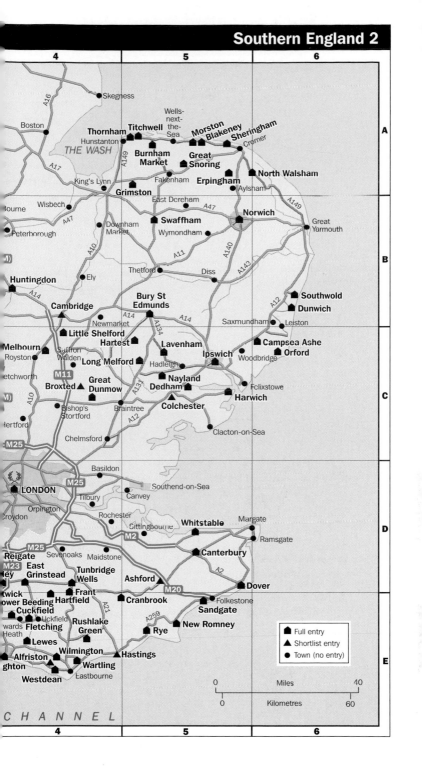

4 **5** **6**

Skegness

Boston

Wells-
next-
the-Sea
Thornham **Titchwell** **Morston** **Blakeney**
Sheringham
Hunstanton Cromer
THE WASH **Burnham** **Great**
Market **Snoring**
King's Lynn **North Walsham**
Fakenham **Erpingham**
Grimston Aylsham
East Dereham

Wisbech A47
Bourne A17
A47 Downham **Swaffham** **Norwich**
Peterborough Market Great
(M) Wymondham Yarmouth
A10
A149

Huntingdon Thetford Diss
Ely
A14
Cambridge **Bury St**
Newmarket **Edmunds** A14 **Southwold**
Dunwich
Little Shelford Saxmundham Leiston
Hartest **Lavenham** **Campsea Ashe**
Melbourn **Ipswich** **Orford**
Royston Saffron **Long Melford** Hadleigh Woodbridge
etchworth Walden **Nayland**
(M) **Broxted** **Great** **Dedham** Felixstowe
A10 **Dunmow** A131 **Harwich**
Bishop's **Colchester**
Hertford Stortford Braintree
A12
M25 Chelmsford Clacton-on-Sea

Basildon
LONDON M25
Southend-on-Sea
Orpington Tilbury Canvey
Croydon
Rochester
Whitstable Margate
Sittingbourne **Canterbury**
M2 **Ramsgate**
Reigate Sevenoaks Maidstone
M23 **East**
ley **Grinstead** **Tunbridge** **Ashford** A2
Wells M20 **Dover**
twick **Frant** **Cranbrook** Folkestone
ower Beeding **Hartfield** **Sandgate**
Cuckfield Uckfield A259
wards **Fletching** **Rushlake** **Rye** **New Romney**
Heath **Green**
Lewes
Alfriston **Wilmington**
ghton **Hastings**
Wartling
Westdean Eastbourne

Full entry
▲ **Shortlist entry**
● **Town (no entry)**

0 Miles 40
0 Kilometres 60

CHANNEL

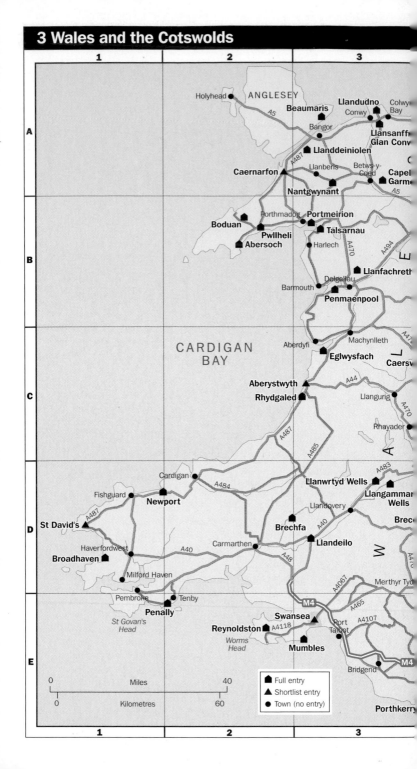

3 Wales and the Cotswolds

A

Holyhead
ANGLESEY
Beaumaris
Llandudno
Colwyn Bay
Conwy
A5
Bangor
Llansanff
Glan Conw
Llanddeiniolen
Llanberis
Betws-y-Coed
Caernarfon
Capel
Garm
A487
Nantgwynant
A5

B

Porthmadog
Portmeirion
Boduan
Talsarnau
Pwllheli
Abersoch
Harlech
A470
A494
E
Llanfachreth
Dolgellau
Barmouth
Penmaenpool

C

CARDIGAN
BAY
Aberdyfi
Machynlleth
Eglwysfach
Caers
Aberystwyth
A44
Rhydgaled
Llangurig
A470
A485
Rhayader
A487

D

Cardigan
A484
Llanwrtyd Wells
A483
Fishguard
Newport
Llangammar
Wells
St David's
A487
Llandovery
A40
Brec
Brechfa
Carmarthen
A48
Llandeilo
W
Haverfordwest
A40
Broadhaven
Milford Haven
A4067
Merthyr Tyd

E

Pembroke
Tenby
M4
A465
Penally
St Govan's
Head
Swansea
Port Talbot
A4107
Reynoldston
A4118
Worms
Head
Mumbles
M4
Bridgend

0 Miles 40
0 Kilometres 60

■ Full entry
▲ Shortlist entry
● Town (no entry)

Porthkerry

1 2 3

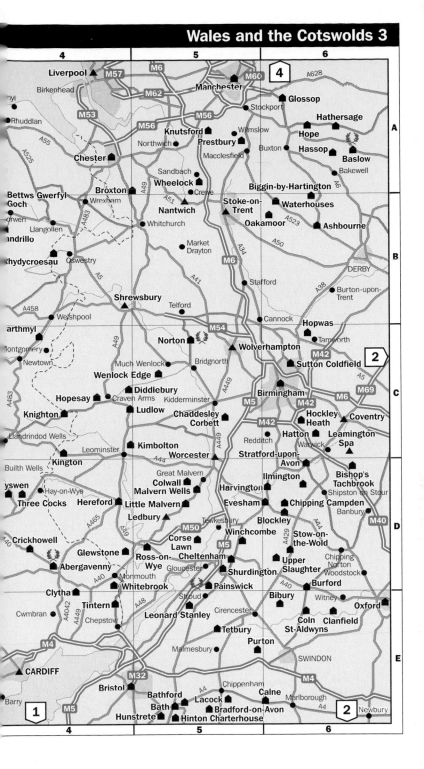

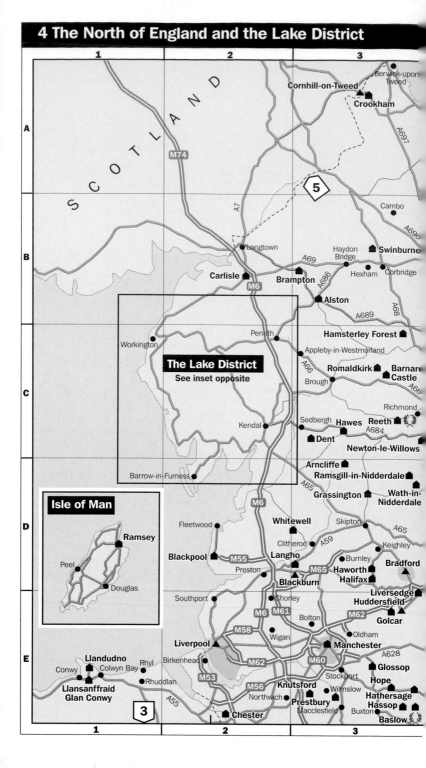

SCOTLAND

M74

A7

Berwick-upon-Tweed

Cornhill-on-Tweed

Crookham

A697

5

Cambo

A696

Longtown

Haydon Bridge

Swinburne

A69

Carlisle

Brampton

A686

Hexham

Corbridge

M6

Alston

A68

A689

Hamsterley Forest

Workington

Penrith

Appleby-in-Westmorland

The Lake District
See inset opposite

A66

Romaldkirk

Barnard Castle

Brough

A66

Richmond

Kendal

Sedbergh

Hawes

Reeth

A684

Dent

Newton-le-Willows

Arncliffe

Ramsgill-in-Nidderdale

Barrow-in-Furness

A65

Grassington

Wath-in-Nidderdale

M6

Whitewell

Skipton

A65

Isle of Man

Fleetwood

Clitheroe

A59

Keighley

Ramsey

Blackpool

M55

Langho

Burnley

Haworth

Bradford

Peel

Preston

M65

Blackburn

Halifax

Douglas

Liversedge

Southport

Chorley

Huddersfield

M6

M61

Bolton

M62

Golcar

Llandudno

Rhyl

M58

Wigan

Oldham

Conwy

Colwyn Bay

Liverpool

Manchester

A628

Llansanffraid Glan Conwy

Rhuddlan

Birkenhead

M62

M60

Glossop

3

A55

M53

Knutsford

Stockport

Hope

M56

Wilmslow

Hathersage

Northwich

Prestbury

Hassop

Chester

Macclesfield

Buxton

Baslow

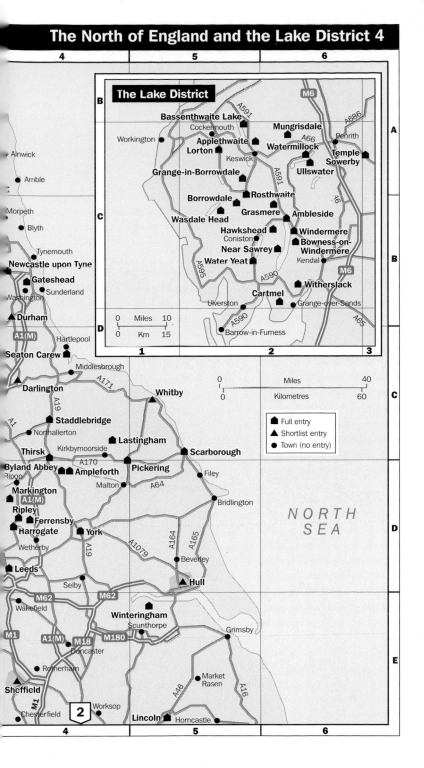

5 Scotland

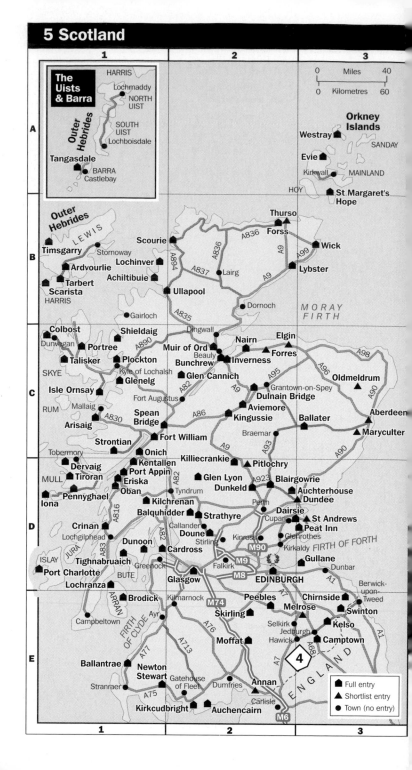